NCLEX-RN® Review

NCLEX-RN® Review

2nd Edition

MARGARET M. DAHLHAUSER, RN, PhD

Professor Emeritus
School of Nursing
Tennessee State University
Nashville, Tennessee

McGRAW-HILL, INC.

Medical Publishing Division

New York   Chicago   San Francisco   Lisbon   Madrid   Mexico City
Milan   New Delhi   San Juan   Seoul   Singapore   Sydney   Toronto

NCLEX-RN® Review, Second Edition

34567890 QPD/QPD 987

Set ISBN # 0-07-144773-3
Book ISBN # 0-07-147024-7
CD-ROM ISBN # 0-07-147025-5

This book was set in Times Roman by TechBooks, Inc.
The editors were Quincy McDonald, Christie Naglieri, and Regina Y. Brown.
The production supervisor was Catherine H. Saggese.
The index was prepared by Jerry Ralya.
The cover designer was Pehrsson Design.
Quebecor World/Dubuque was printer and binder.

Library of Congress Cataloging-in-Publication Data

Dahlhauser, Margaret M.
  NCLEX-RN® Review, 2 ed / Margaret M. Dahlhauser.–2nd ed.
    p. ; cm.
  Includes index.
  ISBN 0-07-147024-7–ISBN 0-07-144773-3 (set)
   1. Nursing–Examinations, questions, etc.   I. Title.
  [DNLM: 1. Nursing–Examination Questions.   WY 18.2 D131c 2006]
RT55.D34   2006
610.73′076—dc22

                                                 2005057687

DEAR STUDENTS,

This package was developed to assist you academically while in college and to help you pass your R.N. State Board Examination.

    With that purpose in mind, allow me to guide you in that direction.

◆ Do not study these questions and rationales *until* you have learned all the medications and diseases in our handbook. This is the most difficult task for you; it takes hours of studying, but remember, we present only the most commonly occurring diseases and the most commonly used medications. Also, study lecture content and answer question per instruction in our booklet before starting to assess what you have learned using this CD-ROM.

◆ When using this CD-ROM, be sure to study the content you miss on each question. Answering questions *will not help you unless you learn the content missed.* I know you will pass your R.N. Board Exam if you follow our directions. We wish you the very best that life has to offer.

Sincerely,

Margaret Dahlhauser, R.N., Ph.D.

Contents

SECTION III TOPICAL OUTLINES, EXAMS, AND RATIONALES

Acknowledgements

I wish to thank my publisher, McGraw-Hill, Inc., and especially Christie Naglieri, Development Editor, Michael Brown, Senior Editor, and Quincy McDonald, Senior Acquisitions Editor.

Particular thanks to all senior and graduate nursing students for their participation in testing new questions.

A special thanks to all student nurses who encouraged me to publish this book.

I especially acknowledge the guidance of the *Holy Spirit* because He knows that I would never have accomplished this task without His constant assistance.

A very special thanks to typists Janet Lester and Glenda Dahlhauser; without their ability and patience in deciphering my handwriting, this project would never have been completed. Also, thanks to Sheila Fairless, who typed material for this project over the past years.

Thanks to Debbie Jones and Karen Roth for contributing their expertise to the writing of this book; without their assistance, this project would have failed.

Last, but not least, thanks to my husband, Arthur, to my children, Doug, Greg, Debbie, Mary, Stephen, Kevin, Bryan, Eric, Tom, Paul, and Lisa, and my 22 grandchildren, whose unfailing love has allowed each individual in our family to grow spiritually and intellectually.

Chapter

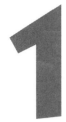

How to Use *NCLEX-RN*® Review

NCLEX-RN® *Review* is divided into three sections: Introduction; Nursing Care for Commonly Occurring Disorders and Diseases; and Topical Outlines, Exams, and Rationales. Section I, "Introduction," covers the computerized testing format and new type of questions. Extensive test-taking tips help readers read questions more carefully and select the correct answer. These tips should increase test-taking ability. This section should be read first and referred to as often as necessary when taking the examinations to reinforce test-taking skills.

Section II, "Nursing Care for Commonly Occurring Disorders and Diseases," covers commonly occurring diseases and injuries in a comprehensive form so that students can easily learn the causes, incidence, signs and symptoms, and treatment for each disease or injury. Most of the commonly occurring diseases and injuries are presented in the corresponding topical outlines (e.g., glomerulonephritis in renal and urinary disorders; spinal cord injury in neurologic disorders).

Section III, "Topical Outlines, Exams, and Rationales," is the most important part of this text. The major areas of nursing study are presented, subject by subject, in outline format. Learning is augmented by examination questions based both on the outlines and *on other information students should know about the particular area*. The rationales review why an answer is correct or best and why the other options are incorrect or less useful. The bonus is that additional information, beyond that given in the outline, is included through the rationales and questions, rounding out and expanding students' knowledge and comprehension.

The outline format helps students focus and comprehend information more quickly. Both outlines and questions are grouped into specific areas (cardiovascular, respiratory, and pediatric). As students review each subject area and complete the related examination, they can ascertain any area of weakness and work to improve on it.

Several matching questions and scenario situations are included in this review, although the NCLEX-RN does not include this question type. Matching and scenario questions are good tools for learning about diagnostic studies and related diseases. Content must be learned before it can be applied. The additional information included with the rationales will help students to better understand medications, diseases, and diagnoses. Many questions are presented in an application process that allows students to apply previously learned knowledge; other questions help students learn new content.

Rationales are provided for all correct answers as well as for all of the other options given. Students sometimes think that there is too much emphasis on questions and too little on rationales. Answering exam questions can be an excellent learning tool if rationales are reviewed for every option. Learning why each option is either correct or incorrect helps students to fully comprehend the question.

Appendix 1, "Simple Math Methods," provides students with a simple mathematical method for calculating drug problems. Those who have difficulty working mathematic problems can master the process and proceed with confidence. Appendix 2 provides a list of laboratory values.

Having administered many NCLEX-RN review courses for 18 years, I have found that most graduates have not adequately mastered academic content in the areas of medications; diseases; and laboratory tests (i.e., their normal values and possible etiologies for abnormal values). That is why students have great difficulty in applying that academic content correctly when answering questions with multiple complex factors seen on RN state board examinations and addressed in Chapter 24 of this book.

Remember *not* to mark answers in this book so that the examinations can be retaken until the content is mastered. Students using this book need to achieve at least an 85 percent on each exam before taking the NCLEX-RN boards. I advise students to go through the material and take each examination three times, and refer to the rationales *after* completing *each* exam.

This book is an excellent academic tool for students preparing for course examinations in class and for graduate nurses preparing for the NCLEX-RN. It is also an excellent reference for RNs who have been practicing for several years.

NCLEX-RN COMPUTERIZED TEST CONTENT

The following describes student's performance on each content area. Any component of the nursing process can be used in these questions (Table 1–1):

TABLE 1–1 ◆ Specific Content on the NCLEX-RN Exam

Physiological Adaptation (12–18% of the test)

◆ Managing and providing care for the clients with acute, chronic, or life-threatening physical health conditions.

◆ Related content includes but is not limited to: Alterations in Body Systems; Fluid and Electrolyte Imbalances; Hemodynamics; Infectious Diseases; Medical Emergencies; Pathophysiology; Radiation Therapy; Respiratory Care; and Unexpected Response to Therapies.

Reduction of Risk Potential (12–18% of the test)

◆ Reducing the likelihood that clients will develop complications or health problems related to existing conditions, treatments, or procedures.

◆ Related content includes but is not limited to: Diagnostic Tests; Laboratory Values; Pathophysiology; Potential for Alterations in Body Systems; Potential for Complications of Diagnostic Tests; Procedure, Surgery, and Health Alterations; and Therapeutic Procedures.

Pharmacological and Parenteral Therapies (5–11% of the test)

◆ Managing and providing care related to the administration of medications and parenteral therapies.

◆ Related content includes but is not limited to: Adverse Effects/Contraindications: Blood and Blood Products; Central Venous Access Devices; Chemotherapy; Expected Effects: Intravenous Therapy; Medication Administration; Parenteral Fluids; Pharmacological Actions; Pharmacological Agents; Pharmacological Interactions; Pharmacological Pain Management; Side Effects; and Total Parenteral Nutrition.

Prevention and Early Detection of Disease (5–11% of the test)

◆ Assisting the client and significant others through the normal expected stages of growth and development from conception through advanced old age.

◆ Related content includes but is not limited to: Advance Directives; Advocacy; Case Management; Client Rights; Concepts of Management; Confidentiality; Consultation with Members of the Health Care Team; Continuity of Care; Continuous Quality Improvement; Delegation Establishing Priorities; Ethical Practice; Incident/Irregular Occurrence/Variance Reports; Informed Consent; Legal Responsibilities; Organ Donation; Referrals; Resource Management; and Supervision.

Psychosocial Adaptation (5–11% of the test)

◆ Managing and providing care for clients with acute or chronic mental illnesses, as well as maladaptive behaviors.

◆ Related content includes but is not limited to: Behavioral Interventions; Chemical Dependency; Child Abuse/Neglect; Crisis Intervention; Domestic Violence; Elder Abuse/Neglect; Psychopathology; Sexual Abuse; and Therapeutic Milieu.

Safety and Infection Control (5–11% of the test)

◆ Protecting clients and health care personnel from environmental hazards.

◆ Related content includes but is not limited to: Accident Prevention; Disaster Planning; Error Prevention; Handling Hazardous and Infectious Materials; Medical and Surgical Asepsis: Standard (Universal) and Other Precautions; and Use of Restraints.

Coping and Adaptation (5–11% of the test)

◆ Promoting clients and/or significant other's ability to cope, adapt, and/or problem solve situations related to illnesses or stressful events.

◆ Related content includes but is not limited to: Coping Mechanisms; End of Life; Grief and Loss; Mental Health Concepts; Religious and Spiritual Influences on Health; Sensory/Perceptual Alterations; Situational Role Changes; Stress Management; Support Systems; Therapeutic Interactions; and Unexpected Body Image Changes.

Basic Care and Comfort (7–13% of the test)

◆ Providing comfort and assistance in the performance of activities of daily living.

◆ Related content includes but is not limited to: Assistive Devices; Eliminations; Mobility/Immobility; Nonpharmacological Comfort Interventions; Nutrition and Oral Hydration; Palliative/Comfort Care; Personal Hygiene; and Rest and Sleep.

ABOUT NCLEX-RN

The National Council of State Boards of Nursing (NCSBN) develops and administers the licensure examination designed to test knowledge, skills, and abilities essential for the safe and effective practice of nursing at the entry level. Unlike a paper-and-pencil test given in the classroom, the computer selects the questions as the test is taken; thus, every candidate's test is different from that of every other candidate. The NCLEX-RN is designed so that previous experience using a computer is not required to take the examination. Only two keys or the mouse is used to record your answers. You will have an opportunity to practice before the test begins. Questions on the NCLEX-RN include many different types of questions. The following are examples:

- ◆ Multiple choice
- ◆ Fill in the blank
- ◆ Use numbers to establish the correct procedure for (e.g.) inserting an IV
- ◆ Check boxes that are related to (e.g.) iron deficiency
- ◆ Which medication will you administer first?
- ◆ A catastrophe has occurred in the area of the hospital, and you are asked to discharge a patient. Which patient will you discharge?
- ◆ You are the RN on a medical/surgical unit, and a pediatric-trained RN is transferred to your unit. Which patient will you assign to the pediatric-trained RN?
- ◆ Which patients can share the same room?
- ◆ A scenario followed by several questions relating to that scenario

To answer these questions, you have to take into consideration the patient's age, disease, disorder, number of days the patient has been in the hospital, etc. You can look at each question for as long as you like, but because you cannot return to previous questions and there are time constraints, it is generally best to mark your first "educated guess" and move on.

All candidates are given a minimum of 75 questions. A candidate can be given a maximum of 265 questions over a 5-hour period. Only a few candidates will take the maximum number of questions or the minimum amount of time. Each student has a separate set of questions. Each question stands alone, and there are no situations related to several questions (no group questions). This is because once you have answered a question and go to the next question, you cannot return to the previous question.

If you answer the first question correctly, you may be given a question that is somewhat more difficult. If you answer that question correctly, you may be given another equally difficult question. If you answer that question incorrectly, you will be given an easier question. This process will continue until you pass or fail your examination.

READ AND TIME EACH QUESTION CAREFULLY

Recognizing which component of the *nursing process* is being used and which *patient need* is being addressed will greatly help you to determine the correct answer for each question. You must answer all of the questions because the computer will not allow you to skip a question. If you are not sure which answer is correct, eliminate as many options as you can and then make an educated guess.

Theoretically, each question is supposed to take you 1 minute to answer. To repeat, you have a maximum of 6 hours to take the 1-day exam. Use your time wisely; there is a mandatory 10-minute break after the first 2 hours of testing, and you can take a 5-minute break at any time during the examination; that time is counted in the 5 hours allowed for testing. Be sure to take a snack (e.g., protein bar) along with you to eat during the break. Take your breaks as needed because your mind will become tired and cause you to miss questions. You should take more time on each question when you first start the exam because you will be the most anxious at the beginning of the test. If you find yourself getting stuck, select an answer and move on. Use the space bar (or mouse) to move a small light to the option you want to choose for the correct answer. When you are sure that you have selected the option you want, push the "Enter" key and your answer is locked in. A new question automatically appears. Because CAT examinations are constructed interactively, testing will stop when the candidate's performance is statistically estimated to be a pass or a fail. This does not occur until a high level of certainty of the candidate's performance is determined. Remember, the CAT examination will stop when the maximum number of items has been taken (265 questions) or when the time limit is reached (6 hours). A calculator (for math problems) will be provided for you at the testing center.

AUTHORIZATION TO TEST

Approximately 1 month after you graduate, notification of your graduation is sent to the RN board from the university or college that you attended. The RN board then sends you an "authorization-to-test" form. This form contains your test authorization number, identification number, and an expiration date. You must schedule your test for a date on or before the expiration date indicated on your authorization-to-test form by calling the telephone number given. You will not be admitted to the examination without this form.

DEVELOPING EXCELLENT TEST-TAKING SKILLS FOR NCLEX-RN

1. *Never* change an answer unless you have misread a part of the question.

2. Answer all of the questions you think you know. *Do not* waste time on questions you do not know, but do not rush. You have time to answer the questions. If you go through too fast, you may fail the examination before you give yourself the opportunity to pass.

3. Concentration during the examination is *crucial*. Your ability to concentrate allows you to note the *key* words and select the correct answers.

4. When taking the examinations in this book, work on concentration skills. Do not allow small distractions to clutter you mind. Keep pushing them away. The more you do this, the stronger your ability to concentrate becomes.

5. Improve your self-confidence by answering every question in this book. Do not mark your answers in the book; use the answer sheets instead. Then take all of the examinations again. Continue to do this until you get at least 85 percent correct on every examination. Just as a boxer prepares for a fight by building his or her muscles, you must prepare for your NCLEX-RN exam by building self-confidence. The harder you work, the better prepared you will be.

6. Read questions carefully.

7. Ask yourself the question before looking at the options. This takes practice. It is hard to break old habits!

8. If you do not know what the question is about, you cannot answer it correctly. A poor test taker wastes time choosing an option before really comprehending the subject of the question. Poor test takers make anxious test takers.

9. Remember to identify critical elements; for example, is the question asking you for an intervention, an assessment, or an evaluation? If the question asks for an evaluation, do not answer with an intervention. If the question deals with a cardiac problem, choose an option that deals with the cardiovascular system. If the problem deals with a renal problem, choose an option the deals with the renal system.

10. When answering questions, remember that this exam is testing to see if you will be a safe caregiver. For example it is more important to monitor blood pressure on a hypertensive patient than it is to monitor caloric intake. Remember, safety for the patient will be the correct answer. Questions are simple and straightforward. Do not try to make them difficult.

11. Try to eliminate at least two options quickly, and then with the remaining two options look for a *global response*. For example, if the options are:

    a. take patient's blood pressure every 3 h.

    b. take patient's vital signs every 3 h.

    Option b probably will be the correct response because blood pressure is included in this global response.

Look for a word or phrase used in both the stem (the clinical scenario of the question) and in the options. For example, if the word "assessment" is used in the stem and the phrase "assess patient for liver failure" is used in one of the options, then that option is likely to be the correct answer.

12. Answer questions as if the situation is ideal; the nurse has all the time necessary and all the resources needed. For example, the stem reads:

    The RN enters Mrs. Jones' room and finds her crying uncontrollably after her physician tells her she has cancer.

    Which of the following responses by the nurse would be *most* appropriate?

    a. It's okay to cry Mrs. Jones; I understand your pain.

    b. I will call your husband; it is no time for you to be alone.

    c. I will be back as soon as I can. We are very busy on the floor today, and we will talk about your concerns later.

    d. Mrs. Jones, I will sit here beside your bed; if you want to talk, I am a good listener.

    Option d: The correct answer. The patient needs someone *now*, not later, to be there for her. Telling the patient that you will sit by her bedside lets her know that the nurse has time for her.

    Option a: The nurse should assure the patient that it is okay to cry, but this response belittles the patient because no one can fully understand another person's pain.

    Option b: Mrs. Jones may not want the nurse to call her husband.

    Option c: A nurse should not tell a patient who is crying that she will be back later. The patient needs the nurse now, not later.

13. When reading *each* question, be sure to determine if the response asks for a *false* response or a *true* response. If the question asks for an answer that is not true, read each option and say to yourself, "Yes, I would do that," or "Yes, that is true," after each option until you come to the option that is not true. That option is the correct answer. This takes practice!

14. Examples of "not true" response stems:

    ◆ Which of the following demonstrates an *unsafe* nursing judgment?

    ◆ Which of the following characteristics would *least likely* contribute to CHF?

    ◆ Which of the following nursing interventions would be the *exception* in this situation?

    ◆ Which of the following statements would indicate

that the client demonstrates a *need for further education*?

◆ Which of the following nursing actions receives the *lowest priority*?

◆ Which of the following demonstrates *incorrect* placement of an NG tube?

15. Look for key words and phrases in the stems.
   ◆ *Early* or *late* signs and symptoms
   ◆ *On the day of* surgery, or admission
   ◆ The *initial* nursing action
   ◆ *Immediately* postoperative
   ◆ *After several days* or *after several hours*
   ◆ The *Most likely* or *Least likely*
   ◆ The *intervention*
   ◆ Stat
   ◆ *Prior* to surgery

16. In considering options (Table 1–2), *do not*:
   ◆ Make decisions for patients.
   ◆ Ask patients why.
   ◆ Tell patients how they feel.
   ◆ Tell patients not to worry.
   ◆ Tell patients to ask their physician.
   ◆ Have psychiatric patient participate in competitive games.
   ◆ Have psychiatric patients become involved in a group activity before a trusting relationship is established between the nurse and the patient.

17. If a question asks whether a male or female patient has a disease and you do not know, choose men; men tend to have more diseases than women.

18. Look for key words in the options. *Correct* options will tend to have the following words.

Accept	Listen
Anticipate	Maintain
Appropriate	Manage
Assess	Monitor
Assuring	Observe
Communicate with	Promote
Compliance	Protect
Consistency	Provide
Discuss	Safety
Encourage	Schedule (a family meeting)
Entire family (when counseling patients)	Share feelings
Evaluate	Share (with me)
Explain	Simple (instructions)
Firmly (when dealing with patients)	Support
Identify	Talk with
Inspect	Tell me more about
It must be difficult	Trusting relationship
	Understanding

19. Look for key words in the options. *Incorrect* options will tend to have the following words.

Absolute	Make
All	Never
Always	Only
Any	Suggest
Entire	Tell
Force	Unrestricted
Insist	Whenever
Limit	

20. Communication is a major tool in the practice of nursing. Therefore, communication skills are an integral part of this exam. *The following key words, phrases are an indication that the option is incorrect in a communication question.*

21. The following terms cause problems and must be read carefully when answering questions.
   ◆ Not indicative: not true.
   ◆ Proximal: nearest to a point of attachment or origin.
   ◆ Contraindicated: something that should not be done.
   ◆ Modified: to make minor changes that can be important changes.
   ◆ Anticipate: give adequate thought, to foresee.
   ◆ Compliance: cooperative in relation to prescribed therapy.
   ◆ Insidious: a disease that develops so slowly the client is unaware of the onset.

TABLE 1–2 ◆ In Answering Questions, Never

Tools	Key Words
Give advice	If I were you, I would.
Show disapproval	You knew that was wrong.
Be defensive	Every nurse on this unit is trying to help you!
Focus on an inappropriate patient response	Have I said something wrong?
False reassurance	Don't worry; it will be all right.
Request an explanation	Why did you do that?
Make a patient wait	Ask your physician about that.
Belittle a patient	Don't be concerned—it's nothing to worry about.

◆ Flank: outside of the thigh, hip, and buttocks.

◆ Inappropriate: should not be done, not appropriate.

◆ Malaise: discomfort, uneasiness, slight illness.

22. Poor test-taking habits are hard to break. After reading the rationale for a question that you got wrong, decide if you answered the question wrong because you did not know the content necessary to answer the question. If that is the situation, learn the content. If you got the question wrong, but you really do not know why, go back to testing-tips and look at them in reference to the question. This will help you to become more test wise.

23. Success on the NCLEX-RN is highly influenced by how effectively you think. You have progressed through many years of formal and informal education to get to this educational level. In the process, you established your own learning techniques and patterns of thinking. You use these skills every time you take an examination.

   ◆ How effective are your learning techniques and your thinking skills?

   ◆ How well do they work?

   ◆ Effective thinking begins with an awareness of your own thinking. Unless you are consciously aware of your own thought process and how it controls your learning and test-taking ability, you cannot take control of what goes on in your own mind when you take a test.

24. The taxonomy of thinking consists of six levels. The first two, *memory* and *comprehension*, are the lower levels of thinking. Although they are the lower levels of thinking, they are the required foundation for higher levels of thinking. The next four higher levels of thinking are part of the nursing process: *analysis*, *synthesis* (assessment), *application* (implementation and planning), and *evaluation*. The NCLEX-RN examination test items are constructed using these four higher levels of thinking.

   ◆ No one likes to fail, especially at something as important as the RN licensure examination.

   ◆ A correlation exists between anxiety and the unknown. As the unknown factor increases, a person's anxiety increases.

Some common unknowns experienced by the graduate preparing for the RN state board examinations are the following:

   ◆ How many questions will I have to answer before the computer shuts off?

   ◆ If the computer shuts off at 75 questions, will that mean I passed or failed?

   ◆ What questions will they ask me?

   ◆ What if they ask me questions I know nothing about?

   ◆ How should I pace myself, fast or slow?

   ◆ How will I know when I am ready for the RN licensure examination?

   ◆ What if I fail the RN licensure examination?

25. You can eliminate most of your fears of the unknown by carefully establishing a well-designed plan to pass the RN licensure examination. You have already started that process by buying this book. A well-designed plan must include a desire, which gives you motivation to reap the rewards of your hard work. Some motivators are:

   ◆ Your RN license

   ◆ Personal satisfaction of achievement

   ◆ Your first RN paycheck

   ◆ Prestige and status

   ◆ The power to help people in ways that no one but a professional nurse can

26. A well-designed plan for test-taking success must include a search to know how you think. To help you in this search, I have identified the following test-taking personalities. Now see if you can identify with one or two of these personalities.

   ◆ The *speed test taker* is an individual who hurries through the entire process of taking an examination in a desperate rush to complete it before essential facts that have been studied are forgotten. The *speed test taker* arrives at the testing room early, waits anxiously, and asks potential test questions to anyone who will listen. The *speed test taker* now has a very high level of anxiety, which makes thinking accurately impossible, and wants to go back and change every option he or she has chosen. The *speed test taker* loves options, so he or she spends the rest of the examination time changing options. The stem of the question is really not important to a speed option lover. On the NCLEX-RN board examination, you cannot physically go back over the questions you have answered but you can mentally go back, and this will interfere with your thinking process.

   ◆ The *low–self-esteem test taker* views examinations as a hurdle to jump, a cross to carry, and a threat to self-esteem, rather than just as a part of learning. Rather than pursuing a plan of ongoing study and preparation for an examination, he or she faces an upcoming test with an attitude of, "I will study tomorrow." This is a defense mechanism of suppression by which the anxiety about the test is put out of mind, at least away from his or her immediate thoughts. The night before the examination is an all-night study session. Morning comes, and the student thinks he or she is ready, until he or she looks at the first two questions. Now, all the student has learned is running together as he or she tries desperately to find the right option. Such a test taker is not concerned about what the question is asking. Yes, another option lover.

◆ The *procrastinating test taker* does nothing fast because he or she cannot make up his or her mind when it comes to testing. The *procrastinating test taker* looks for underlying, hidden meaning in the stem of the question. He or she studies the stem with undue care and caution, searching for a "trick" in the question. The *procrastinator* has no doubt been told by faculty that he or she "reads into" the questions on examination. Yes, you guessed it, this is a stem lover. Let the option wait, because the *procrastinating test taker* needs to find out what is wrong with the stem of the question.

◆ Last, but not least, the *academic-minded test taker* is typically a talented, thoughtful, intelligent student who has enjoyed a successful academic career, mainly as a result of persistence, discipline, well-structured study habits, and high self-esteem. The *academic-minded test taker* knows what the question is asking *before* looking at the options. This test taker has an appreciation of the need to know what the question is asking before he or she tries to answer it. This student is both a stem and an option lover, resulting in high grades for him or her. Yes, you too can become an *academic-minded test taker* by working on improving your test-taking skills and studying until you knows all of the content in this NCLEX package.

Do you recognize yourself in any of these test-taking personalities? Unless you are aware of your learning techniques, you are not in control of your learning.

◆ Are you a visual learner?

◆ Are you an auditory learner?

◆ Is your reading comprehension excellent or poor?

◆ Do you tend to put off studying until the next day?

◆ Can you read and see the whole picture presented, or do you learn in a fragmented way?

27. Nursing students tend to be visual learners. However, most learn best by using more than one method. If your reading comprehension is poor, do not spend hours reading chapters. Use a book like this one that gives you the MOST important information you need to know and learn that. If you have a tendency to put off studying, acknowledge that and make yourself spend 3 to 4 hours each day (time yourself) 5 days per week studying. Reward yourself on your 2 free days. If you tend to learn in fragmented ways, acknowledge that, and work on putting the fragments together so that you can see the whole picture. As you learn about a disease or medication, try to apply it to a clinical situation.

Taking a *good* NCLEX-RN review before taking your RN state board examination will challenge your academic thinking and will also help you retain what you have learned longer. It will make you very aware of what you do not know. If it is a good review, it will give you a step-by-step process so that you will know when you are ready to take the RN state board exam. It will help improve your learning techniques and thinking skills, which will help you develop excellent test-taking skills and make passing the RN state board exam a reality, not a dream.

Note: When reading a long scenario on the NCLEX-RN examination, read the last line in the scenario first; this will allow you to search for the right answer while you are reading.

Chapter

2

Endocrine Disorders

TOPICAL OUTLINE

I. ADRENAL AND PITUITARY DISORDERS

A. Adrenocortical Disorders

1. Major disorders of the adrenal cortex (part of the adrenal gland) are characterized by hypofunction and hyperfunction.

2. Hypofunction of the adrenal cortex results in a deficiency of glucocorticoids, mineralocorticoids, and adrenal androgens. Hypofunction of the adrenal cortex is seen in Addison's disease.

3. Hyperfunction results in excessive production of glucocorticoids, mineralocorticoids, and androgens. Hyperfunction of the adrenal cortex is seen in Cushing's syndrome.

4. Androgens stimulate the development of male characteristics (e.g., testosterone).

B. Addison's Disease (Adrenal Insufficiency)

◆ Adrenocortical hypofunction results in decreased levels of mineralocorticoids (aldosterone), glucocorticoids (cortisol), and androgens.

1. Incidence

◆ Addison's disease is a relatively uncommon disorder that can occur at any age and in both sexes.

2. Etiology

a. Primary adrenal hypofunction (Addison's disease) originates in the gland itself and is caused by

(1) An autoimmune process in which 90 percent of the adrenal gland is destroyed

(2) Bilateral adrenalectomy (e.g., surgery due to neoplasm)

(3) Hemorrhage into adrenal gland

b. Secondary adrenal hypofunction originates outside the gland and is caused by

(1) Abrupt withdrawal of long-term corticosteroid therapy (causing decreased secretion of adrenocorticotropic hormone [ACTH]). Long-term exogenous corticosteroid therapy suppresses pituitary ACTH secretion and results in adrenal atrophy

(2) Removal of an ACTH-secreting tumor

(3) Hypopituitarism disease (causing decreased secretion of ACTH) and melanocyte-stimulating hormone (MSH)

3. Pathophysiology with Signs and Symptoms

a. Adrenal hypofunction results in aldosterone deficiency (aldosterone retains sodium and, consequently, water) and excretion of potassium, which results in

(1) Increased water excretion

(2) Decreased intravascular volume

(3) Hypotension

(4) Decreased cardiac output

(5) The heart becoming smaller as a result of its diminished workload

(6) Weight loss

b. If not treated, signs and symptoms of hypotension become severe and cardiovascular activity weakens, leading to circulatory collapse, shock, and death. Because the body excretes sodium and saves potassium, elevation of the potassium level to more than 7 mEq/L results in arrhythmias and, possibly, cardiac arrest (normal potassium level is 3.5–5.5).

c. Glucocorticoid deficiency causes widespread metabolic disturbances.

d. Remember that the glucocorticoids promote gluconeogenesis and have an anti-insulin effect (decrease the effect of insulin).

e. Consequently, when glucocorticoids become deficient, gluconeogenesis decreases, which causes hypoglycemia.

f. The patient grows weak and exhausted; develops anorexia, weight loss, and nausea; and vomiting occurs.

g. Emotional disturbances can develop, ranging from mild neurotic symptoms to severe depression.

h. Glucocorticoid deficiency causes diminished resistance to stress.

i. Stress from surgery, injury, infection, and pregnancy can cause an addisonian crisis (acute adrenal insufficiency).

   (1) Addison's disease (primary adrenal cortex hypofunction) causes a decrease in secretion of cortisol (the major glucocorticoid), which causes the pituitary gland to simultaneously secrete excessive amounts of ACTH and MSH. Excessive amounts of MSH cause a conspicuous bronze coloration of the skin in patients with Addison's disease. The patient appears to be deeply suntanned.

   (2) Secondary adrenal hypofunction (not Addison's disease) produces similar clinical effects but without hyperpigmentation because the MSH level is low. ACTH also is low. Secondary adrenal hypofunction that results in glucocorticoid deficiency can stem from hypopituitarism (causing a decreased corticotropin secretion), and from abrupt withdrawal of long-term exogenous corticosteroid therapy. Long-term exogenous corticosteroid stimulation suppresses pituitary corticotropin secretion and results in adrenal gland atrophy. Adrenal crisis follows when trauma, surgery, or other physiologic stress exhausts the body's store of glucocorticoids in persons with adrenal hypofunction.

4. Treatment

a. For all patients with primary or secondary adrenal hypofunction, corticosteroid replacement with cortisone or hydrocortisone (both have mineralocorticoid effects) is the primary treatment and must continue for life.

b. Addison's disease may also necessitate the administration of fludrocortisone acetate (Florinef) PO, which acts like aldosterone. These mineralocorticoids prevent dangerous dehydration and hypotension.

c. Patients with Addison's disease will have decreased muscle strength and decreased libido. Testosterone injections may be of benefit but are associated with the unfortunate risk of masculine effects.

5. Nursing Implications

a. Adrenal crisis requires prompt IV bolus administration of 100 mg hydrocortisone. Later a 50- to 100-mg dose is given IV or IM. In adrenal crisis, monitor vital signs carefully, especially for hypotension, volume depletion, and other signs of shock (decreased levels of consciousness and decreased urine output). Watch for hyperkalemia before treatment and/or hypokalemia after treatment (from excessive mineralocorticoid effect).

b. With rapid, efficient intervention, adrenal crisis usually passes by 12 h.

c. Monitor the patient's vital signs while the disease is being diagnosed and during adrenal crisis. Report a drop in blood pressure below the client's baseline.

d. Synthetic steroids are used in adrenal insufficiency (e.g., cortisone [Cortone], dexamethasone [Decadron], hydrocortisone [Cortef], methylprednisolone [Medrol, Solu-Medrol], prednisolone [Delta-Cortef], and prednisone [no trade name]).

e. Fludrocortisone (Florinef), a mineralocorticoid that acts like aldosterone, is used in the management of sodium loss and hypotension associated with adrenocortical insufficiency. Florinef is given with a glucocorticoid. Some glucocorticoid drugs contain mineral cortisone; these include cortisone and hydrocortisone.

f. Assess for signs of sodium and potassium imbalance.

g. Monitor for signs of infections. Remember, a patient with adrenal insufficiency cannot tolerate stress.

h. Arrange for a diet that will aid in maintaining sodium and potassium balances.

i. If patient has anorexia, suggest six small meals per day to increase calorie intake.

j. Ask the dietitian to provide a diet high in protein and carbohydrates.

k. Offer the patient a late-morning and late-evening snack to avoid hypoglycemia reaction.

l. Record weight and intake and output carefully because the patient may have volume depletion.

m. Encourage fluid volume ingestion to replace excessive fluid loss.

n. Educate the patient about

   (1) The need for a Medic Alert bracelet to indicate the diagnosis and/or need for cortisol replacement

   (2) The importance of the availability of hydrocortisone for self-injection, for use when the patient is unable to tolerate oral medications (e.g., due to nausea/vomiting) and during times of acute distress (automobile accident, trauma) because the body is unable to compensate for its need for additional glucocorticoid coverage

   (3) The need for the patient and significant others to have the ability to prepare medications into a syringe and perform injections

(4) The side effects of synthetic steroids, which include depression, flushing, sweating, petechiae, hyperglycemia, hypertension, decreased wound healing, and muscle wasting.

o. Side effects of fludrocortisone (Florinef) include congestive heart failure, edema, arrhythmias, weight gain (due to sodium/water retention), hypokalemia, and negative nitrogen balance.

p. Patients receiving Florinef may require a high-protein diet because of the potential for a negative nitrogen balance.

Note: Glucocorticoid or mineralocorticoid drugs with therapy lasting more than 10 days should not be abruptly stopped.

C. Cushing's Syndrome (Hypercortisolism)

1. Incidence

a. Cushing's syndrome is a relatively rare condition. It occurs mainly in women at an average age of 20 to 40 years but can be seen in women up to age 60 years (Fig. 2–1).

2. Etiology

a. Cushing's syndrome results from excessive production of ACTH from the pituitary (Cushing's disease).

b. Pituitary hypersecretion causes approximately 70 percent of cases of Cushing's syndrome. The remaining 30 percent of cases of Cushing's syndrome are

(1) Ectopic secretion by ACTH-producing tumors in another organ (particularly bronchogenic or pancreatic carcinoma)

(2) Administration of synthetic glucocorticoid or ACTH

(3) Adrenal tumor (cortex) causing increased production of glucocorticoids, mineralocorticoids, and androgens.

3. Pathophysiology with Signs and Symptoms

a. When Cushing's syndrome develops, the classic signs and symptoms of the syndrome emerge.

(1) Persistent hyperglycemia (steroid diabetes).

(2) Protein tissue wasting, which results in

(a) Weakness due to muscle wasting

(b) Capillary fragility, resulting in ecchymosis.

(3) Osteoporosis, resulting in fractures.

(4) Abnormal fat distribution, resulting in a moon-shaped face, a fat pad on the back (buffalo hump), and trunk obesity with slender arms and legs.

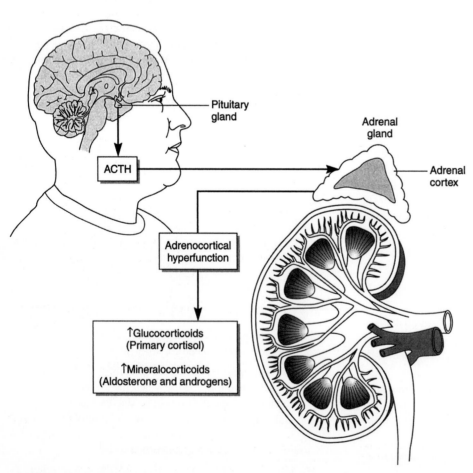

FIGURE 2–1 ◆ Cushing's Syndrome (Hypercortisolism)

Adrenocortical hyperfunction results in increased levels of glucocorticoids (primary cortisol) and, to a lesser extent, mineralocorticoids (aldosterone) and androgens. ACTH = adrenocorticotropic hormone.

(5) Poor wound healing.

(6) Hirsutism (abnormal hairiness) in women (increased androgen production).

(7) Peptic ulcers, resulting from increased gastric secretion.

(8) Irritability, emotional lability ranging from euphoric behavior to depression or psychosis, and insomnia may occur.

(9) Hypertension due to sodium, which causes water retention; left ventricular hypertrophy.

(10) Increased susceptibility to infection due to decreased lymphocyte production and suppression of antibody formation.

(11) Decreased resistance to stress.

(12) Increased potassium excretion (hypokalemia).

4. Treatment

a. The resection of most pituitary tumors causing Cushing's syndrome is performed via transsphenoidal hypophysectomy (removal of the pituitary).

b. When Cushing's syndrome is due to adrenal tumors, an adrenalectomy can be performed to remove the gland containing the tumor. Sometimes the tumor can be removed, leaving the adrenal gland intact.

c. The ectopic ACTH-secreting tumor is totally removed from the organ in which it developed, along with surrounding cancerous tissue.

d. Medications that interfere with ACTH production or adrenal hormone synthesis are available. Mitotane (Lysodren) is a cytotoxic antihormonal agent that inhibits corticosteroid synthesis without destroying cortical cells.

e. Cortisol is essential during and after surgery to help the client tolerate the physiologic stress imposed by removal of the pituitary or adrenal gland. If normal cortisol production occurs in the body, then steroid therapy may be gradually tapered and eventually discontinued. However, bilateral adrenalectomy or total hypophysectomy mandates lifelong steroid replacement therapy.

5. Nursing Implications

a. Clients with Cushing's syndrome require painstaking assessment and vigorous supportive care.

b. Frequent monitoring of vital signs, especially blood pressure, assessing for hypertension.

c. Assess client for cardiac disease.

d. Monitor laboratory reports for hypernatremia, hypokalemia, hyperglycemia, and glycosuria.

e. Assess for edema; monitor weight, intake, and output daily.

f. Remember, Cushing's syndrome produces emotional lability. Offer emotional support.

g. Instruct client to avoid foods high in vanillin (e.g., nuts, coffee, chocolates, and bananas) and to avoid use of salicylates for 2 days before urine collection of vanillylmandelic acid (VMA).

h. Keep the client quiet, especially postoperatively; provide a private room, because excitement may trigger a hypertensive episode. Postoperative hypertension is common because the stress of surgery and manipulation of the adrenal gland stimulate secretion of catecholamines. Monitor blood pressure closely.

D. Adrenomedullary Disorders (Pheochromocytoma)

◆ Pheochromocytoma is a tumor that results in hyperactivity of the adrenal gland. It is a catecholamine-secreting tumor usually found in the adrenal medulla (Fig. 2–2).

1. Incidence

a. Pheochromocytomas are rare, causing approximately 0.1 percent of cases of hypertension. It affects all races and both genders. Although the disease can occur at any age, it is most common in middle age.

2. Etiology

a. The exact cause of pheochromocytomas is unknown.

3. Pathophysiology with Signs and Symptoms

a. Pheochromocytomas usually are benign; less than 10 percent are malignant. The excessive amounts of catecholamines (epinephrine, norepinephrine, and dopamine) secreted by the adrenal medulla produce severe symptoms and can even cause death. Without early intervention, the

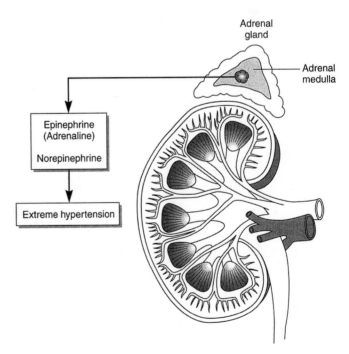

FIGURE 2–2 ◆ Pheochromocytoma

During stressful situations, norepinephrine and epinephrine are released and increase blood glucose levels. A tumor located on the adrenal medulla is known as a *pheochromocytoma*. This causes extreme hypertension due to the release of norepinephrine and epinephrine.

patient is at risk for severe hypertension cerebrovascular accident (CVA) and cardiac failure brought on by acute hypertension. Common signs and symptoms include palpitations, tachycardia, diaphoresis, tremors, excitation, nervousness, feelings of impending doom, and tachypnea.

b. Hyperglycemia (catecholamines increase glucose level).

c. Acute attacks may be associated with profuse diaphoresis, dilated pupils, and cold extremities.

d. Diagnosis includes a history of acute episodes of hypertension and tachycardia.

e. Increased urinary excretion of total free catecholamines and their metabolite, vanillylmandelic acid (VMA), as measured by analysis of 24-h urine collection, confirms pheochromocytoma.

f. Direct assay of total plasma catecholamines may show levels 10 to 50 times higher than normal.

g. X-ray imaging with various radiographic techniques, such as a computerized tomography (CT) or magnetic resonance imaging (MRI), can help to confirm and identify the adrenomedullary tumor location.

h. In the presence of a pheochromocytoma, the basal metabolic rate increases; increased blood glucose level and glycosuria can occur.

4. Treatment

a. Surgical removal of the tumor is the treatment of choice.

b. To decrease blood pressure, alpha-adrenergic blocking agents (phentolamine or phenoxybenzamine) are used to block norepinephrine-induced vasoconstriction. Therapeutic effect is vasodilation and decreased blood pressure.

5. Nursing Implications

a. Assess and control the patient's blood pressure preoperatively.

(1) Administer antihypertensive agents as ordered by physician.

(2) Promote rest and relief from anxiety and stress.

b. To ensure the reliability of urine catecholamine measurements:

(1) Make sure all urine is collected within the 24-h period.

(2) Advise the patient to save all urine voided during the 24-h period.

II. DIABETES MELLITUS

A. Pathophysiology

◆ Diabetes mellitus is the most common endocrine disease.

◆ Diabetes mellitus is a chronic disease of absolute or relative insulin deficiency or resistance.

◆ It is a systemic disease caused by an imbalance between insulin supply and insulin demand.

◆ Insulin is produced by the pancreas and normally maintains the balance between high and low blood glucose levels.

1. Diagnosis

a. Glycosylated hemoglobin (GHb) is a diagnostic test for blood glucose level over a period of 8 to 12 weeks. Therapy choices will be based on the patient's blood and hemoglobin A1C levels. Fasting and postprandial blood glucose measurements indicate the patient's levels throughout each day. The hemoglobin A1C level reveals the big picture of glucose control over the previous 8 to 12 weeks, with the previous 2 weeks most heavily weighted. The following are the recommended targets:

◆ Fasting blood glucose 90 to 130 mg/dL

◆ Postprandial blood glucose less than 180 mg/dL

◆ Hemoglobin A1C less than 7 percent

b. Home glucose monitoring involves obtaining a drop of capillary blood from a finger using a sterile lancet. The blood is placed on a semipermeable membrane that contains a reagent. The amount of blood glucose (in milligrams) can be read using a glucose meter (e.g., Accu-Chek glucometer).

c. Test urine for ketones when blood glucose levels are 240 mg/100 mL in home situations; in the hospital, blood is used to test for ketones.

d. The fasting blood sugar level is used to diagnose diabetes mellitus. Two or more fasting blood glucose levels above 126 mg/100 mL are diagnostic of diabetes mellitus.

Note: Glycosylated hemoglobin cannot be used to monitor control of diabetic clients with chronic renal failure because levels are significantly lower as a result of shortened erythrocyte survival.

2. Classification

a. The term *type 1* is often used and is synonymous with insulin-dependent diabetes mellitus (IDDM). *Type 2* diabetes is considered equivalent to non–insulin-dependent diabetes mellitus (NIDDM). Patients with secondary forms of diabetes may or may not require insulin, depending on the number of beta cells that can still produce insulin.

b. There is no ideal classification because obese patients with apparent NIDDM may become fully insulin dependent and prone to ketoacidosis. Diabetes is a very complicated disease and is not as easily placed into simple classifications as once thought.

3. Types and Incidence

a. IDDM: Patients are prone to ketoacidosis and genetically susceptible to the disease. It usually occurs before age 30 years. The patient usually is thin and requires exogenous insulin and dietary management to achieve control.

b. NIDDM: Usually occurs in obese adults after age 40 years and is most often treated with diet, exercise, and hypoglycemic agents. Treatment includes insulin therapy if oral hypoglycemic agents fail to control blood sugar levels.

c. Secondary diabetes mellitus usually occurs after age 30 years. The patient may develop IDDM or NIDDM depending on the severity of the cause.

- ◆ Diabetes mellitus affects an estimated 10 to 12 million persons in the United States.
- ◆ Incidence is equal in males and females.

4. Etiology

a. The etiology of primary diabetes (type 1 IDDM and type 2 NIDDM) remains unknown. The cause of *secondary* diabetes is known, but its pathophysiology is not completely understood.

5. Pathogenic Sequence for Type 1 Ketoacidosis-Prone Diabetes Mellitus (Primary)

a. By the time insulin-dependent diabetes mellitus (IDDM) appears, most of the beta cells are destroyed. The destructive process is almost certainly autoimmune in nature, although details remain obscure. Characteristically, the plasma insulin level is low or immeasurable. Glucagon levels are elevated, but suppressible with synthetic insulin.

b. Once symptoms have developed, insulin therapy is required.

c. Occasionally, an initial episode of ketoacidosis is followed by a symptom-free interval (the "honeymoon" period) during which no treatment is required. The reason for this phenomenon is unknown.

6. Pathophysiology Sequence for Type 1 IDDM

a. Genetic susceptibility to the disease may be present.

b. Environmental event ordinarily initiates the process in genetically susceptible individuals. Viral infection is believed to be one triggering mechanism, but noninfectious agents also could be involved.

c. Inflammatory response in the pancreas is called an *insult*. The cells that infiltrate the beta cells are monocytes/macrophages and activated T lymphocytes.

d. Alteration of the beta cells such that they are no longer recognized as "self" but are seen by the immune system as foreign cells or "non-self."

e. Development of an immune response. Because the islets are now considered "non-self," cytotoxic antibodies develop and act in concert with cell-mediated immune mechanisms. The end results are the destruction of beta cells and the appearance of diabetes mellitus.

7. Pathophysiology Sequence for Type 2 Ketoacidosis-Resistant NIDDM

a. Patients with type 2 NIDDM have three physiologic defects:

(1) Abnormally low insulin secretion.

(2) Resistance to insulin action in target tissues.

(3) Excess of glucagon.

b. Which of these abnormalities is primary is not known.

c. The alpha-cell population is increased, resulting in more alpha cells than beta cells (alpha cells produce the hormone glucagon). This imbalance accounts for the excess of glucagon (glucose) relative to insulin that characterizes NIDDM and is a feature of all hyperglycemic states. Relative insulin deficiency is present. Glucagon increases the concentration of glucose in the blood. The insulin level is lower than predicted for the level of plasma glucose.

d. In the first phase, the plasma glucose remains normal, despite demonstrable insulin resistance, because insulin levels are elevated.

e. In the second phase, insulin resistance tends to worsen so that, despite elevated insulin concentration, glucose intolerance becomes manifested and the patient experiences hyperglycemia.

f. In the third phase, insulin resistance does not change but insulin secretion declines, resulting in fasting hyperglycemia and overt diabetes.

g. Authorities believe that, in the first phase, a defect in the beta cells causes insulin hypersecretion, which in turn leads to insulin resistance.

h. Most patients with NIDDM are obese.

i. Some beta cells are intact in type 2 NIDDM, but there is a defect in insulin release; this is in contrast to the situation with type 1 IDDM in which no beta cells are intact.

j. For unknown reasons, patients with NIDDM do not develop ketoacidosis.

k. The majority of patients who do not respond to dietary therapy respond to hypoglycemic agents, but improvement of hyperglycemia in many patients is not sufficient for control of diabetes. For this reason, a high percentage of patients with NIDDM are treated with insulin.

l. Instruct the patient to maintain diabetes control during periods of illness or stress.

(1) Call the physician immediately when any unusual symptoms become evident; do not allow diabetes to get out of control.

(2) Make dietary adjustments during illness according to physician's directions.

(3) Continue taking insulin; the physician may increase dosage during illness.

(4) Test blood for sugar and urine for ketones more frequently; keep records.

(5) Monitor blood glucose levels.

(6) Know the conditions that bring about diabetic ketoacidosis:

- ◆ Failure to increase insulin when blood sugar is increasing
- ◆ Failure to take insulin

◆ Stress

◆ Infection

◆ Illness

8. Pathophysiology for Secondary Form of Diabetes

a. The secondary form of diabetes encompasses many conditions. Pancreatic disease, particularly chronic pancreatitis in alcoholic patients, is a common cause. Destruction of beta cell mass is the etiologic mechanism, resulting in hyperglycemia.

b. Hormonal causes include pheochromocytoma, acromegaly, Cushing's syndrome, therapeutic administration of steroid hormones, and "stress hyperglycemia" associated with severe burns, acute myocardial infarction (MI), and other life-threatening illnesses due to endogenous release of glucagon and catecholamines. Mechanisms of hormonal hyperglycemia include varying combinations of impaired insulin release and induction of insulin resistance.

c. A large number of drugs can lead to hyperglycemia "secondary diabetes," for example, steroids and catecholamines.

d. Hyperglycemia and even ketoacidosis can occur in secondary diabetes as a result of abnormalities at the level of the insulin receptors or destruction of beta cells. The pathophysiologic cause will determine whether the client is insulin dependent or oral hypoglycemic medications can be used.

B. Hypoglycemia

1. Signs and Symptoms

a. Early signs of hypoglycemia include vagueness, disorientation, dizziness, weakness, pallor, tachycardia, diaphoresis, and anger.

b. Late signs include loss of consciousness and coma.

2. Incidence

a. The problem of hypoglycemia is common in insulin-dependent diabetics, particularly when aggressive efforts are made to keep fasting plasma glucose levels within normal range.

b. Hypoglycemia may be caused by missing a meal or doing unexpected exercise but can occur in the absence of known precipitating events.

c. Daytime episodes of hypoglycemia usually are recognized by autonomic symptoms such as disorientation, nervousness, tremor, sweating, and hunger.

d. Hypoglycemia during sleep may produce no symptoms or cause night sweats and early-morning headaches.

e. If hypoglycemia is not aborted by counterregulatory hormone (glucagon) response or by ingestion of carbohydrate, then central nervous system symptoms occur and include confusion, anger, agitation, abnormal behavior (e.g., staring at the wall), loss of consciousness, coma, and death.

f. Very early on, the diabetic patient with type 1 IDDM loses the capacity to increase glucagon release in response to hypoglycemia. Thus protection is dependent on catecholamines.

g. Unfortunately, many patients subsequently also lose the capacity to release epinephrine and norepinephrine *in response to hypoglycemia*.

h. Counterregulatory hormone failure is especially dangerous when intensive insulin therapy is prescribed.

i. It must be emphasized that hypoglycemia attacks are dangerous. If they occur frequently, a serious or even fatal outcome can occur.

j. The Somogyi effect (phenomenon) is a rebound phenomenon occurring in diabetes mellitus. Overtreatment with insulin induces hypoglycemia, which initiates the release of epinephrine, ACTH, glucagon, and growth hormone. This release stimulates lipolysis, gluconeogenesis, and glycogenolysis, which in turn results in rebound hyperglycemia and ketosis.

k. It should be suspected whenever wide swings in the plasma glucose occur over short time intervals.

l. The Somogyi phenomenon probably is rare in adults but may be more frequent in children.

3. Treatment

a. An appropriate diet is constructed from the exchange system provided by the American Diabetic Association (ADA).

b. The importance of diet in the management of diabetes varies with the type of disease.

c. In insulin-dependent patients, particularly those on intensive insulin regimens, the composition of the diet is not critically important because adjustment of insulin can cover wide variations in food ingestion.

d. In non–insulin-dependent patients not treated with exogenous insulin, more rigorous adherence to a fixed diet is required because endogenous insulin reserve is limited. Such patients cannot respond to the increased demand produced by excess calories or increased intake of rapidly absorbed carbohydrate. These patients must be on a strict diet or they will become insulin dependent.

e. The initial treatment of serious hypoglycemia (producing confusion or coma) is administration of a 50-mL IV bolus of 50% glucose, followed by constant infusion of glucose until the patient is able to eat a meal.

f. Oral hypoglycemic agents: non–insulin-dependent diabetes that cannot be controlled by dietary management often responds to sulfonylurea (oral hypoglycemic) agents (see *Handbook of Medications for the NCLEX-RN® Review,* Chapter 7).

g. Frequent measurement of capillary glucose concentrations should be carried out (blood glucose finger sticks) to assess the effectiveness of the glucose infusion rate.

h. Early clinical manifestations of an insulin reaction (hypoglycemia) include headache, weakness, irritability, lack of muscle coordination, and diaphoresis. Patients are conscious during this early stage of hypoglycemic reaction and are given food high in sugar to eat and drink.

i. If a patient refuses to eat, glucagon can be administered IM.

j. A patient should have a vial of glucagon available in the home, and a significant other should have the skills needed to administer the glucagon injection.

k. Hypoglycemia is less common with oral agents than with insulin, but when it occurs, it tends to be severe and prolonged. Some patients require massive glucose infusion for days following the last dose of oral hypoglycemic agent.

4. Nursing Implications

    a. Instruct the patient to prevent and treat hypoglycemia.

        (1) Eat prescribed meal plan/snacks as scheduled.

        (2) Eat extra food before periods of vigorous exercise.

        (3) Take the prescribed insulin dose at the same time each day.

        (4) Monitor blood glucose levels daily.

        (5) Emphasize early treatment of hypoglycemia with a simple sugar.

C. Hyperglycemia

1. Sign and Symptoms

    a. Early signs in patients with type 1 diabetes (IDDM) include polyuria, polydipsia, and polyphagia.

        (1) Later signs include weight loss despite increased food intake, extreme fatigue, and pruritus. If not treated, ketoacidosis will develop in patients with IDDM.

    b. Patients with type 2 diabetes (NIDDM) initially may have none of the classic symptoms of the disease. If symptoms of polyuria, polydipsia, or polyphagia do occur, they are less severe than in IDDM.

        (1) Patients usually are obese, have vaginal itching, and usually are older than 40 years at onset of the disease.

        (2) Late signs include polyuria, polydipsia, and polyphagia. If not treated, hyperosmolar coma will develop in patients with NIDDM.

2. Treatment

    a. In planning a hyperglycemia diet, an estimate is made of the total energy intake needed per day based on ideal weight (determined from life insurance tables).

    b. An appropriate diet is constructed from exchange system provided by the American Diabetic Association (ADA).

    c. Hyperosmolar nonketotic coma is a complication of NIDDM.

    d. The importance of diet in the management of diabetes varies with type of disease.

        (1) In insulin-dependent patients, particularly those on intensive insulin regimens, the composition of the diet is not as critically important because adjustment of insulin can cover wide variations in food ingestion.

        (2) In non–insulin-dependent patients not treated with exogenous insulin, more rigorous adherence to a fixed diet is required because endogenous insulin reserve is limited. Such patients cannot respond to the increased demand produced by excess calories or increased intake of rapidly absorbed carbohydrates.

        (3) Insulin is required for treatment of all patients with IDDM and many patients with non–insulin-dependent disease.

        (4) If clients do not respond to oral hypoglycemic agents (see *Handbook of Medications for the NCLEX-RN® Review,* Chapter 7), insulin must be given.

        (5) It is fairly easy to control the symptoms with insulin, but it is difficult to maintain a normal blood sugar level throughout 24 h even if one utilizes injections of regular insulin or insulin infusion pumps.

    e. Insulin and treatment plans vary from physician to physician and with a given physician for different clients. Three treatment regimens are described: (a) conventional, (b) multiple subcutaneous insulin injections (MSI), and (c) continuous subcutaneous insulin infusion (CSII).

        (1) The MSI or CSII regimen is required in an intensive treatment schedule designed to protect against complications.

        (2) *Conventional insulin therapy* involves the administration of one or two injections per day of intermediate-acting insulin such as lente insulin or Novolin insulin (NPH insulin), with or without the addition of small amounts of regular insulin.

        (3) The *MSI* technique most commonly involves administration of intermediate or long-acting insulin in the evening (or morning) as a single dose together with regular insulin prior to each meal.

        (4) *CSII* (also known as insulin infusion pump) involves the use of a small battery-driven pump that delivers insulin subcutaneously into the abdominal wall, usually through a 27-gauge butterfly needle.

        (5) With CSII, insulin is delivered at a basal rate continuously throughout the day, with increased rates programmed prior to meals.

        (6) Adjustments in dosage are made in response to capillary glucose value (blood glucose finger stick), in a fashion similar to that used in MSI, using a sliding scale.

        (7) There is strong belief that CSII can improve diabetic control relative to conventional therapy.

        (8) Most patients using CSII report positive feelings of well-being as control improves.

        (9) The danger of hypoglycemia is real, especially during the night in patients who maintain a plasma glucose level consistently below 100 mg/dL.

        (10) A fall in plasma glucose level of 50 mg/dL may not be important if the starting value is 150 mg/dL but can be fatal if it occurs against a steady-state level of 60 mg/dL.

(11) Several deaths from hypoglycemia have occurred in pump users.

(12) There is also an increased frequency of diabetic ketoacidosis in patients using CSII.

Note: Pumps should be prescribed only for disciplined and motivated patients who are followed by physicians with extensive experience in pump use.

(13) For surgical procedures in diabetic clients, intermediate insulin is omitted, and treatment is carried out with regular insulin alone.

(14) Types of insulin: a variety of insulins are available for treatment of diabetes (see *Handbook of Medications for the NCLEX-RN® Review,* Chapter 7).

(15) Rapid-acting preparations are used in diabetic emergencies, at onset of insulin therapy, and in CSII and MSI programs.

(16) Peak effect and duration vary from patient to patient and depend not only on route of administration but also on dose. Generally accepted peak effect and duration for different types of insulin's are given in the *Handbook of Medications for the NCLEX-RN® Review,* Chapter 7.

(17) Most patients now are treated with synthesized "human" insulin (Humulin). The amino acid sequence is identical to that of the human hormone, and biologic activity appears to be equivalent.

(18) Complications of insulin therapy, such as insulin allergy and fat atrophy, are less common using "human insulin" but can still occur.

f. Self-monitoring glucose: a variety of glucose analyzers are on the market. The cost of equipment is reasonable, and many insurance carriers reimburse for its purchase.

(1) The client needs to have supervised training in the technique, and simultaneous checks of the blood sugar level in a laboratory should be done periodically to test the accuracy of the self-analysis.

(2) Repeated studies show that patients can measure blood glucose accurately using these techniques.

(3) Although urine testing for glucose is no longer used to follow diabetes, the measurement of ketones in the urine remains important.

D. Diabetic Ketoacidosis

◆ In addition to hypoglycemia and hyperglycemia, patients with diabetes are susceptible to two other major acute metabolic complications: diabetic ketoacidosis and hyperosmolar nonketotic coma.

(1) Ketoacidosis is a complication of IDDM and secondary diabetes.

(2) Hyperosmolar nonketotic coma is a complication of NIDDM.

Note: Ketoacidosis rarely, if ever, develops into true NIDDM.

1. Pathophysiology

a. Diabetic ketoacidosis results from insulin deficiency and increases in glucagon concentration.

(1) Ketoacidosis is often caused by a cessation of insulin intake but can result from physical (e.g., infection, surgery) or emotional stress despite continued insulin therapy.

(2) In times of stress, the body releases epinephrine, norepinephrine, dopamine, and glucocorticoids, all of which increase blood glucose levels.

(3) Hyperglycemia induces an osmotic diuresis that leads to volume depletion and dehydration, which is characterized by a state of ketosis.

(4) When the body does not have sufficient insulin to carry glucose into the cells for use as energy, it burns fat for energy. The by-product of fat is ketones.

(5) Overproduction of ketones by the liver is the primary event in the ketotic state and leads to ketoacidosis.

(6) Clinically, ketoacidosis begins with anorexia, nausea, and vomiting, coupled with an increased rate of urine formation.

(7) If untreated, altered consciousness or frank coma may occur.

(8) Initial examination usually shows Kussmaul's respirations, together with signs of volume depletion.

(9) Body temperature is normal or below normal in uncomplicated ketoacidosis: hence, fever suggests the presence of infection.

2. Diagnoses

a. The diagnosis of ketoacidosis in a patient known to have IDDM is not difficult. Its appearance in a patient not previously diagnosed requires differentiation from the other common causes of metabolic acidosis.

b. The first step is to test plasma glucose level, which may be 600 to 800 mg/100 mL (normal is 60–120).

c. The second step is to test the urine for glucose and ketones. If urine ketones are negative, another cause for the acidosis is likely.

3. Nursing Implications

a. Instruct the patient to know the conditions that bring about diabetic ketoacidosis:

(1) Failure to increase insulin when blood sugar level is increasing

(2) Failure to take insulin

(3) Stress

(4) Infection

(5) Illness

b. Instruct the patient to prevent hyperglycemia, which can lead to ketoacidosis.

(1) Encourage the patient to

(a) Avoid overeating

(b) Take prescribed insulin dose at scheduled times

(c) Continue daily exercise levels

(d) Monitor blood glucose levels daily

(e) Monitor urine for ketones if blood glucose levels are elevated

(2) Emphasize early recognition and treatment of hyperglycemia to avoid ketosis.

(3) Advise the patient to contact the physician for change in insulin dosage or additional insulin as indicated by elevated blood glucose and/or presence of urinary ketones.

E. Hyperosmolar Coma

1. Pathophysiology

a. Hyperosmolar, nonketotic diabetic coma usually is a complication of NIDDM. These patients tend to be insulin resistant.

b. It is a state of profound dehydration resulting from sustained hyperglycemic diuresis under circumstances in which the client is unable to drink sufficient water to keep up with urinary fluid losses. Patients can lose 10 to 12 L/day.

c. Commonly, an elderly diabetic patient, often living alone or in a nursing home, develops a stroke or infection, which worsens hyperglycemia and prevents adequate water intake.

d. Therapy for hyperosmolar coma requires regular insulin IV and a large amount of IV fluids.

e. A patient with NIDDM does not have the signs and symptom of nausea, vomiting, and Kussmaul's breathing that an IDDM patient will have when Ketoacidosis is developing. Such a protective mechanism is not operative in a ketoacidosis-resistant NIDDM patient. Therefore the patients will become severely dehydrated before hyperosmolar coma is diagnosised.

f. Interestingly, hyperosmolar coma can occur in IDDM patients given sufficient insulin to prevent ketosis but insufficient to control hyperglycemia.

g. The reason for the absence of ketoacidosis in NIDDM is not known.

2. Nursing Implications

a. Instruct the patient to maintain diabetes control during periods of illness or stress.

(1) Call the physician immediately when any unusual symptoms become evident; do not allow diabetes to get out of control.

(2) Make dietary adjustments during illness according to physician's directions.

(3) Continue taking oral hypoglycemic agent; the physician may increase dosage during illness or may prescribe regular insulin.

(4) Monitor blood glucose levels.

(5) Know the conditions that bring about diabetic hyperosmolar coma:

(a) Failure to increase oral hypoglycemic agent when blood sugar level is increasing

(b) Failure to take oral hypoglycemic agent

(c) Stress

(d) Infection

(e) Illness

b. Instruct the patient to prevent hyperglycemia, which can lead to hyperosmolar coma.

(1) Encourage the patient to

(a) Avoid overeating

(b) Take prescribed oral hypoglycemic agent dose at scheduled times

(c) Continue daily exercise levels

(d) Monitor blood glucose levels daily

(2) Emphasize early recognition and treatment of hyperglycemia to avoid hyperosmolar coma.

(3) Advise the patient to contact the physician for change in oral hypoglycemic dosage or additional insulin as indicated by elevated blood glucose levels.

F. Hyperosmolality (Hyperglycemic Nonketotic Coma)

1. Signs and Symptoms

a. Extreme hyperglycemia and volume depletion, coupled with central nervous system signs ranging from clouded sensorium (awareness) to coma.

b. Seizure activity and transient hemiplegia may be seen.

c. Infection, particularly pneumonia, and gram-negative sepsis, are common and indicate a poor prognosis.

2. Treatment

a. Treatment includes IV normal saline used to hydrate and Humulin R insulin in another bag of normal saline to lower blood sugar level.

G. Late Diabetic Complications

◆ The diabetic patient is susceptible to a series of complications that cause morbidity and premature mortality. Although some patients may never develop these problems and others recognize their onset early, on average, complications develop 15 to 20 years following the appearance of overt hyperglycemia.

1. Circulatory abnormalities

a. Atherosclerosis occurs more extensively and earlier than in the general population. The cause of accelerated atherosclerosis is not known.

(1) Atherosclerotic lesions produce symptoms in a variety of sites. Peripheral deposits may cause intermittent claudication, gangrene, and, in men, organic impotence on a vascular basis.

(2) Coronary artery disease and strokes are common.

(3) Silent MI is thought to occur with increased frequency in diabetic patients and should be suspected when symptoms of left ventricular failure appear suddenly. Silent MI is thought to occur because of sensory defect caused by diabetic neuropathy.

b. Diabetic retinopathy is a leading cause of blindness in the United States.

(1) The frequency of diabetic retinopathy appears to vary with the age of onset and the duration of the disease.

(2) It is estimated that 85 percent of patients eventually develop retinopathy.

(3) Treatment of diabetic retinopathy is photocoagulation. Such treatment decreases the incidence of hemorrhage and scarring. Photocoagulation is the use of a laser beam for treatment of bleeding from the retina or for treatment of retinal detachments.

c. Diabetic nephropathy is a renal disease that is a leading cause of death and disability in diabetics. About half of end-stage renal disease cases in the United States are now due to diabetic nephropathy.

(1) It is estimated that 35 percent of patients with IDDM develop nephropathy complications.

(2) There is no specific treatment for diabetic nephropathy.

(3) Hypertension must be treated aggressively whenever present.

(4) Angiotensin-converting enzyme inhibitors (see *Handbook of Medications for the NCLEX-RN® Review,* Chapter 5) appear to be useful in slowing the progression of diabetic nephropathy.

d. Based on experimental studies in animals and humans, a low-protein diet may be useful.

e. Chronic dialysis and renal transplantation are routine in patients with renal failure due to diabetes.

f. Diabetic neuropathy can affect every part of the nervous system, with possible exception of the brain. It is rarely a direct cause of death; however, it is a major cause of morbidity.

(1) The most common clinical picture of peripheral polyneuropathy usually is bilateral presentation and symptoms that include numbness, paresthesias, severe hyperesthesias (increased sensitivity to sensory stimuli), and pain.

(2) Pain may be severe and often is worse at night. The extreme pain syndrome lasts only a few months to a few years. Patients may experience a painless neuropathy characterized by an inability to perceive pain.

(3) Treatment of diabetic neuropathy is unsatisfactory in most respects.

(4) When pain is severe, it is easy for the patient to become habituated or addicted to narcotics or nonnarcotic analgesics such as pentazocine (Talwin).

g. Development of ulcers of the feet and lower extremities is a special problem in the diabetic patient.

(1) The ulcers appear to be primarily due to abnormal pressure distribution secondary to diabetic neuropathy. The client does not perceive prolonged body pressure because of sensory deficit and, therefore, does not change position. Ischemia develops, followed by ulceration.

(2) Ill-fitting shoes cause blister formation in patients whose sensory deficits preclude recognition of pain.

(3) Cuts and punctures from foreign objects, such as needles, tacks, and glass, are common, and foreign objects, of which the patient is unaware, may be found in soft tissue.

(4) For this reason, all diabetic patients with ulcers should have x-ray films taken of their feet.

h. Vascular disease with diminished blood supply contributes to development of lesions. Infection is common, often with multiple organisms.

i. Patients with diabetes are susceptible to infections of many types.

(1) Infections are difficult to treat once they occur. Infected areas heal slowly because the damaged vascular system cannot carry sufficient oxygen, white blood cells, nutrients, and antibodies to the injured site.

(2) Infections increases the need for insulin.

III. DIABETES INSIPIDUS

A. Deficiency of Vasopressin

◆ Diabetes insipidus results from a deficiency of circulating vasopressin, also called antidiuretic hormone (ADH) (Fig. 2–3).

1. Etiology

a. This uncommon condition occurs equally among both genders, usually between the ages of 15 and 20 years.

2. Pathophysiology with Signs and Symptoms

a. Primary diabetes insipidus (50 percent of patients) is familial or is a primary disease without apparent cause (idiopathic in origin).

b. Secondary diabetes insipidus results from metastatic lesions, hypophysectomy, or other neurosurgery.

c. The lack of ADH allows filtered water to be excreted in the urine instead of being reabsorbed.

d. The hypothalamus synthesizes vasopressin, which is stored in the posterior pituitary gland and released into circulation. It causes the kidneys to reabsorb water by making the distal and collecting tubule cells water permeable.

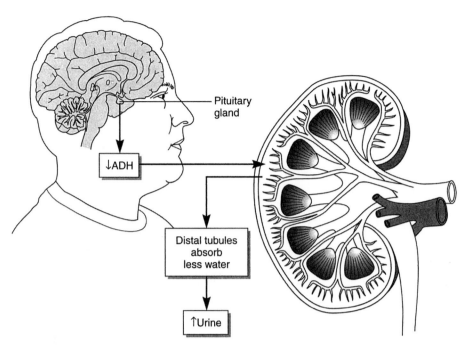

FIGURE 2-3 ◆ Diabetes Insipidus

Antidiuretic hormone (ADH) decreases water reabsorption by the distal tubules of the kidney, thus increasing urine output. A decrease in ADH causes diabetes insipidus.

e. Symptoms include

(1) Polyuria, as much as 30 L/day or urine may be excreted. The urine is dilute with a specific gravity of 1.005 or less.

(2) Polydipsia secondary to increased thirst.

3. Treatment

a. Administration of a vasopressin stimulant such as pitressin tannate (duration SC 2–8 h) can control fluid balance and prevent dehydration. When the deficiency is total, ADH replacement therapy is required. The primary agents include the following:

◆ Desmopressin (duration nasal 5–21 h) is the agent of choice for treating diabetes insipidus because of its prolonged action, ease of administration, and lack of significant side effects. Response to treatment is rapid, and urinary volume quickly drops to normal levels.

◆ Pitressin is an aqueous preparation that is administered SC or IM several times per day because effectiveness lasts for only 2 to 8 h. Often used in acute disease.

◆ Vasopressin tannate (pitressin tannate) is an oil preparation administered IM only. It is effective for 24 to 96 h. Warm the vial of vasopressin tannate between hands.

(1) Shake vial vigorously to mix the active ingredients, which settle as brown specks at the bottom of vial.

(2) When ADH replacement is required, treatment usually is lifelong.

(3) Major side effects of ADH replacement agents include pain at IM site, chest pain, and MI.

(4) When the deficiency is only partial, medication other than ADH may be used. The primary agents is chlorpropamide (Diabinese), which promotes ADH release and increases renal responsiveness. Diabinese is also used to treat type 2 NIDDM2.

4. Nursing Implications

a. Nursing interventions for the patient with diabetes insipidus focus on maintenance of fluid and electrolyte balance, provision of rest, and teaching.

b. Assess intake and output, urine specific gravity, and vital signs.

c. Provide teaching for diagnostic tests, procedures, and required monitoring (e.g., ECG).

d. Instruct the patient in self-management of drug therapy.

IV. PARATHYROID DISORDERS

A. Hyperparathyroid

1. Etiology

a. The parathyroid gland produces one hormone: parathyroid hormone (PTH). This hormone is continually synthesized.

b. Two factors influence parathyroid function: calcitonin levels and serum phosphorus levels; both decrease serum calcium.

c. Calcitonin and etidronate (Didronel) are hypocalcemic peptide hormone that, in many ways, act as the physiologic antagonist to PTH.

d. The hypocalcemic activity of calcitonin is accounted for by inhibition of osteoclast-mediated bone resorption and by stimulation of renal calcium clearance.

e. The major role of PTH is regulation of the blood levels of calcium and phosphorus by acting on three sites:

   (1) In the gastrointestinal tract, PTH enhances absorption of calcium in the presence of normal vitamin D levels

   (2) In the kidney, PTH increases the reabsorption of calcium and promotes the excretion of phosphorus in the renal tubules

   (3) In bone, PTH is believed to stimulate osteoclastic activity to release calcium into the blood

2. Incidence

   a. Primary hyperparathyroidism is a relatively common disorder that arises within the gland itself.

   b. It is accompanied by parathyroid gland enlargement and increased secretion of PTH.

   c. Solitary adenomas account for 90 percent of primary hyperparathyroidism cases.

   d. Other causes include multiple adenomas, carcinoma, and hyperplasia of all four parathyroid glands.

3. Pathophysiology with Nursing Implications

   a. In hyperparathyroidism, PTH is overproduced. The excess hormone results in hypercalcemia secondary to increased intestinal calcium absorption, reduced renal calcium clearance, and increased bone calcium release.

   b. The signs and symptoms that result from high circulating levels of calcium and low phosphorus levels include

   (1) Nausea and vomiting

   (2) Recurring kidney stones (nephrolithiasis), which may lead to renal insufficiency; as a result of kidney stones, the patient experiences renal colic (pain), recurrent urinary tract infections, and polyuria; polyuria is secondary to the kidney's decreased ability to concentrate urine

   (3) The patient experiences low back pain, bone tenderness, bone deformities, and pathologic fractures due to generalized bone demineralization

   (4) Marked proximal muscle weakness and atrophy are caused by decreased muscle contractility; serum calcium levels greatly elevate the resting membrane potential of muscle cells, thereby decreasing excitability of nerve and muscle cell membrane

   (5) Mild to severe psychomotor or behavioral disturbances may be observed; disorientation, confusion, memory loss, and psychosis may occur

   (6) Cardiac changes include bradycardia with bursts of tachycardia; atrioventricular block also may ensue

   (7) Calcification of the cornea of the eye and decreased auditory activity

4. Treatment

   a. Surgical removal of the parathyroid tumor in the case of adenomas or carcinomas is often required.

   b. A portion of parathyroid gland must be left to supply sufficient amounts of PTH.

   c. If surgery is contraindicated and hypercalcemia is marked, the patient can be managed with hydration and etidronate (Didronel). Didronel decreases bone resorption and promotes new bone development.

   d. Didronel generally must be given IV to be effective. At times, the continuation of oral Didronel after IV therapy is useful for controlling hypercalcemia.

   e. Etidronate (Didronel) blocks the growth of calcium hydroxyapatite crystals by binding calcium phosphate. The therapeutic effects are decreased bone resorption and turnover.

   f. For acute management, plicamycin (Mithracin) is used for management of hypercalcemia, which inhibits bone resorption.

   g. The first principle of treatment is to restore normal hydration. Many hypercalcemic patients are dehydrated because of vomiting and hypercalcemia-induced defects in urinary concentration ability.

   h. Fluid volume helps to correct these abnormalities by increasing calcium and sodium excretion.

B. Hypoparathyroid

1. Causes and Incidence

   a. Hypoparathyroidism may be acute or chronic and is classified as idiopathic, acquired, or reversible.

   b. Idiopathic hypoparathyroidism may result from an autoimmune genetic disorder or the congenital absence of the parathyroid glands.

   c. Acquired hypoparathyroidism often results from accidental removal of, or injury to, one or more parathyroid glands during thyroidectomy or other neck surgery, or from massive thyroid irradiation.

   d. It also may result from ischemic infarction of the parathyroids during surgery, or from neoplasms or trauma.

   e. An acquired, reversible hypoparathyroidism may result from hypomagnesemia-induced impairment of hormone synthesis, from suppression of normal gland function due to hypercalcemia, or from delayed maturation of parathyroid function.

2. Parathyroidectomy (Postoperative)

   a. When surgery is performed, postoperative care is similar to that for the patient with thyroidectomy.

   b. A tracheostomy set is kept at the patient's bedside should edema or hemorrhage cause airway obstruction.

c. As with patients with thyroidectomy, a semi-Fowler's position is recommended along with prevention of head and neck movement; support of head and neck should be provided. This will decrease the edema, thus minimizing the risk of tracheal occlusion.

d. Assessments of the degree of respiratory distress and swelling at the operative site are important interventions.

e. Monitoring laboratory data for low serum calcium concentration can alert the nurse to potential postoperative problems.

f. Early signs resulting from tetany include complaints of tingling in the hands and face. These symptoms may subside or progress to severe neuromuscular irritability with seizures.

g. Early manifestation of hypocalcemia (e.g., tetany) should be reported immediately, and intravenous calcium gluconate should be available for emergency administration.

3. Diagnostic evaluation for hypocalcemia

a. Trousseau's sign: inflation of blood pressure cuff on arm will cause the hand to adduct if hypocalcemia is present.

b. Chvostek's sign: hyperirritability of the facial nerve when tapped; exists when the patient is in a state of hypocalcemia.

4. Treatment of hypocalcemia

a. Treatment may require adjusting diet to allow for adequate intake of calcium and vitamin D.

b. Acute hypocalcemia is an emergency situation that must be corrected immediately by IV administration of calcium gluconate or calcium chloride. Acute hypocalcemia can occur after a thyroidectomy because of trauma to the parathyroid glands (glands are unable to produce calcium for several days due to surgical trauma) or after surgery to remove a portion of the parathyroid gland due to cancer in the area. Once calcium levels have been restored, an oral calcium salt (e.g., calcium carbonate) can be given for maintenance.

c. Early in the postoperative course, patient ambulation is encouraged; pressure on long bones will increase bone recalcification.

V. THYROID DISORDERS

◆ Disorders of the thyroid gland are relatively common endocrine problems.

◆ They are second to diabetes mellitus in frequency of occurrence.

◆ Alterations in the thyroid gland may be associated with hypersecretion, hyposecretion, or normal secretion of thyroid hormone.

A. Hyperthyroidism (Graves' disease)

◆ Hyperthyroidism, also called *thyrotoxicosis,* is a condition that results when tissues are stimulated by excessive thyroid-stimulating hormone (TSH).

◆ Hyperthyroidism is also known as *Graves' disease.*

1. Incidence

a. The incidence of Graves' disease is highest between the ages of 30 and 40 years, especially in patients with a family history of thyroid abnormalities.

b. Only 5 percent of hyperthyroid patients are younger than age 15 years.

2. Etiology

a. The cause is unknown, but the disease may result from genetic and immunologic factors.

3. Pathophysiology with Signs and Symptoms

a. It is possible that no single factor is responsible for the entire syndrome.

b. With respect to hyperthyroidism, although the basic cause in not understood, it is believed that the central disorder is a disruption of a homeostatic mechanism that normally adjusts hormone secretion to meet the needs of peripheral tissues. This homeostatic disruption results from the presence of an abnormal thyroid stimulator in plasma.

c. Common manifestations of Graves' disease include nervousness, emotional lability, inability to sleep, tremors, excessive sweating, and heat intolerance.

d. Weight loss occurs despite increased appetite.

e. Muscle weakness is present, as are dyspnea, palpitations, tachycardia, and hypertension.

f. Separation of fingernails from the nail bed (Plummer's nail) is common.

g. The hair is fine and silky.

h. A fine tremor of the fingers and tongue may occur.

i. Ocular signs include exophthalmos eyes, which is produced by the combined effects of accumulation of fat and fluid behind the eyeball; lid lag; infrequent blinking; and staring gaze.

j. Goiter is the most common sign.

k. When severe, Graves' disease presents little difficulty in diagnosis. Laboratory tests document elevated serum triiodothyronine (T_3) and thyroxine (T_4) levels. Presence of goiter makes the diagnosis of hyperthyroidism likely.

4. Treatment

a. The major treatments are directed to limiting the quantity of thyroid hormones produced by the gland.

b. Antithyroid agents interpose a chemical blockade to hormone synthesis, the effect of which is operative only as long as the drug is administered.

c. Iodide (e.g., Lugol's solution) inhibits the release of hormones (T_3 and T_4) from the hyperfunctioning thyroid gland, and its effects are more rapid than those agents that inhibit hormone synthesis. Hence, it is mainly use in patients with actual or impending thyrotoxic crisis (e.g., thyroid surgery) and in patients with severe cardiac disease.

d. The second major approach is ablation (removal of part) of thyroid tissue, thereby limiting hormone production. This can be achieved either by surgery or by radioactive iodine.

e. Because these procedures induce permanent anatomical alterations of the thyroid, they can control the active phase and are more likely to prevent later exacerbation or recurrence.

f. Radioactive iodine 131 is more likely to lead to hypothyroidism, either shortly after treatment or with the passage of years. Each therapy has advantages and disadvantages and indications and contraindications.

g. Antithyroid therapy is desirable in children, adolescents, young adults, and pregnant women but also may be used in older patients.

h. Indications for ablative procedures include

    (1) Relapse or recurrence following drug therapy

    (2) Large goiter

    (3) Drug toxicity

    (4) Failure to follow a medical regimen

i. Radioactive iodine (see *Handbook of Medications for the NCLEX-RN® Review,* Chapter 7) is the ablative procedure of choice for older patients, for those who have undergone previous thyroid surgery, and for those in whom systemic disease contraindicates surgery.

j. A single PO dose of iodine 131 is picked up by the thyroid gland as it would pick up regular iodine. Radioactivity destroys cells that normally concentrate iodine and produce thyroxine, thus decreasing the production of thyroid hormones. This may cause myxedema. The patient may leave the hospital the same day that iodine 131 is given, unless the dosage is very high. Instruct the patient to use rubber gloves when handling his or her urine and to flush the toilet three times.

k. In patients selected for long-term antithyroid therapy, satisfactory control can almost always be achieved if sufficient amount of an antithyroid drug is administered (see *Handbook of Medications for the NCLEX-RN® Review,* Chapter 7).

l. Most patients can be managed with propylthiouracil, 100 to 150 mg every 6 to 8 h.

m. During pregnancy, antithyroid medications are kept at the minimum dosage required to keep maternal thyroid function normal until delivery and to minimize the risk of fetal hypothyroidism even though most infants of hyperthyroid mothers are born with mild and transient hyperthyroidism. Neonatal hyperthyroidism may even necessitate treatment with antithyroid drugs for 2 to 3 months. Throughout neonatal antithyroid therapy, the mother should not breast-feed, as this can cause neonatal hypothyroidism.

5. Nursing Implications

a. Inform the patient to avoid stimulants such as coffee, caffeine, and alcohol.

b. Offer measures to help the patient relax.

c. Include the family in discussions.

d. Decrease known stressors; explain all interventions, and listen to patient.

e. Balance periods of activity with rest.

f. Administer prescribed drugs and monitor therapeutic response.

g. Report any changes to the physician.

h. Control environmental temperature for the patient's comfort.

i. Encourage adequate fluid intake and monitor fluid losses.

j. Assess vital signs, especially heart rate and rhythm, at least qid; if the patient worsens, assess qh.

k. Instruct the patient to report palpitations, chest pain, and dizziness.

l. Assess weight, intake, and output daily; assess for signs of edema, jugular vain distention, and pulmonary congestion every 8 h.

m. Assess visual activity, ability to close eyes, and photophobia.

n. Protect eyes from irritants.

o. Use patches of glasses when in high wind, if exophthalmia is present.

p. Keep the patient in the semi-Fowler's position at night.

q. Instruct the patient not to lie prone, if exophthalmos is present.

r. If eyes do not close completely, inquire about using shields at night.

s. Use artificial tears, if prescribed, for exophthalmia.

B. Thyrotoxic Crisis (Severe Hyperthyroidism)

◆ Thyrotoxic crisis, or thyroid storm (also called *medical storm*), causes a fulminating increase in the signs and symptoms of thyrotoxicosis. In the past, this disturbance usually occurred postoperatively in clients poorly prepared for surgery. With the preoperative use of antithyroid drugs and iodine and with appropriate therapy for controlling metabolic factors, postoperative crisis should not occur.

◆ At present, medical storm (thyroid storm) occurs in untreated or inadequately treated clients. It is precipitated by surgical emergency or complicating illness, usually sepsis.

◆ The syndrome is characterized by extreme irritability, fever to 106°F, tachycardia, hypertension, arrhythmias, profuse diapiresis, vomiting, and diarrhea. If not treated, delirium or coma ensues.

◆ Treatment consists of administration of large doses of antithyroid therapy to decrease thyroid synthesis of thyroid hormone and iodide to block release of thyroid hormone. An adrenergic antagonist, usually propranolol (Inderal), is administered.

C. Simple Goiter

1. Incidence and Etiology

   a. Any enlargement of the thyroid gland is called a *goiter.*

   b. If the enlargement is not associated with hyperthyroidism or hypothyroidism, cancer, or inflammation, it is referred to as a *simple goiter.* In most instances, the cause of a simple goiter is unknown.

2. Etiology with Classifications and Incidence

   a. *Endemic goiter* (hypothyroidism) is a goiter that occurs in a particular geographic region and from a common cause such as iodine deficiency.

   (1) Endemic goiter caused by environmental iodine deficiency is found in all continents except North America and is estimated to affect more than 200 million people.

   (2) In the United States, regions such as the Great Lakes Basin previously had a high incidence of endemic goiter but no longer do because of education about the use of iodized salt.

   (3) Iodine is needed for the thyroid gland to synthesis T_3 and T_4.

   (4) When an iodine deficiency is present, the thyroid cannot secrete enough thyroid hormone to meet metabolic requirements. As a result, the thyroid mass increases (goiter) to compensate for inadequate hormone synthesis.

   b. *Sporadic goiter* (hypothyroidism) is caused by the ingestion of large amounts of goitrogenic foods or drugs. Goitrogenic foods contain agents that decrease thyroxine production. They include rutabagas, cabbage, soybeans, peanuts, peaches, peas, strawberries, spinach, and radishes. Goitrogenic drugs include propylthiouracil, iodides, phenylbutazone, cobalt, and lithium.

   c. Autoimmune disorder appears to be a major factor in goiter development. Thyroid-stimulating immunoglobulins (TSIs) and autoantibodies react to a component of the thyroid cell membrane, somehow stimulating the thyroid gland (mimicking TSH) to secrete excess thyroid hormone. As a result, a goiter develops.

3. Pathophysiology with Signs and Symptoms

   a. The underlying pathophysiologic involved in simple goiter formation is an increase in TSH. It is believed that when factors inhibit normal thyroid hormone production, hypersecretion of TSH occurs because of a lack of negative feedback. The increase in TSH results in an increase in thyroid mass.

   b. The increase in TSH increases the turnover of iodine, and the T_3/T_4 ratio in thyroid secretion is increased. The patient remains euthyroid at the expense of the elevated TSH and an enlarged gland.

   c. Thyroid enlargement (simple goiter), which varies greatly, is the cause of symptoms.

   d. The primary sign may be disfigurement, and the primary symptom may be patient's complaints of tightening of garments worn around the neck.

   e. If the goiter is very large, it may displace or compress the esophagus or trachea and cause dysphagia, choking sensation, or inspiratory stridor.

   f. Compression of the laryngeal nerve can lead to hoarseness.

4. Treatment

   a. Medical management is directed at removing the stimulus causing the increased thyroid mass.

   b. If extrinsic factors such as goitrogenic drugs or foods are the cause, they are eliminated. Iodine deficiency, although rare, is ruled out and replacement is instituted if appropriate.

   c. Only small doses of iodide, such as saturated solution of potassium iodide (SSKI) or Lugol's solution, are needed.

   d. In most instances, the cause of goiter is unknown and therapy is directed at supplying exogenous hormone, which will inhibit TSH secretion.

   e. Levothyroxine (Synthroid) usually is necessary (see *Handbook of Medications for the NCLEX-RN® Review,* Chapter 7). The adequacy of the dosage in suppressing TSH secretion is verified by a radioactive iodine uptake (RAIU) test.

D. Autoimmune Thyroiditis (Hashimoto's Thyroiditis)

   ◆ There are three types of thyroiditis (inflammation of the thyroid):

   ◆ Acute

   ◆ Subacute

   ◆ Chronic

1. Incidence

   a. Hashimoto's thyroiditis is the most common form of chronic thyroiditis.

   b. It is most common in women, with peak incidence in middle age.

   c. Acute thyroiditis is rare. It results from infections of the thyroid by pyogenic organism.

2. Etiology

   a. Autoimmune thyroiditis is due to the development of antibodies to thyroid antigens in the blood. It is the cause of Hashimoto's thyroiditis.

3. Pathophysiology with Signs and Symptoms

   a. Autoimmune thyroiditis is the most prevalent cause of spontaneous hypothyroidism. The major finding in Hashimoto's thyroiditis is diffuse thyroid enlargement, found as a goiter on examination. The thyroid is firm and smooth, moves freely, and usually is painless.

   b. Some patients may experience dysphagia or choking.

c. The patient may have transient periods of hyperthyroidism early in the disease. The patient may be euthyroid (normal) for several years. As the disease progresses, the gland is destroyed, and the signs and symptoms of hypothyroidism occur.

4. Treatment

a. No treatment for mild asymptomatic disease.

b. Thyroid hormone replacement with levothyroxine (Synthroid) for goiter or hypothyroidism (see *Handbook of Medications for the NCLEX-RN® Review,* Chapter 7).

c. Surgery if the goiter is unresponsive to thyroid hormone, is pressing on adjacent structures, or is disfiguring.

5. Nursing Implications

a. Nursing care focuses primarily on teaching the patient about the disease process, diagnostic tests, and treatment.

E. Hypothyroidism (Myxedema)

◆ Hypothyroidism is a relatively common metabolic state caused by a deficiency in circulating thyroid hormone.

◆ Adult onset of severe hypothyroidism is sometimes known as *myxedema.*

◆ Hypothyroidism occurring in infancy is termed *congential hypothyroidism* or *cretinism.*

1. Incidence

a. Hypothyroidism is most prevalent in women. In the United States, the incidence is rising significantly in persons aged 30 to 50 years.

2. Etiology

a. In adults, inadequate production of thyroid hormone is caused by dysfunction of the gland as a result of

(1) Surgery (thyroidectomy)

(2) Irradiation (particularly radioactive iodine therapy)

(3) Chronic autoimmune thyroiditis (Hashimoto's thyroiditis)

(4) Pituitary failure to produce TSH

(5) Hypothalamic failure to produce thyrotropin-releasing hormone (TRH)

(6) Inability to synthesize the hormone because of iodine deficiency (usually dietary)

(7) Use of antithyroid medications, such as propylthiouracil

(8) Excess ingestion of food goitrogens

b. In infants, hypothyroidism results from

(1) Congenital absence or underdevelopment of the thyroid gland

(2) Severe iodine deficiency suffered by the mother during pregnancy

(3) Less frequently, an enzymatic defect in thyroxine synthesis is inherited as an autosomal recessive trait

3. Pathophysiology with Signs and Symptoms

a. Typically, the early clinical signs and symptoms of hypothyroidism are vague and insidious: forgetfulness, fatigue, intolerance to cold, unexplained weight gain (obesity), and constipation.

b. As the disease progresses and the metabolic process slows, characteristic myxedematous symptoms appear: puffy face with periorbital edema; upper eyelid droops; dry, sparse hair due to hair loss; thick, brittle nails; decreased mental stability; dry, flaky inelastic skin; intentional tremors; cardiovascular involvement leading to decreased cardiac output; bradycardia; and poor peripheral circulation.

c. Irregular menstrual periods and severe menorrhagia are common in young women.

d. Decreased libido occurs in both genders.

e. Fertility usually is diminished but pregnancy is possible.

f. Client has unusually slow intellectual functioning. Agitation and psychosis can occur, however, and are accompanied by paranoid ideation, suicidal tendencies, and hallucinations.

g. With the failure of the metabolic processes along with hepatic and renal impairment, life-threatening coma (myxedema coma) ensues.

h. It usually develops gradually with progressive stupor, hypotension, and hypothermia.

i. Usually, clinical signs of hypothyroidism in infancy occur at age 3 to 6 months and may be delayed in the breast-fed infant because some thyroid hormone is contained in breast milk.

j. Usually, the baby is described as a "good baby" who sleeps excessively with only an occasional hoarse cry.

k. The baby's development, both mental and physical, is delayed.

l. The infant's reflexes are diminished, and the infant makes slow awkward movements.

m. The infant has feeding problems and has constipation.

n. Liver impairment interferes with conjugation of bilirubin, and the infant may become jaundiced.

o. The tongue is enlarged, making breathing noisy and sometimes causing airway obstruction.

p. The classic physical features include wide-set puffy eyes, short forehead, broad flat nose, dull sparse hair, and cold, dry skin.

q. Mental retardation typically is profound but may be limited, depending on how soon thyroid hormone replacement therapy begins.

4. Treatment

a. Therapy for hypothyroidism consists of gradual thyroid replacement with levothyroxine (Synthroid) and liothyronine (Cytomel) (see *Handbook of Medications for the NCLEX-RN® Review,* Chapter 7).

b. Dosage varies with age, the severity of hypothyroidism, general medical condition (particularly cardiovascular disorders), and the patient's response to medical treatment.

c. Patients with cardiac complications must be started on small doses of levothyroxine (Synthroid). Large doses could precipitate heart failure or MI by increasing body metabolism, myocardial oxygen requirements, and, consequently, the workload of the heart.

d. Myxedema coma is corrected by immediate intravenous administration of levothyroxine (Synthroid) or liothyronine (Cytomel) with maintenance doses every 8 to 12 h.

e. Despite prompt and appropriate therapy, the mortality of myxedema coma remains approximately 50 percent.

5. Nursing Implications

a. Nursing interventions for the client with hypothyroidism consist of (a) restoring a normal metabolic state, (b) preventing complications of the disease, and (c) strengthening long-term coping resources to better handle the chronic nature of the disease.

b. Maintain a warm environment.

c. Provide good skin care by avoiding daily bathing and the use of soap. Blot skin dry with a soft towel, and use oil or lotion after bath. Provide a diet high in protein, carbohydrates, and vitamins. Teach the patient and family members how to identify skin breakdown.

d. Prevent constipation by encouraging high fluid intake and a diet high in foods with fiber, such as fruits and raw vegetables. Encourage adequate exercise to the level of the patient's tolerance.

e. Monitor cardiovascular performance, evaluate blood pressure and pulse, and assess for signs of congestive heart failure (pulmonary crackles, etc.).

F. Thyroid Neoplasm

◆ One of the most common abnormalities of the thyroid gland is the development of a nodule, a localized area of enlargement.

◆ Benign adenomas usually are not dangerous, although they can grow large enough to cause respiratory symptoms by pressing against the trachea.

◆ Occasionally, malignant transformation occurs, and the benign nodules become cancerous.

1. Incidence

a. Malignant tumors of the thyroid are relatively rare.

b. Thyroid cancer accounts for approximately 0.4 percent of cancer deaths.

c. It develops mainly in patients between the ages of 40 and 60 years and affects twice as many women as men.

2. Etiology

a. Thyroid cancer occurs more frequently among patients who have received large doses of radiation to the head and neck.

3. Pathophysiology with Nursing Implications

a. The major manifestation of thyroid cancer is the appearance of a hard, painless nodule in the thyroid gland.

b. The nodule typically is solitary and does not take up radioactive iodine (cold spot) when radioisotope scanning using iodine 131 is performed.

c. If the tumor has already metastasized, the lymph nodes are sometimes palpable.

d. There are three major types of thyroid cancer: (a) *Papillary cancer* accounts for half of all thyroid cancers in adults. It metastasizes slowly and is the least virulent form of thyroid cancer. (b) *Follicular carcinoma* is less common (30 percent of all cases) but is more likely to recur and metastasize to the regional nodes, and through blood vessels into the rest of the body. (c) *Medullary (solid) carcinoma* is even less common (10 percent of all cases) and originates in the parafollicular cells. It can produce calcitonin, histamines, and ACTH (producing Cushing's syndrome).

e. Thyroid cancer is familial.

f. It is a relatively rare form of cancer and completely curable when detected before symptoms occur. Untreated, it grows rapidly, frequently metastasizing to bones, liver, and kidneys.

G. Thyroidectomy (Preoperative)

1. Treatment

a. Thyroidectomy is the surgical removal of all or part of the thyroid gland as treatment of hyperthyroidism or cancer of the thyroid gland.

b. Thyroidectomy (removal of the thyroid gland) can be total or partial.

c. Total thyroidectomy is performed to remove thyroid cancer.

d. Patients who undergo this operation must take thyroid hormone on a permanent basis.

e. Subtotal thyroidectomy is performed to correct hyperthyroidism and for extreme cases of simple goiter.

f. Approximately five-sixths of the gland is removed; however, because one-sixth of the functioning gland usually is left intact, hormonal replacements may not be necessary.

g. Preoperative preparation for a subtotal thyroidectomy is extremely important.

h. The patient must be euthyroid (normal thyroid functioning) before the operation, if possible.

i. If the patient is not euthyroid, the risk of postoperative thyroid storm is greatly increased.

2. Nursing Implications

   a. Preoperative

   ◆ Preoperative care of clients with Graves' disease includes administration of:

   (1) Antithyroid drugs (e.g., Lugol's solution, SSKI) to suppress secretion of thyroid hormone (propylthiouracil).

   (2) Iodine preparations (potassium iodide) to reduce the size and vascularity of the organ, thereby diminishing the chance of hemorrhage. Adequate preoperative preparation may take as long as 1 to 2 months.

   b. Postoperative

   (1) Check vital signs as needed.

   (2) Identify signs and symptoms of hemorrhage and respiratory obstruction, such as vital sign changes, frequent swallowing, dyspnea, and gasping.

   (3) Observe for signs of parathyroid damage and laryngeal nerve damage, such as tetany (low calcium), hoarseness (laryngeal nerve damage), and respiratory difficulty (swelling at operative site).

   (4) Look for early signs of thyroid crisis (thyrotoxicosis), such as fever, restlessness, tachycardia, sweating, and pulmonary edema.

   (5) Auscultate lung sounds and heart sounds.

   (6) Assess for pain, noting intensity, duration, and relief methods.

   (7) Instruct the patient to support his or her head when moving in the bed.

   (8) Apply an ice collar and place the patient in semi-Fowler's position.

   (9) Monitor vital signs, looking for subtle changes reflecting complications.

   (10) Have the patient speak every 2 h to determine voice quality.

   (11) Administer humidified oxygen.

   (12) Check the dressing every 1 to 2 h for edema and bleeding for the first 24 h.

   (13) Evaluate the patient frequently for restlessness; irritability; numbness; tingling of the fingers, toes, ears, and circumoral area; muscle twitching; or a positive Chvostek's sign or Trousseau's sign.

   (14) Keep equipment for emergency tracheotomy as well as calcium gluconate and parenteral administration available at the bedside.

   (15) Surgical treatment is effective in most people with Graves' disease.

   (16) A small percentage of patients remain hyperthyroid, and some develop hypothyroidism.

   (17) Rarely, vocal cord paralysis or hypoparathyroidism develops as a result of nerve damage.

Chapter

3

Hematologic Disorders

◆ Aplastic anemia results from injury or destruction of stem cells of the bone marrow or bone marrow matrix, causing anemia, thrombocytopenia, and marrow hypoplasia. Total red blood cells (RBCs) are very low (1,000,000 or less). This is a life-threatening disease. Platelet, white blood cell (WBC), and RBC counts are decreased. The disease can produce fatal bleeding, infection, or anemia. RBCs are excessively varied in size and larger than normal.

1. Etiology and Incidence

   a. Agents that in an adequate dose will predictably produce marrow depression (aplastic anemia) include antineoplastic agents (cancer chemotherapy) and immunosuppressive drugs, along with ionizing radiation.

   b. Marrow depression also may be induced by excessive use of x-rays.

   c. Benzene-induced aplastic anemia may result from both industrial and domestic use of benzene-containing products. The severity of aplastic anemia depends on the dose and rate of exposure.

2. Signs and Symptoms

   ◆ Progressive weakness, headache, pallor, shortness of breath, tachycardia, and congestive heart failure. Thrombocytopenia leads to ecchymosis, petechiae, and hemorrhage, especially from the mucous membranes (gingival, nasal, vaginal, and rectal).

3. Treatment

   a. Administration of packed red cells and platelets. Marrow transplant is the treatment of choice for anemia due to severe aplastic anemia and for clients who need continual RBC transfusions.

   b. Removal of causative agents is very important.

   c. Other treatments may include administration of corticosteroids.

4. Nursing Implications

   a. If the platelet count is less than 20,000/mm^3 (normal 150,000–400,000/mm^3), prevent hemorrhage by avoiding IM injections; suggest use of soft toothbrush; promote regular bowel movements through use of stool softener and high-fiber diet.

   b. Detect bleeding early by close assessment for blood in urine or stool.

   c. Avoid IM injection because of bleeding at the site. If bleeding occurs, apply pressure for 10 to 15 min. If bleeding persists, notify physician immediately.

   d. Maintain reversed isolation if WBC count is decreased and administer prophylactic antibiotics.

   (1) Clients with low WBC counts need special measures to prevent infection

B. Sickle Cell Anemia

◆ Chronic hemolytic disorder characterized by sickle-shaped erythrocytes and accelerated hemolysis. RBCs lyse easily when oxygen is low.

1. Etiology and Incidence

a. Sickle cell anemia is a congenital hemolytic anemia that occurs mainly in the black population.

2. Signs and Symptoms

a. Sickle cell anemia results in dyspnea on exertion, swollen joints, and fatigue; destruction of sickled cells (RBCs); and infections because of destruction of WBCs.

b. Thrombosis and infarction from sludging (clotting) of sickled cells.

c. Elevated bilirubin levels; bilirubin is produced from the hemoglobin of destroyed RBCs, leading to jaundice.

d. Liver and spleen enlarge and result in decreased function.

e. Leg ulcers caused by vascular occlusion; skin ulcers occur in 75 percent of clients.

f. Marrow attempts to compensate for blood cell destruction; when it fails, osteoporosis occurs.

g. Cerebral hemorrhage or shock cause death.

3. Treatment

a. Currently accepted management of sickle cell anemia is primarily supportive and conservative.

b. Early detection of infections and prompt administration of appropriate antibiotic therapy.

c. Painful crisis should be treated promptly with adequate analgesia and hydration.

d. Bone marrow transplant may be performed.

e. Oxygen should be administered during acute pain crisis if the client has arterial hypoxemia.

f. Analgesics are administered as needed for pain.

g. Blood transfusions play a limited role in the management of sickle cell anemia. Between crises, clients do not derive much subjective benefit from blood transfusions. However, IV hydration is an effective way to prevent a vascular occlusion crisis.

4. Nursing Implications

a. Administer IV fluid as ordered to prevent vascular occlusion crisis.

b. If the patient is scheduled for a bone marrow transplant, he or she should be taught about the procedure and be given time to ask questions.

c. Maintain reverse isolation to prevent infection if the patient has a low leukocyte count.

d. Administer oxygen and blood transfusions as ordered for patients with low hemoglobin concentration.

e. Administer sedation, analgesics, and antibiotics as ordered by the physician.

f. Evaluate results of patient's laboratory tests.

II. DISORDERS OF COAGULATION

A. Disseminated Intravascular Coagulation

◆ Disseminated intravascular coagulation occurs when there is accelerated clotting throughout the body.

◆ Depletion of circulating clotting factors and platelets can provoke severe hemorrhage.

1. Etiology and Incidence

a. Occurs in adults of either gender.

b. DIC is generally an acute condition. Chronic conditions are seen secondary to malignancy.

c. Although a long list of diseases are associated with DIC, the most frequent are obstetric catastrophes, metastatic malignancy, massive trauma, and bacterial sepsis.

d. Regardless of how DIC begins, the typical accelerated clotting results in an abnormal increase in prothrombin production. This causes excessive clotting throughout the body until the prothrombin is used up and hemorrhage occurs.

2. Signs and Symptoms

a. Early stages of the disease produce no symptoms (an increase in hematocrit may be an incidental laboratory finding).

b. The clinical presentation varies with the severity of the syndrome.

c. Most patients have extensive skin and mucous membrane bleeding and hemorrhage from multiple sites, usually surgical incisions or venipuncture or catheter sites. Some patients, particularly those with chronic DIC secondary to malignancy, have laboratory abnormalities without any evidence of thrombosis or hemorrhage.

3. Treatment

a. Attempt to correct a reversible cause of DIC.

b. Measures to control the major symptoms, either thrombosis or bleeding.

c. Treatment varies with the clinical presentation.

4. Nursing Implications

a. Monitor the patient for thrombosis and bleeding.

b. Administer frozen plasma as ordered to replace depleted clotting factors.

c. Administer platelet concentrates as ordered to correct thrombocytopenia.

d. Administer heparin as ordered to prevent clotting.

e. If bleeding occurs in a joint (e.g., leg), immediately elevate the affected joint.

f. Closely monitor prothrombin time (PT) and partial thromboplastin time (PTT).

g. Prevent injury.

h. Avoid IM injections because of bleeding and possible hematoma formation at the injection site.

i. Check all IV and venipuncture sites frequently for bleeding. Apply pressure to bleeding site for at least 10 to 15 min; notify the physician immediately if bleeding persists.

j. Explain all diagnostic tests and procedures to the patient and allow time for questions.

k. Monitor intake and output hourly in acute DIC, especially when administering blood products.

l. Assess for signs of fluid overload.

B. Idiopathic Thrombocytopenic Purpura

◆ Idiopathic thrombocytopenic purpura (ITP) results from immunologic platelet destruction; it can be acute or chronic. (Remember: "Only an idiot would attack and destroy his or her own platelets.")

◆ Platelet count less than 20,000/mm^3 and a prolonged bleeding time suggest ITP.

1. Etiology and Incidence

    a. Chronic ITP mainly affects adults younger than 50 years, especially women between age 20 and 40 years. Acute ITP usually affects children between age 2 and 8 years.

    b. Acute ITP usually follows a viral infection, such as rubella or chickenpox, and can follow immunization with a live virus vaccine.

2. Signs and Symptoms

    ◆ ITP produces clinical features common to all forms of thrombocytopenia: ecchymoses, petechiae, easy bruising, bleeding from mucous membranes, hematuria, menorrhagia, epistaxis, and bleeding gums.

3. Treatment

    a. Corticosteroids, the initial treatment of choice, promote capillary integrity but are only temporarily effective in chronic ITP.

    b. Steroids may be administered IV (intravenously), IM (intramuscularly), or PO (by mouth) as ordered by the physician.

    c. Calcium and vitamin K may be administered (catalysts in blood clotting).

    d. Transfusion of platelets or whole blood.

    e. Immunosuppression agents may be administered; splenectomy, which reduces the destruction of platelets, is also performed in adults (85 percent successful).

C. Thrombocytopenia

◆ It is the most common cause of hemorrhage. It is characterized by deficiency of platelets in circulating blood.

◆ Coagulation tests show diminished platelet count of 20,000/mm^3 in adults, and prolonged PT.

◆ Platelets play a vital role in coagulation. Prognosis is excellent in drug-induced thrombocytopenia. If the drug causing the problem is no longer used, recovery may be immediate.

◆ Prognosis of thrombocytopenia from other causes depends on the response to treatment of the underlying cause.

1. Etiology and Incidence

    a. Can be congenital or acquired; acquired thrombocytopenia is more common.

    b. Either the congenital or acquired case usually results from decreased or defective production of platelets in the bone marrow (e.g., leukemia, aplastic anemia, or toxicity from certain drugs). It also can occur from increased destruction from outside the marrow caused by underlying disorder (e.g., cirrhosis of the liver, DIC, or severe infection).

    c. An idiopathic (unknown cause) form of thrombocytopenia commonly occurs in children.

2. Signs and Symptoms

    a. Sudden onset of petechiae or ecchymoses in the skin or bleeding into any mucous membrane.

    b. As a result of bleeding, the patient may experience feelings of general weakness or lethargy.

    c. If bleeding is severe, the patient will develop tachycardia, shortness of breath, loss of consciousness, and will die.

3. Treatment

    a. Treatment varies with the underlying cause and may include steroids or lithium carbonate to increase platelet production.

    b. Remove offending agents in drug-induced thrombocytopenia or treat the underlying cause, when possible.

    c. Platelet transfusions are helpful only when treating complications of severe hemorrhage.

4. Nursing Implications

    a. Be alert for bleeding from orifices (e.g., rectal and oral cavity).

    b. Administer steroids and vitamin K as ordered.

    c. Monitor for pale skin, tachycardia, and hypotension.

    d. Monitor for tarry stools (blood in stools) and hematuria.

    e. Transfuse platelets or whole blood as ordered; take the patient's vital signs as needed.

    f. Assess for blood transfusion reaction.

    g. Use gentle care when working with the patient.

    h. Monitor results of the patient's laboratory tests.

III. HEREDITARY BLEEDING DISORDERS

A. Hemophilia

◆ Hemophilia is a hereditary bleeding disorder resulting from deficiency of specific clotting factors.

1. Etiology and Incidence

    a. Deficiency of factor VIII, classic hemophilia, accounts for 80 percent of cases; also called hemophilia A.

b. Deficiency of factor IX (B) accounts for 15 percent of cases; called hemophilia B (Christmas disease).

c. Hemophilia may result from nonfunctioning factors VIII and IX, rather than from their deficiency.

2. Transmission

a. Mother to son: sex-linked recessive disorder. Mother is the carrier; she does not have the disease but inherits the trait.

b. Each son has a 50 percent chance of getting the disease.

c. Each daughter has a 50 percent chance of becoming a carrier.

d. One in 10,000 males is born with deficiency or dysfunction of factor VIII.

3. Signs and Symptoms

a. Abnormal bleeding into muscles, joints, and body cavities hours or days after injury.

b. Can be mild, moderate, or severe. Mild may go undiagnosed until adulthood.

c. Spontaneous bleeding after minor trauma can produce large subcutaneous and deep intramuscular hematomas. Bleeding into joints and muscles causes pain, swelling, and possibly permanent deformity.

d. Bleeding near peripheral nerves can cause peripheral neuropathies, pain, paresthesias, and muscle atrophy.

e. If bleeding impairs blood flow through a major vessel, it can cause ischemia and gangrene.

4. Treatment

a. Hemophilia is not curable; it is a lifelong condition.

b. In hemophilia (A) VIII, cryoprecipitated or lyophilized antihemophilic factor, or both, is given in doses large enough to raise clotting factor levels to approximately 25 percent of normal, which permits normal homeostasis.

c. In hemophilia (B) IX, factor IX concentrate is administered during bleeding episodes to raise clotting factor.

d. Early treatment can prevent crippling deformities and prolong life expectancy. Treatment can quickly stop bleeding by increasing plasma levels of deficient clotting factors.

5. Nursing Implications

a. Administer clotting factors or plasma as ordered, and check IV site frequently for bleeding.

b. Apply pressure to bleeding site for 10 to 15 min; notify physician immediately if bleeding persists.

c. Assess for pain and administer analgesics as ordered.

d. Educate the patient about the need to restrict activity for 48 h after bleeding is under control.

e. If bleeding occurs in joint, immediately elevate the joint.

f. Restart range-of-motion exercises at least 48 h after the bleeding is controlled to maintain joint mobility.

g. Closely monitor PTT and PT.

h. Teach parents special precaution to prevent bleeding episode.

i. Teach parents to avoid aspirin and aspirin-containing medications because they decrease platelet adherence and can increase bleeding.

j. Avoid IM injections because of bleeding and possible hematoma formation at the injection site.

B. Polycythemia Vera

◆ Polycythemia is characterized by an increase in RBC mass, leukocytosis, thrombocytosis, and increased hemoglobin concentration.

1. Etiology and Incidence

a. Usually occurs between ages 40 and 60 years; most common among males of Jewish ancestry; rarely affects children or blacks; does not appear to be familial.

b. Cause is unknown.

2. Pathophysiology with Signs and Symptoms

a. Erythrocyte, leukocyte, and platelet counts are increased.

b. Increased RBC mass results in hyperviscosity and inhibits blood flow to microcirculation.

c. Thrombocytosis promotes intravascular occlusion.

d. Early stages of the disease produce no symptoms. (An increase in hematocrit may be an incidental laboratory finding).

e. Paradoxically, hemorrhage can be a complication of polycythemia vera; it may be due to defective platelet function or to hyperviscosity exerting pressure on distended venous and capillary walls.

f. Altered circulation secondary to increased RBC can produce symptoms.

3. Treatment

a. Phlebotomy, the primary treatment, can reduce red cell mass promptly. The frequency of phlebotomy and the amount of blood removed each time depend on the patient's condition.

b. After repeated phlebotomies, the patient develops an iron deficiency anemia, which reduces RBC count and reduces the need for phlebotomy.

c. Radioactive phosphorus (^{32}P1) or cancer chemotherapeutic agents can satisfactorily control the disease in most cases. However, these agents can cause leukemia, so they usually are reserved for patients with severe problems not controlled by phlebotomy.

4. Nursing Implications

a. Explain phlebotomy procedure; reassure the patient that it will relieve distressing signs and symptoms.

b. Monitor vital signs before, during, and after phlebotomy.

c. Monitor laboratory values before, during, and after phlebotomy.

d. Keep the patient active and walking to prevent thrombosis.

e. Observe for signs of thrombocytosis.

Chapter

4

Diseases

TOPICAL OUTLINE

I. INFECTIOUS DISEASE

A. Infectious Mononucleosis

◆ Infectious mononucleosis is an acute infectious disease.

1. Incidence

   a. Infectious mononucleosis is fairly common in the United States, Canada, and Europe; both genders are affected equally.

   b. It is most common in children and young adults.

2. Etiology

   a. Infectious mononucleosis is caused by Epstein-Barr virus (EBV). It probably spreads by the oropharyngeal route, as approximately 80 percent of clients carry EBV in the throat during acute infection.

   b. It occurs most often in young people; the highest incidence occurs between the ages of 15 and 30 years.

3. Pathophysiology with Signs and Symptoms

   a. The symptoms of mononucleosis mimic those of many other infectious diseases. Symptoms develop after an incubation period of approximately 10 days in children and approximately 30 to 50 days in adults.

   b. Typical symptoms include sore throat, cervical lymph node enlargement, and temperature fluctuations.

   c. Leukocyte count increases 10,000 to 20,000/mm^3 during the second week of illness. Sometimes a maculopapular rash that resembles rubella develops early in the illness. Jaundice occurs in approximately 5 percent of patients.

   d. Major complications are rare but may include Guillain-Barré syndrome, idiopathic thrombocytopenic purpura, hepatitis, and aseptic meningitis.

4. Treatment

   a. Treatment includes antimicrobial agents, bed rest during the acute febrile period, and analgesics for headache and sore throat.

   b. If throat inflammation is severe, steroids may be given.

5. Nursing Implications

   a. Because uncomplicated infectious mononucleosis does not require hospitalization, patient teaching is essential.

   b. Stress bed rest during acute illness and avoidance of contact sports and heavy physical labor until after recovery is completed.

   c. Instruct the patient to complete prescribed prophylactic antibiotic therapy.

II. RICKETTSIA

A. Rocky Mountain Spotted Fever

◆ The organism *Rickettsia* is transmitted through the skin by a tick bite and can occur at any age. Fatal in approximately 5 percent of patients.

1. Signs and Symptoms

   a. Incubation period is 7 days but can range from 2 to 14 days; onset of symptoms usually is abrupt, producing a persistent temperature of 102°F to 104°F, with excruciating headache and aching of bones, joints, and muscles throughout the body.

   b. The tongue is covered with a thick white coating that generally turns brown as the fever persists and rises. Initially, the skin may be flushed; in 3 to 6 days, eruptions begin on the wrists, ankles, or forehead; within 2 days after eruption begins, they cover the entire body, including the scalp, palms, and soles.

   c. By the third week, the skin may become gangrenous and peel.

2. Treatment

   a. Treatment requires careful removal of the tick and administration of antibiotics such as tetracycline. Symptoms are treated to make the client as comfortable as possible.

   b. Ticks usually are removed at home; the tick may be pulled off, leaving the head of the tick in the skin. If the tick is a carrier of Rocky Mountain spotted fever, the person may develop the disease.

3. Nursing Implications

   a. Carefully monitor the patient's intake and output. Watch closely for decreased urine output, which is a possible indicator of renal failure.

   b. Monitor for vital signs, and watch for hypotension and shock.

   c. Instruct the patient to report any recurrent symptoms to the physician at once so that treatment measures may resume immediately.

Chapter

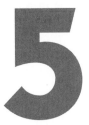

Integumentary Disorders (Common Skin Disorders)

TOPICAL OUTLINE

I. INFLAMMATORY SKIN DISEASES

A. Acne Vulgaris

◆ Acne is a very common inflammatory disease of the sebaceous follicles; acne vulgaris primarily affects adolescents.

1. Incidence

   a. Acne strikes boys more often and more severely; it usually occurs in girls at an earlier age and tends to affect them for a longer period, sometimes into adulthood.

   b. Prognosis is good with treatment.

2. Etiology

   a. The cause of acne is still unknown, but it is thought to be multifactorial.

   b. Some of the common causes that have been postulated are endocrine effects, heredity, and infection.

3. Pathophysiology with Signs and Symptoms

   a. At puberty, sebaceous glands undergo enlargement due to androgen stimulation.

   b. Expression of the disease is increased sebum release by sebaceous glands after puberty.

   c. Small cysts, called *comedones,* form in hair follicles due to blockage of the follicular orifice by retention of sebum and keratinous material. The action of lipophilic yeast and bacteria within the comedones releases free fatty acids from sebum, causes inflammation within the cyst, and results in rupture of the cyst wall.

   d. An inflammatory reaction develops as a result of extrusion of oily and keratinous debris from the cyst.

   e. Exogenous and endogenous factors can alter the expression of acne vulgaris. Friction (vigorous scrubbing) and trauma may rupture preexisting microcomedones and elicit inflammatory acne.

   f. Factors that predispose to comedone formation include topical agents in cosmetics or hair preparations such as lanolin, petrolatum, and oleic acid.

   g. Glucocorticoids, applied topically or administered systemically, also elicit acne.

   h. Other systemic medication, such as estrogenic oral contraceptives, isoniazid (INH), phenytoin (Dilantin), and other phenobarbital agents, may produce acne from eruption or aggravate preexisting acne.

4. Treatment

   a. Treatment is directed toward eliminating comedones, decreasing the population of lipophilic bacteria and yeast, and decreasing inflammation.

   b. Areas affected with acne should be kept clean; removal of surface oils does not play an important role in therapy. Vigorous scrubbing may aggravate acne due to mechanical rupture of comedones.

   c. Oral tetracycline or erythromycin in doses of 250 to 1000 mg/day to decrease bacterial growth until the patient is in remission. A lower dosage is used for long-term maintenance.

d. Tetracycline is contraindicated during pregnancy because it discolors the teeth of the fetus.

e. Topical agents such as retinoic acid, benzoyl peroxide, and salicylic acid may prevent the formation of comedones and assist in the resolution of preexisting cysts.

f. Severe acne may be treated with systemic isotretinoin. Women are (a) screened for pregnancy prior to initiating therapy, (b) told to maintain a fail-safe method of birth control during treatment, and (c) screened for pregnancy during treatment. Side effects of isotretinoin are hypertriglyceridemia and bone overgrowth of vertebrae.

g. Cryosurgery may be used to destroy acne tissue by rapid freezing.

5. Nursing Implications

a. Assist the patient in identifying predisposing factors that can eliminate or modify acne.

b. Review the patient's drug history because medications, such as oral contraceptives, can cause acne flare-up.

c. Explain predisposing factors to the patient and family.

d. Make sure that the patient understands that prescribed medications will improve acne to some degree if taken as prescribed. Help the patient to understand that strict diet and over-the-counter medications are not helpful.

e. Instruct the patient receiving isotretinoin to apply it at least 30 min after washing the face, neck, shoulders, and at least 1 h before bedtime.

f. Warn the patient against using it around eyes or lips. After the treatment, the skin should look pink and dry.

g. If skin becomes red or starts to peel, notify physician.

h. Advise the patient to avoid exposure to sunlight or to use a sunscreen agent while using tretinoin.

i. Instruct the patient to take tetracycline on an empty stomach and not to take it with antacids or milk because they cause poor absorption.

j. Inform the patient that acne takes a long time to clear and may take years for complete resolution.

k. Assist the patient in dealing with perceptions of his or her physical appearance by offering emotional support.

B. Herpes Zoster (Shingles)

◆ Herpes zoster is an acute unilateral and segmental inflammation of the dorsal root ganglia.

1. Incidence

a. Infection usually occurs in adults or immunosuppressed patients.

2. Etiology

a. Herpes zoster, or shingles, is a common viral disease that affects the peripheral nervous system. *It is caused by the same virus that causes varicella (chickenpox).* Although herpes zoster is far less communicable than chickenpox, persons who have not had chickenpox can develop it after exposure to the vesicular lesions of persons with herpes zoster.

b. For this reason, susceptible persons should not care for patients with herpes zoster.

c. Herpes zoster often occurs in persons with AIDS, Hodgkin's disease, or reduced cell-mediated immunity.

3. Pathophysiology with Signs and Symptoms

a. Onset of herpes zoster is characterized by fever and malaise.

b. Clusters of small vesicles usually follow the course of the peripheral sensory nerve and often are unilateral.

c. Because they follow nerve pathways, the lesions never cross the midline of the body.

d. Nerves on both sides of the body can be involved, however.

e. Lesions commonly spread unilaterally around the thorax or vertically over arms and legs.

f. The first symptom is small red nodular skin lesions, which quickly become vesicles filled with clear fluid or pus.

g. Approximately 10 days after vesicles appear, they dry and form scabs.

h. Malaise, fever, itching, and pain over the involved area may precede the eruption of the lesions.

i. Discomfort from pain and itching is the major problem with herpes zoster.

j. It is one of the most drawn out and exasperating conditions found in the elderly and may lead to discouragement and depression. Discomfort from pain usually persists for up to 4 weeks. In approximately 50 percent of persons older than 60 years, the pain can last for months or years.

4. Treatment

a. Acyclovir (Zovirax) accelerates healing and reduces acute pain.

b. Analgesics are prescribed for pain relief.

c. Aspirin with or without codeine or meperidine (Demerol) may be used for pain.

d. Local discomfort may be relieved by calamine lotion.

5. Nursing Implications

a. Keep the patient comfortable, maintaining meticulous hygiene to prevent lesion infection.

b. Instruct the patient to avoid scratching the lesions.

c. When vesicles rupture, apply a cold compress, as ordered, to reduce pain.

d. Instruct the patient to use a soft toothbrush, eat foods low in spices, and use saline mouthwash to reduce the pain of oral lesions.

e. Explain to the patient the need to take prescribed medication before pain becomes severe.

II. SKIN LESIONS

A. Keloids

1. Incidence

    a. Some people, especially those with brown or black skin, are prone to excessive scar formation.

    b. Keloids occur most often in young adults and may require many years to reach full growth.

2. Etiology and Pathophysiology

    a. Keloids are hard, raised, shiny growths of collagen tissue that usually originate from a scar and then grow beyond the wound, often with projections.

3. Signs and Symptoms

    a. Keloids may cause disfigurement or undergo malignant degeneration, so they usually are excised surgically.

    b. Keloids occur most frequently on the sternum, mandible, ear, and neck.

    c. Keloids may occur after simple excision; therefore, surgery is followed by intralesional steroid therapy, radiation therapy, or electron beam therapy.

B. Psoriasis

   ◆ Psoriasis is a chronic, recurrent disease marked by epidermal proliferation.

1. Incidence

    a. Psoriasis, one of the most common dermatologic diseases, affects approximately 3 percent of US population. The incidence is higher among Caucasians than other races.

    b. Psoriasis is most common in adults, but it can strike at any age, including infancy.

2. Etiology

    a. Psoriasis is a genetically determined, chronic, epidermal proliferative disease. It is not infectious or contagious.

3. Pathophysiology with Signs and Symptoms

    a. Epidermal proliferation appears as erythematous papules and plaques covered with silvery scales; they vary widely in severity and distribution.

    b. The most common complaint of the patient with psoriasis is itching and, occasionally, pain from dry, cracked, encrusted lesions.

    c. Widespread shedding of scales is common in the acute stage and may also develop in chronic cases of psoriasis.

    d. Many patients with psoriasis develop arthritis symptoms.

4. Treatment

    a. No permanent cure exists, and all methods of treatment are merely palliative.

    b. Removal of psoriatic scales increases the effectiveness of topical glucocorticoids.

    c. Scales are removed by softening them with petrolatum, salicylic acid preparations, or preparations containing urea. These medications soften scales, which then can be removed by scrubbing them carefully with a soft brush while bathing.

    d. Crude coal tar (1–5% ointment base) is an old but useful method of treatment in conjunction with ultraviolet light.

    e. Ultraviolet light is useful for widespread psoriasis. It is effective alone or in combination with coal tar.

    f. Natural sunlight or an artificial light source can be used.

    g. Other agents can be used for associated disease. For example, methotrexate is useful in patients with associated arthritis.

5. Nursing Implications

    a. Teach the patient about the disease process and treatment, including side effects of drug therapy.

    b. Make sure that the patient understands prescribed therapy; provide written instructions (especially for the elderly) to avoid confusion.

    c. Teach correct skin care; for example, a steroid cream should be applied in a thin film and rubbed gently into skin until the cream disappears.

    d. Teach the patient to reduce episodes of rapid-spreading psoriasis (flare-ups) by avoiding skin trauma (injury, sunburn, infection) and extremes of temperature and stress.

    e. Shampoo hair frequently to remove scales. If the scalp has plaque, use tar shampoo (Polytar, Sebutone) for 10 min before rinsing. Presoften thick plaques with mineral oil the night before a morning shampoo; use a fine-toothed comb or brush to removed loose scales.

    f. Instruct client to seek medical follow-up during periods of exacerbation.

Chapter

6

Autoimmune Disorders

TOPICAL OUTLINE

I. HUMAN IMMUNODEFICIENCY VIRUS

A. Acquired Immunodeficiency Syndrome

◆ Currently one of the most publicized diseases, acquired immunodeficiency syndrome (AIDS) is characterized by progressive weakened cell-mediated (T-cell) immunity that makes patients susceptible to opportunistic infections and cancers.

1. Incidence and Etiology

a. AIDS has become a worldwide epidemic. The cause is the human immunodeficiency virus (HIV). More than 50 percent of the reported cases of HIV infection and AIDS have been in homosexuals and bisexual men. The greatest identified risk factor for HIV transmission in this group is anal intercourse.

b. Transmission of HIV by vaginal heterosexual intercourse is increasing. Associated risk factors for heterosexual transmission include anal intercourse and multiple sexual partners who may be infected but not symptomatic.

c. Studies on nonsexual household contact, sharing of eating utensils and bathroom facilities, and close personal contact have failed to demonstrate transmission of HIV by casual contact.

d. Other risk groups include intravenous drug abusers and hemophiliacs, especially those who have received multiple blood transfusions or been treated with factor VIII concentrate (cryoprecipitated).

e. Although the risk of HIV infection to health care workers is low, it remains a potential risk for those workers exposed to body secretions such as blood, saliva, urine, and stool.

f. Exposure to HIV can occur by accidental needle stick or mucous membrane exposure by a splash of blood in the mouth, nose, or an open cut.

g. The three major methods of HIV transmission are: (a) intimate contact with body secretions, including semen and vaginal secretions that occur during sexual intercourse; (b) contact with infected blood through blood transfusions or the sharing of needles during drug use; and (c) maternal–infant transfer via placental exchange or breast milk.

2. Pathophysiology with Signs and Symptoms

a. Infection with HIV renders the immune system severely compromised.

b. HIV, which selectively strikes T_4 (helper) lymphocytes, gradually depletes their numbers and impairs their function. HIV also invades other components of the immune system, including B cells, macrophages, and nerve cells.

c. The decrease in helper T cells, lymphocytes, B cells, and macrophages profoundly impairs cell-mediated immunity.

d. The latest method for diagnosing AIDS is determining the amount of HIV present in the blood. This information is also used to establish medication regimen.

e. Some patients with AIDS are asymptomatic until they develop an opportunistic infection, for example, Kaposi's sarcoma, which is typified by purple skin nodules.

f. Most often, the patients have a recent history of nonspecific signs and symptoms, such as fatigue, afternoon fevers, night sweats, weight loss, diarrhea, or cough. Patients may be asymptomatic and have no opportunistic infections for years.

g. HIV infection can remain dormant for several years, producing no symptoms. This prolonged incubation period is of great concern because individuals may be asymptomatic but contagious.

h. Others infected with the virus experience transient acute symptoms of muscle aches, rashes, fever, gastrointestinal cramps, and diarrhea.

i. Other patients harboring HIV antibodies exhibit chronic symptoms of diffuse noncancerous lymph node enlargement, or persistent generalized chills, fever, night sweats, and weight loss.

j. Others have what is sometimes referred to as *full-blown AIDS*. They have all of the above symptoms, but the symptoms are more severe. They have opportunistic infections or cancer.

k. The most common opportunistic infections include the following:

    (1) Bacterial: *Mycobacterium tuberculosis*—TB, respiratory

    (2) Fungal: *Candida albicans*—GI, mouth, vaginal

    (3) Protozoal:*Pneumocystis carinii*—respiratory; *Toxoplasma gondii*—generalized infection; *Cryptosporidium*—gastrointestinal (severe diarrhea)

    (4) Viral: *herpes simplex virus*—mouth, genital, perianal; *varicella zoster*—integumentary; *cytomegalovirus*—encephalitis, hepatitis, pneumonitis

    (5) Neoplastic disease: *Kaposi's sarcoma*—skin and mucous membrane; *Hodgkin's disease*—lymph system: *chronic lymphocytic leukemia*—white blood cells

3. Multidrug Regimens Offer Promise and a Challenge

◆ Multidrug regimens offer promise; unfortunately, interactions between HIV drugs and other drugs pose health risks. Adverse drug effects can make therapy especially difficult, even for the most compliant patients. Support groups can help patients stick with the program.

◆ With the following range of agents, antiretroviral therapy now can target HIV at different stages of replication. As a result, HIV infection has evolved from an inevitably fatal disease to a chronic disease that is life threatening but treatable.

◆ The antiretroviral agents currently approved for treatment of HIV fall into the following major categories:

a. Protease inhibitors keep infected cells from producing new viruses (e.g., nelfinavir [Viracept], ritonavir [Norvir])

b. Nucleoside reverse transcriptase inhibitors (NRTIs), also known as *nucleoside analogues,* inhibit HIV replication in both T cells and monocytes (e.g., abacavir [Ziagen])

c. Nonnucleoside reverse transcriptase inhibitors (NNRTIs), as their name implies, block the action of reverse transcriptase (e.g., efavirenz [Sustiva], delavirdine [Rescriptor])

d. Nucleotide analogue reverse transcriptase inhibitors represent a new class of HIV medication, first introduced with the approval of tenofovir (Viread) in 2002. The drug, which is approved for use in combination therapies, is chemically similar to the nucleotides required for viral replication and thus inhibits reverse transcriptase (e.g., tenofovir [Viread])

e. See *Handbook of Medications for the NCLEX-RN Reviews* (Chapter 12) for more information about drug therapy, AIDS, and opportunistic disease.

    ◆ Patients with HIV usually receive at least three drugs spanning two of the classes in one of several regimens known as "highly active antiretroviral therapy" (HAART).

    ◆ These regimens can effectively reduce the virus to undetectable levels in the plasma, preventing or delaying the progression of HIV infection to full-blown AIDS.

    ◆ There is no one specific HAART prescription. The mix of drugs depends on many factors, including the patient's condition, current medication, which antiretroviral agents the patient has already tried, and the strain of the virus.

    ◆ In recent years, the availability of drug formulations combining two antiretroviral agents in one pill has helped to reduce the number of pills taken by patients in 1 day.

    ◆ Studies performed in the early 1990s showed zidovudine (AZT) effectively reduced the spread of HIV from mother to child when given to the mother from the second trimester of pregnancy through delivery and to the baby for 6 weeks after birth.

    ◆ This course of treatment costs approximately $1000, which explains why 95 percent of the 1000 infants infected daily with HIV by their mothers live in the developing world.

4. Nursing Implications

a. In addition to health education strategies, infection control is one of the most important areas of concern for nurses caring for patients known to have AIDS and others who may have AIDS and may not be symptomatic.

b. Hand washing is critical, not only for self-protection but to protect immunocompromised patients.

c. Gloves should be used whenever there is contact with body secretions, such as during care of lesions, giving IM injections, drawing blood, starting an IV line, changing dressings, cleaning a patient incontinent of urine or stool, changing soiled linens, and performing oral care.

d. Gloves are not necessary for casual contact, such as bathing (without the presence of lesions), feeding, or ambulating a patient.

e. Soiled dressings, wet linens, and respiratory equipment should be discarded in heavy plastic bags.

f. Needles should be disposed of promptly, *without recapping*, because recapping is the most frequent cause of accidental needle sticks.

g. Dispose of needles in a puncture-resistant needle disposal container, which should be in each patient room and wherever needles are discarded.

h. Instruct patients that the use of condoms offers some protection against the transmission of HIV infection, but they are not absolute protection. Abstinence from sexual activities is the only absolute protection against HIV infection.

i. Teach the patient that some factors that increase the risk of sexual transmission include multiple sexual partners, receptive anal intercourse, the presence of open lesions in the genital area, and sexual activity without some form of barrier, such as a condom.

II. CHRONIC SYSTEMIC INFLAMMATORY DISEASES

A. Rheumatoid Arthritis

◆ Rheumatoid arthritis (RA) is a chronic systemic inflammatory disease that primarily attacks peripheral joints, surrounding muscles, ligaments, and blood vessels. It causes bone erosion.

1. Incidence

a. RA is believed to be an autoimmune disease that occurs worldwide, affecting females three times more often than males.

b. RA can occur at any age, but the prevalence increases with age; gender differences diminish in the older age group.

c. Onset is more frequent during the fourth and fifth decades of life.

2. Etiology

a. The cause is unknown. Family studies indicate a genetic predisposition.

b. Currently, it is believed that genetically susceptible individuals develop abnormal or altered antibodies when exposed to antigens.

3. Pathophysiology

a. Continued inflammation leads to thickening of the synovium, particularly where it joins the articular cartilage.

b. The rheumatoid synovium has a number of secreted products of activated lymphocytes, macrophage-activated antigens, autoantibody rheumatoid factor, and other cell types.

4. Signs and Symptoms

a. Signs and symptoms include joint pain and swelling; generalized stiffness is frequent and usually is greatest after periods of inactivity.

b. The majority of clients experience symptoms such as weakness, early fatigability, anorexia, and weight loss.

5. Diagnosis

a. No tests are specific for diagnosing rheumatoid arthritis RA. Rheumatoid factor, however, which is autoantibody reactive, is found in more than two-thirds of adults with the disease. The presence of rheumatoid factor does not establish the diagnosis of RA but can be of prognostic significance because patients with high titers tend to have more severe and progressive disease with extraarticular (outside the joint) manifestation.

b. The erythrocyte sedimentation rate is increased in nearly all clients with active RA.

c. Synovial fluid analysis confirms the presence of inflammatory arthritis.

d. The synovial fluid is usually cloudy with reduced viscosity and increased protein content.

6. Treatment

a. The goals of therapy for RA are (a) relief of pain, (b) reduction of inflammation, (c) preservation of functional joints, (d) resolution of the pathogenesis process, and (e) facilitation of healing.

b. Currently, medications are available that are capable of providing pain relief and some reduction of inflammation. None of the therapeutic interventions are curative; therefore, all must be viewed as palliative, aimed at relieving signs and symptoms of the disease.

c. The medical management of RA involves three general approaches. The first is the use of aspirin and other nonsteroidal antiinflammatory drugs (NSAIDs), mild analgesics, and, if necessary, low-dose glucocorticoids to control the symptoms and signs of local inflammatory process.

d. The second line of therapy includes a variety of agents that have been classified as disease-modifying antirheumatic drugs (DMARDs) (see *Handbook of Medications for the NCLEX-RN® Review,* Chapter 8).

e. The third approach involves the use of experimental modalities, such as immunosuppressive agents.

f. The immunosuppressive drugs azathioprine (Imuran) and cyclosporine (Sandimmune) have been shown to be effective in the treatment of RA and to exert therapeutic effects similar to those of the DMARDs (see *Handbook of Medications for the NCLEX-RN® Review,* Chapter 8).

g. These agents appear to be no more effective than other DMARDs. Moreover, they cause a variety of toxic side effects, and cyclosporine appears to predispose the patient to the development of malignant neoplasms. Therefore, use of these drugs is reserved for patients who have clearly failed therapy with other disease-modifying drugs (DMARDs).

h. Methotrexate is considered by many physicians to be the first-choice drug among the DMARDs.

i. Recent trials documented the efficacy of methotrexate and indicated that its onset of action is more rapid than that of other DMARDs. Patients tend to remain on methotrexate therapy longer than they remain on other disease-modifying drugs (DMARDs) because of better clinical response and less toxicity.

j. More drugs used to treat RA are presented in the *Handbook of Medications for the NCLEX-RN® Review* Chapter 8.

B. Systemic Lupus Erythematosus

◆ Systemic lupus erythematosus (SLE) is a disease of unknown cause in which tissue and cells are damaged by pathogenic autoantibodies and immune complexes. The body produces antibodies against its own cells.

1. Incidence

a. Ninety percent of cases are women, usually of childbearing age, but children, men, and the elderly can be affected.

b. It is more common in African Americans than in whites. The Hispanic and Asian populations also are susceptible. The annual incidence of SLE averages 75 cases per 1,000,000 people.

2. Etiology

a. The exact cause of SLE is unknown but probably results from interaction between susceptibility genes and the environment.

b. This interaction results in abnormal immune response with T- and B-lymphocyte hyperactivity, which is not suppressed by the usual immunoregulatory circuits.

c. The antigen–antibody complexes can suppress the body's normal immunity and damage tissues.

d. One significant feature is the ability of patients with SLE to produce antibodies against red blood cells, platelets, lymphocytes, and almost any other organ or tissue in the body.

e. SLE can be triggered by physical or mental stress; streptococcal or viral infections; immunization; pregnancy; certain drugs such as anticonvulsants, procainamide, hydralazine, and oral contraceptives; or exposure to sunlight or ultraviolet light.

3. Pathophysiology with Signs and Symptoms

a. The onset of SLE can be acute or insidious.

b. Symptoms commonly include fatigue, weight loss, fever, malaise, skin rash, and polyarthritis (inflammation in more than one joint).

c. In 90 percent of patients, joint involvement is similar to that of rheumatoid arthritis.

d. Skin lesions most commonly are erythematous (diffuse redness over the skin) in areas exposed to light. The classic butterfly rash over the nose and cheeks occurs in less than 50 percent of patients.

e. Vasculitis can develop (especially in the digits), possibly leading to vascular occlusion, causing digital ulcers or gangrene.

f. Thrombosis in vessels of any size can be a major problem.

g. Approximately 50 percent of SLE clients develop signs of cardiopulmonary abnormalities, such pericarditis, myocarditis, endocarditis, and pleuritis; pneumonitis can also occur.

h. Renal effects include hematuria and proteinuria; renal involvement may progress to kidney failure.

i. Convulsive disorders and mental dysfunction may indicate neurologic damage. CNS involvement can produce emotional instability such as psychosis.

4. Diagnosis

a. Diagnostic tests for clients with SLE include a complete blood count (CBC), which may show a decrease in red blood cell (RBC) count (anemia); a decrease in white blood cell (WBC) cell (susceptible to infections); and decrease in platelet count (susceptible to bleeding).

b. Specific tests for SLE include anti-deoxyribonucleic acid (DNA) and anti-Smith antibodies. These tests are positive in most patients with active lupus erythematosus.

c. Because the anti-DNA test is rarely positive in other conditions, it is the most specific test for SLE. If a patient is in remission, however, anti-DNA can be reduced or absent.

d. Blood studies showing decreased serum complement (C3 and C4) levels indicate active disease.

e. Kidney biopsy determines disease stage and extent of renal involvement.

5. Treatment

a. There is no cure for SLE. Complete remissions are rare. Approximately 25 percent of SLE patients have mild disease with no life-threatening manifestations, although pain and fatigue can be disabling. These patients should be managed without glucocorticoids.

b. Arthritis, myalgias, fever, and mild serositis (inflamed serous membranes) may improve with NSAIDs, including salicylates. NSAID toxicities, such as elevated liver enzyme levels, aseptic meningitis, and renal impairment, however, are especially frequent in patients with SLE.

c. The dermatitides of SLE and, occasionally, lupus arthritis may respond to antimalarial agents such as chloroquine or hydroxychloroquine. Skin lesions may improve in a few weeks. Because hydroxychloroquine and chloroquine can cause retinal damage, such treatment requires ophthalmologic examinations every 6 to 8 months.

d. Other therapies for rash include sunscreens with an SPF rating of 15 or higher. Topical corticosteroid creams such as flurandrenolide (Cordran) are recommended for acute lesions.

e. Corticosteroids remain the treatment of choice for acute systemic symptoms of SLE.

f. Diffuse proliferative glomerulonephritis, a major complication of SLE, requires treatment with large doses of steroids.

g. If renal failure occurs, dialysis may be necessary.

h. Photosensitive patients should wear protective clothing (hat, sunglasses, long sleeves, slacks) and use a sunscreen agent.

i. SLE usually afflicts women of childbearing age; a woman can have a safe, successful pregnancy if she has no serious renal or neurologic impairment. These patients will have a much higher rate of fetal loss and an increase in congenital heart defects and hypertension.

j. Patchy alopecia may occur.

k. Some manifestations of SLE do not respond to immunosuppression, including clotting disorders and some behavioral abnormalities.

l. Anticoagulation is the therapy of choice for prevention of clotting.

6. Nursing Implications

a. Assess for joint pain and stiffness, weakness, fever, fatigue, and chills.

b. Note the size and locations of skin lesions.

c. Check urine for hematuria, scalp for hair loss, and digits for ulcers.

d. Apply heat packs to relieve joint pain and stiffness. Encourage regular exercise to maintain full range of motion and prevent contractures.

e. Teach range-of-motion exercises.

f. Explain the expected benefit of prescribed medications and side effects, especially when the patient is taking high doses of steroids.

g. Teach the patient to monitor hypertension, weight gain, and other signs of renal involvement.

h. Refer the patient to the Lupus Foundation of America and the Arthritis Foundation.

Chapter

7

Neoplastic Skin Disorders

TOPICAL OUTLINE

I. CANCER

A. Basal Cell Carcinoma

1. Incidence

   a. Basal cell carcinoma is the most common malignant tumor affecting light-skinned people older than 40 years. It is uncommon among blacks and Asians.

   b. Skin cancers are the most frequently occurring of all neoplasms.

   c. They represent 30 to 40 percent of all cancers.

   d. Approximately 80 percent of these cancers are basal cell carcinomas. Basal cell cancer almost never metastasizes.

2. Etiology

   a. The risk factors for the whole category of skin cancer are so similar that a general discussion is used as an introduction and is not repeated in discussions of other skin cancers in this section.

   b. Although hereditary factors and chemical exposures are definite contributors in the development of skin cancer, the most important is exposure to the sun.

   c. It is the cumulative effects of long-term exposure to the sun, particularly the ultraviolet B rays, that causes the development of premalignant and malignant skin lesions.

   d. Skin most exposed is the prime target for sun damage; this includes the head, neck, back, forearms, and hands.

   e. Certain hereditary factors are considered indicative of high risk for skin malignancies, especially light skin, blue or gray eyes, and red or blonde hair.

   f. People with darker skin have higher protective melanin and are much less likely to develop skin neoplasms resulting from sun exposure.

   g. Chemical exposures are thought to contribute to the development of skin malignancies.

   h. Arsenic found in certain insecticides is considered a common chemical source of skin cancer.

   i. Chronic exposure to polycyclic aromatic hydrocarbons, which may be found in hair spray and other chemical products, may cause skin cancer.

   j. People with a history of previous skin malignancy are at high risk for repeated skin malignancy.

   k. Areas of radiation dermatitis and burn scars are especially at high risk.

3. Pathophysiology with Signs and Symptoms

   a. There are five different types of basal cell carcinomas: noduloulcerative, pigmented, superficial, sclerosing, and recurrent.

   b. The noduloulcerative lesions are the most common type and this is the only basal cell carcinoma discussed here.

   c. The growth initially has a characteristic translucent appearance; dilated blood vessels usually are present around the lesion.

   d. The center of the lesion may form an ulcer crater and frequently bleeds with minor trauma.

e. The main manifestation of basal cell carcinomas is the appearance of skin lesions as described above.

f. There usually is a history of frequent bleeding in the involved area.

4. Treatment

a. Treatment of basal cell carcinoma depends on the site and extent of the tumor. The five treatment modalities include the following:

(1) Curettage

(2) Electrodesiccation

(3) Cryosurgery

(4) Radiation therapy

(5) Topical chemotherapy

b. Curettage is the scraping out of superficial lesions with a curette, which is a spoon-shaped, sharp-edged instrument.

(1) A local anesthetic usually is injected around the lesion before curettage.

(2) Bleeding is controlled by a chemical styptic (astringent action), such as ferric chloride, or by electrocoagulation.

c. Electrodesiccation (electrosurgery) is the drying of tissue by means of a monopolar current through the needle electrode. The needle is held close to the tissue, thus spraying the area with sparks.

(1) Bipolar current is used for electrocoagulation, which coagulates the tissue and curtails capillary bleeding, and for electrosection, which cuts the tissue.

(2) Electrosurgery usually is performed under local anesthetic.

(3) Following most uses of electrosurgery, the wound is left exposed for air drying.

d. In cryosurgery, tissue can be destroyed by rapid freezing with substances such as liquid oxygen, carbon dioxide snow, liquid nitrogen, or nitrous oxide.

(1) Carbon dioxide snow and liquid nitrogen are used most frequently.

(2) The rapid freezing causes formation of intracellular ice, which destroys the cell membranes and produces cell dehydration.

(3) Local anesthesia may be necessary.

(4) Tissue necrosis may not be evident until 24 h after cryosurgery.

e. Radiation therapy is often used around the eyes and the tip of the nose because other methods may be dangerous and cause excessive deformities.

(1) Because of the danger of additional malignancy occurring later in these areas, this treatment mode usually is confined to elderly clients.

(2) The treated area may become reddened and blistered for several days.

f. Topical chemotherapy (e.g., fluorouracil) is used to destroy the malignant cells.

(1) This treatment usually involves at least a daily application of the medication for several weeks.

(2) With the possible exception of topical chemotherapy, the treatment modes discussed have well-documented success rates; all are more than 90 percent successful. Lesions caught early in their development have an excellent prognosis.

5. Nursing Implications

a. Careful inspection of the skin must be included in the assessment of all patients. Suspicious area should be examined closely and the patient questioned about its history.

b. Bleeding or ulcerating tendencies of the area should be determined.

c. Educate the patient about the cancer therapy to be used and the care of the involved area after treatment.

d. After superficial skin surgery, the patient should be instructed not to remove the crust (scab), which acts as a protection (healing occurs under crust). The crust should be kept as dry as possible.

e. Teach the patient about the cumulative effect of sun radiation; instruct on the need to wear protective clothing (e.g., hat, long-sleeved shirt) and to use and apply frequently sunscreen lotions with high levels of para-aminobenzoic acid (PABA).

f. Patients who are at risk for skin cancer should be taught to inspect the skin frequently and to seek medical advice whenever they notice any suspicious skin changes.

B. Kaposi's Sarcoma

1. Incidence

a. Kaposi's sarcoma was a rare disorder in older men in the United States until recently. The disorder now is commonly seen as one of the opportunistic disorders occurring in conjunction with acquired immunodeficiency syndrome (AIDS), especially in homosexual men.

b. Kaposi's sarcoma was first described in 1969 and has always been considered a disease primarily affecting men, usually African Americans and men of Jewish descent.

2. Etiology

a. The etiology is not known, although genetics have always been considered a prime factor.

b. The disease is linked with people having a compromised immune system.

3. Pathophysiology

a. The lesions of Kaposi's sarcoma usually begin in the mid-dermis and extend upward into the epidermis. They can appear anywhere, including the mucous membranes, and are frequently found on the lower extremities.

b. The lesions arise as either patches or nodules. They frequently first appear as a red, dark, or purple macules.

c. The lesions are the first manifestation of the disease. As the disease progresses, the lesions increase in number and form large plaques, which become ulcerated or eroded.

d. Frequently, edema of the lower extremities occurs, indicating invasion into the lymphatics.

e. Patients complain of pain and itching.

f. Kaposi's sarcoma metastasizes to the gastrointestinal system, spleen, liver, bone, lung, pleura, adrenals, and kidneys.

4. Treatment

a. Antineoplastic agents such as vincristine or alpha-interferon are used to treat Kaposi's sarcoma.

b. Radiation and laser therapy are palliative measures for local lesions.

5. Nursing Implications

a. After diagnosis, review the physician's explanation of treatments with the patient.

b. Before chemotherapy is started, explain the side effects and how to minimize them.

c. Control and prevent pain.

d. Provide a supportive environment through active listening and therapeutic counseling.

e. Individual and group counseling is needed to help patients and significant others cope with a diagnosis of terminal cancer. Refer the patient to a hospice organization.

C. Squamous Cell Carcinomas

◆ Squamous cell carcinomas occur less frequently than basal cell carcinomas. Their etiology, medical management, and nursing management have many similarities to those of basal cell carcinomas, although there are a few differences.

1. Etiology and Pathophysiology with Signs and Symptoms

a. Squamous cell tumors arise in the keratinizing cells of the epidermis.

b. The most common sites for squamous cell lesions are the lower lip, tongue and floor of mouth, cheek region, and dorsum (back) or hand.

c. Squamous cell lesions also develop on mucous membranes exposed to chronic irritation, such as from tobacco smoked in pipes, cigars, and cigarettes, or chewed or "dipped" tobacco.

d. Evidence linking oral syphilitic lesions and oral candidiasis with oral cancer is circumstantial, but a growing body of data indicates roles for the herpes simplex virus and human papillomavirus.

e. The most common precancerous lesions in the oral cavity present as leukoplakia, a white patch on the mucosa that cannot be rubbed off.

f. All chronic ulcerative lesions that fail to heal within 1 to 2 weeks should be considered potentially malignant and must be biopsied to make a definitive diagnosis.

g. Squamous cell carcinomas are rarely painful, in contrast to similar-appearing inflammatory lesions.

h. As with basal cell carcinoma, these cells are slow growing. Squamous cell carcinoma can metastasize to the lymph node region. Patients with carcinoma of the tongue have a poorer prognosis because the carcinoma can spread to underlying bone.

2. Treatment

a. The diagnosis, treatment, and nursing implications of squamous cell carcinoma are similar to those of basal cell carcinomas.

b. The primary difference lies in the slight variation in treatment modalities. Surgical excision may be a bit more extensive, with wider margins taken to ensure complete removal of the malignant cells.

c. Systemic antineoplastic chemotherapy may be used earlier in the disease process than with basal cell carcinoma.

3. Nursing Implications

a. Nursing implications have many similarities to those of basal cell carcinomas (see section on Basal Cell Carcinoma).

D. Malignant Melanoma

◆ Malignant melanoma originates from melanocytes (pigment cells present normally in epidermis and sometimes dermis).

1. Incidence

a. Malignant melanoma is slightly more common in women than in men. The tumor affects approximately 32,000 individuals per year in the United States and results in 6700 deaths.

b. The incidence has increased dramatically (300 percent increase in the past 40 years). It can affect adults of all ages, even younger individuals (onset from mid-teens). Peak incidence is between ages 40 and 50 years.

2. Etiology

a. The reason for the increased incidence is uncertain but may stem from increased recreational sun exposure, especially early in life.

b. Individuals most susceptible to development of melanoma are those with fair complexions, red or blonde hair, blue eyes, and freckles; and those who are poor tanners and easily sunburned.

c. Other factors associated with increased risk include a family history of melanoma.

3. Pathophysiology with Signs and Symptoms

a. There are four types of cutaneous melanoma. Three of these are superficial spreading melanomas are not discussed here.

b. The fourth type, *nodular melanoma,* usually presents as a dark-brown, black, or grayish atypical mole, which looks like a blackberry. It is a deep invasive lesion, fully capable of early metastasis. Up to 70 percent arise from a preexisting nevus (mole).

c. A skin biopsy with histologic examination can distinguish malignant melanoma from a benign nevus; tumor thickness can also be determined.

d. As in breast cancer, recurrence of melanoma may be seen after many years.

e. Melanomas can spread by lymph channel or the bloodstream. Liver, lung, bone, and brain are common sites for metastasis.

4. Treatment

a. Any suspicious lesions should be biopsied.

b. Examination of lymph nodes and palpation of the abdominal viscera are part of the staging examination for suspected melanoma.

c. If either melanoma or atypical moles are present in the patient, family members should be advised to undergo screening.

d. A patient with malignant melanoma always requires surgical resection to remove the tumor. The extent of resection depends on the size and location of the primary lesion.

e. Closure of a wide resection may necessitate a skin graft.

f. Surgical treatment may also include regional lymphadenectomy (surgical removal of lymph nodes).

g. Radiation therapy and chemotherapy usually are reserved for metastatic disease.

h. Regardless of treatment, melanomas require close long-term follow-up to detect metastasis and recurrence.

i. Statistics show that 13 percent of recurrences develop more than 5 years after surgery.

5. Nursing Implications

a. After diagnosis, review the explanation of treatment alternatives with the patient.

b. Explain to the patient what to expect before and after surgery.

c. Encourage the patient to discuss his or her feelings and concerns about diagnosis, surgery, and treatment.

d. After surgery, prevent wound infection. Check dressing for drainage and foul odor.

e. Check wound for redness, exudate, and swelling.

f. Before chemotherapy is started, explain to the patient what side effects to expect and how to minimize them. For example, antiemetics will reduce nausea and vomiting.

g. Control and prevent pain with the use of a patient-controlled analgesic (PCA) pump; the physician will usually order one.

h. Emphasize the need for close follow-up to detect recurrences early.

i. Make referrals for home care, social service, and spiritual and financial assistance, as needed.

j. Advise the patient to use sunscreen with an SPF greater than 15, wear protective clothing, and avoid intense mid-day ultraviolet exposure.

Chapter

Neoplasms

TOPICAL OUTLINE

I. CANCER OF LYMPHOID TISSUE AND PLASMA CELLS

A. Hodgkin's Disease

◆ Hodgkin's disease is one of a group of neoplastic tumors that affect the lymphoid tissue and, as such, is termed a *lymphoma*.

1. Incidence and Etiology

   a. Approximately 7500 new cases of Hodgkin's disease are diagnosed annually in the United States. The cause of Hodgkin's disease is unknown.

   b. It is most common in young adults, with a higher incidence in males than in females. It occurs in all races but is slightly more common in whites. The incidence of Hodgkin's disease peaks in the age groups from 16 to 35 years and after age 50 years.

   c. In the United States, Hodgkin's disease occurs in approximately 2 of every 100,000 persons.

2. Pathophysiology with Signs and Symptoms

   a. Hodgkin's disease is characterized by a progressive, *painless enlargement of the lymph nodes*. It also can affect the spleen and liver.

   b. Eventually, tissues and organs throughout the body can be involved.

   c. Two systems of classification are used with each patient: histologic classification and clinical staging.

   d. *Histologic classification* and prognosis are based on the cellular composition of the infiltrate in the lymph nodes.

   e. In *clinical staging,* the four clinical stages (I, II, III, and IV) are based on the number, location, and degree of involved lymph nodes.

   f. Possible etiologies for Hodgkin's disease include viral, genetic, and immunologic factors and exposure to gamma radiation. Much inconclusive evidence supports these etiologic factors, with the exception of genetics. There is some tendency for clustering of Hodgkin's disease in families.

   g. Like other neoplastic blood disorders, Hodgkin's disease is characterized by the proliferation of one type of cell, in this case the Reed-Sternberg cell. The Reed-Sternberg cell is a giant connective tissue cell with one or two large nuclei that is characteristic of Hodgkin's disease.

   h. An early and characteristic indication of Hodgkin's disease is pruritus, which is mild at first and becomes acute as the disease progresses.

   i. The most common presenting feature is an *enlarged, painless cervical node*. Other frequent symptoms include fatigue, malaise, and weakness. The lymph nodes may "wax and wane," but they usually do not return to normal.

   j. Diagnosis for confirming Hodgkin's disease includes medical history, complete physical, and biopsy checking for Reed-Sternberg cells.

3. Treatment

   a. Radiotherapy may cure more than 80 percent of clients with localized Hodgkin's disease and chemotherapy may cure more than 50 percent of those with disseminated disease.

b. The choice of treatment regimen is totally dependent on the stage of disease. Management includes high-dose radiation therapy for stages I and II, and radiation and chemotherapy for stages III and IV.

4. Nursing Implications

a. Monitor for acute and late complications of external radiation therapy. Early effects of radiation include nausea, vomiting, anorexia, diarrhea, and blanching and erythema of the skin and mucous membranes, possibly progressing to desquamation (shedding of the epidermis).

(1) Recovery after desquamation usually takes 2 to 4 weeks, and the skin returns to normal in 2 to 3 months.

(2) Other side effects of external radiation include itching, tingling, burning sensation, oozing, and sloughing of skin.

(3) Radiation therapy causes depression of the hematopoietic system and, in turn, a low white blood cell count, predisposing the patient to infection.

(4) Pulmonary effects include cough, dyspnea, fatigue, and sore throat.

b. Late effects of radiation may be apparent month or years after therapy. Genital tissue, muscles, and kidneys may be affected, resulting in painful radionecrosis (disintegration of tissue due to exposure to radiant energy). Radiation causes destruction of fine vasculature, and the skin may show signs of atrophy (thinning and blanching), pigmentation, and telangiectasis (a vascular lesion formed by dilation of a group of small blood vessels). If vascular damage is severe, bleeding may occur and the irradiated tissues may fail to heal.

(1) Alopecia may occur.

(2) Teach the patient the early and late signs and symptoms of radiation therapy.

(3) Advise the patient to wear loose clothing (no girdle, tight pantyhose, tight trousers, or belts) during treatment to trunk area and for several weeks thereafter.

(4) Avoid excess heat or cold to skin during treatment period.

(5) Avoid using cosmetics if radiation is applied to facial area.

(6) Suggest wig or cap to the patient if alopecia occurs.

(7) Advise avoidance of sunbathing or extremes of temperature if blanching or discoloration of skin occurs.

(8) Do not wash off skin marks placed by radiologists.

(9) Use sponge bath instead of shower or tub bath after skin marks are placed.

(10) Prevent skin breakdown by applying ointments (if ordered).

(11) Promote healing of irritated skin after therapy by gently cleaning area with a solution of 30 mL hydrogen peroxide in 100 mL water.

(12) Use saline soaks, antibiotic ointments, or steroid cream for desquamation per physician's order.

(13) Provide antiemetics and analgesics as prescribed.

(14) Prevent infection using a private room and protective isolation if white blood count is low.

(15) Administer prophylactic antibiotics as prescribed during or after treatment.

(16) Use sterile technique when giving skin care around injection site.

(17) Chemotherapeutic agents are given orally, intravenously, intraarterially, intramuscularly, and by local instillation (i.e., intrapleurally within the pleural cavity and intrathecally within the spinal canal).

(18) The route of administration is based on which route will deliver the optimal amount of drugs to the tumor.

(19) Many cytotoxic drugs are given in pill form. Because they may be prescribed to be taken on a daily basis at home, careful instructions must be given topatients.

II. INTRAVENOUS AND INTRAARTERIAL CATHETERS

A. Catheters Used for Different Types of Therapy

◆ To extend the life of a peripherally inserted central catheter (PICC) and the midline catheter, the insertion site must stay free of microorganisms and free of complications. Many nurses prefer a transparent dressing, such as Tegaderm, for these catheters because they allow visualization of the site. The Tegaderm should be changed every 7 to 10 days or PRN (as needed). If purulent drainage is seen at the insertion site or the patient develops a fever, the drainage must be cultured, and 10 mL of blood should be obtained from the line. This helps to determine if the line is the source of infection. If the patient with a PICC line hears a gurgling sound in his or her ear or has chest pain when you flush the catheter, the catheter may have migrated. The PICC is kept patent with 100 U/mL heparin (Heplock). The midline catheter is kept patent with 25 U/mL heparin. A 10-mL syringe should be used when flushing catheters because this small-barrel syringe results in less pressure. Pressure should never be used when flushing catheters.

1. Both the PICC and midline catheter are used for long-term IV therapy. The PICC is a true central line because the tip of the catheter is located in the vena cava. The PICC lines are approximately 20 inches long and have been known to remain in place for up to 1 year.

a. A midline catheter line ranges from 3 to 8 inches in length and is placed just below the axilla (armpit) depending on the length. It can remain in place for approximately 2 to 4 weeks. Patients with midline catheters should not receive vancomycin HCl or phenytoin (Dilantin) because these drugs have a very low pH. Likewise patients should not receive hyperosmolar solutions such as total parental nutrition (TPN), blood products, or potentially irritating infusions such as antibiotics or chemotherapy.

b. In contrast, you can infuse all of the above products when using a PICC because the line empties into the superior vena cava, which contains a large volume of blood to dilute these products.

2. The Hickman catheter is available as single, double, or triple lumen and is irrigated daily with 5 mL of a heparin/saline solution (10 U heparin/mL) to prevent clotting. The distal end of the catheter is located in the *right atrium*. Meticulous aseptic technique following established protocols is observed when changing the dressing around the insertion site. Complications include catheter displacement or occlusion and infection. When withdrawing blood, discard the first 5 to 10 mL of blood, draw the blood sample, then replace heparin/saline solution to keep the lumen patent. Complications include catheter or vascular occlusion and infection.

3. The Groshong catheter is available as single, double, or triple lumen. The closed distal end of the catheter has a pressure-sensitive two-way valve that *eliminates the need for heparin/saline flushing*. The two-way valve prevents blood from backing into catheter. Care of the catheter is similar to that of other central venous lines in terms of dressing changes and aseptic technique. *Avoid using acetone during site care because acetone can weaken the catheter*. Other differences include the following:

a. Irrigated briskly with 5 mL normal saline every 7 days.

b. After administration of viscous liquids (e.g., lipids), flush briskly with 20 mL normal saline.

c. When withdrawing blood, discard the first 5 to 10 mL of blood, draw the sample, then flush briskly with 20 mL of normal saline.

d. Complications include catheter or vascular occlusion and infection.

4. Implantable vascular access systems (Port-a-Cath) can be implanted under the skin with the catheter inserted in the subclavian vein or bronchial artery. There is less danger of blood vessel or catheter occlusion, catheter displacement, or infection compared to an externally inserted catheter, but these complications can occur. Special needles (e.g., Huber needles) must be used to prevent perforation of the infusion port. The nurse must

a. Inspect the skin over the catheter for redness, swelling, or drainage

b. Monitor patients for signs of systemic infection

c. Irrigate the catheter daily with 3 mL heparin/saline solution (10 U heparin/mL)

5. Vascular access graft is a subcutaneous arteriovenous (AV) shunt frequently used for dialysis. This shunt is used in patients without readily accessible veins. The AV graft is inserted into the upper arm or groin area, sutured to an artery, and then run subcutaneously for approximately 7 inches and sutured to a vein.

Needles are inserted into the graft to draw blood and give IV fluids. Problems associated with the graft include thrombosis, hematoma formation, extravasation (escape of fluids into surrounding tissue from use of large needles that have torn the graft), and graft infection.

6. Assessment of the client receiving chemotherapy includes the following regimen:

a. Identify marrow depression.

b. Monitor WBC, platelet count, hemoglobin, and hematocrit.

c. Monitor for signs of bleeding, infection, and anemia. Prevent infection by meticulous aseptic technique when caring for a patient with open wound; use sterile gloves for procedures.

d. Observe for signs of urinary toxicity, which include monitoring urine for blood, signs of cystitis, elevated renal function data such as serum creatinine or 24-h urine for creatinine clearance.

e. Assess for gastrointestinal (GI) toxicity, including ulcer in mouth or rectum; monitor weight loss, fluid, and electrolytes.

B. Multiple Myeloma

◆ Multiple myeloma represents a malignant proliferation of plasma cells.

◆ The disease results from the uncontrolled proliferation of plasma cells that infiltrate bone, producing osteolytic lesions throughout the skeletal flat bones (vertebrae, skull, pelvis, and ribs) in late stages.

◆ It also infiltrates the body organs (liver, spleen, lymph nodes, lung, adrenal glands, kidney, skin, and GI tract).

1. Incidence

a. It is rare in persons younger than 40 years; it occurs most frequently in men older than 40 years.

b. Incidence of multiple myeloma increases with age.

2. Etiology

a. The cause of myeloma is not known.

b. In those exposed to radiation of nuclear warheads used in World War II, myeloma occurred with increased frequency after a 20-year latency.

c. Myeloma has been seen more commonly than expected among farmers, wood workers, leather workers, and those exposed to petroleum products.

3. Pathophysiology with Signs and Symptoms

a. Bone pain is the most common symptom in persons with myeloma.

b. The pain usually involves the back and ribs and often is worse at night.

c. The bone lesions of myeloma are caused by the proliferation of tumor cells and the activation of osteoclasts, which destroy the bone.

d. Arthritic symptoms, such as aching and swelling of the joints, can occur.

e. Other effects include fever, malaise, and pathologic fractures.

f. Severe recurrent infection, such as pneumonia and pyelonephritis.

g. Anemia occurs in 80 percent of myeloma clients.

h. Kidney stones as a result of hypercalcemia are common due to bone demineralization.

4. Treatment

a. Systemic chemotherapy to control the progression of myeloma and symptomatic supportive care to prevent serious morbidity from the complications of the disease.

b. Hypercalcemia is managed with hydration, diuretics, corticosteroids, and oral phosphate.

5. Nursing Implications

a. Encourage the patient to drink 3000 to 4000 mL fluids daily, particularly before an intravenous pyelogram (IVP) used to assess renal involvement. Monitor fluid intake and output (daily output should not be less than 1500 mL).

b. Encourage the patient to walk because pressure on the long bones is necessary for calcium absorption.

c. Administer analgesics as ordered to decrease pain.

d. Observe for signs of infections, such as fever or malaise.

e. Provide needed emotional support for the patient and his or her family.

f. Explain diagnostic procedures, such as marrow biopsy, to the patient.

g. Discuss effects and side effects of drug treatment.

C. Malignant Lymphomas (Non-Hodgkin's Lymphomas)

◆ Malignant lymphomas are a group of malignant diseases originating in lymph glands.

1. Incidence

a. Up to 8000 new cases of malignant lymphomas occur annually in the United States.

b. They are two to three times more common in males than in females and occur in all age groups.

c. Although rare in children, non-Hodgkin's lymphomas occur three times more often and cause twice as many deaths as Hodgkin's disease in children younger than 15 years.

2. Etiology

a. The cause of malignant lymphomas is unknown.

3. Signs and Symptoms

a. Usually, the first indication of malignant lymphoma is swelling of the lymph glands, enlarged tonsils and adenoids, and painless, rubbery nodes in the cervical and supraclavicular areas.

b. As the disease progresses, the patient develops symptoms of fatigue, malaise, weight loss, fever, and night sweats.

4. Prognosis

a. Nodular lymphomas yield a better prognosis than the diffuse form of the disease, but prognosis is less hopeful than in Hodgkin's disease.

b. Malignant lymphomas are classified into four stages ranging from stage I (involvement of a single lymph node) to stage IV (disseminated involvement of one or more body organs).

5. Treatment

a. Biopsy differentiates malignant lymphoma from Hodgkin's disease.

b. Treatment of malignant lymphomas may include radiotherapy, chemotherapy, or the bioengineered cancer treatment Rituxan. Rituxan is the first class of compounds known as monoclonal antibodies to be approved for treating cancer. Monoclonal antibodies work by targeting cell proteins believed to have a role in development of cancer. Monoclonal antibodies are less toxic to patients than chemotherapy.

D. Breast Cancer

1. Incidence

a. The United States has one of the highest rates of breast carcinoma in the world. One in eight American women will develop breast cancer in her lifetime. Breast cancer deaths occur in women age 50 years and older (84 percent of cases), and 77 percent of new breast cancer cases occur in this age group. However, it may develop any time after puberty. It occurs in men but only rarely; male cases of breast cancer account for less than 1 percent of all cases.

2. Clinical Manifestations and Diagnosis

a. Breast cancer in its earliest from usually is detected on a mammogram before it can be felt by the woman or her health care provider. However, it is estimated that 90 percent of all breast lumps are detected by the client. Of this 90 percent, only 20 to 25 percent are malignant.

b. More than half of all lumps are discovered in the upper outer quadrant of the breast.

c. The most common initial symptom is a lump or thickening of the breast. The lump may feel hard and fixed or soft and spongy. It may have well-defined or irregular borders. It may be fixed to the skin, thereby causing dimpling to occur. A nipple discharge that is bloody or clear may be present.

d. Monthly breast self-examination (BSE), routine screening mammography, and yearly breast examinations by practitioners are recommended for early detection of breast cancer.

3. Risk Factors for Breast Cancer

a. Age 50 and older

b. Previous history of breast cancer

c. Family history of breast cancer, especially a mother or sister (particularly significant if cancer was diagnosed pre-menopausally)

d. Previous history of ovarian, endometrial, colon, or thyroid cancer

e. Early menarche (before age 12 years)

f. Late menopause (after age 55 years)

g. Nulliparity or first pregnancy after age 30 years

h. Prolonged use of estrogen replacement therapy

i. Daily alcohol use

j. Obesity after menopause

k. Previous history of benign breast disease with fibrocytic changes

l. Race (Caucasian women have highest incidence)

m. High socioeconomic status

n. Sedentary lifestyle

o. Never having been pregnant

Note: Risk factors are cumulative—the more risk factors present, the greater the likelihood of breast cancer occurrence.

4. Treatment

a. Segmental, modified radical, lumpectomy, and radical mastectomy are the most common surgical procedures used to treat breast cancer, although lumpectomy and radiation may be an alternative for stage I and II disease and for tumors 4 cm or smaller.

b. Adjuvant chemotherapy is most helpful for premenopausal women with breast cancer that has spread to the lymph nodes. Tamoxifen, along with other new drug therapies, may provide the first real hope for preventing breast cancer.

c. Tamoxifen has potent antiestrogenic effects by competing with estrogen for binding sites in target tissue such as the breast.

Chapter 9

Pediatrics

A. Asthma

◆ Asthma is a disorder of the bronchial airways characterized by periods of bronchospasms. It is a hypersensitivity response.

1. Incidence

   a. Asthma is a common disorder occurring in approximately 9 percent of children. It is slightly more common in males than in females.

   b. It tends to occur before age 5 years but can occur at any age.

2. Etiology

   a. Asthma may result from sensitivity to specific external allergens (extrinsic) or from internal, nonallergenic factors (intrinsic).

   b. Extrinsic allergens include inhalation of known allergens such as animal hair, house dust or mold, pollen, feather pillows, cigarette smoke, and certain foods.

   c. Intrinsic asthma is triggered by a severe respiratory infection and may result from hypersensitivity to specific bacteria.

   d. Irritants, emotional stress, temperature, and humidity changes can aggravate intrinsic asthma.

3. Pathophysiology with Signs and Symptoms

   a. Asthma primarily affects the small airways and involves three separate processes: bronchospasm, increased bronchial secretions (mucus), and edema of the bronchial tubes.

   b. All three processes reduce the size of the lumen of the airway, leading to distress.

   c. Bronchial constriction occurs because of stimulation of the parasympathetic nervous system, which causes smooth muscle constriction.

   d. Typically, an acute asthmatic attack causes sudden dyspnea, wheezing, tightness in the chest, and a nonproductive cough or clear sputum. Patients feel as if they will suffocate during an acute attack and may not be able to speak more than a few words. Other signs include audible wheezing on expiration, use of accessory muscles, and profuse respirations. Tachypnea may develop as the disease progresses; the chest may become barrel shaped, and patients must purse their lips to exhale air.

   e. Status asthmaticus is an asthmatic attack that is acute and resistant to therapy. Status asthmaticus is an emergency situation often requiring respiratory assistance.

4. Treatment

   a. Identify and avoid precipitating factors, if possible.

   b. Drug treatment usually includes bronchodilators, which are most effective if started right after onset of symptoms.

   c. Drugs include epinephrine, aminophylline, montelukast (Singulair), and corticosteroids.

   d. After an attack, arterial blood gas studies will help determine the severity of an asthmatic attack.

B. Cerebral Palsy

◆ Cerebral palsy (CP) is divided into four separate types based on neuromuscular involvement; (1) spastic (approximately 70 percent of affected children), (2) dyskinetic (approximately 15 percent), (3) ataxia (approximately 5 percent), and (4) mixed (10 percent).

1. Incidence

   a. It is the most common cause of crippling in children. Incidence is highest in premature infants who are small for gestational age and have a low Apgar score at 5 min.

   b. The spastic form of CP affects approximately 70 percent of patients.

   c. CP occurs in an estimated 17,000 live births each year.

2. Etiology

   a. The cause is unknown. CP comprises a group of neuromuscular disorders associated with prenatal or postnatal CNS damage.

3. Pathophysiology with Signs and Symptoms

   a. Spasticity means an increased tone in voluntary muscle (loss of upper motor neurons).

   b. Patients with spastic CP have increased muscle tone, abnormal clonus (spasms in which rigidity and relaxation alternate in rapid succession), exaggeration of deep tendon reflexes, and abnormal reflexes such as a positive Babinski reflex. In a positive Babinski reflex, the toes extend instead of flexing when the sole of the foot is stimulated. This reflex is normal in infants younger than 6 months.

   c. CP is suspected whenever an infant exhibits the following signs and symptoms:

   (1) Has difficulty sucking or keeping nipple in mouth.

   (2) Seldom moves voluntarily or has leg and arm tremors with voluntary movement.

   (3) Crosses legs when lifted from behind rather than pulling legs up as healthy infant would do.

   (4) Legs are difficult to separate.

   (5) Persistently uses only one hand or uses hands but not legs.

   (6) Associated defects, seizures, speech disorders, and mental retardation are common.

4. Treatment

   a. Although there is no cure for CP, patients can be made comfortable and quality of life improved with the following assistance:

   (1) Braces, splints, specially designed eating utensils, and orthopedic surgery

   (2) Phenytoin (Dilantin) or other anticonvulsant agents to control seizures

5. Nursing Implications

   a. Maintain nutrition by

   (1) Assessing feeding problems

   (2) Providing high-calorie diet for children with constant movement

   (3) Allowing children adequate time to eat without feeling hurried

   (4) Providing soft food and liquid if chewing is uncoordinated and difficult

   b. Protect muscle and joint function for patient on bed rest by

   (1) Repositioning every 2–3 h to prevent contractures

   (2) Providing passive range of motion two times daily

   (3) Maintaining good body alignment

   (4) Using tennis shoes to prevent foot drop

   c. Promote safety by

   (1) Using protective head gear when beginning to walk

   (2) Supervising while eating to avoid aspiration

   (3) Assessing if leg braces are too tight and are interfering with circulation

   d. Promote communication and self-esteem by

   (1) Listening to child and allowing child time to communicate

   (2) Making referral for speech therapy if needed

   (3) Praising the child for goal attained

   (4) Encouraging the child to be as independent as possible

C. Cystic Fibrosis

◆ Cystic fibrosis (CF) is generalized dysfunction of the exocrine glands, affecting multiple organ systems in varying degrees of severity.

1. Incidence and Etiology

   a. CF is a common inherited recessive disorder and is the most common fatal genetic disease of white children. When both parents are carriers, with each pregnancy there is a one in four chance that the child will have CF. Reaching adulthood is now a realistic expectation for infants with CF.

   b. The average life expectancy is 24 years with a maximum survival of 30 to 40 years.

   c. The major contributing factors to increased life expectancy include early diagnosis and improved therapeutic interventions.

2. Pathophysiology with Signs and Symptoms

   a. Pancreas

   (1) The acinar cells of the pancreas normally produce lipase, trypsin, and amylase, enzymes that flow into the duodenum to digest fat, protein, and carbohydrate. Lipase breaks down fat, trypsin breaks down protein, and amylase breaks down starches.

(2) With cystic fibrosis, these enzyme secretions become so tenacious that they plug the ducts and create back pressure on the acinar cells, which causes cells to atrophy and destroys their ability to produce enzymes. Therefore, amylase, lipase, trypsin, and amylase cannot reach the duodenum.

(3) Islets of Langerhans, which produce insulin, remain unaffected by the disease process because they are endocrine (ductless secretion). However, as pancreatic fibrosis occurs and the disease progresses, they may be destroyed, resulting in diabetes mellitus.

(4) Without pancreatic enzymes, children are unable to digest fat and protein. Quantities of fat and protein pass undigested through the intestinal tract, causing large, bulky, greasy stools (steatorrhea).

b. Intestinal

(1) *Meconium ileus appears in newborns immediately after birth.* The lumen of the small bowel is blocked with thick mucus, which causes symptoms of intestinal obstruction.

(2) Intestinal bacteria increase because of the undigested food and, combined with fat, gives stool an extremely foul odor.

(3) The bulk of feces in the intestines may cause abdominal distention.

(4) Because children benefit from only approximately 40 percent of the food they ingest, they show signs of malnutrition, such as emaciated extremities.

(5) As the disease progresses and pancreatic enzymes are not secreted into the duodenum, nutritional absorption decreases, producing malnutrition. Common deficiency of fat-soluble vitamins A, D, E, and K develops, as does anemia.

(6) Hunger is constant because of poor food absorption.

(7) Nondigested food is excreted as unabsorbed fat and protein, causing the following symptoms:

(a) Steatorrhea (excessive fat in stool)

(b) Excessive protein in stool

(c) Increased bulk of fecal material (two to three times normal amount)

(d) Smelly stools

(e) Large stools causing rectal prolapse, which can result in internal obstruction or impaction.

c. Respiratory

(1) Pulmonary congestion exists in almost all children with CF because the large amount of mucus in the lungs is a serious threat to life.

(2) Respiratory tract infections are common. The child will have wheezing and great difficulty breathing, with a productive cough and dyspnea, barrel chest, and cyanotic clubbing of digits.

(3) Repeated episodes of bronchitis and bronchial pneumonia, primarily caused by *Streptococcus, Pneumococcus, Staphylococcus,* and *Haemophilus*, will occur.

(4) Hemoptysis occurs when a blood vessel is eroded as a result of repeated respiratory infections.

(a) The child may expectorate as much as 200 to 300 mL of blood in 24 h.

(b) When a child with a pulmonary disease such as CF has an uncontrollable urge to cough, this is sign that usually indicates blood in the airway from hemoptysis.

(5) The child will develop anemia due to blood loss.

(a) The child will be very anxious and should not be left alone.

(6) As the airway becomes progressively plugged with mucus, atelectasis may occur.

(7) Cor pulmonale (right-sided heart failure) can be expected to develop as accumulation of thick secretions in the lung increases, causing barrel chest, cyanosis, pneumonia, emphysema, and atelectasis. Atelectasis is usually the cause of death.

3. Diagnosis

a. History of disease in family

b. Absence of pancreatic enzymes

c. Increased sodium (Na) in sweat; electrolyte abnormality

d. Chronic pulmonary involvement

4. Treatment

a. CF is managed with diet and oral administration of pancreatic enzymes and fat-soluble vitamins.

b. Reduce dietary fat: institute a low-fat diet but use homogenized milk; infant cannot be given skim milk because of the need for lecithin, which occurs in whole milk.

c. Regulate diet according to severity of pancreatic defect. A pancreatic enzyme (pancrelipase [Viokase]) is given in conjunction with meals and snacks (see *Handbook of Medications for the NCLEX-RN® Review* Chapter 10, Pancreatic Enzymes).

d. Give vitamins A, D, E, and K in twice the normal daily dosage.

e. Give salt tablets as ordered.

f. Provide simple sugars, which are a good source of energy because of direct absorption.

g. Manage pulmonary congestion by suctioning PRN (as required) and prophylactic antibiotics (penicillin; if the child is allergic to penicillin, erythromycin is prescribed).

h. Administer oxygen and IV fluids to prevent dehydration and keep mucus moist.

i. Postural drainage is administered PRN.

j. Bed rest PRN because child becomes easily fatigued.

D. Galactosemia

1. Incidence and Etiology

   a. There are three main disorders of galactose metabolism. The most well known is transferase deficiency (classic) galactosemia. Galactosemia is an inborn error of galactose metabolism—lack of the enzyme needed to digest lactose.

   b. Incidence of the severe form is variable but is estimated to be 1 in 60,000. Some states include galactosemia in newborn screening programs.

2. Pathophysiology with Signs and Symptoms

   a. Deficient transferase activity causes the accumulation of galactose-1-phophate, galactose, and galactitol.

   b. Consequences include cataracts, liver damage, and neurologic impairment.

   c. Affected neonate may die without appropriate intervention.

3. Diagnostic Assessment

   a. Because of the morbidity and mortality resulting from classic galactosemia, prompt recognition of the clinical signs and immediate treatment are imperative.

   b. Shortly after birth, drops of blood are drawn from the heel and tested for lactose enzyme.

   c. If enzyme is not present, the infant will be given a soy-based formula.

   d. In severe cases, the symptoms begin within the first day of life.

   e. The signs of galactosemia tend to mimic other diseases, with vomiting, lethargy, and failure to thrive beginning after feeding with breast milk or lactose-containing formula.

   f. Development of jaundice provides an additional clue. If the neonate remains untreated, progressive liver damage will occur. Coma and death may follow.

   g. Untreated children who survive the neonatal period usually have neurologic deficits and mental retardation.

4. Treatment

   a. Early implementation of treatment quickly changes the course of the disease.

   b. *Galactose is eliminated from the diet by removing milk and milk products.*

   c. Formulas that do not contain lactose, such as soy formulas, are used.

   d. An affected infant begins to show improvement after starting the galactose-free diet.

   e. Vomiting and diarrhea subside, weight gain occurs, and cataracts regress.

   f. Lactose and galactose restriction are lifelong in children with classic galactosemia.

   g. Warn parents to *read medication and food product labels carefully to avoid foods containing lactose.*

E. Acute Leukemia

◆ Leukemia, which is the uncontrolled proliferation of leukocytes (white blood cells), is the most common form of cancer in children.

1. Incidence and Etiology

   a. Acute lymphocytic leukemia (ALL) is the most frequent type of leukemia in children, accounting for one third of all leukemia cases. The exact cause of leukemia is unknown.

   b. The highest frequency of ALL occurs in children between the ages of 2 and 8 years; they have the best survival rate.

   c. The prognosis for children younger than 12 months and older than 10 years at the time of first occurrence is poor.

   d. Acute leukemia is more common in males than in females.

   e. Acute myelogenous leukemia (AML) accounts for approximately 20 percent of all childhood leukemia cases. It is more frequent in late adolescence, and it is the most common type of leukemia in adulthood.

   f. In AML there is an overproduction of granulocytes that grow so rapidly that they often are forced out into the bloodstream while they are still in blast stage. This limits the production of red blood cells and platelets.

   g. *In AML, the average survival rate is only 1 year* after diagnosis, even with aggressive treatment.

2. Pathophysiology with Signs and Symptoms

   a. The malignant cell involved is an immature lymphocyte, the lymphoblast. With rapid proliferation of lymphocytes, the production of red blood cells and platelets falls, and the invasion of body organs by rapidly increasing white blood cells begins.

   b. The leukocyte count may be over 100,000 at the time of diagnosis.

   c. ALL and AML: sudden onset of low-grade fever accompanied by thrombocytopenia and abnormal bleeding, such as nosebleeds, petechiae, easy bruising after minor trauma, and prolonged menses; anemia; fatigue; malaise; tachycardia; and palpitations.

3. Treatment

   a. As many as 95 percent of children with ALL achieve remission with chemotherapy.

   b. ALL was the first of the human cancers to be cured by combination of chemotherapy (see *Handbook of Medications for the NCLEX-RN® Review,* Chapter 13, Cancer Chemotherapy).

   c. Radiation therapy may be administered as an adjunct to chemotherapy when leukemic cells infiltrate the CNS, skin, rectum, and testes, or when a large mediastinal mass is noted at diagnosis.

   d. Current treatment modalities for cancer destroy both normal and cancer cells.

e. Therapy is aimed at preventing or controlling side effects of cancer therapy, such as anemia, infections, and bleeding.

4. Nursing Implications

a. The nurse should institute good hand washing techniques for everyone coming in contact with the patient.

b. The patient should be in a private room with reverse isolation.

c. Monitor laboratory values frequently.

d. Minimize the side effects of chemotherapy by administering antiemetics as needed.

e. Teach the patient and family how to recognize infection (chills, fever, cough, sore throat) and abnormal bleeding (petechiae, bruising) and to report complications to the physician immediately.

f. Explain the side effects of chemotherapy, such as oral cavity and rectal ulcerations, anorexia, weight loss, susceptibility to infection, and bleeding.

g. Avoid using Foley catheters and giving IM injections because they provide easy avenues for infection.

h. Avoid taking rectal temperatures because bleeding may occur due to rectal irritation.

i. The mouth and rectum have a high turnover of cells, resulting in many immature cells that are attacked as cancer cells by cancer drugs.

j. Daily stool softeners are ordered to reduce the risk of anal fissures.

k. Provide frequent mouth care and saline rinses. Advise the patient to use a soft toothbrush and to avoid spicy foods.

l. Provide psychological support to family by establishing a trusting relationship to promote communication.

m. Provide the opportunity for religious counseling, if appropriate.

n. Discuss with parents the option of home hospice care.

F. Meningitis (Bacterial)

◆ Bacterial meningitis is a serious CNS infection caused by an invasion of the meninges by bacteria.

1. Incidence

a. Bacterial meningitis remains a common disease worldwide. The incidence of bacterial meningitis is between 5 and 10 per 100,000 people per year in the United States.

b. More than 2000 deaths are due to bacterial meningitis.

c. Approximately 25,000 cases of bacterial meningitis occur annually, of which approximately 70 percent occur in children younger than 5 years.

2. Etiology

a. *Escherichia coli, Pseudomonas*, and group B *Streptococci* are the causes during the neonatal period.

b. *Haemophilus influenza, Neisseria meningitidis, Streptococcus*, and *E. coli* are the major causes in children older than 1 month.

3. Pathophysiology with Signs and Symptoms

a. The pathogen process includes the following:

(1) Nasopharyngeal colonization

(2) Nasopharyngeal epithelial cell invasion

(3) Bloodstream invasion

(4) Bacteria with intravascular survival

(5) Survival and replication within the subarachnoid space

b. One of the major pathophysiologic consequences of bacterial meningitis is increased permeability of the blood–brain barrier, which leads to vasogenic cerebral edema.

c. Signs and symptoms in children include headache, fever, chills, malaise, increased intracranial pressure (ICP) causing headache, vomiting, and muscle (back and neck) rigidity, which results in a positive Brudzinski's sign and Kernig's sign.

d. To test for Kernig's sign, place the patient in a supine position, flex the hip and knee, then straighten the knee. Pain or resistance can indicate meningitis.

e. To test for Brudzinski's sign, place the patient in a dorsal recumbent position and place hands behind the patient's neck, bending forward. Pain and resistance can indicate meningeal inflammation. If the patient flexes the hips and knees in response to this manipulation, the possibility that he or she has meningitis is increased.

f. The neonate may not manifest many of the classic signs and symptoms of bacterial meningitis. Neurologic signs and symptoms and/or fever are commonly absent.

g. The only clinical clues may be listlessness, high-pitched crying, refusal to feed, irritability, or other nonspecific manifestations.

4. Treatment

a. Therapy for bacterial meningitis is IV antibiotics given for at least 2 weeks, followed by oral antibiotics. Dexamethasone has been shown to be effective as adjunctive therapy in the treatment of meningitis caused by *H. influenzae* type B and in pneumococcal meningitis if given before the first dose of antibiotic.

b. If the child is allergic to penicillin, anti-infective therapy will be given (e.g., tetracycline).

c. Other drugs include mannitol to decrease cerebral edema, an anticonvulsant such as phenytoin (Dilantin), and acetaminophen to relieve headache and fever.

d. The patient must be kept in isolation.

5. Nursing Implications

a. Assess neurologic function frequently.

b. Institute seizure precautions.

c. Test for Kernig's sign and Brudzinski's sign.

d. Maintain a quiet environment by reducing light and noise levels.

e. Monitor intake and output.

f. Assess vital signs frequently.

g. Observe for signs of increased ICP.

h. Change position gradually.

i. Administer stool softener to prevent straining during bowel movement.

G. Mumps

1. Incidence and Etiology

a. Mumps is an acute viral disease caused by paramyxovirus. The mumps paramyxovirus is found in the saliva of an infected person and is transmitted by droplets or by direct contact.

b. It is most common in children older than 5 years but younger than 10 years.

2. Signs and Symptoms

a. Symptoms include malaise, headache, earache, temperature 101°F to 104°F, tenderness and swelling of parotid gland, and pain when chewing.

3. Complications

a. A complication of mumps is epididymoorchitis (inflammation of the testes and epididymis), which can cause sterility.

b. Inflammation produces testicular swelling and tenderness, scrotal erythema, lower abdominal pain, nausea and vomiting, fever, and chills.

4. Treatment

a. Treatment includes analgesics for pain, antipyretics for fever, and adequate fluid intake to prevent dehydration from fever and anorexia.

b. Bed rest during the febrile period can be helpful.

H. Phenylketonuria (Classic)

1. Incidence

a. In the United States, phenylketonuria (PKU) occurs in 1 of approximately 14,000 births. The incidence of PKU is low in Finland, Japan, and in African Americans.

b. This is a lifelong condition.

c. Approximately 1 in every 70 persons in the United States is a carrier of PKU, an autosomal recessive disorder.

2. Etiology

a. PKU is an inborn error in phenylalanine metabolism. In this disorder, phenylalanine is not metabolized to tyrosine because of a deficiency or inactivity of phenylalanine hydroxylase.

b. Various degrees of PKU are caused by differences in amount of enzyme activity. It can be thought of as a continuum, with classic PKU (severe enzyme deficiency) at one end and benign mild enzyme deficiency at the other end.

c. High levels of phenylalanine affect brain development.

d. Currently, most states have newborn screening programs for PKU.

3. Signs and Symptoms

a. Arrested brain development and mental retardation, which can be prevented with early detection.

b. Phenylalanine levels can be normal at birth but will increase after intake of dietary protein (milk).

c. Infants in whom the condition is detected and treated before age 6 weeks will not become mentally retarded.

d. If the infant is not identified by testing, the first conspicuous sign of PKU is the child's inability to sit unassisted at the normal age; motor development is slowed.

4. Treatment

a. Treatment begins the first week of life to prevent brain damage. The objective is to balance the amino acid needs for normal growth and development against the danger of amino acid accumulation. Lofenalac powder is substituted for milk. It contains regular amounts of amino acids.

b. Phenylalanine is an essential amino acid; therefore, sufficient amounts must be supplied to ensure protein synthesis, but accumulation of excess phenylalanine must be avoided.

c. Dietary management includes the use of special formula and restricted phenylalanine intake in other foods.

d. The infant's metabolic pattern is determined by frequently measuring serum phenylalanine levels and keeping detailed records of intake.

e. Close follow-up is required and dietary adjustments are needed throughout infancy and childhood to allow for growth needs.

f. Solid foods are started at the usual time in infants with PKU.

g. The solid foods gradually become the source of needed phenylalanine.

h. Parents and children must recognize appropriate sources of this amino acid.

i. *Foods allowed on the diet include measured amounts of fruits, vegetables, cereal, and grains.*

j. Parents and child (at appropriate age) are taught to measure and calculate the amount of these foods to match the dietary prescription, which is based on age, weight, and serum phenylalanine levels. Cookbooks that feature low-phenylalanine foods are available.

k. Studies have shown that discontinuing the diet at any age can cause a decrease in IQ level.

5. Nursing Implications

a. Educate parents to recognize appropriate sources of amino acids.

b. Teach parents how to calculate appropriate dietary intake for child.

c. Stress the importance of close follow-up, which includes phenylalanine levels, weight, and dietary adjustment if necessary.

d. Provide resources for parents, such as educational materials, parent support groups, newsletters, and availability of cookbooks with low-phenylalanine foods.

I. Roseola Infantum

1. Incidence and Etiology

a. Roseola infantum is an acute, benign, presumably viral, infection. It affects infants and young children aged 8 months to 4 years.

2. Signs and Symptoms

a. The initial sign is high fever followed by rash, an abrupt drop in temperature, then a return of temperature to normal. This is the most common inflammatory skin eruption in children.

3. Treatments

a. Because roseola is self-limiting, treatment is supportive and symptomatic.

b. Antipyretics are used to reduce fever; parents are educated to dress child in light clothing and to give tepid baths to reduce fever.

J. Rubella (German Measles)

◆ Rubella is an acute, mildly contagious viral disease that produces a distinctive 3- to 4-day rash and lymphadenopathy.

1. Incidence

a. It occurs most often among children aged 5 to 9 years, adolescents, and young adults.

2. Etiology

a. The rubella virus is transmitted through contact with the blood, urine, stool, or nasopharyngeal secretions of infected persons.

b. *Transplacental transmission, especially in the first trimester of pregnancy, can cause serious birth defects.*

3. Pathophysiology with Signs and Symptoms

a. In children, after an incubation period of 15 to 17 days, a maculopapular rash (discolored red spots or patches on the skin) erupts abruptly. In adults, lymph node enlargement is a hallmark of rubella. *Typically, the rubella rash begins on the face.* The maculopapular eruptions spread rapidly, often covering the entire body within hours.

b. Small red, petechial macules on the soft palate may precede or accompany the rash.

c. Complications seldom occur in children with rubella. However, when they occur, they appear as hemorrhagic problems such as thrombocytopenia.

d. Two to three days after the rash appears, a temperature of 103°F to 105°F, severe cough, puffy red eyes, and rhinorrhea develop.

e. Approximately 6 days after the rash appears, other symptoms disappear and communicability ends.

4. Treatment and Prevention

a. Bed rest, with vaporizer, helps to reduce respiratory irritation.

b. Cough preparation, antibiotics, and antipyretics usually are administered.

c. Rubella vaccine (measles, mumps, rubella [MMR]) for infants is given after 12 months.

d. Many schools and colleges now require proof of MMR immunization before enrollment. Rubella vaccine is contraindicated in pregnant women and in persons who are immunocompromised.

5. Nursing Implications

a. Teach parents supportive measures, and stress the need for isolation, plenty of rest, and increased fluid intake.

b. Instruct parents to monitor temperature and to give medications as ordered.

c. Teach parents to assess for early signs of complications, such as pneumonia, and to seek medical help immediately.

K. Rubeola (Measles)

◆ Rubeola is an acute, highly contagious infection. It is one of the most serious of all communicable childhood diseases.

1. Etiology

a. Measles is spread by direct contact or by contaminated airborne respiratory droplets.

b. It is one of the most serious of all communicable childhood diseases.

2. Pathophysiology with Signs and Symptoms

a. Incubation period is 10 to 15 days.

b. Initial symptoms begin and greatest communicability occurs approximately 12 days after exposure to the virus.

c. This phase lasts from 3 to 5 days; symptoms include fever, anorexia, malaise, hoarseness, and hacking cough.

d. Before the rash appears, Koplik's spots appear in the mouth. Koplik's spots are small red spots with bluish-white center on the oral mucosa opposite the molars; they are the hallmark of rubeola (measles).

e. Approximately 5 days after Koplik's spots appear, temperature rises sharply, spots slough off, and rash appears.

f. This characteristic rash starts as faint macules behind the ear and on the neck and cheeks.

g. The macules develop into diffused redness over the skin.

h. They rapidly spread over the entire face, neck, eyelids, arms, back, chest, abdomen, and thighs.

i. When the rash reaches the feet (2–3 days), it begins to fade in the same sequence as it appeared, leaving brownish discoloration that disappears in 8 to 10 days.

j. Two to three days after the rash appears, the patient develops temperature of 103°F to 105°F, severe cough, puffy red eyes, and rhinorrhea.

k. Approximately 5 days after the rash appears, other symptoms disappear and communicability ends.

l. Severe infections may lead to secondary bacterial infection and to autoimmune reactions or organ invasion by the virus, resulting in pneumonia and encephalitis.

3. Treatment and Prevention

a. Bed rest and respiratory isolation throughout the communicable period.

b. A vaporizer may help reduce respiratory irritation but cough preparations are usually administered.

c. Antibiotics may be used prophylactically, and antipyretics can be given to reduce fever.

d. Measles vaccine is generally not administered to children younger than 12 months because of circulating maternal antibodies.

e. MMR vaccine is given between 15 and 18 months of age.

f. Avoid giving the vaccine to pregnant women (ask date of last menstrual period). Warn women to avoid pregnancy for at least 3 months following vaccination.

g. Children cannot receive the vaccine if they have immunodeficiency, leukemia, or untreated tuberculosis.

h. If children are exposed to the virus and have not been vaccinated, they should receive gamma-globulin (it may not prevent the measles but will lessen its severity).

i. Delay vaccination from 8 to 12 weeks after administration of whole blood, plasma, or gamma-globulin because measles antibodies in these products may neutralize the vaccine.

j. Watch for anaphylaxis for 30 min after vaccination. Have epinephrine available.

k. Generally, once an individual has measles, immunity is established.

4. Nursing Implications

a. Teach parents supportive measures, and stress the need for isolation, plenty of rest, and increased fluid intake.

b. Advise parents to monitor temperature and to assess for early complications such as pneumonia.

c. Advise parents of the importance of having the child receive the measles vaccine.

d. Warn the patients that possible side effects of the measles vaccine are anorexia, malaise, rash, mild thrombocytopenia or leukopenia, and fever.

e. Ask parents about known allergies to *neomycin* or *gelatin*. If allergic, the vaccine is not given and the physician is notified. *Patients who are allergic to eggs can receive the vaccine because only minimal amounts of albumin and yolk component are present in the vaccine.*

L. Varicella (Chickenpox)

◆ Varicella is a common, acute, highly contagious infection.

1. Incidence

a. Can occur at any age, but occurs most often in children aged 2 to 8 years.

b. Chickenpox has worldwide distribution.

c. An estimated 4,000,000 Americans, mostly children, suffer from the disease every year.

2. Etiology

a. Chickenpox is caused by the herpes virus varicella-zoster, *the same virus that, in its latent stage, causes herpes zoster (shingles).*

3. Pathophysiology with Signs and Symptoms

a. Varicella infection is transmitted by direct contact, primarily secretions from the respiratory tract, saliva, and, frequently skin lesions.

b. The incubation period last from 10 to 20 days.

c. Chickenpox is communicable 1 day before the rash to 5 to 6 days after appearance of the rash, when vesicles have all crusted.

d. Contracting the disease offers lasting natural immunity to chickenpox.

e. Pruritic rash on trunk, scalp, and face (rarely on extremities), slightly elevated fever, malaise, and anorexia; erythematous macules progress to papules then to clear vesicles, which break easily and form scabs.

4. Treatment

a. The Food and Drug Administration (FDA) approved a chickenpox vaccine called Varivax. Approval came in 1995 after 29 years of research.

b. Varivax is 70 to 80 percent effective at preventing chickenpox, and those who develop chickenpox after taking the vaccine have a much milder disease according to the FDA report.

c. The vaccine cannot be given to children younger than 1 year, even though 5 percent of infants develop chickenpox.

d. Children aged 1 to 12 get a single vaccination; teenagers and adults who have never had chickenpox get two vaccinations, 4 to 8 weeks apart.

5. Nursing Implications

a. If the disease develops, prevent scratching of vesicles, which causes infection, scarring, impetigo, and furuncles. Patients with chickenpox are isolated until all vesicles and most scabs disappear (usually 1 week after onset of rash). Generally, treatment consists of local or systemic antipruritics, such as cool baths with bicarbonate of soda, calamine lotion, or antihistamines.

b. Advise parents of the importance of having their child vaccinated with Varivax. Susceptible patients may need special treatment, especially if the child has immunodeficiency. When given 72 hours after exposer to varicella-zoster, immunoglobulin may provide positive immunity.

M. Wilms' Tumor (Nephroblastoma)

1. Etiology

    a. The cause is unknown. It is the most frequent intraabdominal tumor of childhood. Increased incidence among siblings and identical twins, reflecting evidence of genetic inheritance.

2. Incidence

    a. Occurs in children of either gender.

3. Signs and Symptoms

    a. Swelling or mass within the abdomen; mass is firm, nontender, and located deep within the flank area.

    b. Intermittent hematuria and anemia secondary to hemorrhage within the tumor.

    c. Hypertension from increased secretion of renin.

    d. Weight loss and fever.

    e. If metastasized to the lungs, then dyspnea, cough shortness of breath, and chest pain develop.

    f. Adrenal mass should not be palpitated because of the possibility of spreading the cancer.

4. Treatment

    a. Radiotherapy when client is older than 18 months with stage I disease.

    b. Infants are extremely radiosensitive; devastating skeletal and soft-tissue destruction can result from radiotherapy.

    c. Chemotherapy agents used are dactinomycin and vincristine. The most common site of metastasis is to the lungs.

N. Lyme Disease

    ◆ Lyme disease is a multisystemic disorder caused by a spirochete that is carried by a tick.

1. Incidence and Etiology

    a. Initially, Lyme disease was identified in a group of children diagnosed with arthritis around Lyme, Connecticut.

    b. According to the Centers for Disease Control and Prevention, more that 99,000 cases of Lyme disease have been reported since 1982, and the annual number has been increasing every year.

    c. Although cases have been reported in nearly every state, most of them occur in the Northeast, the upper Midwest (particularly Minnesota and Wisconsin), and northern California.

    d. People are more likely to become infected during the spring and summer, but it is possible to contact Lyme disease at any time of the year.

2. Signs and Symptoms

    a. The first stage of the disease is the appearance of a red macule or papule, usually at the site of the tick bite. This lesion often feels hot and itchy and may grow to over 50 cm in diameter.

    b. The second stage, which occurs weeks or months later, begins with neurologic abnormalities. Facial palsy is especially noticeable.

    c. The third stage begins weeks or years later and is characterized by arthritis with marked swelling in the large joints; arthritis can become chronic.

3. Nursing Implications

    a. Tick on a patient's body should be removed using a pair of tweezers.

    b. Grasp the tick as close to the skin as possible.

    c. After tick is removed, clean the bite with antiseptic.

    d. Place tick in a covered container of alcohol to preserve for examination by a physician.

4. Treatment

    a. Oral tetracycline is the treatment of choice for adults, administered for approximately 15 to 20 days. Penicillin and erythromycin are alternates and usually prescribed for children.

    b. When given in the early stages of the disease, these drugs can minimize later complications.

O. Respiratory Syncytial Virus Infection

    ◆ Respiratory syncytial virus (RSV) is a highly contagious pathogen. Its primary effect is on the lower respiratory tract.

1. Incidence and Etiology

    a. Antibody titers indicate that few children younger than 4 years escape contracting some form of RSV, even if it is mild.

    b. RSV is the only viral disease that has its maximum impact during the first few months of life (incidence peaks at age 2 months).

    c. The organism is transmitted from person to person by respiratory secretions and has an incubation period of 4 to 5 days.

2. Signs and Symptoms

    a. Otitis media is a common complication of RSV in infants. Severe respiratory distress may occur.

3. Treatment

    a. Treatment of this viral infection is supportive and based on the severity of symptoms.

    b. In mild cases, humidified oxygen and intravenous fluids are administered.

    c. Children with severe respiratory distress require endotracheal intubation and mechanical ventilation.

    d. Ribavirin or other antiviral drugs may be administered.

P. Muscular Dystrophy

1. Etiology

   a. Muscular dystrophy is a group of congenital disorders characterized by progressive symmetric wasting of skeletal muscles.

   b. These wasted muscles tend to enlarge because of connective tissue and fat deposits, giving a false impression of muscle strength.

   c. There are four main types of muscular dystrophy.

   d. This chromosome recessive disorder is transmitted by both sexes.

2. Incidence

   a. Duchenne's muscular dystrophy accounts for 50 percent of all cases and is an X-linked recessive disorder.

   b. Affects males most often.

3. Signs and Symptoms

   a. Begins insidiously, between ages 3 and 5 years.

   b. It affects leg and pelvic muscles, but eventually spreads to the voluntary muscles.

   c. Muscle weakness produces a waddling gait, toe walking, and lordosis (abnormal anterior convexity of the spine).

   d. Children with this disorder have difficulty climbing stairs and running, they fall down often, and their arms "wing out" when they raise their arms.

   e. Calf muscles become enlarged and firm.

   f. Muscle deterioration progresses rapidly and contractures develop.

   g. Usually these children are confined to wheelchairs by age 9 to 12 years.

   h. Within 10 to 15 years after onset of the disease, the electrocardiogram shows abnormalities. Tachycardia occurs due to progressive weakening of cardiac muscles.

   i. Death commonly results from sudden heart failure, respiratory failure, or infections within 10 to 15 years after onset of the disease.

4. Treatment

   a. No treatment can stop the progressive degeneration of muscles.

   b. Orthopedic appliances, exercise, physical therapy, and surgery to correct contractures can help preserve mobility and independence.

   c. Family members who are carriers of muscular dystrophy should receive genetic counseling regarding the risk of transmitting this disease.

Q. Down Syndrome

1. Etiology and Incidence

   a. Down syndrome usually results from trisomy 21, an error in which chromosome 21 has three copies instead of the normal two because of faulty meiosis of the ovum or sometimes sperm.

   b. Down syndrome occurs in 1 of 650 live births, but the incidence increases with maternal age, especially after age 35 years.

2. Signs and Symptoms

   a. As infant grows older, mental retardation becomes obvious.

   b. Child has craniofacial anomalies, such as

   - Slanting, almond-shaped eyes
   - Protruding tongue
   - Small, open mouth
   - Single transverse crease (simian crease)
   - Small skull
   - Flat bridge across the nose
   - Slow dental development or absent teeth
   - Flattened face
   - Short neck

3. Treatment

   a. Down syndrome has no cure. Surgery may be performed to correct heart defects and other congenital abnormalities.

   b. Antibiotic therapy for recurrent infections has improved life expectancy.

   c. Plastic surgery may be performed to correct the facial anomalies, especially the protruding tongue, which may improve speech.

4. Nursing Implications

   a. Teach parents the need for patience while feeding the infant who may have difficulty sucking.

   b. Assist parents in setting realistic goals for their child.

   c. Refer parents to national Down syndrome organizations.

R. Tay-Sachs Disease

- Tay-Sachs disease is the most common of *lipid diseases*. Tay-Sachs disease results from a congenital enzyme deficiency. It is characterized by progressive mental and motor deterioration and is always fatal, usually before age 5 years.

- Tay-Sachs disease is quite rare, occurring in fewer than 100 infants born each year in the United States.

- It strikes persons of Jewish ancestry approximately 100 times more often than the general population, occurring in approximately 1 in 3600 live births in this ethnic group.

Note: Because this disease is rare, it is not discussed further.

Chapter
10

Sensory Disorders

TOPICAL OUTLINE

I. EYE DISORDERS

A. Cataract

◆ A cataract is a clouding or opacity of the lens that leads to gradual painless blurring of vision and eventually loss of sight.

1. Incidence

a. Cataracts are classified as *senile,* those associated with aging; *traumatic,* those associated with injury; *congenital,* those that occur at birth; or *secondary,* those that occur following other eye diseases.

b. Cataracts are most prevalent in persons older than 70 years, occurring as part of the aging process.

2. Etiology and Pathophysiology

a. Research suggest cataracts in the elderly are related to long exposure to the sun's ultraviolet light. Also may be related to vitamin C deficiency.

b. Senile cataracts in the elderly may result from changes in the chemical state of protein in the lens.

c. Congenital cataracts occur in newborns as genetic defects or due to maternal rubella during the first trimester.

d. Traumatic cataracts develop after a foreign body injures the lens with sufficient force to allow aqueous or vitreous humor to enter the lens capsule.

e. Secondary cataracts occur secondary to uveitis (inflammation of the iris, ciliary body, and choroids), glaucoma, retinitis, detached retina, in the course of systemic disease (e.g., diabetes mellitus), or galactosemia.

3. Signs and Symptoms

a. Typically, a patient with cataracts experiences painless, gradual blurring and loss of vision.

b. Both eyes may develop cataracts, but they usually develop at different rates.

4. Treatment

a. Operative treatment is the only method for treating cataracts.

b. Surgery can restore vision loss by removing the cataract.

c. Between 90 and 95 percent of all cataract operations are successful.

d. Cataracts are removed whenever the decreased vision interferes with the person's activities of daily living or when the cataracts may lead to other complications such as glaucoma.

e. Cataracts usually are removed with local anesthetic dropped in the patient's eye and a small amount of sedative hypnotic (e.g., midazolam [Versed]) administered by IV. The surgery is done on an inpatient or outpatient basis.

f. The most popular method of cataract removal is extracapsular cataract extraction.

g. In this method, only the anterior portion of the lens capsule plus the capsule contents are removed, using techniques such as irrigation and aspiration or phacoemulsification (ultrasonic vibration to break up the lens).

h. Cataracts also can be removed within their capsule (intracapsular cataract extraction) using a freezing (cryo) probe that adheres to the surface of the lens.

5. Corrective Lenses

a. Because the lens has been removed, something is needed to replace the lost focusing power.

b. The intraocular lens is the most commonly used. When this is not possible, cataract glasses or contact lenses are necessary.

c. The intraocular lens is implanted within the eye at the time of surgery.

d. The intraocular lens is the primary form of lens replacement today because it restores vision to near 20/20.

6. Nursing Implications

a. Most cataract surgery is now performed in ambulatory surgery centers; few patients require hospitalization.

b. Before surgery, the pupil of the operative eye is well dilated.

c. The patients usually can go home the same day as the surgery.

d. General anesthesia may be necessary for patients who cannot hold still during surgery.

e. Following any cataract operation, a dressing may be applied to the eye, and the eye is covered with a metal shield to protect the eye from injury. The dressing usually is removed the day after surgery, but the eye shield is worn at night for a few weeks until the eye is healed to avoid accidental scratching of the operative site during sleep.

B. Chronic Open-Angle Glaucoma

1. Incidence

a. Occurs in persons older than 40 years. Highest incidence is among the black population.

b. Glaucoma is the third major cause of blindness in the United States, affecting approximately 3 percent of the population. Diabetes mellitus is the number one cause of blindness in the United States.

2. Etiology

a. Inherited, recessive trait.

3. Pathophysiology with Signs and Symptoms

a. The most common form of primary glaucoma is open-angle glaucoma, which usually occurs bilaterally, either simultaneously or consecutively.

b. Chronic open-angle glaucoma results from overproduction of aqueous humor or obstruction to its outflow through trabecular meshwork. This causes an increase in intraocular pressure (IOP).

c. It usually is bilateral, with insidious onset and a slow progressive course. Symptoms appear late in the disease and include mild pain in the eyes, loss of peripheral vision, visual disturbances such as seeing halos around lights, and reduced visual acuity (especially at night).

4. Treatment

a. Decrease production of aqueous humor with beta-blockers such as timolol and pilocarpine (mitotic eye drops), which are used to increase aqueous humor outflow (see *Handbook of Medications for the NCLEX-RN* Chapter 2).

b. If the patient is unresponsive to drug therapy, trabeculectomy can be performed, creating an opening for aqueous outflow, or a trabeculoplasty is performed, using a laser beam to open the trabecular mesh so that aqueous humor can flow out at a faster rate and reduce IOP.

C. Acute Closed-Angle Glaucoma

1. Etiology and Incidence

a. Glaucoma is an inherited, recessive trait.

b. It affects 3 percent of the US population over age 40 and accounts for 12 percent of all cases of blindness in the United States.

2. Pathophysiology with Signs and Symptoms

a. The obstruction to outflow of aqueous humor is due to obstruction in a part of the outflow channel that results in backup of fluid and increased IOP.

b. Acute angle-closed glaucoma typically has a rapid onset, constituting an ophthalmic emergency. Symptoms include acute pain in a unilaterally inflamed eye, pressure over the eye, moderate pupil dilation that is nonreactive to light, cloudy cornea, blurring visual acuity, and seeing halos around lights. Increased IOP may induce nausea and vomiting. Unless treated promptly, this acute form of glaucoma produces blindness in 3 to 5 days.

3. Treatment

a. Acute closed-angle glaucoma is an ocular emergency requiring immediate treatment to lower IOP.

b. If IOP does not decrease with drug therapy, a laser iridotomy or surgical iridectomy (trabeculectomy) must be performed to save vision. The procedures create an opening for aqueous outflow.

4. Nursing Implications

a. Stress the importance of compliance with prescribed drug therapy to prevent increased IOP and loss of vision.

b. For patients having laser iridotomy or surgical trabeculectomy, give medications as ordered and prepare the patient physically and psychologically.

c. Stress the importance of glaucoma screening for early detection and prevention.

d. Inform the patient that all persons older than 35 years, especially those with family histories of glaucoma, should have an annual diagnostic testing that includes peripheral vision test to determine changes in the field of vision or possible retinal changes. If changes are noted, a tonometric examination for early detection of IOP may be administered.

D. Retinal Detachment

1. Incidence

   a. Retinal detachment is more common in adult males than females; it is rare in children.

   b. Retinal detachment may occur from major or minor trauma. More males than females are involved in traumatic activities, which may explain why retinal detachment is twice as common in males.

2. Etiology

   a. In adults, retinal detachment usually results from degenerative changes of aging, myopia degeneration, cataract surgery, and trauma.

3. Pathophysiology with Signs and Symptoms

   a. Any retinal tear or hole allows the liquid vitreous to seep between the retinal layers, separating the retina from its blood supply.

   b. The patient complains of floating spots and recurrent flashes of light. As detachment progresses, gradual, painless visual loss may be described as a veil, curtain, or cobweb that comes down over the eye and eliminates a portion or all of the visual field.

4. Treatment

   a. The retinal breaks are sealed off with photocoagulation or cryotherapy.

   b. For retinal detachment, scleral buckling procedure is used to push the choroids and retina together.

5. Nursing Implications

   a. Administer eye medications as ordered. Mydriatics are used to produce dilation of the pupil; cycloplegics, which cause paralysis of ciliary muscle and also cause dilation of pupil, are used.

   b. Keeping the pupil dilated puts less pressure on the repaired retinal area.

   c. Instruct the patient to avoid jerking motions of the head (sneezing, coughing, and vomiting).

   d. Administer cough medication as required.

E. Artificial Eye

1. Care of artificial eye

   a. Remove daily for cleansing

   b. Cleanse with mild detergent and water

   c. Dry and store in water or contact lens soaking solution

   d. Remove before general surgery

   e. Insertion method

      (1) Raise upper lid and slip eye beneath it

      (2) Release lid

      (3) Support lower lid and draw it over the lower edge of eye

   f. Removal method

      (1) Draw lower lid downward

      (2) Slip eye forward over lower lid and remove

      (3) Instill eye drops (artificial eye drops)

II. EAR DISORDERS

A. Ménière's Disease

   ◆ Ménière's disease is a labyrinthine dysfunction that produces severe vertigo, sensorineural hearing loss, and tinnitus.

1. Incidence

   a. Symptoms begin between the ages of 20 and 60 years. Usually one ear is involved; however, 20 to 30 percent of patients have bilateral involvement.

2. Etiology

   a. The etiology of the disease is unknown, but the disturbance is related to the cerebellum.

3. Pathophysiology with Signs and Symptoms

   a. The patient's attacks of vertigo are sudden and without warning, possibly caused by autonomic nervous or metabolic system dysfunction, local allergy, or vascular disturbance.

   b. Prior to the vertigo attacks, the patient experiences fullness in the ear.

   c. The patient complains that the environment is whirling about him or her and feels a need to lie down.

   d. The duration may last from 10 min to several hours, and attacks occur several times per year. Remission may last as long as several years.

   e. During an acute attack, other symptoms include severe nausea, vomiting, sweating, and giddiness.

   f. Initially, the associated hearing loss fluctuates, but gradually it becomes permanent and worsens over years.

4. Treatment

   a. During an acute attack, rest is the most effective treatment; the patient usually can find a position in which vertigo is minimal. The nurse should educate the patient to not move suddenly because this will increase symptoms.

   b. Dimenhydrinate (Dramamine), an antiemetic, may be necessary in a severe attack. Long-term management includes use of a diuretic and restricted sodium intake and meclizine HCl (Antivert).

   c. Prophylactic antihistamines or mild sedatives (phenobarbital, diazepam) may be helpful.

   d. Usually the deafness is unilateral and progressive; when it is complete, the vertiginous attacks cease. The course is variable, however, and if the attacks persist in a severe manner, permanent relief can be obtained by surgical destruction of the labyrinth or section of the vestibular portion of the eighth cranial nerve.

5. Nursing Implications

   a. Advise the patient against reading and exposure to glaring light to reduce dizziness.

   b. If hospitalized, instruct the patient to ask for assistance when getting out of bed to walk.

   c. Instruct the patient to avoid sudden position changes, which may cause an attack.

   d. Administer antiemetics and diuretics as ordered.

   e. Instruct the patient to follow a sodium-restricted intake.

   f. Record intake and output carefully.

B. Otitis Media

   ◆ The most prevalent disease of the middle ear are infections resulting in otitis media. Otitis media is caused by various types of bacteria and viruses.

1. Incidence

   a. Acute and chronic otitis media are common in children; incidence increases during the winter months, paralleling bacterial respiratory tract infections.

2. Etiology

   a. Otitis media results from respiratory tract infection and allergic reaction. Predisposing factors include a more horizontal or short eustachian tube and increased lymphoid tissue in children.

   b. Another predisposing factor is holding or laying an infant supine during bottle feeding. This allows nasopharyngeal bacteria to reflux into the eustachian tube and colonize in the middle ear.

3. Pathophysiology with Signs and Symptoms

   a. When infections recur, usually causing drainage and perforation, the problem is called *chronic otitis media*. Between periods of otitis media, the middle ear may form fluid (serous otitis media). Serous otitis media with suppurative chronic infection is a leading cause of hearing loss in children.

   b. Negative pressure in the middle ear promotes transudation of sterile serous fluid from blood vessels in the membrane of the middle ear, causing obstruction of the eustachian tube.

   c. Infection causes swelling of the mucous membranes throughout the middle ear and eustachian tube.

   d. Signs and symptoms of *acute otitis media* include severe, deep throbbing pain (from pressure behind the tympanic membrane); mild to very high fever; dizziness; nausea; and vomiting.

   e. The tympanic membrane may be bulging, or there may be purulent drainage in the ear canal from tympanic membrane rupture. In acute secretory otitis media, the tympanic membrane is retracted due to inflammation.

4. Treatment

   a. In acute otitis media, antibiotic therapy includes trimethoprim or amoxicillin.

   b. Severe, painful bulging of the tympanic membrane usually necessitates myringotomy (incision of the tympanic membrane), and aspiration of middle ear fluid is necessary.

   c. If infusion is chronic, it is followed by insertion of a polyethylene tube into the tympanic membrane for immediate and prolonged equalization of inner ear pressure.

   d. The tube falls out spontaneously after 9 to 12 months.

   e. In acute secretory otitis media, the Valsalva maneuver is performed several times per day and decongestant therapy is used. If this fails, a myringotomy and aspiration of middle ear fluid are necessary.

5. Nursing Implications

   a. After myringotomy, maintain drainage flow.

   b. Do not place cotton in the ear canal to absorb drainage because damp cotton in the ear is a good medium for infection.

   c. Stress the need to complete the prescribed course of antibiotic treatment.

   d. Advise the parents to seek medical assistance if the child has fever or ear pain.

Chapter

11

Diseases, Medications, and Nutrition

QUESTIONS AND RATIONALES FOR CHAPTERS 2 THROUGH 10

EXAMINATION

1. The nurse would expect a patient with hyperparathyroidism to have which of the following characteristics?
   1. Increased bone reabsorption, elevated serum calcium levels, and decreased serum phosphate levels.
   2. Decreased bone reabsorption, decreased serum calcium levels, and increased phosphate levels.
   3. Increased serum calcium levels and increased vitamin D absorption.
   4. Decreased bone resorption, depressed urine excretion of calcium, and increased calcium levels.

2. A female patient is admitted to the hospital with a diagnosis of Addison's disease. She exhibits signs and symptoms of hypotension, hypoglycemia, and low sodium. She asks the nurse why she is hypotensive. The nurse is correct when she tells the patient that hypotension is caused by a decrease in production of
   1. Glucocorticoids.
   2. Androgens.
   3. Mineralocorticoids.
   4. Estrogen.

3. The nurse should observe a patient with Addison's disease for signs of infection because which one of the following processes will NOT function properly?

1. Hormonal process.
2. Antiinflammatory process.
3. Metabolic process.
4. Electrolytic process.

4. The nurse explains to a patient with Addison's disease that emaciation, muscular weakness, and fatigue are due to
   1. Protein catabolism and decreased gluconeogenesis.
   2. Electrolyte imbalance and increased gluconeogenesis.
   3. Calcium deficiency and increased protein excretion.
   4. Iron deficiency and increased gluconeogenesis.

5. The nurse preparing a patient for an organ transplant will anticipate giving an immunosuppressant drug that would include
   1. Cromolyn (Intal) and cortisol (Cortef).
   2. Indomethacin (Indocin) and diazepam (Valium).
   3. Cyclosporine (Sandimmune) and azathioprine (Imuran).
   4. Liothyronine (Cytomel) and methotrexate (Rheumatrex).

6. The nurse caring for a patient with tuberculosis (TB) would observe for signs and symptoms of TB, which are
   1. Persistent cough, weight loss, anorexia, night sweats, and fever.
   2. Muscle weakness, increased susceptibility to infection, and diarrhea.
   3. Diarrhea, dehydration, hyponatremia, hyperkalemia, and fever.

4. Dyspnea, hemoptysis, wheezing, chest pain, and hoarseness.

7. The nurse explains to a patient suspected of having TB that the diagnostic tests for TB are

1. Hemoglobin (Hb) concentration study, endoscopy, and x-ray film.
2. X-ray film, lung scan, and pulmonary function test.
3. Mantoux test, chest x-ray film, and sputum analysis.
4. Blood culture, endoscopy, and lung biopsy.

8. The nurse educates the patient about TB agents that may be used in his treatment. They include

1. Allopurinol (Zyloprim), aminophylline (Amoline), and amyl nitrate (Amyl Nitrate Aspirols).
2. Guanethidine (Ismelin), interferon, meclizine (Antivert), and isosorbide dinitrate (Isordil).
3. Ibuprofen (Motrin), immune serum globulin (gamma globulin), and indomethacin (Indocin).
4. Isoniazid (INH), rifampin (Rifadin), ethambutol (Myambutol), and streptomycin.

9. The nurse explains to a patient suspected of having TB that the method of transmission of TB is by

1. Blood, spinal fluid, and semen.
2. Coughing, sneezing, and unpasteurized milk.
3. Physical contact, sexual contact, and blood.
4. Urine, stool, and semen.

10. When administering the following drugs, the nurse knows that which of the following drugs must be protected from light?

1. Nipride (nitroprusside).
2. Procardia (nifedipine).
3. Isoptin (verapamil).
4. Cardizem (diltiazem).

QUESTIONS 11 TO 14

In assessing an *adult patient*, the nurse associates the following signs and symptoms with which disease?

11. ___ Bronze-colored skin and weight loss
12. ___ Moon face and buffalo hump
13. ___ Hypertension
14. ___ Hypothyroidism

1. Cushing's disease
2. Addison's disease
3. Primary aldosteronism
4. Cretinism
5. Myxedema

End of Case

15. When administering the following medications, the nurse knows that which one of the following combinations is classified as a peripheral vasodilator?

1. Captopril (Capoten) and enalapril (Vasotec).
2. Metoprolol (Lopressor) and acebutolol (Sectral).
3. Atenolol (Tenormin) and diazoxide (Hyperstat).
4. Hydralazine (Apresoline) and nitroprusside (Nipride).

16. A male patient with glaucoma asks the nurse which of the drugs he is taking decreases the production of aqueous humor and which one increases the aqueous humor outflow. The nurse is correct when she tells him that

1. Acetazolamide (Diamox) decreases aqueous humor production and pilocarpine (Pilocar) increases aqueous humor outflow.
2. Epinephrine decreases aqueous humor production and carteolol (Cartrol) increases aqueous humor outflow.
3. Dipivefrin (Propine) increases humor aqueous humor outflow and pilocarpine (Pilocar) decreases aqueous humor production.
4. Physostigmine (Antilirium) decreases aqueous humor production and metoprolol increases aqueous humor outflow.

17. The nurse describes closed-angle glaucoma correctly to a female patient when she tells the patient that there is an

1. Increased flow of aqueous humor, causing increased intraocular pressure (IOP).
2. Abnormal decrease in IOP caused by vasoconstriction.
3. Obstruction of vitreous humor causing IOP.
4. Abnormal increase in IOP caused by obstruction of aqueous humor outflow.

18. A female patient is admitted to the hospital with pronounced weakness of the left facial muscles and difficulty swallowing. Physical examination reveals a small, pale patient with ptosis of the left eyelid. She is diagnosed as having myasthenia gravis. The nurse will assess a client with myasthenia gravis for which of the following symptoms?

1. Weight loss and smooth muscle weakness.
2. Skeletal muscle weakness and ptosis.
3. Tingling sensation in the fingers and weak trembling.
4. Irritability, anxiety, and hoarseness.

19. ALL of the following statements are true about myasthenia gravis *except*

1. A thymectomy will not produce remissions in myasthenia gravis.
2. Myasthenia gravis may cause respiratory failure.
3. Some families may be predisposed to myasthenia gravis.
4. Generally, myasthenia gravis follows a chronic and progressive course, with occasional spontaneous remissions.

20. A nurse advises a 50-year-old female patient with a diagnosis of chronic open-angle glaucoma to have her eyes checked annually. The nurse explains to the client that the signs, symptoms, and damage that occurs with chronic open-angle glaucoma are
    1. Asymptomatic with insidious onset caused by overproduction of aqueous humor or from obstruction of aqueous humor outflow; it progressively destroys peripheral vision.
    2. Symptomatic with severe ocular pain, headache, and "halo vision" caused by IOP.
    3. Asymptomatic with intraocular tension, severe enough to cause nausea and vomiting.
    4. Rapid onset with an increase in the production of aqueous humor, which progressively destroys the retina.

21. A female patient is under a lot of stress related to unemployment and a recent divorce. She asks the nurse, "What effect will this have on my health?" The nurse answers correctly when she states she may develop hypertension and tachycardia due to an increase in
    1. Cortisol, epinephrine, glucagon, and growth hormone (GH).
    2. Thyroid-stimulating hormone (TSH), sodium, and GH.
    3. Potassium, glucagon, calcium, and epinephrine.
    4. Glucagon, insulin, and epinephrine.

22. While preparing a male patient for surgery, the patient says to the nurse, "I think I'm going to die." What is the MOST appropriate nursing response?
    1. Don't worry, you have a good doctor.
    2. This procedure is not as difficult as you think.
    3. Whatever gave you that idea?
    4. You think you're going to die?

23. The intravenous pyelogram (IVP) reveals that a female patient has a renal calculus. To increase the chance of passing the stone, the nurse should
    1. Teach her to strain all urine, and keep all stones for the physician to examine.
    2. Have her ambulate and increase fluid intake.
    3. Keep her on bedrest until the stones have passed.
    4. Give medication to relax her, which will help her pass the stones.

24. A male patient diagnosed with a brain tumor asks the nurse why his hand shakes when he reaches for an object. The nurse is correct when she tells him intentional tremors usually are associated with a tumor located on the
    1. Cerebrum.
    2. Frontal lobe.
    3. Hypothalamus.
    4. Cerebellum.

25. The MOST common highly malignant, rapidly growing brain tumor that occurs twice as often in adult males than in females is
    1. An oligodendroglioma.
    2. A medulloblastoma.
    3. An astrocytoma.
    4. A glioblastoma multiforme.

26. Before giving chlorpromazine (Thorazine), the nurse should first check the patient's
    1. Pulse and temperature.
    2. Apical pulse.
    3. Pupillary reflexes.
    4. Blood pressure.

27. The nurse explains to a patient with chronic alcoholism that he is being started on a regimen of disulfiram (Antabuse) to
    1. Decrease his depression so that he can decrease his consumption of alcohol.
    2. Deter the consumption of alcohol by producing nausea when he drinks alcoholic beverages.
    3. Create a feeling of well-being and thus eliminate the need for alcohol.
    4. Create a nerve block so that the effects of alcohol are not felt.

28. Before administering medication, the nurse explains to the patient that adverse effects such as jaundice, photosensitivity, and parkinsonism may occur in patients receiving
    1. Diazepam (Valium).
    2. Amitriptyline (Elavil).
    3. Meprobamate (Miltown).
    4. Chlorpromazine (Thorazine).

29. The nurse explains to a patient with a brain tumor that chemotherapy given systemically for intracranial cancer is of limited use because
    1. Chemotherapeutic drugs are inactive against brain tumors; these tumors are sealed off in capsules.
    2. Many of the commonly used agents cannot pass the blood–brain barrier in sufficient quantities to be effective.
    3. Chemotherapeutic drugs tend to destroy surrounding tissues; destruction of brain tissue leads to retardation.
    4. Chemotherapeutic drugs tend to increase intracranial pressure (ICP).

30. According to a blood test, an 82-year-old woman has an elevated blood glucose level, but her urine specimen is negative when tested for the presence of glucose. She is taking an oral hypoglycemic agent. When evaluating the phenomenon of hyperglycemia without glucosuria, the nurse should consider

1. The client's need for glucose most probably has increased with advanced age.
2. The client's renal threshold for glucose most probably has risen with advanced age.
3. The client's exercising program most probably has become too strenuous because of her advanced age.
4. The client's response to the stress of her surgery most probably has been excessive because of her advanced age.

31. A female patient's oral hypoglycemic agent is discontinued and isophane insulin suspension (NPH insulin) is prescribed. She takes the insulin daily at 8:00 AM. The nurse tells the patient that the time of the day she is MOST likely to experience hypoglycemia is
    1. 11:00 AM, shortly before lunch.
    2. 2:00 PM, shortly after lunch.
    3. 6:00 PM, shortly before dinner.
    4. 11:00 PM, shortly before bedtime.

32. The nurse caring for patients with many different disorders must know that a phenothiazine is most often given to a client with
    1. Severe agitation and confusion due to psychosis.
    2. Extrapyramidal signs due to Parkinson's disease.
    3. Psychomotor retardation due to extrapyramidal signs.
    4. Tendencies toward addiction due to genetic tendency.

33. The nurse knows that all of the following are side effects of antipsychotic medication *except*
    1. Anticholinergic effects.
    2. Sedation.
    3. Agranulocytosis.
    4. Hypertension.

34. A patient is accidentally given an overdose of heparin. The nurse anticipated the physician ordering an antidote for heparin, which is
    1. Insulin zinc suspension (Lente/Iletin).
    2. Vitamin K.
    3. Protamine sulfate.
    4. Protamine zinc.

35. Foods that should not be eaten when a patient is taking monoamine oxidase (MAO) inhibitors are
    1. Cabbage, spinach, liver, bacon, milk, coffee, tea, cola, and cheese.
    2. Beer, wheat products, yeast, green beans, liver, and milk products.
    3. Hamburger, bacon, wheat products, yeast, and canned meats.
    4. Wine, yeast products, chocolate, bologna, pepperoni, and cream cheese.

36. The nurse caring for a patient with a head injury will assess for signs and symptoms of increased ICP, which include
    1. Distended neck veins, pruritus, paresthesia, and nausea and vomiting.
    2. Widening pulse pressure, headache, and change in level of consciousness.
    3. Decreased respirations, bradycardia, malaise, fever, and vomiting.
    4. Narrow pulse pressure, headache, fever, tachycardia, and vomiting.

37. A patient who becomes forgetful, is unable to concentrate, has a short attention span, and has increased irritability before each hemodialysis treatment shows signs of
    1. Fear of treatment.
    2. Fear of dying.
    3. Accumulation of end-products of metabolism.
    4. Fluid volume overload.

38. Following regional perfusion of a neoplasm with mechlorethamine (nitrogen mustard), a patient's blood studies show evidence of bone marrow depression. The interpretation and action that are indicated are that this finding is
    1. Indicative of a serious adverse reaction; preparations should be made for a transfusion of whole blood.
    2. A common development; no action is indicated.
    3. An expected response; the client should be protected from infection.
    4. Most likely an allergic response; desensitization procedures should be started.

39. When administering antineoplastic drugs for the treatment of isolated neoplasms, regional perfusion is the preferred method because
    1. It is easier to administer and to control drug dosage.
    2. Higher dosage can be given to a specific area, with a lower systemic toxicity.
    3. There are fewer and less serious administration problems.
    4. It is cost efficient, and medication can be administered with a peripheral IV.

40. A male patient is hospitalized with diabetes mellitus. The nurse is reviewing a diabetic diet with the client. Which of the following statements concerning the diabetic diet is MOST accurate?
    1. Dietetic foods (e.g., nonfat cookies) may be eaten as free foods.
    2. A regular meal pattern need not be followed because the patient is not taking insulin.
    3. Complex carbohydrates, such as whole grain bread and cereal, should be included in the diet.
    4. Research indicates that fats should be eliminated from a diabetic person's diet.

41. When administering furosemide, cortisol, and calcium, the nurse should keep in mind that these drugs will cause
    1. Hypertension.
    2. Stomatitis.
    3. Potassium depletion.
    4. Hypoglycemia.

42. Diagnosis of venereal disease must be reported to the local health department. The MAIN purpose for this is
    1. Adequate treatment of those with a venereal disease necessitates that the sexual partner be treated as well.
    2. The sexual contacts of those infected may need treatment.
    3. To decrease the incidence of venereal disease.
    4. Such reporting usually causes those with venereal disease to limit the number of sexual contacts.

43. Which of the following statements made by the nurse to a 60-year-old patient BEST describes acute closed-angle glaucoma? It usually
    1. Has rapid onset with pressure pain over the eye, blurring, and decreased visual acuity.
    2. Is asymptomatic with insidious onset and is bilateral.
    3. Has insidious onset with blurred vision and headaches.
    4. Is asymptomatic and caused by overproduction of aqueous humor.

44. Which one of the following accounts for 50 percent of cases of thyroid cancers in adults and usually is associated with a prolonged survival rate?
    1. Follicular.
    2. Papillary.
    3. Wilms' tumor.
    4. Medullary.

45. Which one of the following disorders is characterized as a rare, inherited, degenerative, generalized disease of connective tissue, characterized by long bones and fingers that are very long and slender?
    1. Tay-Sachs disease.
    2. Amyotrophic lateral sclerosis (ALS).
    3. Marfan's syndrome.
    4. Galactosemia.

46. Parents of a child with acute lymphocytic leukemia (ALL) ask the nurse about the progression of this disease. The BEST response would be
    1. It is a fatal disease, but medications provide long periods when the child is free from symptoms.
    2. With treatment, most children go into remission quickly and may remain symptom-free for a year or 5 years; there is no way of knowing how long.
    3. There is no way to predict how an individual will respond to treatment; we'll just have to hope and pray all will be OK.

4. Children generally have short periods (3–4 days) of feeling well and then a return of symptoms, and this cycle keeps repeating until the disease is cured.

47. People with acquired immunodeficiency syndrome (AIDS) have a decreased T-cell count and are susceptible to opportunistic infections. Which of the following will be MOST life threatening?
    1. Actinomycosis, meningococcal infection, and *Haemophilus influenzae*.
    2. *Pneumocystis carinii* pneumonia, Kaposi's sarcoma, toxoplasmosis, and TB.
    3. Aspergillosis, blastomycosis, and histoplasmosis.
    4. Spirochetosis, coccidioidomycosis, and respiratory syncytial viral infection.

48. A patient asks the nurse, "What did my doctor mean when he said an autotransfusion would be done during my surgery?" Which of the following statements by the nurse is MOST accurate?
    1. A collection and reinfusion of a patient's own blood or blood components.
    2. Freezing of a patient's own blood for future use by the patient.
    3. Transfusion to the patient of his or her own blood type.
    4. Transfusion to the patient of a family member's blood type.

49. The nurse would anticipate that a patient in stage III of breast cancer would receive which of the following combinations of chemotherapeutic drugs?
    1. Mechlorethamine (Mustargen), vincristine (Oncovin), prednisone (Deltasone), and doxorubicin (Adriamycin).
    2. Cyclophosphamide (Cytoxan) and fluorouracil (5-FU) with methotrexate (Methotrexate LPF) or doxorubicin (Adriamycin).
    3. Cyclophosphamide (Cytoxan), azathioprine (Imuran), and radiation.
    4. Interferon-alpha, vincristine (Oncovin), and prednisone (Deltasone).

50. Which one of the following adverse effects is associated with use of doxorubicin as a chemotherapeutic agent?
    1. Cirrhosis of the liver.
    2. Meningitis.
    3. Hypertension.
    4. Cardiomyopathy.

51. Which of the following are considered aplastic anemias?
    1. Sickle cell anemia and folic acid anemia.
    2. Iron deficiency anemia and pernicious anemia.
    3. Sickle cell anemia and hemolytic anemia.
    4. Thrombocytopenia and leukopenia.

52. A 3-year-old female patient is admitted to the hospital for rheumatic fever. This connective tissue disease will affect the

1. Joints, mitral valve, and myocardium.
2. Liver, gallbladder, and kidneys.
3. Joints, liver, and neurologic system.
4. Pancreas, lungs, and heart.

53. A female patient, aged 40 years, is admitted to the hospital with petechiae, ecchymosis, and bleeding from the oral mucous membranes and gastrointestinal (GI) tract; her platelet count is very low. These are signs and symptoms of

1. Pernicious anemia.
2. Disseminated intravascular coagulation (DIC).
3. Thrombocytopenic purpura.
4. Sickle cell anemia.

54. A male patient has been taking INH (isoniazid) for treatment of TB for the previous 18 months. He recently developed peripheral neuropathy and a slight fever. The nurse's evaluation of the situation is that the patient

1. Is developing hepatitis from INH (isoniazid) toxicity.
2. Has been taking INH (isoniazid) for too many months and dosage should be reduced.
3. Is having an adverse reaction to INH (isoniazid) and his physician will add vitamin B_6 to his medication regimen.
4. Is demonstrating late signs of drug hypersensitivity to INH (isoniazid).

55. The nurse anticipates the therapeutic regiment for thyroid cancer will include

1. Doxorubicin (Adriamycin) and cisplatin (Platinol).
2. Radiation (iodine-131) and external radiation.
3. Fluorouracil (5-FU) and vincristine (Oncovin).
4. Levothyroxine (Synthroid) and phenobarbital (Barbita).

56. When caring for a patient with *P. carinii* pneumonia and toxoplasmosis, the nurse will anticipate the doctor ordering which of the following medications?

1. Pentamidine, Bactrim, and Septra.
2. Methotrexate, doxorubicin, and vincristine.
3. Septra, acyclovir, and nystatin.
4. Meperidine, dextran, and mannitol.

57. It is very important for a male patient who has TB to understand and comply with the need to be on INH (isoniazid) and Rifadin (rifampin) for 1 year, years, or possibly longer. The nursing measure that would be most helpful in obtaining the patient's compliance with his plan of treatment is to

1. Involve the patient in teaching sessions.
2. Teach the patient about his prescribed medications.
3. Ask the social worker to talk with the patient.
4. Refer the patient to the American Lung Association.

58. The nurse caring for a neonate born to an alcoholic mother would assess for which of the following signs and symptoms?

1. Rigid extremities, elevated temperature, tremors, and extreme lethargy.
2. Diarrhea, decreased Moro reflex, vomiting, elevated temperature, seldom cries, and tremors.
3. Rigid extremities, tremors, vomiting, diarrhea, extreme sleepiness, and tremors.
4. Poor sucking reflex, convulsions, irritability, tremors, apnea, and sweating.

59. The nurse caring for a neonate born to a mother addicted to drugs would assess the neonate for which of the following signs and symptoms?

1. Lethargy, sleeping for most of the time, poor sucking reflex, and infrequent cries.
2. Disturbed sleep, convulsions, tremors, lethargy and sleepiness, and poor sucking reflex.
3. Convulsions, tremor, sleeping most of the time, and poor sucking reflex.
4. Respiratory distress, sleeping for short intervals, diarrhea, high-pitched cry, poor sucking reflex, and bulging fontanelle at rest.

60. Mary, an 18-month-old girl, is admitted to the pediatric unit with Kawasaki disease. Mary's mother asks the nurses, "What is Kawasaki disease?" and "Is it serious?" The nurses' MOST correct response is

1. It is an acute disease of unknown origin that produces inflammation of the coronary arteries, and it can damage the heart muscle.
2. It is an acute disease that causes inflammation of the lymph nodes and kidney. If this disease is not treated, the child will have to receive hemodialysis to remove the waste products that the kidney can no longer remove.
3. It is an acute disease that causes inflammation of the central nervous system (CNS) and especially affects the upper body.
4. It is a rare acute disease of unknown cause that usually is self-limiting, with no known treatment.

61. The nurse explains to the mother of a child with Kawasaki disease that the child will be treated with which of the following drugs?

1. High dosage of intravenous (IV) gamma-globulin in conjunction with salicylate therapy.
2. High dosages of antibiotics in conjunction with salicylate therapy.
3. IV antibiotics and steroids in conjunction with salicylate therapy.
4. No known treatment is available.

62. A female client admitted to the hospital with Cushing's disease asks the nurse what caused the disease.

Which of the following statements would be MOST accurate?

1. Excessive secretion of adrenocorticotropic hormone (ACTH) causing the adrenal cortex to oversecrete glucocorticoid and mineralocorticoids.
2. Excessive secretion of ACTH causing adrenal cortex to oversecrete aldosterone.
3. Decreased secretion of ACTH causing the adrenal medulla to decrease the production of catecholamines.
4. Decreased secretion of antidiuretic hormone causing an increase in urinary output, which decreases the potassium level.

63. Which of the following results from Cushing's disease?

1. Postural hypotension, decreased tolerance for stress, and a weak irregular pulse.
2. Psychosis, diabetes mellitus, osteoporosis, and hypertension.
3. Polyuria, extreme fatigue, and postural hypotension.
4. Excessive thirst, polyuria, and diabetes mellitus.

64. A patient with Addison's disease asks the nurse to discuss with him the characteristics of the disease. Which of the following statements by the nurse is MOST accurate? "Addison's disease is characterized by

1. Decreased mineralocorticoid, glucocorticoid, and androgen secretion."
2. Increased mineralocorticoid, glucocorticoid, and androgen secretion."
3. An increase in synthetic ACTH causing the adrenal gland to stop secreting catecholamines."
4. Excessive administration of cortisol, causing destruction of the adrenal gland."

65. The nurse knows that the patient understands the signs and symptoms of Addison's disease when he states

1. Hyperglycemia, muscle weakness, bone demineralization, purple-like striae, and glucosuria.
2. Bronze coloration of the skin, postural hypotension, decreased tolerance to minor stress, poor coordination, hypoglycemia, and a craving for salt.
3. Hypertension, increased susceptibility to infection, decreased resistance to stress, and muscle weakness.
4. Decreased glucose tolerance, hyperglycemia, hypokalemia, and muscle weakness.

66. Agnes Miller stops treatment with Premarin PO because of hypertension. She is unable to tolerate estrogen patches because of skin irritation. The physician then places her on

1. Yutopar (IM).
2. Xanax (PO).
3. Theelin Aqueous (IM).
4. Prostigmin.

67. When comparing midazolam hydrochloride (Versed) to diazepam (Valium) for use as a preoperative sedative. Versed

1. Has a longer sedative effect and fewer side effects than Valium.
2. Can be combined with most other preoperative agents. Versed decreases mental recall.
3. Cannot be combined with preoperative medications but has fewer side effects and will not decrease mental recall.
4. Has fewer side effects and longer sedative effects.

68. Which of the following are nonsteroidal antiinflammatory drugs (NSAIDs)?

1. Butazolidin, aspirin, Advil, Motrin, Indocin, Nuprin, and Dolobid.
2. Aspirin, testolactone, Nuprin, Advil, danazol (Cyclomen), and fluoxymesterone.
3. Nuprin, codeine, pentazocine, aspirin, and Android-5.

69. The nurse tells the patient that sources of vitamin D include

1. Hamburger, veal, tuna, and fortified foods.
2. Cheese, peanut butter, and fortified foods.
3. Liver, fish, eggs, and fortified foods.
4. Fortified foods, whole wheat bread, potatoes, and baked beans.

70. The nurse would use which of the following gauge needles to administer blood?

1. 18 gauge.
2. 20 gauge.
3. 22 gauge.
4. 25 gauge.

71. A patient wants to know what medication is being given to her by the nurse. The most appropriate response by the nurse would be

1. This is the medicine the doctor ordered.
2. You will have to ask your doctor the next time she comes in.
3. This is the antibiotic the doctor told you she was going to order for you.
4. It is Keflex, an antibiotic to help fight the infection in your lungs.

72. The nurse knows that the most essential part of pain assessment is

1. Checking all vital signs.
2. Consulting the physician.
3. Doing a complete physical examination.
4. Interviewing the client.

73. The nurse tells the patient on a low-sodium diet that which one of the following foods is lowest in natural sodium?
    1. Meat.
    2. Milk.
    3. Canned vegetables.
    4. Fresh fruit.

74. A patient tells the nurse, "My doctor said I didn't have to take this anymore." The nurse's BEST initial action would be to
    1. Recheck the medication sheet.
    2. Check the physician's orders.
    3. Call the physician.
    4. Assure the patient that the medication is correct.

75. A patient is involved in a serious automobile accident and is at risk for suffering serious complications. The assessment characteristic of a fat embolus after a long-bone fracture is
    1. Severe stabbing chest pain 12 days post fracture, tachycardia, and hypertension.
    2. Frothy sputum, tachycardia, tachypnea, cyanosis, fever, and a petechial rash.
    3. Pulmonary edema, seizures, circulatory overload, and coarse crackles.
    4. Respiratory depression, cardiac arrhythmias, and neuromuscular irritability.

76. The nurse advises the patient that calcium decreases the absorption in the GI tract when combined with
    1. Tetracycline.
    2. Thiamin.
    3. Ranitidine.
    4. Penicillin G.

77. An 80-year-old patient with hepatitis B wants to know why his physician will only give him a small amount of pain medication. The nurse would explain that the body system mainly responsible for the metabolism of drugs is injured. The nurse is referring to the
    1. Kidneys.
    2. Liver.
    3. Cardiovascular.
    4. Lymph.

78. Bill Robb is on IV procainamide (Pronestyl). As soon as severe arrhythmias are under control, his physician changes the medication to PO Pronestyl 600 mg every 4 h. The nurse advises the patient that reactions to this drug are
    1. Hypertension, increased serum creatinine level, or dyspnea.
    2. Confusion, hypotension, ventricular arrhythmias, or heart block.
    3. Fainting, drowsiness, and nervousness.
    4. Hallucinations, blurred vision, or mydriasis.

79. The nurse needs to be aware that which of the following will increase urinary excretion of magnesium?
    1. Haldol and cabbage.
    2. Keflex and alcohol.
    3. Iodine and diarrhea.
    4. Lasix and alcohol.

80. The signs and early symptoms of retinal detachment are
    1. Floating spots in field of vision, recurrent flashes of light, and a curtain falling over the visual field.
    2. Painful, unilateral loss of vision (partial or complete) with pupils dilating, and flashes of light.
    3. Gradual blurring, pupil turning milky white, and pain.
    4. Recurrent painless peripheral vision loss, and bright flashing light in field of vision.

81. A nurse instructing a patient consuming foods high in vitamin C would list which of the following?
    1. Broccoli, potatoes, cabbage, tomatoes, and citrus fruit.
    2. Breakfast cereals, salmon, tuna fish, and fortified milk.
    3. Cheese, meat, eggs, cabbage, and fruits.
    4. Green beans, Brussels sprouts, strawberries, and citrus fruit.

82. A female patient with glaucoma asks the nurse to give her the name of her eye medications and to explain how they help her glaucoma. The nurse's MOST correct reply is
    1. Epinephrine (Epinephrine) and physostigmine salicylate (Antilirium) decrease IOP by increasing the outflow of aqueous humor.
    2. Betaxolol (Betoptic) and metoprolol tartrate (Lopressor) increasing aqueous outflow.
    3. Acetazolamide (Diamox) and betaxolol (Betoptic) of aqueous humor and thereby reduce IOP.
    4. Epinephrine (Epinephrine) and physostigmine (Eserine) are used to constrict the pupil and contract ciliary musculature. This reduces IOP by increasing aqueous humor outflow.

83. Which one of the following drugs slows conduction of impulses through the atrioventricular (AV) node?
    1. Digitalis.
    2. Nitroglycerin.
    3. Quinidine.
    4. Lidocaine.

84. A patient's medication order is to take digoxin 0.125 mg PO qd. The nurse has on hand Lanoxin 0.25-mg tablet. The best course of action is to
    1. Dispense 1½ tablets.
    2. Dispense ½ tablet.
    3. Dispense 2 tablets.
    4. Return the medication to the pharmacy.

85. A client develops severe bradycardia; the nurse anticipates the physician ordering
    1. Atropine.
    2. Morphine.
    3. Lidocaine.
    4. Isoproterenol.

86. The nurse should advise a male patient to have sex counseling because of the side effects caused by
    1. Guanethidine monosulfate (Ismelin) and reserpine (Serpasil).
    2. Captopril (Capoten) and metaraminol (Aramine).
    3. Hydralazine hydrochloride (Apresoline) and vincristine (Oncovin).
    4. Codeine and hydromorphone hydrochloride (Dilaudid).

87. A patient's laboratory study showed an erythrocyte count of 3,200,000/mm^3. The nurse would anticipate that the patient had which of the following disorders?
    1. Pernicious anemia.
    2. Cirrhosis of the liver.
    3. Sickle cell anemia.
    4. DIC.

88. When giving Nipride by IV infusion to patients with hypertensive emergencies, the nurse should be aware that Nipride is given to reduce
    1. Afterload and preload.
    2. Heart rate.
    3. Contractility of the heart.
    4. Pulmonary edema.

89. The MOST important assessment of a patient receiving streptomycin is to evaluate
    1. Cardiac rate prior to and throughout the course of therapy.
    2. Eye coordination prior to and throughout the course of therapy.
    3. Facial spasms and pain throughout the course of therapy.
    4. Nerve function of CN VIII by audiometry prior to and throughout the course of therapy.

90. A patient develops cardiogenic shock. The nurse would anticipate administering which of the following drugs?
    1. Sodium bicarbonate, epinephrine, and atropine.
    2. Epinephrine, sodium bicarbonate, and Lasix.
    3. Dobutamine, dopamine, and epinephrine.
    4. Atropine, metaraminol (Aramine), and digoxin.

91. The physician orders a stool sample from a patient to be checked for amoeba. The nurse knows that the correct procedure for obtaining a stool specimen for examination for amoeba is to

1. Deliver the specimen immediately to the laboratory while it is warm and fresh.
2. Mix the specimen with chlorinated lime solution before taking it to the laboratory.
3. Store the specimen in the refrigerator until time for delivery to the laboratory.
4. Store the specimen at room temperature or in warm water until it is picked up by a laboratory technician.

92. When preparing a patient for an autotransfusion, the nurse knows that contraindications to the use of autotransfusion blood products include
    1. Bowel obstruction or gastroenteritis.
    2. Electrical burns or electrical shock.
    3. Radiation exposure or multiple trauma.
    4. Malignant neoplasms, pulmonary or respiratory infections.

93. During the nurse's hourly intake and output (I&O) rounds, the nurse notes that Mr. Robert's total parenteral nutrition (TPN) is not infusing, and 200 mL remains in the bag. The nurse's BEST initial action would be to
    1. Check the tubing for kinks, twists, or clots.
    2. Hang a new bottle of TPN.
    3. Assess the stability of the client's vital signs.
    4. Irrigate the line to establish patency.

94. Mr. Meyer asks why he is receiving Tagamet at 8:00 AM and an antacid at 10:00 AM. The nurse's explanation should include the information that
    1. Tagamet is a hydrogen adrenergic that is activated by an antacid; the drugs must be given at different times.
    2. The antacid minimizes the side effects of Tagamet if given 2 h after Tagamet.
    3. The antacid increases the pH of gastric contents, and Tagamet absorbs the gastric acid; therefore, they are given at different times.
    4. Antacids and Tagamet should be taken at different times because the antacid may absorb the Tagamet.

95. When talking with the nurse about her health problem, Mrs. Little says that she has been taking Zantac to relieve gastric discomfort. The nurse should explain to her that Zantac
    1. Neutralizes HCl acids so it is readily absorbed from the GI tract.
    2. Provides a coating for a peptic ulcer and decreases epigastric pain.
    3. Absorbs gastric juice and relieves GI distention.
    4. Slows the production of HCl acid in the stomach and duodenum.

96. The nurse would anticipate using which of the following drugs in the management of hepatic encephalopathy (it is also used for chronic constipation of the elderly)?

1. Lactulose (Cephulac).

2. Docusate sodium (Correctol Extra Gentle).

3. Docusate calcium (Surfak).

4. Docusate sodium (Colace).

97. The nurse would anticipate which one of the following drugs for the treatment of abdominal distention and diabetes insipidus?

1. Mannitol.

2. Mandol.

3. Pitressin.

4. Allopurinol.

98. A patient in the cardiac care unit is having premature ventricular contractions (PVCs). Which of the following drugs would the nurse administer?

1. Digoxin (Lanoxin) and propranolol (Inderal).

2. Quinidine gluconate (Duraquin), procainamide (Pronestyl), and lidocaine (Xylocaine).

3. Isoproterenol hydrochloride (Isuprel hydrochloride), dopamine (Intropin), and diltiazem (Cardizem).

4. Metaraminol (Aramine) and nifedipine (Procardia).

99. A 4-week-old infant has cold feet, dyspnea, and a lower blood pressure in legs than in arms and delayed pulse in legs. The nurse would suspect

1. Atrial septal defect.

2. Patent ductus arteriosus.

3. Coarctation of aorta.

4. Tetralogy of Fallot.

100. The nurse assesses a patient closely when he or she is taking Lanoxin and has which of the following conditions?

1. Hyponatremia.

2. Hypercalcemia.

3. Hypokalemia.

4. Hyperkalemia.

ANSWERS AND RATIONALES

1. **①** Hyperparathyroidism is characterized by increased bone resorption, elevated serum calcium levels, and depressed serum phosphate levels, which will increase renal and GI absorption of calcium. Signs and symptoms of primary hyperparathyroidism result from hypercalcemia, which usually is present in several body systems, and include the following:

◆ Renal nephrocalcinosis (deposits of calcium in renal tubules) is due to elevated levels of calcium.

◆ Skeletal effects are low back pain and easy fracturing due to bone degeneration.

◆ GI effects include pancreatitis, causing constant severe gastric pain radiating to the back, and peptic ulcers.

◆ A neuromuscular effect is muscle weakness.

◆ CNS effects include psychomotor and personality disturbance, depression, and overt psychosis.
(2, 3, 4) These options are incorrect as seen in rationale (1).

2. **③** Addison's disease (adrenal insufficiency) is characterized by decreased production of mineralocorticoids, glucocorticoids, and androgens. The disturbance in the production of mineralocorticoids from the adrenal cortex is significant because the primary mineralocorticoid is aldosterone. Aldosterone retains sodium and sodium retains water. If insufficient aldosterone is secreted, the patient may experience hypotension because of low fluid volume. The patient will also have a high potassium level; when sodium is lost, potassium is retained. Signs and symptoms of Addison's disease typically include hypotension, weakness, fatigue, weight loss, and GI disturbances such as nausea and vomiting, anorexia, and chronic diarrhea.

Treatment is replacement of corticosteroids, usually with cortisone or hydrocortisone, which have a mineralocorticoid effect. The patient may also be treated with fludrocortisone acetate (Florinef Acetate) PO, a synthetic drug that acts as a mineralocorticoid and prevents dehydration and hypotension.

1. The primary glucocorticoid is cortisol, a steroid produced by the adrenal cortex. Cortisol suppresses the normal immune response and inflammation. Cortisol also increases blood glucose through increased gluconeogenesis. Decreased production of cortisol causes the pituitary gland to secrete excessive amounts of ACTH and melanocyte-stimulating hormone (MSH), a skin pigmentation hormone.

Excessive MSH causes darkening of scars and absence of pigmentation in some areas of the skin and increased pigmentation in other areas. Excessive amounts of MSH in a patient with Addison's disease will cause a bronze coloration of the skin.

2, 4. The adrenal cortex secretes both male (androgens) and female (estrogens and progesterone) sex hormones. The adrenal sex hormones are relatively insignificant compared with those produced by the testes and ovaries.

3. **②** A patient with Addison's disease should be monitored closely for signs of infectious complications because of dysfunction in the antiinflammatory process. The patient must be treated with steroids because the normal immune and inflammation responses are decreased, which puts the patient at risk for infection.
(1, 3, 4) These options are incorrect as seen in rationale (2).

4. **①** When a client does not have normal amounts of androgens, protein will break down. Androgen has a protein anabolic (building-up) effect; for example, athletes take androgen to increase muscle mass.

Cortisol promotes the process of gluconeogenesis. Consequently, when glucocorticoid production (e.g., cortisol) results in deficiency, gluconeogenesis decreases, resulting in hypoglycemia and liver glycogen deficiency. Signs and symptoms include weakness and exhaustion, anorexia, weight loss, and nausea and vomiting.
(2, 3, 4) These options are incorrect as seen in rationale (1).

5. ❸ Cyclosporine (Sandimmune) and azathioprine (Imuran) are immunosuppressant drugs used to prevent rejection in renal, cardiac, and hepatic transplants.

1. Cromolyn (Intal), is antasthmatic (prophylactic). It inhibits the allergen-triggered release of histamine and is used in prophylaxis of allergic disorders, including rhinitis, conjunctivitis, and asthma. Cortisol (Cortef) is an antiinflammatory.

2. Diazepam (Valium), a sedative hypnotic, is used in the management of anxiety and as a preoperative sedative. An NSAID (e.g., indomethacin [Indocin]) is used in the management of rheumatoid arthritis, osteoarthritis, and acute gouty arthritis.

4. Liothyronine (Cytomel), a thyroid preparation hormone, is used to replace diminished or absent thyroid function. Methotrexate (Folex), an antineoplastic immunosuppressant, is used for the treatment of cancer.

6. ❶ Signs and symptoms of TB are persistent cough, weight loss, anorexia, night sweats, and fever. Many of these signs and symptoms also occur in a person infected with the AIDS virus. Incidence of TB is increasing because of AIDS (human immunodeficiency virus [HIV]). When the immune system is weakened, susceptibility to opportunistic diseases (including TB) increases. Another cause of the worldwide increase in TB is the increase in numbers of people living in overcrowded conditions because of poverty and war.

(2, 3, 4) These options are incorrect as seen in rationale (1).

7. ❸ Diagnostic tests for TB include Mantoux test, chest x-ray film, and sputum analysis.

The skin Mantoux test is the most common diagnostic test, often administered and read by nurses. Proper technique in administering the test is very important. The Mantoux test is administered using purified protein derivative (PPD), available in three strengths (two of which are 1 tuberculin unit (TU) and 5 TU). The weakest, 1 TU, is used only for people with previous reactive skin tests. The 5 TU preparation is the standard strength used for intradermal (Mantoux) screening for TB.

The nurse marks the area on the arm where the Mantoux injection is given so that the skin can be observed for a reaction. If the skin reacts, the person has been infected with TB, and further assessment is needed (chest x-ray film, sputum analysis for acid-fast bacteria [AFB]). DNA verification is now available.

(1, 2, 4) These options are incorrect as seen in rationale (3).

8. ❹ Agents used to treat TB include isoniazid (INH), rifampin (Rifadin), ethambutol (Myambutol), and streptomycin. As a result of the long-term nature of drug therapy, patients may need support in maintaining the therapeutic regimen and managing the side effects of drugs used to treat TB.

If peripheral neuritis (a side effect of the antitubercular drugs) occurs, it is important to teach patients precautionary strategies to avoid injury until an alteration in sensory sensation is remedied.

1. Allopurinol (Zyloprim) is an antigout agent. Aminophylline (Amoline) is a bronchodilator.

Amyl nitrate (Amyl Nitrite Aspirols) is an antianginal agent and an antidote for cyanide poisoning.

2. Guanethidine (Ismelin), an antihypertensive, is a peripherally acting antiadrenergic agent.

Interferon (Intron A) is an antineoplastic and a immunomodulatory agent. It is used for the treatment of hairy cell leukemia, AIDS-associated Kaposi's sarcoma, and chronic hepatitis B.

Meclizine (Antivert), an antiemetic and an antihistaminic agent, is one of the agents used for the treatment of Ménière's disease. Isosorbide dinitrate (Isordil), a coronary vasodilator, is used for the treatment of acute anginal attacks, long-term prophylactic management of angina pectoris, and treatment of congestive heart failure (CHF).

3. Ibuprofen (Motrin), an NSAID, is used in the management of inflammatory disorders.

Immune serum globulin (gamma-globulin) provides passive immunity to infections such as measles (rubeola) and hepatitis A and hepatitis B.

Gamma-globulin is used when there is insufficient time for active immunization to take place. For example, gamma-globulin is given to the nurse when she has cared for a client with hepatitis and was not aware that the client had the disease.

Indomethacin (Indocin), an NSAID, is used to treat inflammation.

9. ❷ TB is transmitted by air current (coughing or sneezing) or by unpasteurized milk.

(1, 3, 4) These options are incorrect as seen in rationale (2).

10. ❶ Nipride, an antihypertensive vasodilator, must be protected from light. This agent may cause cyanide poisoning with symptoms such as blurred vision, dyspnea, dizziness, headache, syncope, and metabolic acidosis.

Treatment for Nipride toxicity is inhalation of amyl nitrate and infusion of sodium nitrate.

(2, 3, 4) These drugs do not have to be protected from light.

11. ❷ A patient with Addison's disease will have bronze-colored skin, weight loss, weakness, nausea and vomiting, anorexia, chronic diarrhea, hypotension, a weak and irregular pulse rate, and decreased tolerance for minor stress because of cortisol deficiency.

(1, 3, 4, 5) These options are incorrect as seen in rationale (2).

12. ❶ A patient with Cushing's disease will have a moon face and buffalo hump because of excessive production of cortisol by the adrenal cortex.

Other signs and symptoms of Cushing's disease are hyperglycemia, hypokalemia, hypernatremia, loss of muscle mass, peptic ulcer, irritability, emotional lability (ranging from euphoric behavior to depression), and increased susceptibility to infections because of high cortisol levels.

Cortisol reduces inflammation; therefore, white blood cells (WBCs) will not defend the body against infections.

(2, 3, 4, 5) These options are incorrect as seen in rationale (1).

13. ❸ Clients with primary aldosteronism will have hypertension. Aldosterone, a mineralocorticoid, regulates the reabsorption of sodium and the excretion of potassium by the kidneys. Sodium causes water retention, and excessive fluid volume causes hypertension.

(1, 2, 4, 5) These options are incorrect as seen in rationale (3).

14. ❺ Hypothyroidism is called *cretinism* in children and *myxedema* in adults. Typically, an infant with cretinism sleeps excessively, seldom cries, and is generally inactive; parents often describe the infant as a "good baby, no trouble at all." Such behavior actually results in reduced metabolic rate and progressive mental impairment.

(1, 2, 3, 4) These options are incorrect as seen in rationale (5).

15. ❹ Peripheral vasodilators are hydralazine (Apresoline) and nitroprusside (Nipride). Apresoline given in combination with a diuretic is used in the management of moderate to severe hypertension.

Nipride is used in the management of hypertensive crisis. Nipride must be covered from light during administration, and the patient must be monitored for cyanide poisoning, as discussed in answer 10, rationale 1. Nipride administered IV must be monitored every 5 to 15 min to prevent hypotension.

1. Captopril (Capoten), an antihypertensive agent, is used alone or in combination with other drugs for the treatment of CHF. Enalapril (Vasotec), an antihypertensive agent, is used in combination with other drugs for the treatment of CHF.

2. Metoprolol (Lopressor), a beta-blocker, is used alone or in combination with other agents for the treatment of hypertension and angina pectoris. An apical pulse rate should be taken before giving a beta-blocker because these agents slow conduction at the AV node. Acebutolol (Sectral), an antihypertensive agent and beta-blocker, is used for the treatment of ventricular tachyarrhythmias. Beta-blockers decrease heart rate and blood pressure and constrict bronchioles; therefore, they should not be used for the treatment of asthma.

3. Atenolol (Tenormin), a beta-blocker, is used for the treatment of hypertension and in the management of angina pectoris.

Diazoxide (Hyperstat), an antihypertensive agent and vasodilator, is used for emergency treatment of malignant hypertension. It also is used for the treatment of hypoglycemia associated with hyperinsulinism (hypoglycemic crisis).

16. ❶ Acetazolamide (Diamox) decreases the production of aqueous humor, thereby decreasing IOP; pilocarpine (Pilocar) reduces IOP by increasing aqueous humor outflow.

(2, 3, 4) These options are incorrect as seen in rationale (1) (for more information, see Unit II, Section 12).

17. ❹ Closed-angle glaucoma can best be described as an abnormal increase in IOP because aqueous humor *outflow is obstructed;* this does not occur because there is an increased production of aqueous humor. Medication is used to decrease aqueous humor production as a means of reducing IOP, and surgery must be performed.

It usually is unilateral and can progress to complete blindness without ever producing an acute attack. Those with a family history of glaucoma should have their eyes checked yearly.

(1, 2, 3) These options are incorrect as seen in rationale (4).

18. ❷ The dominant symptoms of myasthenia gravis are skeletal muscle weakness and fatigability. Myasthenia gravis causes a failure in transmission of nerve impulses at the neuromuscular junction, with ineffective acetylcholine (ACh) release at the neuromuscular junction. Onset is insidious or sudden; early signs are weak eye closure and ptosis (eyelid droop).

Treatment for myasthenia gravis is symptomatic. Anticholinesterase drugs, such as neostigmine (Prostigmin) and pyridostigmine bromide (Mestinon), counteract fatigue and muscle weakness. Anticholinesterase drugs inhibit the breakdown of ACh, which then accumulates at the myoneural junction and has a prolonged action.

When the disease involves the respiratory system, it can be life threatening.

Remember that neostigmine (Prostigmin) is also used for the treatment of postoperative bladder distention and urinary retention or ileus.

(1, 3, 4) These options are incorrect as seen in rationale (2).

19. ❶ Option (1) states that a thymectomy will not produce remissions; therefore, this option is the one that is not true about myasthenia gravis. A thymectomy can cause remission in some cases of adult-onset myasthenia gravis. The reason for this is unknown.

(2, 3, 4) These options are true; (2) myasthenia gravis may cause respiratory failure because of muscle weakness, (3) some families seem to be predisposed to myasthenia gravis, and (4) generally, myasthenia gravis follows a chronic, progressive course with occasional spontaneous remissions. Remember this is a negative question and must be read carefully.

20. ❶ Chronic open-angle glaucoma, the most common form of glaucoma, usually is asymptomatic with insidious onset, which progressively destroys peripheral vision. It is caused by overproduction of aqueous humor or obstruction of the trabecular meshwork and Schlemm's canal. It usually is bilateral and can progress insidiously to complete blindness without ever producing an acute attack.

(2, 3, 4) These options are incorrect as seen in rationale (1).

21. ❶ Physiologic or emotional stress cause prolonged elevation of cortisol, epinephrine, glucagon, and growth hormone (GH). Stress increases the production of ACTH, which stimulates the adrenal cortex to release cortisol (steroid).

Cortisol increases gluconeogenesis and thereby increases glucose and the storage of glucagon. Stress causes anxiety, which causes the adrenal medulla to release epinephrine and norepinephrine.

Epinephrine speeds the heart rate and dilates the bronchioles because of the beta-receptors in the heart and lungs. Norepinephrine vasoconstricts peripherally because of the alpha-receptors in the periphery.

GH is also released under stress; the cause is not understood. (2, 3, 4) These options are incorrect as seen in rationale (1).

22. ❹ When being prepared for surgery, the patient says, "I think I am going to die." The nurse's most appropriate response should be, "You think you are going to die?" This allows the patient to discuss his fears, and it lets the nurse know if the physician should be notified. If a patient is afraid of dying during surgery, the surgeon will cancel the surgery. Studies performed in 1991 show that if patients really believe they will die during surgery, they may die.

(1, 2, 3) These options are incorrect as seen in rationale (4).

23. ❷ If a patient has a stone that may pass spontaneously, the nurse should increase the patient's fluid intake and encourage ambulation. Walking will increase urethral peristalsis, and gravity will be increased in an upright position, which should help pass the renal calculus.

1. Straining the patient's urine will indicate if she passes the stone but will not help pass the stone.

3. Keeping the patient on bedrest will decrease the chances of passing the calculus.

4. Giving the patient medication to relax may make her feel better but will not help pass the stone.

24. ❹ Intentional tremors usually are associated with a tumor on the cerebellum. Cerebellar function as it relates to tremor can be assessed by asking a person to move the hand so as to touch the nose with a finger. The functions of the cerebellum are smooth, coordinated, skillful movement. When the cerebellum is damaged, these functions are impaired.

(1, 2, 3) These options are incorrect as seen in rationale (4).

25. ❹ The most common highly malignant brain tumor is a glioblastoma, which grows rapidly and occurs twice as often in adult males as in adult females. Symptoms of increased ICP may occur and include nausea and vomiting, headache, and papilledema. Other symptoms include mental changes, behavioral changes, and widened pulse pressure. Children will also have projectile vomiting and irritability.

1. Oligodendrogliomas are malignant brain tumors that are more common in women than in men. They are slow growing.

2. A medulloblastoma is a rare malignant brain tumor, and it is more common in males than in females.

3. An astrocytoma, the second most common malignant brain tumor, occurs more often in males than in females at any age. Signs and symptoms are increased ICP, mental and behavioral changes, and decreased visual acuity.

26. ❹ Before giving chlorpromazine (Thorazine), the nurse should take the client's blood pressure. Thorazine possesses significant alpha-adrenergic blocking activity and may cause hypotension.

(1, 2, 3) These options are incorrect as seen in rationale (4).

27. ❷ Antabuse is used for the treatment of alcoholics to deter consumption of alcohol. Antabuse produces an uncomfortable "sick feeling" (e.g., nausea and vomiting and vertigo) following alcohol ingestion.

(1, 3, 4) These options are incorrect as seen in rationale (2).

28. ❹ Jaundice, photosensitivity, and parkinsonism may occur in clients who receive Thorazine. All are side effects of the drug.

1. Side effects of Valium are dizziness, lethargy, mental depression, and headache. Valium is used to treat anxiety.

2. Side effects of Elavil are drowsiness, sedation, lethargy, fatigue, hypotension, and constipation. Elavil is used for the treatment of depression.

3. Side effects of Miltown are drowsiness, ataxia, blurred vision, hypotension, pruritus, rashes, and nausea. Miltown, a sedative hypnotic, is used as a sedative in the management of anxiety disorders.

29. ❷ Chemotherapy given systemically for intracranial cancer is limited because many of the commonly used agents cannot pass the blood–brain barrier in sufficient quantities to be effective. Sometimes, a catheter is inserted through the skull so that chemotherapy can be given directly to the tumor.

(1, 3, 4) These options are incorrect as seen in rationale (2).

30. ❷ The elderly (65 years and older) patient's renal threshold for glucose has increased, not allowing glucose to spill into the urine as easily.

(1, 3, 4) These options are incorrect as seen in rationale (2).

31. ❸ NPH is an intermediate-acting insulin. The time onset of action is from 1 to 2 h; the peak action is from 8 to 12 h; and the duration of action is 18 to 24 h. If a client took NPH insulin at 8:00 AM, it would peak at 6:00 PM (which is 10 h), shortly before dinner. When peak action occurs, the patient may experience hypoglycemia (an insulin reaction).

(1, 2, 4) These options are incorrect as seen in rationale (3).

32. ❶ Phenothiazine, one of the most powerful classes of tranquilizers, is most often given to patients with severe agitation and confusion due to psychosis. The phenothiazine most often used is chlorpromazine (Thorazine).

(2, 3, 4) These options are incorrect as seen in rationale (1).

33. ❹ Hypertension is not a side effect of antipsychotic drugs; orthostatic hypotension is a side effect of antipsychotic drugs.

(1, 2, 3) Side effects of antipsychotic medications are anticholinergic effects (dry mouth, dry eyes, blurred vision, constipation, ileus, urinary retention), hypotension, sedation, and agranulocytosis (an acute disease in which the WBC count drops to an extremely low level).

34. ❸ Protamine sulfate is an antidote for heparin toxicity. Partial thromboplastin time (PTT) is used to monitor heparin therapy.

1. Lente Iletin is an intermediate-acting insulin. It peaks at 8 to 12 h, and it is at this time that the patient may develop hypoglycemia (insulin reaction).

2. Vitamin K is an antidote for warfarin (Coumadin) toxicity. Prothrombin time (PT) is used to monitor Coumadin.

4. Protamine zinc is a slow-acting, long-lasting insulin. Onset is 4 to 8 h, peak is 16 to 18 h, and duration is 36 h.

35. ❹ Foods that should not be eaten when a client is taking MAO inhibitors are wine, yeast products, chocolate, meat, chicken, bologna, pepperoni, and cream cheese. MAO inhibitors are not prescribed as often as they were several years ago. They have been replaced with newer drugs that have fewer side effects, but they still are prescribed for some patients.

(1, 2, 3) These options are incorrect as seen in rationale (4).

36. ❷ The general signs of increased ICP are widened pulse pressure, nausea, vomiting, headache, change in the level of consciousness, and subtle behavior changes. The area of the brain most affected by increased ICP will dictate which signs and symptoms occur.

Identification of increased ICP is difficult until signs and symptoms of compromised brain function become apparent. Unfortunately, these may not appear or may not be recognized until significant brain damage has occurred. Continuous ICP monitoring and computed tomography (CT) scans can help to identify people with impending ICP, which is not clinically identifiable.

A disadvantage of intracranial catheter monitoring is that the catheter gives access to brain tissue and increases the chances of infection. The catheter can also become occluded with tissue or fluid and give a false ICP reading.

Another method of measuring ICP is the subarachnoid screw. A screw (bolt) is placed through the skull into the subarachnoid space and a measurement of ICP is transmitted through brain tissue. This method is less accurate than direct intraventricular monitoring; volume pressure cannot be measured, and if the screw becomes occluded with fluid or tissue, a false ICP reading will be obtained. An advantage of this method is that access is easy, and there is less risk of infection because the screw does not penetrate the brain tissue.

(1, 3, 4) These options are incorrect as seen in rationale (2).

37. ❸ Patients often become forgetful, are unable to concentrate, have a short attention span, and have increased nervous irritability before each hemodialysis treatment, due to the accumulation of end-products of metabolism.

Metabolic acidosis occurs because of the inability of the kidneys to excrete hydrogen ions and a decreased reabsorption of sodium bicarbonate. The patient who shows these signs and symptoms will have very high blood urea nitrogen (BUN) and creatinine levels.

The four basic goals of dialysis are to remove the end-products of protein metabolism, such as urea and creatinine, from the blood; maintain a safe concentration of serum electrolytes; correct acidosis and replenish the blood's bicarbonate buffer system; and remove excess fluid from the blood.

(1, 2, 4) These options are incorrect as seen in rationale (3).

38. ❸ The interpretation is that the side effect of nitrogen mustard, or any other chemotherapeutic agent, is bone marrow depression. The action is that the client needs to be protected from infection because of a low WBC count. This side effect must be monitored closely; chemotherapy may have to be discontinued for a period of time to allow the bone marrow to recover.

(1, 2, 4) These options are incorrect as seen in rationale (3).

39. ❷ In comparison with other methods of administering antineoplastic drugs for the treatment of isolated neoplasms, regional perfusion has the advantage of higher dosage to a specific area and lower systemic toxicity.

Regional perfusion is done by using a Groshong-Hickman catheter or Port-a-Cath access system, which delivers chemotherapy directly to a malignant tumor.

Less chemotherapy is used because the medication needed to destroy the tumor is delivered directly to the tumor and not systemically. The side effects of chemotherapy are reduced.

1. The administration of chemotherapy by regional perfusion is not easier than systemic administration, and the Hickman catheter and Port-A-Cath can be used to deliver chemotherapy systemically or regionally. The only difference is catheter placement. When used systemically, the catheter usually is placed in the right atrium of the heart. The dosage is controlled the same way in both methods of administration.

3. The administration problems are different, but not fewer or less serious.

4. Cost is not a number one concern for the nurse, and a peripheral IV delivers medication systemically.

40. ❸ Complex carbohydrates have value in the diabetic diet; they are a good source of energy and maintain a more stable blood sugar level.

1. Dietetic foods are not recommended by the American Diabetic Association (ADA), and they definitely cannot be eaten as free food. Free foods are foods that do not need to be counted as part of daily intake (e.g., raw vegetables); no-fat cookies may have high sugar content.

2. A diabetic patient must always be on an ADA diet and must eat regular meals at about the same time each day, even if the person is not required to take insulin.

4. Fats cannot be removed totally from anyone's diet; fat is important for the absorption of fat-soluble vitamins.

41. ❸ Furosemide and calcium increase urinary excretion of potassium.

(1, 2, 4) These options are incorrect. Furosemide and cortisol will not cause hypertension, stomatitis, or hypoglycemia. Cortisol will increase fluid retention and over several weeks may increase blood pressure.

42. ❷ The main reason for reporting cases of venereal disease to the local health department is that sexual contacts of the infectious person may need to be treated. This is one of the best ways to control venereal disease.

1. A person can be adequately treated without a partner receiving treatment.

3. Contacting the infected partner will not decrease the incidence of venereal disease.

4. Reporting venereal cases to the health department does not cause people with venereal disease to limit the number of sexual contacts.

43. ❶ Acute *closed-angle* glaucoma usually has rapid onset, with severe pain, red eye, nausea and vomiting, blurring, and decreased visual activity. A typical attack is *unilateral* and occurs either in a darkened environment (which causes pupil dilation) or during emotional stress. Acute closed-angle glaucoma is a medical emergency.

The aim of treatment is to open the closed chamber angle and permit outflow of aqueous humor and decrease aqueous humor production. Although this goal can sometimes be achieved with medication, surgery usually is eventually required.

If IOP is not relieved, complete and permanent blindness results within 3 to 5 days after symptoms appear.

Before surgery, IOP is reduced by topical miotics such as pilocarpine (Pilocar) to increase aqueous outflow as often as every 5 to 10 min; acetazolamide (Diamox) IV or IM reduces production of aqueous humor.

(2, 3, 4) These options are incorrect as seen in rationale (1).

44. ❷ Papillary cancer accounts for 50 percent of thyroid cancer in adults and usually is associated with prolonged survival rates.

1. Follicular carcinoma is a less common thyroid cancer (occurs in 30 percent of all cases) and is more likely to recur and metastasize.

3. Wilms' tumor occurs primarily in children and is a tumor of the kidney.

4. Medullary is a malignant thyroid cancer; it is rare and metastasizes.

45. ❸ Marfan's syndrome is a rare, inherited, degenerative, generalized disease of connective tissue. It is characterized by long bones. The person is taller than average for the family height and has fingers that are very long and slender.

1. Tay-Sachs disease, the most common of the lipid storage diseases, results from a congenital enzyme deficiency. It is characterized by progressive mental and motor deterioration and is always fatal, usually before age 5 years.

2. Lou Gehrig's disease (amyotrophic lateral sclerosis [ALS]) is the most common motor neuron disease causing muscular atrophy. It affects men four times more often than women and usually is fatal within 3 to 10 years after onset, usually as a result of aspiration pneumonia. Mental status remains intact while progressive physical degeneration occurs; the patient acutely perceives these changes.

4. Galactosemia is any disorder of galactose metabolism. It produces symptoms ranging from cataracts and liver damage to mental retardation. Although a galactose-free diet relieves most symptoms of galactosemia, induced mental impairment is irreversible.

It is an inherited autosomal-recessive defect that occurs in 1 of 60,000 births in the United States.

Signs are evident at birth or begin a few days after milk ingestion and include failure to thrive, vomiting, and diarrhea. Other clinical effects are liver damage (which causes jaundice, hepatomegaly, cirrhosis, ascites), galactosuria, and proteinuria. Cataracts may be present at birth or develop later.

Treatment is elimination of galactose and lactose from the diet, which causes most side effects to subside. Soybean formula is used for infants. As the child matures, a balanced galactose-free diet must be maintained.

46. ❷ The best response by the nurse would be, "With treatment, most children go into remission quickly and may remain symptom-free for a year or five years; there is no way of knowing how long." Acute lymphocytic leukemia (ALL) is the most frequent type of leukemia in children, accounting for one third of all cases of leukemia. The highest frequency of ALL occurs in children between the ages of 2 to 8 years. The prognosis for infants younger than 12 months or children older than 10 years at the first occurrence is not as good as for those between 12 months and 10 years.

After diagnosis, chemotherapy often begins with doxorubicin (Adriamycin) and cytarabine (Cytosine). During their administration, the patient generally receives allopurinol (Alloprin) to help the kidneys manage the uric acid created by the large amount of destroyed cells being evacuated from the blood. Usually, a full remission state can be reached within 1 to 2 months. A child is said to be in remission when bone marrow shows fewer than 5 percent blast cells.

After the remission phase, the sanctuary phase begins. Maintenance therapy is continued indefinitely. Remission is more difficult to achieve in children with acute myelogenous leukemia (AML) than in those with ALL; if achieved, the period usually is very brief.

(1, 3, 4) These options are incorrect as seen in rationale (2).

47. ❷ People with AIDS will have a *decreased* T-cell count and a high HIV count, and they are most susceptible to opportunistic infections such as *P. carinii*, Kaposi's sarcoma, toxoplasmosis, and TB. Pentamidine and sulfamethoxazole (Gantanol) are used prophylactically and for treatment of *P. carinii*. Kaposi's sarcoma (cancer of the skin) is treated with radiation and chemotherapy.

Toxoplasmosis is spread by cat litter and infected tissue cysts in raw, uncooked meat (heating, drying, of freezing destroys these cysts). Treatment consists of pyrimethamine (Daraprim) and sulfadiazine.

Treatment for TB consists of isoniazid (INH), rifampin, ethambutol, streptomycin, and pyrazinamide (PZA).

(1, 3, 4) These options are incorrect as seen in rationale (2).

48. ❶ An autotransfusion is the collection and reinfusion of a patient's own blood or blood components. This process is very helpful for a patient losing a large amount of blood during surgery. Patients who have AIDS or other diseases that can be transmitted by blood are not candidates for autologous transfusion. It is best for them to receive donated blood that is not infected.

(2, 3, 4) These options are incorrect as seen in rationale (1).

49. ❷ In stage III of breast cancer, the chemotherapy drugs commonly used are cyclophosphamide (Cytoxan) and fluorouracil (5-FU) with methotrexate (Methotrexate LPF) or doxorubicin (Adriamycin). The major side effects of chemotherapy are nausea and vomiting and bone marrow depression.

1. Mustargen is used for the treatment of Hodgkin's disease and lung cancer. Vincristine is used for the treatment of Hodgkin's disease and acute leukemia. Prednisone is a steroid

used for antiinflammatory purposes. Doxorubicin is used for the treatment of acute leukemia and is also used for breast cancer.

3. Imuran is used to prevent rejection of renal transplants. Radiation therapy is a local treatment modality for cancer that can be used externally. It is estimated that more than 50 percent of patients with cancer are treated with radiation therapy. Radiation is the emission of tiny particles or waves of energy from a radioactive source that destroys cancer cells.

External radiation therapy is the delivery of a high dose of radiation to a small amount of tissue in a short period of time. Cells are destroyed by an inflammatory response. As more cells are destroyed, cells may slough, causing the tissue to become thin and ulcerated. Side effects of external radiation include nausea and vomiting, diarrhea, cystitis, alopecia (hair loss), leukopenia, thrombocytopenia, and sterility.

4. Interferon-alpha is used for the treatment of hairy cell leukemia and other cancers. Interferons are a natural body protein formed in response to viral infections and stimulated by the immune system and certain chemical substances.

50. ❹ Doxorubicin has the usual chemotherapeutic side effects associated with most antineoplastic agents. This drug also is used to treat cardiomyopathy.

(1, 2, 3) Cirrhosis of the liver, meningitis, and hypertension are not side effects of doxorubicin.

51. ❹ Thrombocytopenia and leukopenia are forms of aplastic anemia. Leukopenia is abnormal decrease of WBCs. Thrombocytopenia is abnormal decrease in the number of blood platelets.

(1, 2, 3) None of these anemias are forms of aplastic anemia.

52. ❶ Rheumatic fever is a connective tissue disease that affects joints, the mitral valve, and myocardium.

(2, 3, 4) These options are incorrect as seen in rationale (1).

53. ❸ Thrombocytopenia commonly occurs in children and is characterized by a deficiency of circulating platelets. Because platelets play a vital role in coagulation, this disease poses a serious threat to hemostasis.

Prognosis is excellent in drug-induced thrombocytopenia if the offending drug is withdrawn; in such cases, recovery can be immediate.

Purpura is a condition characterized by hemorrhages into the skin, mucous membranes, internal organs, and other tissues. Hemorrhage into the skin shows red darkening to purple and then to brownish yellow; finally, the hemorrhages disappear within 2 to 3 weeks.

1. Pernicious anemia is discussed in answer 87, rationale 1.
2. DIC is discussed in answer 87, rationale 4.
4. Sickle cell anemia is discussed in answer 87, rationale 3.

54. ❸ Peripheral neuropathy is an adverse reaction to INH (isoniazid). The physician will add vitamin B_6 to the patient's regimen of medications to reduce and possibly eliminate the symptoms of neuropathy.

2. It is not unusual for a patient to be treated with INH for 18 months or longer because of the length of time it takes to destroy

the gram-negative bacteria TB. Some patients stop taking the medications before all bacteria are destroyed and then must be treated again with INH and other medications for TB. These patients tend to develop TB-resistant bacterial strains, which are difficult to cure.

It is extremely important for patients with TB to remain on medications, such as INH and other antituberculin drugs, for the length of time recommended by the physician.

The x-ray film and sputum culture must be clear of any signs of tuberculin bacteria before the patient can stop taking the antiinfective agent. DNA testing for TB is now available. Noncompliant patients remaining infected with the bacteria will continue to spread TB.

(1, 4) These options are incorrect as seen in rationales (3) and (2).

55. ❷ Treatment of thyroid cancer consists of radiation (iodine-131) and external radiation. The thyroid gland will be destroyed and the patient must take Synthroid (levothyroxine), a thyroid hormone, regularly for life.

1. Doxorubicin (Adriamycin) is an antineoplastic agent; it is not used for treatment of thyroid cancer. Side effects of doxorubicin are cardiomyopathy, bone marrow depression, alopecia, stomatitis, esophagitis, nausea and vomiting, leukopenia, and thrombocytopenia.

Cisplatin is an antineoplastic agent and is not used for treatment of thyroid cancer. Side effects of cisplatin are tinnitus (ringing in the ears), hypoglycemia, nausea and vomiting, nephrotoxicity, anemia, and thrombocytopenia.

3. Fluorouracil (5-FU) and vincristine are antineoplastic agents and are not used for the treatment of thyroid cancer. Side effects of 5-FU are alopecia, nausea, vomiting, stomatitis, diarrhea, anemia, leukopenia, and thrombocytopenia.

4. Synthroid (levothyroxine) is a thyroid hormone used for the treatment of hypothyroidism. Phenobarbital is an anticonvulsant, barbiturate, sedative, hypnotic agent.

56. ❶ Drugs used for the treatment of *P. carinii* pneumonia and toxoplasmosis are pentamidine, Bactrim, and Septra.

2. Methotrexate doxorubicin and vincristine are cancer chemotherapeutic agents.

3. Septra, an antibiotic, is commonly used for urinary tract infections and is also used to treat *P. carinii*. Acyclovir is commonly used to treat herpes zoster of the eyes and skin.

4. Meperidine, a narcotic analgesic, is used to relieve pain. Dextran, a plasma volume expander, is used to treat cerebral edema, to decrease IOP, and to improve renal function in acute renal failure and in chemical poisoning.

57. ❶ It is important that patients comply with TB therapy, as discussed in answer 54, rationale 2. The nursing measures that would be most helpful in obtaining the patient's compliance with his treatment would be to involve the client in teaching sessions.

(2, 3, 4) These options are incorrect as seen in rationale (1).

58. ❹ Signs and symptoms of fetal alcohol syndrome (FAS) are seizures, poor sucking reflex, apnea, increased respiratory effort, irritability, hyperactivity alternating with lethargy, increased muscle tone, and diaphoresis. Infants born to drug abusers are harder to hold, less cuddly, and more difficult to control. They show a depressed visual response and an exaggerated auditory response. Deformities of the head and face (e.g., microcephaly, small eyes, flattened maxilla, and thin upper lip) are also found.

Characteristic anomalies seen in FAS include microcephaly, cleft palate, altered palmar creases, and joint and cardiac defects. There may be severe mental retardation with depressed sucking and swallowing reflexes or slight retardation, not detected until later when developmental problems occur.

(1, 2, 3) These options are incorrect as seen in rationale (4).

59. ❹ Signs and symptoms of fetal drug addiction are respiratory distress, tremors, vomiting, diarrhea, a high-pitched cry, poor sucking reflex, no cough, bulging fontanelle at rest, and fixation of gaze without blinking. Cocaine can cause mental retardation. Observe neonate for seizures.

(1, 2, 3) These options are incorrect as seen in rationale (4).

60. ❶ Kawasaki disease, an acute disease of unknown cause, produces inflammation of the coronary arteries and damages the heart muscle. It is the leading cause of acquired heart disease in children in the United States. In many cases, the disease is self-limited.

(2, 3, 4) These options do not describe Kawasaki disease.

61. ❶ Kawasaki disease is treated with a high dose of IV gamma-globulin in conjunction with salicylate therapy.

(2, 3, 4) These are not treatments for Kawasaki disease.

62. ❶ Cushing's disease is caused by excessive ACTH and consequent hyperplasia of the adrenal cortex. An exogenous cause of Cushing's syndrome is excessive administration of steroids.

Cushing's disease is caused by oversecretion of glucocorticoids and, to a lesser extent, androgens and aldosterone. This causes rapidly developing adiposity (excessive fat) of the face (moon face), neck, and trunk. Purple striae appear on the skin. The disease is most commonly found in women.

(2, 3, 4) These options are incorrect as seen in rationale (1).

63. ❷ Cushing's disease results in psychosis, diabetes mellitus, osteoporosis, and hypertension.

(1, 3, 4) There are not symptoms of Cushing's disease.

64. ❶ Addison's disease is characterized by decreased mineralocorticoid, glucocorticoid, and androgen secretions.

(2, 3, 4) These are not characteristics of Addison's disease.

65. ❷ Addison's disease results in a bronze coloration of the skin, postural hypotension, decreased tolerance for stress, poor coordination, hypoglycemia, and a craving for salt.

(1, 3, 4) These are not the results of Addison's disease.

66. ❸ If a patient cannot take oral Premarin (estrogen) or use estrogen patches because of hypertension or skin irritation, respectively, the physician will place her on Theelin Aqueous (estrogen) IM. A signed consent form may be required before administering Theelin Aqueous IM.

1. Yutopar is used to stop preterm labor.

2. Xanax is used for the treatment of anxiety.

4. Prostigmin is used to increase muscle strength in symptomatic treatment of myasthenia gravis. It also is used for the prevention and treatment of bladder distention or urinary ileus.

67. ❷ Versed may be used in the place of Valium preoperatively because it can be combined with most preoperative agents. Valium cannot be combined with any other medications.

(1, 3, 4) These options are incorrect as seen in rationale (2).

68. ❶ The following are NSAIDS agents: Butazolidin, aspirin, Advil, Motrin, Indocin, Nuprin, and Dolobid.

(2, 3, 4) These options were not the best response because some but not all of the agents in each option are NSAIDS.

69. ❸ There are several sources of vitamin D in the diet; sources high in vitamin D are liver, fish, eggs, and fortified foods.

(1, 2, 4) These options were not the best response because some but not all foods in each option were high in vitamin D.

70. ❶ Diameter of IV needles is given in gauge numbers. The larger the gauge number, the smaller the lumen. To administer blood, an 18-gauge needle is used to prevent breaking of red blood cells (RBCs) as they pass through the lumen of the needle.

(2, 3, 4) The 20-, 22-, and 25-gauge needles are too small to use for administration of blood.

71. ❹ If a patient asks the nurse what medication he or she is receiving, the nurse should tell him or her the name and action of the medications. The only time a nurse would not tell a patient the name of the medication he or she were given is if the patient was addicted to a drug.

The physician may order the same drug to which the patient is addicted, and it would be given alternately with a placebo. If the patient then asks what medication he or she is receiving, the nurse would reply, "What did your physician order?" If addicted to Demerol, the patient would probably say Demerol. In this way, the nurse is not being dishonest with the patient.

1. Telling a patient "this is the medication your doctor ordered" is telling the patient nothing. He or she may be taking several medications and may not know what medications the physician ordered.

2. The nurse is a professional and should answer the patient's question and not refer the patient to the physician. Referring a patient to the physician usually is not the right answer on an NCLEX-RN exam.

3. Telling the patient "This is the antibiotic your doctor ordered for you" assumes that the doctor told the patient about the antibiotic. Many times patients do not understand what their physician has told them about medications. The nurse is a professional and should discuss the medication with the patient.

72. ❹ The most important part of pain assessment is interviewing the patient. The patient is the only one who feels the pain, so she or he will know where the pain is located and the severity of the pain.

(1, 2, 3) These options are incorrect as seen in rationale (4).

73. **④** The food group lowest in natural sodium is fresh fruit.

(1, 2, 3) Meat, milk, and canned vegetables are high in sodium.

74. **②** If a patient tells the nurse, "My doctor said I didn't have to take this anymore," the nurse's best initial action would be to check the physician's orders to see if the medication was discontinued (DC). It is possible that the nurse failed to see the DC order. Rechecking the medication sheet will not help if the DC order has not been taken off the client's chart and written on the medication sheet.

(1, 3, 4) These options are incorrect as seen in rationale (2).

75. **②** The signs and symptoms of fat embolus are frothy sputum, tachycardia, tachypnea, cyanosis, fever, and a petechial rash. Indications of fat embolism usually develop within 72 h of trauma. Assessment findings also include progressive hypoxemia, sudden drop in hematocrit, diffuse infiltration visible on chest x-ray film, CNS disturbances, oliguria, elevated serum lipase, and fat globules in the blood vessels of the retina.

Treatment includes support with oxygen and administration of steroids.

1. Severe chest pain does *not* occur with fat embolus; it would be unusual for emboli to occur 12 days post fracture. Hypertension is not a symptom of fat embolus.

3. Pulmonary edema, seizures, circulatory overload, and coarse crackles are *not* signs and symptoms of fat embolus.

4. Respiratory depression, cardiac arrhythmias, and neuromuscular irritability are *not* signs of fat embolus.

76. **①** Calcium will decrease the absorption of tetracycline in the GI tract when taken together. Calcium contained in foods or dairy products decreases absorption of tetracycline by forming an insoluble compound.

(2, 3, 4) Calcium will not decrease the absorption of thiamin, ranitidine, or penicillin G. Thiamin is vitamin B and is required for carbohydrate metabolism. Ranitidine (Zantac) reduces production of HCl in the stomach and duodenum, and it is used for the treatment of ulcers. Penicillin G, an antibiotic, is used for the treatment of infections.

77. **②** The liver is mainly responsible for metabolism of drugs. If the patient is in liver failure, the liver cannot break down drugs; therefore, overdosing a patient with medications, such as analgesics, is easily done.

(1, 3, 4) These options are incorrect as seen in rationale (2).

78. **②** A patient is taken off IV Pronestyl and given IM or PO Pronestyl as soon as severe arrhythmias are controlled. When converting from an IV dose to an oral dose regimen, allow 3 to 4 h to lapse between the last IV dose and administration of the first oral dose. Side effects of Pronestyl are confusion, hypotension, ventricular arrhythmias, heart block, and nausea and vomiting.

(1, 3, 4) These are not signs of Pronestyl toxicity.

79. **④** Alcohol and furosemide (Lasix) will increase the urinary excretion of magnesium; usually alcoholic patients have low levels of magnesium and Lasix will decrease levels even more.

(1, 2, 3) These combinations will not increase the urinary excretion of magnesium.

80. **①** The signs and symptoms of retinal detachment include complaints of floating spots and recurrent flashes of light. As detachment progresses, the patient may describe a veil, curtain, or cobweb that eliminates a portion of the visual field.

2. Retinal detachment is painless (not painful) with unilateral vision loss; the pupils do not dilate, but flashing light does occur.

3. There is no gradual blurring of vision with a detached retina, and the pupil does not turn milky white.

4. Retinal detachment does not cause recurrent, painless, peripheral vision loss; the patient will complain of flashes of light but not bright flashing light.

81. **①** Foods high in vitamin C are broccoli, potatoes, cabbage, tomatoes, and citrus fruits.

(2, 3, 4) These foods are not high in vitamin C.

82. **④** Epinephrine and physostigmine are used to constrict the pupil (miosis) and to contract ciliary musculature to reduce IOP by increasing aqueous humor outflow.

1. Epinephrine and physostigmine reduce IOP by increasing aqueous humor outflow, *not* by increasing absorption.

2. Betoptic and Lopressor are beta-blockers; they decrease IOP by decreasing production, *not* outflow, of aqueous humor.

3. Diamox and Betoptic decrease IOP by decreasing production, *not* outflow, of aqueous humor.

83. **①** Before administering digitalis, it is important to take an apical pulse because digitalis slows conduction of impulses at the AV node. Digitalis is not given if the pulse is less than 60 bpm in an adult, less than 70 bpm/min in a child, and less than 90 bpm in an infant.

2. Nitroglycerin is a coronary vasodilator.

3. Quinidine is a dysrhythmic agent used in the management of various arterial and ventricular arrhythmias.

4. Lidocaine is the agent of choice for the treatment of ventricular arrhythmias.

84. **②** If the order is digoxin 0.125 mg PO qd and the nurse has on hand Lanoxin 0.25-mg tablet, the nurse would give $\frac{1}{2}$ of a tablet. Half of 0.5 mg is 0.25 mg, and half of 0.25 mg is 0.125 mg.

(1, 3, 4) These options are incorrect as seen in rationale (2).

85. **①** The drug of choice for the treatment of sinus bradycardia is atropine or epinephrine.

2. Morphine is an analgesic, and a side effect of morphine is respiratory depression. Stadol (butorphanol tartrate) is similar to morphine but does not cause respiratory depression. Both can be used in the management of severe and moderate pain, and both are narcotic analgesics.

3. Lidocaine (Xylocaine), given either IV or IM, is used for treatment of ventricular arrhythmias. It is also used as a local anesthetic.

4. Isuprel (isoproterenol) usually is not recommended as a bronchodilator because of its severe side effects, which include

nervousness, restlessness, insomnia, tremors, headache, paradoxical bronchospasm (with excessive use), hypertension, arrhythmias, angina, nausea and vomiting, and hyperglycemia.

86. ❶ Patients receiving guanethidine monosulfate (Ismelin) and reserpine (Serpasil) should have sex counseling because these agents can cause penile dysfunction, such as impotence (inability of the male to achieve or maintain erection).

Ismelin, a peripherally acting antiadrenergic agent, is used for the treatment of moderate to severe hypertension.

Reserpine, a peripherally acting antihypertensive, antiadrenergic agent, is used in combination with other antihypertensives (thiazide diuretics) in the management of hypertension.

2. Captopril (Capoten) is an antihypertensive agent used alone or in combination with other antihypertensive agents in the management of hypertension and CHF.

Metaraminol (Aramine) is a vasopressor used in the management of hypotension and circulatory shock, which may occur as a consequence of hemorrhage, drug reaction, or anesthesia. This treatment is used when the patient is unresponsive to fluid volume replacement.

3. Hydralazine hydrochloride (Apresoline) is an antihypertensive agent used alone or in combination with other antihypertensive agents in the management of moderate to severe hypertension.

Vincristine (Oncovin), an antineoplastic agent, is used in combination with other treatment modalities (surgery or radiation therapy) for the treatment of Hodgkin's disease, leukemia, neuroblastoma, and Wilms' tumor.

4. Codeine, a narcotic analgesic, is used in the management of moderate or severe pain. It acts as an antitussive when used in smaller doses.

Hydromorphone hydrochloride (Dilaudid), a narcotic analgesic, is used as an antitussive when given in low doses, and it is considered a powerful analgesic.

87. ❸ Sickle cell anemia is a congenital hemolytic anemia. The RBCs become rigid, rough, and elongated, and form a sickle shape. Such sickling can produce hemolysis (cell destruction), resulting in anemia.

1. Pernicious anemia results from lack of the intrinsic factor in the stomach, which is necessary for absorption of vitamin B_{12}. Vitamin B_{12} is necessary for the production of RBCs. A normal erythrocyte count for an adult is 4,500,000 to 6,000,000 /mm^3; an erythrocyte count of 3,2000,000/mm^3 is extremely low and would indicate RBC destruction or hemorrhage.

2. Cirrhosis of the liver is a chronic hepatic disease characterized by diffuse destruction and fibrotic generation of hepatic cells. As normal tissue yields to fibrosis, this disease alters liver structure, causing impairment of blood and lymph flow and, ultimately, hepatic insufficiency. It is twice as common in men as in women and is especially prevalent among malnourished chronic alcoholics older than 50 years. (Portal hypertension occurs when blood flow meets increased resistance. As portal pressure rises, blood backs up into the spleen and flows through collateral channels, causing esophageal varices, hemorrhoids, and ascites.)

4. DIC occurs as a complication of diseases and conditions that accelerate clotting, causing small blood vessel occlusion, organ necroses, and depletion of circulatory clotting factors and platelets. This, in turn, can provoke severe hemorrhage after clotting factors are depleted.

88. ❶ Nipride may be given as an IV infusion to patients in hypertensive emergencies to decrease afterload (systolic) and preload (diastolic). Nipride must be covered with aluminium foil or placed into a paper bag to prevent chemical breakdown. Blood pressure must be monitored every 15 min because Nipride acts rapidly and can drop blood pressure too rapidly, causing severe hypotension.

(2, 3, 4) These options are incorrect as seen in rationale (1).

89. ❹ The most important assessment of a client receiving streptomycin is evaluating function of cranial nerve (CN) VIII by audiometer prior to and throughout the course of therapy. Prompt recognition and intervention are essential to prevent permanent damage to this nerve.

(1, 2, 3) These options are incorrect as they are not side effects of streptomycin.

90. ❸ The drugs of choice for the treatment of cardiogenic shock include dopamine IV, a vasopressor, to increase cardiac output, blood pressure, and renal flow; dobutamine IV, to increase myocardial contractility; and norepinephrine or dopamine when a more potent vasoconstrictor is necessary.

(1, 2, 4) These drugs are not used in cardiogenic shock. Digoxin usually is not used in cardiogenic shock because it slows conduction at the AV node. Atropine usually is not used because the force of the contraction, and not the rate, must be increased; the latter may cause arrhythmias. Lasix is never given to clients in cardiogenic shock because there is no fluid overload.

91. ❶ The correct procedure for obtaining a stool specimen for examination for amoeba is the delivery of the specimen immediately, while it is warm and fresh, to the laboratory. Stool samples for amoeba must be tested while they are warm and fresh or the amoeba will die.

(2, 3, 4) These options are incorrect as seen in rationale (1).

92. ❹ Autotransfusion of blood products is not used if the patient has pericardial or systemic infections, pulmonary or respiratory infections, coagulopathy (defect in blood clotting mechanism), or malignant neoplasms. Autotransfusion involves collecting the patient's blood that is lost during surgery, filtering it, and transfusing it back into the patient.

(1, 2, 3) These options are incorrect as seen in rationale (4).

93. ❶ When the nurse finds an IV bag of TPN hanging but not infusing, the nurse should check the tubing for kinks, twists, or clots. If these are not causing a problem, then the physician must be notified because only a physician can reinsert a central line. The RN can discontinue (DC) the central line but cannot reinsert it. The physician will DC the order on the central line and reinsert another central line.

2. The problem of TPN not infusing will not be solved by changing the IV bottle (or bag).

3. The problem of TPN not infusing will not be solved by assessing the vital signs.

4. It is not a safe procedure to irrigate a TPN or any IV line; a blood clot may be pushed into the vein or right atrium and cause an infarct to the heart, brain, or kidney.

94. **4** Antacids and Tagamet must be taken at different times of the day because the antacid may absorb the Tagamet.

(1, 2, 3) These options are incorrect as seen in rationale (4).

95. **4** Zantac and Tagamet are used for the treatment of ulcers of the stomach and duodenum because they slow the production of HCl.

(1, 2, 3) These options are incorrect as seen in rationale (4).

96. **1** Lactulose (Cephulac) increases water content in the intestines, softens the stool, and inhibits the diffusion of ammonia from the colon into the blood, thereby reducing blood ammonia levels. Lactulose is used in the management of encephalopathy and is also used for chronic constipation of the elderly.

(2, 3, 4) Correctol Extra Gentle, Docusate Calcium (Surfak), and Docusate sodium (Colace) are all stool softeners and laxatives.

97. **3** Pitressin is used for the treatment of abdominal distention and diabetes insipidus.

1. Mannitol is an osmotic diuretic used for the treatment of acute oliguric renal failure, edema, and reduction of ICP.

2. Mandol is an antiinfective agent (not to be confused with Mannitol).

4. Allopurinol is an antigout agent.

98. **2** Quinidine, procainamide (Pronestyl), and lidocaine (Xylocaine) are used for the treatment of PVCs.

1. Digoxin (Lanoxin) is used to increase cardiac contractions and, thus, increase cardiac output. Propranolol (Inderal), a beta-blocker, is used for the treatment of hypertension, angina pectoris, and arrhythmias.

3. Isoproterenol hydrochloride (Isuprel hydrochloride) is a bronchodilator used for ventricular arrhythmias due to AV block. Dopamine (Intropin) is used in the management of hypotension; it causes peripheral vasoconstriction. Cardizem, a calcium blocker, is used in the management of angina pain and hypertension.

4. Metaraminol (Aramine), a vasopressor, is used in the management of hypotension and circulatory shock when the patient is unresponsive to fluid volume replacement. Nifedipine (Procardia), a calcium blocker, is used for the treatment of angina pain and in the management of hypertension.

99. **3** Signs and symptoms of coarctation of the aorta in infants are cold feet, dyspnea, leg cramps, lower blood pressure in the legs than in the arms, delayed pulse in legs, and symptoms of CHF.

1. Signs and symptoms of atrial septal defect in a child are frequent respiratory tract infection, dyspnea, feeding difficulty, soft early midsystolic murmur, and a fixed, widely split S2 sound.

2. The ductus arteriosus is a vascular connection that, during fetal life, directs blood flow from the pulmonary artery to the aorta, bypassing the lungs. Functional closure of the ductus occurs within hours or days after birth but in some cases takes 6 months to several years. If the ductus remains patent and is large, the direction of blood flow is reversed right to left, causing cyanosis.

4. Signs and symptoms of tetralogy of Fallot after 3 to 6 months are cyanosis, dyspnea, deep sighing respiration, bradycardia, fainting, seizures, and loss of consciousness. In older children, signs and symptoms include decreased exercise tolerance, increased dyspnea on exertion, growth retardation, eating difficulties, squatting when short of breath (tet spells), and clubbing of fingers and toes.

100. **3** The most common cause of digitalis toxicity is hypokalemia (low potassium level). The first sign of digitalis toxicity is bradycardia; other signs include fatigue, yellow blurred vision, headache, and nausea and vomiting.

1. Hyponatremia (decreased serum sodium) does not cause digitalis toxicity. Signs and symptoms of hyponatremia include headache, tachycardia, weakness, lethargy, restlessness, confusion, convulsions, and anorexia. Nausea and vomiting are common.

2. Hypocalcemia (decreased serum calcium) does not cause digitalis toxicity. Signs and symptoms of hypocalcemia include facial muscle hyperirritability. Nurse checks for Chvostek's sign: tap facial nerves; if facial muscle twitches, potential for tetany. To check for Trousseau's sign: constrict circulation in an arm (usually with a blood pressure cuff) for 3 to 5 min. If spasm of lower arm and hand muscle (carpal spasm), hypocalcemia is present, potential for tetany.

4. Hyperkalemia will not cause digitalis toxicity; it will cause cardiac arrhythmias. Hyperkalemia is treated with Kayexalate PO or by enema.

Chapter

12

Fluid and Electrolyte Disorders

TOPICAL OUTLINE

I. NORMAL VALUES

A. Intracellular Fluid = two thirds of body fluid. Major intracellular electrolytes are potassium (K), phosphorus (PO_4), and magnesium (Mg).

B. Extracellular Fluid = one third of body fluid. Major extracellular electrolytes are sodium (Na), chloride (Cl), and bicarbonate (HCO_3).

C. Serum Values

1. Na: 135 to 145 milliequivalents per liter
2. K: 3.5 to 5.0 mEq/L
3. Cl: 95 to 105 mEq/L
4. Mg: 1.5 to 2.5 mEq/L
5. PO_4: 2.8 to 4.5 mg/dL
6. Ca: 9 to 11 mg/dL *or* 4.5 to 5.5 mEq/L

D. Homeostatic Mechanisms

1. Antidiuretic hormone (ADH) results in water retention.
2. Adrenocorticotropic hormone (ACTH) stimulates the adrenal cortex to release cortisol and aldosterone causing sodium retention.
3. Parathormone elevates the serum calcium level and promotes phosphorus excretion.
4. Kidneys regulate acid–base balance by excreting either hydrogen or bicarbonate ions.

II. IMBALANCES IN FLUIDS AND ELECTROLYTES

A. Fluid Volume Deficit

1. Causes
   a. Vomiting
   b. Diarrhea
   c. GI suction
   d. Decreased fluid intake
   e. Hemorrhage
   f. Third-space fluid shifts (fluid moves from vasculature into interstitial spaces and is unavailable for use).

2. Signs and Symptoms
   a. Acute weight loss (unless third spaces)
   b. Decreased skin turgor
   c. Oliguria
   d. Concentrated urine
   e. Weak, rapid pulse
   f. Decreased blood pressure (orthostatic hypotension)
   g. Elevated blood urea nitrogen (BUN) level and hematocrit (unless fluid loss is due to hemorrhage)

3. Treatment and Nursing Implications
   a. Isotonic intravenous fluids (e.g., normal saline, Ringer's lactate)
   b. Treatment of shock
   c. Monitor urinary output, blood pressure
   d. Daily weights

B. Fluid Volume Excess

1. Causes

   a. Renal failure

   b. Congestive heart failure (CHF)

   c. Cirrhosis/liver failure

   d. Rapid excessive infusion of intravenous fluids

2. Signs and Symptoms

   a. Acute weight gain

   b. Edema

   c. Distended neck veins

   d. Rales (moist crackles)

   e. Decreased BUN level and hematocrit (due to dilution)

3. Treatment and Nursing Implications

   a. Administer diuretics as ordered; monitor for electrolyte imbalance (e.g., hypokalemia, hypernatremia, hyponatremia)

   b. Restrict fluid intake; strict intake and output (I&O)

   c. Low-sodium diet (avoid processed meats, canned soups and vegetables, table salt)

   d. Maintain in semi-Fowler's position (for maximum lung expansion to improve gas exchange)

   e. Assess breath sounds frequently

   f. Check for pitting edema

   g. Daily weights

C. Sodium Deficit (Hyponatremia)

1. Causes

   a. Diuretics

   b. Vomiting

   c. GI suction

   d. Diarrhea

   e. Syndrome of inappropriate antidiuretic hormone secretion (SIADH)

   f. Excessive water replacement

2. Signs and Symptoms

   a. Headache

   b. Anxiety

   c. Nausea and vomiting

   d. Muscle cramps

   e. Lethargy

   f. Confusion

   g. Seizures

3. Treatment and Nursing Implications

   a. Monitor serum sodium level

   b. Administer isotonic intravenous solution (e.g., 0.9% NaCl); if serum sodium is <118 mEq/L, administer hypertonic sodium intravenous solution (e.g., 3% NaCl) at a very slow rate

   c. Reorient client as needed and provide safety measures

   d. Seizure precautions

D. Sodium Excess (Hypernatremia)

1. Causes

   a. Water deprivation

   b. Diabetes insipidus

   c. Watery diarrhea

2. Signs and Symptoms

   a. Thirst

   b. Elevated body temperature

   c. Sticky mucous membranes

   d. Lethargy

   e. Disorientation

   f. Seizures

3. Treatment and Nursing Implications

   a. Administer oral fluids.

   b. Administer hypotonic intravenous solutions (e.g., D_5W, 0.2% NaCl, or 0.45% NaCl)

   c. Maintain seizure precautions

   d. Administer desmopressin acetate (DDAVP) nasal spray to slow diuresis of diabetes insipidus

E. Potassium Deficit (Hypokalemia)

1. Causes

   a. Diarrhea

   b. Vomiting

   c. GI suction

   d. Diuretics

2. Signs and Symptoms

   a. Fatigue

   b. Muscle weakness

   c. Nausea and vomiting

   d. Dysrhythmias

   e. Flat T wave accompanied by ST-segment depression on electrocardiogram (ECG)

   f. Predisposed to digitalis toxicity

3. Treatment and Nursing Implications

   a. Administer potassium supplements PO (oral) or IV (maximum 20mEq/h in diluted IV solution); *never* give IV push (bolus)

   b. Encourage potassium-rich foods (apricots, cantaloupe, bananas, oranges, nuts, dark leafy greens, dried fruits)

   c. Monitor ECG

   d. If patient is receiving digoxin, assess for digitalis toxicity (bradycardia, confusion, dysrhythmias, blurred or " white, green, yellow" vision)

   e. Provide for safety when ambulating, due to weakness

F. Potassium Excess (Hyperkalemia)

1. Causes

   a. Renal failure

   b. Acidosis

   c. Burns

   d. Salt substitute

2. Signs and Symptoms

   a. Muscle weakness to flaccid paralysis

   b. Intestinal colic

   c. Elevated T wave on ECG

3. Treatment and Nursing Implications

   a. Administer sodium polystyrene sulfonate (Kayexalate) by mouth or enema

   b. Administer calcium gluconate (IV)

   c. Administer $D_{10}W$ (10% dextrose in water) and regular insulin IV

   d. Dialysis

   e. Monitor ECG pattern for dysrhythmias

   f. Restrict potassium in diet

   g. Monitor for adequate urinary output

G. Calcium Deficit (Hypocalcemia)

1. Causes

   a. Hypoparathyroidism

   b. Incidental removal of or trauma to parathyroid glands during thyroidectomy or radical neck surgery

   c. Malabsorption

   d. Vitamin D deficiency

2. Signs and Symptoms

   a. Circumoral tingling

   b. Numbness in fingers and toes

   c. Trousseau's sign

   d. Chvostek's sign

   e. Seizures

3. Treatment and Nursing Implications

   a. Administer calcium gluconate PO (oral) or slow IV (intravenously); give oral form before meals with milk

   b. Administer alendronate (Fosamax), which slows abnormal and normal bone reabsorption without inhibiting bone formation and mineralization. It is used for treatment and prevention of osteoporosis in postmenopausal women and osteoporosis in men.

   c. Observe seizure precautions

   d. Assess for positive Trousseau's and Chvostek's signs

H. Calcium Excess (Hypercalcemia)

1. Causes

   a. Hyperparathyroidism

   b. Malignant neoplastic disease

   c. Prolonged immobilization

   d. Excess calcium supplements

2. Signs and Symptoms

   a. Muscle weakness

   b. Constipation

   c. Nausea and vomiting

   d. Cardiac dysrhythmias

   e. Renal calculi

3. Treatment and Nursing Implications

   a. Encourage fluids

   b. Administer 0.9% NaCl IV (intravenous) with furosemide (Lasix)

   c. Encourage weight bearing when allowed

   d. Administer phosphorus PO or IV

   e. Administer calcitonin subcutaneously or IV

   f. Monitor ECG pattern

   g. Encourage high-fiber diet to prevent constipation

   h. Assess for renal colic

I. Magnesium Deficit (Hypomagnesemia)

1. Causes

   a. Alcoholism

   b. Chronic malnutrition

   c. Diabetic ketoacidosis

2. Signs and Symptoms

   a. Neuromuscular irritability

   b. Disorientation

   c. Hallucinations

3. Treatment and Nursing Implications

   a. Administer magnesium sulfate deep IM (intramuscular) or IV

   b. Observe seizure precautions

J. Magnesium Excess (Hypermagnesemia)

1. Causes

   a. Renal failure

   b. Medications containing magnesium

2. Signs and Symptoms

   a. Flushing

   b. Hypotension

   c. Hypoactive reflexes

   d. Depressed respirations

   e. Cardiac arrest

3. Treatment and Nursing Implications

   a. Administer calcium gluconate IV

   b. Dialysis

   c. Monitor blood pressure, respiratory rate/depth, and ECG pattern

   d. Avoid antacids containing magnesium

III. NORMAL ARTERIAL BLOOD GASES

A. pH = 7.35 to 7.45

B. PO_2 = 80 to 100 mm Hg

C. PCO_2 = 35 to 45 mm Hg

D. O_2 saturation = 95% to 100%

E. Bicarbonate = 22 to 26 mEq/L

IV. ACID–BASE IMBALANCES

A. Metabolic Acidosis

1. Causes

   a. Diabetes mellitus (fat used for energy, ketones produced)

   b. Starvation (fat used for energy, ketones produced)

   c. Shock, myocardial infarction (lack of oxygen results in anaerobic metabolism producing lactic acid and hypotension)

   d. Renal failure (potassium and hydrogen ions retained)

   e. Acetylsalicylic acid overdose (acid producing)

   f. Diarrhea (bicarbonate base lost)

   g. Intestinal fistulas (bicarbonate base lost)

2. Signs and Symptoms

   a. Confusion

   b. Drowsiness

   c. Headache

   d. Kussmaul's respirations

   e. Decreased cardiac output

   f. pH <7.35

   g. PCO_2 normal or <35 mm Hg, if compensating

   h. Bicarbonate level <22 mEq/L

3. Treatment and Nursing Implications

   a. Maintain in Fowler's position

   b. Monitor ECG pattern

   c. Assess for hyperkalemia

   d. Administer sodium bicarbonate IV

B. Respiratory Acidosis

1. Causes

   a. Chronic obstructive pulmonary disease (COPD)

   b. Any condition that interferes with O_2/CO_2 exchange in the lungs

   c. Drug overdose (respiratory depression)

2. Signs and Symptoms

   a. Dizziness

   b. Palpitations

   c. Headache

   d. Drowsiness

   e. Confusion

   f. Ventricular fibrillation

   g. Decreased cardiac output

   h. pH <7.35

   i. PCO_2 >45 mm Hg

   j. Bicarbonate level normal or >26 mEq/L, if compensating

3. Treatment and Nursing Implications

   a. Administer oxygen (low flow [2 L] with COPD)

   b. Administer sodium bicarbonate IV

C. Metabolic Alkalosis

1. Causes

   a. Vomiting (loss of HCl)

   b. GI suction (loss of HCl)

   c. Diuretics (loss of bicarbonate)

   d. Hyperaldosteronism (aldosterone retains sodium; potassium is excreted in the urine and hydrogen ions always follow potassium, thus possibly causing metabolic acidosis)

   e. Cushing's syndrome (too much steroids)

2. Signs and Symptoms

   a. Increased muscle irritability

   b. Tetany

   c. Slow, shallow respirations

   d. Disorientation

   e. Seizures

   f. pH >7.45

   g. PCO_2 normal or >45 mm Hg, if compensating

   h. Bicarbonate level >26 mEq/L

3. Treatment and Nursing Implications

   a. Administer Ringer's solution IV

   b. Administer acetazolamide (Diamox)

D. Respiratory Alkalosis

1. Causes

   a. High fever with rapid respiratory rate

   b. Hyperventilation

2. Signs and Symptoms

   a. Lightheadedness

   b. Palpitations

   c. Increased muscle irritability

   d. pH >7.45

   e. PCO_2 <35 mm Hg

   f. Bicarbonate level normal or <22 mEq/L, if compensating

3. Treatment and Nursing Implications

   a. Rebreathing bag

   b. Control elevated temperature with antipyretics

Chapter

13

Renal and Urinary Disorders

TOPICAL OUTLINE

I. RENAL FUNCTION

A. Regulation of pH

Kidneys excrete either hydrogen ions or bicarbonate ions to maintain acid–base balance.

B. Maintenance of Blood Pressure

1. Renin is released by the kidney in response to decreased blood pressure. Renin reacts with angiotensinogen (a plasma protein formed by the liver) to form angiotensin I, which is converted in the lungs to angiotensin II. Angiotensin II increases the blood pressure by causing vasoconstriction and stimulating the release of aldosterone (from the adrenal cortex).

2. Aldosterone causes sodium retention, and sodium retains water. Therefore, as blood volume increases, blood pressure increases.

3. Antidiuretic hormone (ADH), secreted by the posterior pituitary gland, causes the kidney to reabsorb water, thereby increasing blood volume and blood pressure.

II. URINARY TRACT DIAGNOSTIC STUDIES

A. Urine Specimens

1. Clean-catch midstream: Patient washes perineal area, then catches urine in a sterile container midstream. Used to detect bacterial infection. Normal result: no bacterial growth or less than 100,000/dL.

2. Double-void specimen: Patient voids and discards first specimen. Second specimen is used to check for glucose and acetone. Normal result: negative for glucose and acetone.

3. Catheterized specimen: When a sterile specimen is required, urine is collected through the catheter.

4. Twenty-four–hour specimen: Patient voids, discards urine, and notes time. All urine for next 24 h is collected and kept in a container with chemical additives and/or placed on ice. May be ordered for measurement of creatinine clearance to evaluate glomerular filtration rate. Normal creatinine clearance: 15 to 25 mg/kg body weight/24 h.

B. Serum Creatinine

Used to diagnose impaired renal function. Level increases as renal function decreases. Normal level: 0.6 to 1.2 mg/dL.

C. Blood Urea Nitrogen

Used to detect declining renal function. Level increases as renal function decreases. May also be elevated with dehydration, excessive protein intake, starvation, and gastrointestinal bleeding. Normal level: 11 to 23 mg/dL.

D. Intravenous Pyelography

1. Description: X-ray with contrast dye injected intravenously to visualize the kidneys, renal pelvis, ureters, and bladder.

2. Purpose: Diagnosis of renal calculi or structural abnormalities.

3. Patient preparation: Check for allergies to shellfish or iodine. Withhold fluids for 8 to 10 h before the x-ray to increase the dye concentration for better visualization. Elderly patients may not tolerate this and, with a physician's approval, may be given water the hour before the test. Cathartics or enemas may be ordered to clear the bowel for better visualization.

4. Postprocedure care: Ensure adequate hydration to eliminate dye from the kidneys. Assess for allergic reaction to dye (e.g., itching, hives, rash, tight feeling in the throat, shortness of breath, and anaphylaxis).

E. Retrograde Pyelography

1. Description: X-ray with contrast dye injected through a catheter into the bladder and retrograde into the ureters and renal pelvis.

2. Purpose: May be used when intravenous pyelography (IVP) is inconclusive and if patient is hypersensitive to intravenous (IV) contrast medium.

3. Patient preparation: Same as for IVP.

4. Postprocedure care: Assess patient's ability to void. May complain of dysuria and pink-tinged urine. Assess for infection.

5. Ensure adequate hydration.

F. Cystoscopy

1. Description: Endoscopy that provides direct visualization of the urethra, the bladder, and, in males, the prostate gland.

2. Purpose: Permits identification of the cause of hematuria (e.g., infection, tumor, or trauma).

3. Patient preparation: Laxatives and/or enemas may be ordered to clear the bowel. Increase fluids PO or IV to maintain continuous flow of urine for collection and to prevent infection. If procedure is done under general anesthesia, patient is NPO.

4. Postprocedure care: Encourage fluid intake. Assess ability to void. Patient may complain of dysuria, pink-tinged urine, or bladder spasms. Administer belladonna and opium (B&O) suppositories or antispasmodics such as propantheline bromide (Pro-Banthine) as ordered. Advise patient that urine may be discolored from dyes used during the procedure. Notify physician of bright red urine or clots. Monitor for bacteremia (severe fever and chills).

G. Renal Arteriography

1. Description: X-ray with contrast dye injected through a femoral artery catheter into the renal artery.

2. Purpose: Permits visualization of the renal artery. May reveal cause of diminished renal blood flow (e.g., stenosis of the artery).

3. Patient preparation: Same as for IVP. Usually performed under local anesthesia with preprocedure sedation. Inform patient that a feeling of heat may be sensed briefly along the course of the vessel when contrast medium is injected.

4. Postprocedure care: Palpate peripheral pulses. Note color and temperature of affected leg and compare with those of uninvolved leg. Institute bed rest with affected extremity straight. Apply pressure dressing to catheter insertion site *to control bleeding*.

5. Ensure adequate hydration of 2000 to 2500 cc.

H. Renal Biopsy

1. Description: May be performed as a needle aspiration, percutaneous punch biopsy, or open surgical tissue excision.

2. Purpose: Used to diagnose renal disease and differentiate tumor type. Allows for microscopic examination of tissue.

3. Patient preparation: Usually performed under local anesthesia with little to no premedication. Patient is placed in prone position with sandbag or pillow under abdomen.

4. Postprocedure care: Monitor vital signs and biopsy site every 5 to 10 min. Bed rest and avoid straining for 24 h. Obtain serial urine specimens to assess bleeding. Encourage large fluid intake. At discharge, advise patient to avoid strenuous activity for 2 weeks and continue monitoring for hemorrhage.

III. URINARY RETENTION

Urine production continues, but the urine remains in the bladder. The patient is unable to void or to completely empty the bladder. To determine urine residual, an in-and-out catheter can be used or a bladder scan performed.

A. Causes

Spinal anesthesia, atonic bladder after surgery, neurogenic bladder (spinal cord injury), and benign prostatic hypertrophy.

B. Diagnosis

1. Have client void (if possible), then catheterize for residual urine remaining in the bladder.

2. Palpate above symphysis pubis for bladder distention.

C. Consequences of Urine Retention

1. Infection

2. Inflammation

3. Urolithiasis (calculi)

D. Treatment

1. Nursing measures to facilitate voiding (e.g., provide privacy, assist to sitting or standing position, run water in sink or toilet).

2. Administer bethanechol (Urecholine) subcutaneously as ordered to stimulate bladder contraction. *Never* administer if mechanical obstruction is a possible cause of urine retention.

3. Catheterize as ordered.

4. Medtronic InterStim Therapy for Urinary Control

    a. Indications: InterStim Therapy for Urinary Control is indicated for treatment of urinary retention and symptoms of overactive bladder, including urinary urge incontinence and significant symptoms of urgency frequency alone or in combination, in patients who have failed or could not tolerate more conservative treatments.

    b. Contraindications: Implant of the InterStim System is contraindicated if patients have not demonstrated an appropriate response to test stimulation or are unable to operate the neurostimulator. Also, the use of diathermy (e.g., short-wave diathermy, microwave diathermy, or therapeutic ultrasound diathermy) is contraindicated because diathermy's energy can be transferred through the implanted system (or any of the separate implanted components), which can cause tissue damage and result in severe injury or death. Diathermy can damage parts of the neurostimulation system; therefore, assessment of the patient for appropriate response to test stimulation and the patient demonstrating the ability to operate the neurostimulator are very important.

c. Precautions/Adverse Events: Safety and effectiveness have not been established for bilateral stimulation; patients with neurologic diseases such as multiple sclerosis; use during pregnancy and delivery; or use in pediatric patients younger than 16 years. System may be affected by, or adversely affect, cardiac pacemakers or therapies, cardioverter-defibrillators, electrocautery, external defibrillators, ultrasonic equipment, radiation therapy, magnetic resonance imaging (MRI), theft detectors, and screening devices. Adverse effects related to the therapy, device, or procedure can include pain at the implant sites, lead infection, skin irritation, technical or device problems, transient electric shock, adverse change in bowel or voiding function, numbness, nerve injury, seroma at the neurostimulator site, change in menstrual cycle, and undesirable stimulation or sensations.

Note: Warning: This therapy is not intended for patients with mechanical obstruction such as benign prostatic hypertrophy, cancer, or urethral stricture.

IV. PROSTATE DISORDERS

A. Benign Prostatic Hyperplasia

1. Benign prostatic hyperplasia (BPH) is a nonmalignant increase in proliferation of glandular and intercellular tissue of the prostate.

1. Incidence

   a. BPH is common in men older than 40 years (mean age 65 years).

   b. The incidence of BPH increases with age from the fifth decade of life through the end of life; more than 90 percent of men in their 80s have BPH.

   c. The incidence is highest is African-Americans and lowest in Asians, with the Japanese showing an appreciably lower incidence.

2. Etiology

   a. Most men older than 50 years have some prostatic enlargement in benign prostatic hypertrophy or hyperplasia (BPH). The prostatic gland enlarges sufficiently to compress the urethra and cause some overt urinary obstruction.

3. Pathophysiology with Signs and Symptoms

   a. The pathogenesis is not well understood, but two features necessary for the process are (a) aging and (b) the presence of testes.

   b. The active androgen that mediates prostatic growth at all ages is dihydrotestosterone. It now is believed that dihydrotestosterone levels in the prostate increase with aging, which might explain prostatic hyperplasia.

   c. BPH usually develops slowly; therefore, it may be overlooked and attributed solely to the aging process.

   d. Signs and symptoms of BPH depend on (a) the extent of prostatic enlargement and (b) the lobes affected.

   e. With increasing urethral obstruction, the following signs and symptoms occur: hesitancy in initiating voiding, postvoiding dribbling, sensation of incomplete emptying, and occasionally urinary retention.

   f. These obstructive symptoms must be distinguished from irritative symptoms such as dysuria, frequency, and urgency, which result from inflammation, infection, or neoplastic causes.

   g. As the amount of residual urine increases, nocturia, overflow incontinence, and palpable bladder may be present.

   h. Eventually, the manifestations of chronic urinary retention and obstruction occur, or acute urinary retention can be precipitated by infection, tranquilizing drugs, or alcohol.

4. Diagnosis

   a. Diagnosis is made by rectal examination and ultrasonography with a rectal probe.

   b. The presence of upper urinary tract reflux and the extent of bladder emptying can be documented by IVP with postvoiding film or renal sonogram of bladder residual.

5. Treatment

   a. Many patients who receive no therapy experience no progression in symptoms over many years.

   b. Several forms of medical or surgical treatment are available for men with more advanced symptoms.

   c. Treatment with luteinizing hormone-releasing hormone (LHRH), finasteride (Proscar), and terazosin hydrochloride (Hytrin) shrinks prostatic glandular hyperplasia by lowering tissue dihydrotestosterone levels.

   d. Therapy with alpha-adrenergic antagonists are used to lower bladder, neck, and urethral resistance but is not approved by the US Food and Drug Administration for this purpose. A research study financed by Merck & Co., the maker of Proscar, and Abbott Laboratories, Inc., the maker of Hytrin (1997), discovered that Hytrin eased discomfort in only one third of men and that Proscar was no better than a placebo.

   e. Surgery has been and still is the benchmark treatment. Indications for surgery include decrease in urine flow of sufficient magnitude to cause discomfort, persistent residual urine, acute urinary retention due to obstruction with no reversible precipitating cause, and hydronephrosis.

f. Transurethral prostatectomy (TURP) is the usual procedure of choice for BPH.

g. Open prostatectomy is used for cancer; massive glands may require retropubic, suprapubic, or perineal approaches.

h. Newer surgical alternatives for BPH include simple transurethral incision prostatectomy and transurethral laser-induced prostatectomy.

i. Nonsurgical interventional therapies for BPH that are undergoing intense study include indwelling urethral stent and balloon dilation of the prostate.

6. Nursing implications

a. Preoperative care includes (a) administering enema as ordered and assessing urinary output, vital signs, and laboratory values, and (b) ensuring that the preoperative permit is signed by patient.

b. Postoperative care includes

(1) Monitoring serum electrolytes and reporting abnormal results to the physician

(2) Assessing for signs of urethral catheter obstruction or increased bladder spasms, pain, or absence of urine

c. If three-way continuous, bladder irrigation is used, check the patient frequently (every 15 min for the first 2 to 4 h, and every 2 h until irrigation is discontinued) for

(1) Bladder distention

(2) Amount of bloody drainage

(3) Shock and hemorrhage

(4) Bladder spasms

Check urinary catheter patency and observe the catheter for blood clots or kinked tubing. Observe the patient for signs of hyponatremia, which include restlessness, disorientation, hypotension, and nausea. Administer B&O suppositories.

d. After the catheter is removed, patients may experience frequency, dribbling, and occasional hematuria. Reassure them that they gradually will regain urinary control, and most symptoms will subside within 2 or 3 weeks.

e. Instruct patients to follow the prescribed oral antibiotic drug regimen and explain the reasons for using a gentle laxative (to prevent straining that may precipitate bleeding).

f. Urge patients to seek medical care immediately if they cannot void, if they are still passing bloody urine (3 weeks after surgery), or if they develop fever.

B. Prostatic Carcinoma

1. Incidence

a. Cancer of the prostate is the most common malignancy in men in the United States and is the second most common cause of death in men older than 55 years (after carcinoma of the lungs and colon).

b. The disease is more common among African-Americans than whites; the reason for this is not known.

2. Diagnosis

a. The posterior surface of the lateral lobe, where carcinoma begins most often, is easily palpable on digital rectal examination.

b. Carcinoma characteristically is hard, nodular, and irregular.

c. It is important that rectal examination be a routine part of the physical examination of men.

d. Elevation of serum prostate-specific antigen (PSA) level is the most sensitive test for early detection of prostatic cancer. PSA level is increased in patients with BPH but does not continue to increase as the disease progresses; in contrast, PSA level continues to increase in patients with prostate cancer.

e. Transrectal prostatic sonography reveals carcinoma but is not specific enough for use as a screening test. Ultrasonography is useful for directing needle biopsy and for documenting the degree of extension of the tumor into the bladder and seminal vesicles.

f. Biopsy of the prostate is essential for establishing the diagnosis and is indicated when an abnormality is detected by palpation or elevation of serum PSA level.

3. Etiology

a. The cause is unknown.

4. Pathophysiology and Signs and Symptoms

a. The majority of cancers occurring in the prostate are adenocarcinomas. These are slow-growing tumors that originate in the posterior portion of the prostate and eventually involve the entire gland.

b. Undetected, the tumor spreads to the seminal vesicles, bladder, urethra, and pelvic region. The bones and lymph nodes, as well as the ileum, are common sites of metastasis.

c. Both early and advanced carcinoma of the prostate may be asymptomatic at the time of diagnosis.

d. In symptomatic patients, common presenting complaints (in descending order) include dysuria, difficulty voiding, increased urinary frequency, complete urinary retention, back or hip pain, and hematuria.

5. Treatment

a. Total prostatovesiculectomy is the oldest treatment for cancer of the prostate.

b. The standard staging scheme (stage A) represents cancer not detectable by rectal examination but found in a surgical specimen obtained during operation for prostatic hyperplasia.

c. Surgical staging is the common modality for assessing lymph node involvement and determining therapy, with A representing the first stages of cancer and D representing the metastatic disease.

d. Treatment varies with each stage of the disease and generally includes radiation, removal of testes to reduce androgen production, and hormone therapy with synthetic estrogen diethylstilbestrol (DES) to decrease androgen production.

e. Androgen deprivation by means of bilateral orchiectomy (removal of testes), DES, or combined orchiectomy plus DES was a standard form of treatment for years. Subsequently, in prospective control studies, the effectiveness of high-dose DES or orchiectomy, alone or in combination, in enhancing survival in any stage of prostate cancer was not successful. Furthermore, death from cardiovascular disease was more frequent in clients treated with large doses of DES. Leuprolide (Lupron) antineoplastic hormone has largely replaced estrogen therapy because of its safer cardiovascular profile. This drug inhibits luteinizing hormone (LH) secretion, thereby lowering plasma testosterone levels.

f. Each of the above forms of androgen ablation still leaves a small amount of circulating adrenal androgen that may be detrimental in controlling advanced prostatic cancer.

g. Androgen depletion beyond that achieved by surgical removal of testes, antineoplastic hormone therapy, or estrogen administration can be accomplished by adrenalectomy or hypophysectomy.

h. Adrenalectomy can be accomplished by either surgical ablation or therapy with drugs such as exogenous glucocorticoids, which block the synthesis of adrenal androgen.

i. Although proof of efficacy is lacking, the current trend is for adrenal and testes androgen ablation in advanced prostate cancer.

j. Interstitial radiation involves retropubic or perineal implantation of seeds ^{125}I or ^{198}Au. Successful seed implantation requires a well-defined primary tumor with a diameter less than 5 cm.

k. Potency is preserved in more than 90 percent, and early complications are fewer and less severe than those after external radiation. External radiation causes impotence, and frequent morbidity follows either form of radiation.

l. Current data suggest that radiation therapy may be less curative than radical prostatectomy.

6. Nursing Implications

a. A primary diagnosis for a client diagnosed with prostatic cancer could be anxiety, related to diagnosis and treatment plan.

V. LOWER URINARY TRACT INFECTION: CYSTITIS AND URETHRITIS

Cystitis and urethritis, the two forms of lower urinary tract infection (UTI), are more common in women than in men. Lower UTI is a prevalent bacterial disease in children, with girls most commonly affected. The nurse must be aware that UTI in children (girls) can be the result of sexual abuse.

A. Causes

1. Most lower UTIs result from ascending infection by a single gram-negative enteric bacterium, such as *Escherichia coli*, *Pseudomonas*, or *Klebsiella*.

2. In patients with an indwelling Foley catheter or fistula between the intestine and bladder, a lower UTI may result from simultaneous infection with multiple pathogens.

B. Signs and Symptoms

1. Dysuria

2. Frequency

3. Urgency

4. Cloudy urine

5. Hematuria

6. Low back and suprapubic pain

7. Fever

8. Malaise

C. Treatment/Nursing Implications

1. Administer antibiotics such as trimethoprim and sulfamethoxazole (Bactrim, Cipro, Septra), nitrofurantoin (Macrodantin), and cephalexin (Keflex), and an analgesic such as phenazopyridine (Pyridium), as ordered.

2. Increase fluid to 2–3 L/day to flush out bacteria.

3. Encourage acid-ash diet (cranberries, meats, eggs, cheese, prunes, plums, whole grains). No carbonated beverages.

4. Teach female client perineal hygiene (cleanse from front to back).

5. Encourage frequent emptying of bladder.

6. Pyridium is given to relieve symptoms of urinary frequency but will turn urine an orange-red color.

VI. ACUTE GLOMERULONEPHRITIS

Usually caused by beta-hemolytic streptococci. Occurs 2 to 3 weeks after a sore throat or skin infection. May persist for months. Recovery usually begins in approximately 2 weeks. Can progress to a chronic state and renal failure.

A. Cause

Immunological reaction: Trapping of antigen–antibody complexes in the glomerulus, resulting in glomerular inflammation.

B. Signs and Symptoms

1. Fever

2. Nausea and vomiting

3. Abdominal and flank pain

4. Generalized edema

5. Moderate to severe hypertension

6. Headache

7. Hematuria and proteinuria

8. Increased serum blood urea nitrogen (BUN) and creatinine levels

9. Oliguria and anuria

C. Treatment/Nursing Implications

1. Complete bed rest. Provide diversionary activities.

2. Assess for skin breakdown caused by edema, prolonged bed rest, and lack of protein.

3. Administer prescribed antibiotics, diuretics, antihypertensives, corticosteroids, and immunosuppressants.

4. Restrict fluids. Relieve thirst with hard candies and ice chips. Strict intake and output (I&O).

5. High-calorie, low-sodium, low-protein diet to allow kidney to rest and decrease edema.

6. Plasmapheresis.

7. Daily weights.

8. Restrict visitors with obvious illness because patient's immune system is depressed.

VII. NEPHROTIC SYNDROME

Protein wasting condition that results from glomerular damage and abnormal increased permeability of the glomerulus to protein molecules.

A. Causes

1. Glomerulonephritis

2. Diabetes mellitus

3. Systemic lupus erythematosus (SLE)

4. Hepatitis B

5. Allergic reactions

6. Medication reactions

7. Sickle cell disease

8. Congestive heart failure (CHF)

B. Signs and Symptoms

1. Proteinuria

2. Hypoalbuminemia

3. Generalized edema

C. Treatment/Nursing Implications

1. Administer steroids as ordered to decrease glomerular inflammation.

2. Administer anticoagulants and antiplatelet agents as ordered. (Decreased blood volume predisposes to blood clots and renal vein thrombosis.)

3. Administer loop diuretics as ordered to decrease edema. Monitor for electrolyte imbalances such as hypokalemia.

4. Administer salt-poor albumin as ordered to increase colloid osmotic pressure and decrease edema.

5. Institute high-biologic-value protein, high-calorie, low-sodium diet.

VIII. RENAL CALCULI

◆ Renal calculi or nephrolithiasis (common only called *kidney stones*) may form anywhere in the urinary tract but usually develop in the renal pelvis or the calyces of the kidney. Calculi formation follows precipitation of substance normally dissolved in the urine, such as calcium oxalate, calcium phosphate, magnesium ammonium phosphate, or occasionally urate or cystine. Renal calculi vary in size and may be solitary or multiple.

◆ Calcium calculi are the most common, accounting for more than 75% of all calculi, but they may be composed of uric acid, cystine, oxalate, or struvite.

◆ Usually appears between ages 20 and 30 years.

◆ Two to three times more common in males.

A. Causes

1. Dehydration

2. Stasis of urine

3. Protein, bacteria, or inflammatory products in the urine

4. Immobility

5. Metabolic factors that may predispose to renal calculi include extremely high doses of vitamin D administered to patients with hypoparathyroidism, and patients with hyperparathyroidism, renal tubular acidosis, elevated uric acid level (usually gout).

6. Infection (injured site serves as a site for calculus development)

7. Obstruction caused by urinary stasis (as in immobility from spinal cord injury) allows calculi constituents to collect and adhere, causing an obstruction. Obstruction causes infection, which compounds the obstruction.

B. Signs and Symptoms

1. Sudden sharp, severe flank pain; testicular pain in men

2. Pallor and diaphoresis

3. Nausea and vomiting

4. Hematuria

C. Treatment/Nursing implications

1. Administer narcotic analgesics and antiemetics (first priority).

2. Ambulate patient.

3. Encourage fluids (after IVP is completed).

4. Strain all urine. Check for stones.

5. Extracorporeal shock wave lithotripsy (ESWL), percutaneous ultrasonic lithotripsy (PUL), ureteral basket extraction via cystoscopy, or open surgical removal of stones (ureterolithotomy, pyelolithotomy, or nephrolithotomy).

D. Postprocedure Nursing Care

1. Encourage increased fluid intake (3–4 L/day).

2. Assess for hemorrhage (increasing flank pain, bloody urine, decreased blood pressure, decreased hematocrit), infection (increased temperature, cloudy urine, increased white blood cell count), and urinary retention (palpable bladder, absence of voiding).

3. Strain all urine for stone fragments.

4. Ensure patency of nephrostomy tube (following PUL or open surgical procedure). This should be draining continuously, a minimum of 30 cc/h.

5. Change sterile dressing around Penrose drain frequently (following open surgical procedure). Keep dressing dry and protect skin against urinary drainage.

E. Discharge Diet Teaching

1. If calcium stone: Acid-ash and calcium-restricted diet (limit dairy products).

2. If uric acid stone: Alkaline-ash and low-purine diet (limit cheeses, wine, and organ meats); allopurinol (Lopurin, Zyloprim).

3. If oxalate stone: Low-oxalate diet (avoid tea, instant coffee, chocolate, colas, citrus fruits, peanuts).

4. If cystine stone: Alkaline-ash and low-protein diet; penicillamine (Cuprimine, Penicillamine); reduce excessive cystine, resulting in a substance more soluble than cystine that is readily excreted.

IX. HYDRONEPHROSIS

Distention of the renal pelvis as a result of obstruction.

A. Causes

1. Renal calculi

2. Tumor

3. BPH

B. Signs and Symptoms

1. Pyelonephritis

2. Decreasing renal function

C. Treatment/Nursing Implications

1. Relieve obstruction (removal of stone, tumor). Watch for large urine output indicating postobstructive reflex diuresis.

2. Administer antibiotics as ordered to treat infection.

3. Encourage increased fluid intake.

X. RENAL CANCER

May be advanced with metastasis before diagnosed.

A. Signs and Symptoms

1. Painless hematuria

2. Dysuria

3. Local obstruction from blood clots (caused by prothrombin deficiency). Nursing implication: administer vitamin K.

4. Fistula formation (fistula can also be a sign of anemia)

B. Treatment

1. Surgical kidney removal

C. Nursing Implications after Surgery

1. Measure urine output hourly for early detection of renal failure.

2. Maintain meticulous catheter care. Prevent infection.

3. Manage pain with narcotic analgesics or nonsteroidal antiinflammatory drugs (NSAIDs), as ordered.

4. Institute aggressive respiratory care (turn, cough, deep breathe, incentive spirometry) to reestablish effective breathing patterns.

5. Maintain sterile wound care.

XI. BLADDER CANCER

Most frequent neoplasm of the urinary tract.

A. Possible Causes

1. Cigarette smoke

2. Bladder calculi

3. Chronic cystitis

4. Industrial exposure to chemicals

5. High phenacetin intake

B. Signs and Symptoms

1. Painless hematuria

2. Dysuria

3. Obstruction

4. Fistula formation

C. Treatment

1. Systemic chemotherapy

2. Radium implant

3. External radiation

4. Hydrostatic distention (compression of the tumor with large balloon-tipped catheter to produce ischemic necrosis of tumor)

5. Cystectomy

D. Care Following Cystectomy

1. Partial cystectomy: Closely monitor urinary catheter output. Bladder capacity may be as little as 60 mL.

2. Total cystectomy with urinary diversion (ileal conduit or continent urostomy) (Kock's pouch—same as ileal conduit with nipple valves at junction of ureters and pouch and at stomal opening, which prevents reflux of urine from pouch back into ureters and prevents flow of urine through stoma; requires catheterization of stoma at least every 6 h). Closely monitor urinary output (expect pink-tinged urine with mucus). Inspect stoma for color and patency. Watch for peritonitis, hemorrhage, and urine leakage into abdomen.

E. Nursing Implications after Surgery

1. Measure urine output hourly for early detection of renal failure.

2. Maintain meticulous catheter care. Prevent infection.

3. Manage pain with narcotic analgesics, as ordered.

4. Institute aggressive respiratory care (turn, cough, deep breathe, incentive spirometry) to reestablish effective breathing patterns.

5. Maintain sterile wound care.

XII. RENAL FAILURE

A. Causes

1. Trauma

2. Shock (hemorrhage, burns, or cardiogenic)

3. Toxins

4. Drug overdose

5. Glomerulonephritis

6. Renal artery obstruction

7. Diabetes mellitus

8. Hypertension

B. Signs and Symptoms

1. Elevated serum creatinine and BUN levels

2. Oliguria/anuria (may be preceded by a period of polyuria)

3. Azotemia

4. Metabolic acidosis

C. Major Consequences

1. Fluid overload (or deficit during polyuria stage), hyperkalemia, hypocalcemia, hypermagnesemia, and hyperphosphatemia

2. Metabolic acidosis

3. Anemia as a result of decreased erythropoietin and decreased red blood cell lifespan

4. Anorexia, nausea and vomiting, diarrhea

5. Platelet dysfunction

6. Increased incidence of pericarditis

7. Tremors, convulsions, coma

D. Treatment

1. Restrict fluids based on fraction of urine output (if any) plus 400 cc to cover insensible losses of body fluid.

2. Restrict potassium intake.

3. Administer diuretics (e.g., mannitol [Osmitrol]), as ordered.

4. Institute low-protein (high-biologic-value) diet.

5. Peritoneal dialysis: Instill by gravity approximately 1 L of sterile dialysate at room temperature. Roll patient from side to side to remove fluid. Strict I&O. Common complication is peritonitis.

6. Hemodialysis: May use external shunt or surgically constructed internal arteriovenous fistula for long-term access. The shunt can be used as soon as implanted. Fistula must mature 4 to 6 weeks. Danger with shunt is exsanguination. Check fistula for bruit, indicating it is functional. There is danger of infection with both accesses. Common complication of hemodialysis is viral hepatitis type B. Hepatitis B is transmitted by contaminated blood and by human secretions and feces. As a result, nurses, physicians, laboratory technicians, and dentists are frequently exposed to type B hepatitis, in many cases as a result of wearing defective gloves.

XIII. RENAL TRANSPLANTS

A. Donor

Most donors are cadavers. Criteria for acceptable donor include age younger than 60 years, normal renal function, no malignancies outside of central nervous system, no systemic infection, no hypertension, negative hepatitis B antigen, negative human immunodeficiency virus (HIV), no abdominal or renal trauma, and continuous ventilation and heartbeat until the kidneys are surgically removed from the donor. The most desirable donor is a living, related donor who matches the patient closely for ABO blood group and tissue type.

B. Major Complications

1. Infection: Most serious in early transplant period. Common sites include urinary tract, lungs, and blood. Early signs are masked by immunosuppressive medications.

2. Rejection: May be acute (usually occurring within 6 weeks of transplant) or chronic (occurring slowly over months to years and mimicking chronic renal failure). Signs of rejection include fever, malaise, anemia, and graft tenderness. Maintenance doses of immunosuppressive agents and corticosteroids are required lifelong. Serious consequences of immunosuppressive therapy include increased susceptibility to infection, increased risk of malignancy, and degenerative bone disease.

3. Hypertension: Occurs in approximately half of recipients as a result of renal artery stenosis, acute tubular necrosis, graft rejection, steroids, and antirejection medications.

EXAMINATION

1. Which of the following causes proteinuria, hypoalbuminemia, hyperlipidemia, and edema?
   1. Nephrotic syndrome.
   2. Cystinuria.
   3. Renal tubular acidosis.
   4. Chronic renal failure.

2. Azotemia will occur if
   1. The glomerular filtration rate increases.
   2. Nitrogenous substances increase in the plasma.
   3. The blood urea level drops.
   4. Edema develops rapidly.

3. A patient with a BUN level of 90 would most likely display
   1. Hematuria and dysuria.
   2. Confusion and disorientation.
   3. Oliguria and increased respirations.
   4. A fruity odor of breath.

4. When a patient goes into shock, which of the following substances is secreted to aid in maintenance of blood pressure and glomerular filtration?
   1. Renin and aldosterone.
   2. Angiotensin and sodium.
   3. Renin and parathormone.
   4. ADH and corticosteroids.

5. In acute glomerulonephritis, protein appears in the urine because of significant alterations in the permeability of the
   1. Distal convoluted tubules.
   2. Proximal convoluted tubules.
   3. Glomerulus.
   4. Loop of Henle.

6. Billy Adams, a 16-year-old boy, visited his physician because he had developed swelling of his face, eyes, and ankles. In checking the patient's blood pressure, the physician noted hypertension. A urine specimen showed 3+ albumin. The admitting diagnosis is acute glomerulonephritis. A complete history would most likely reveal that Billy recently had
   1. A sore throat.
   2. UTI.
   3. Viral pharyngitis.
   4. A generalized infection.

7. A low-protein diet is ordered for the patient with acute glomerulonephritis because it
   1. Acts as an antidiuretic.
   2. Allows the kidneys to rest.
   3. Decreases antigen–antibody reaction.
   4. Decreases the colloid osmotic pressure in the renal system.

8. The patient with reversible acute renal failure passes through two phases before renal function returns to normal. These two phases are
   1. Polyuria and dysuria.
   2. Anuria and pyuria.
   3. Oliguria and diuresis.
   4. Nocturia and enuresis.

9. Hyperkalemia is the most dangerous electrolyte imbalance resulting from acute renal failure. Which of the following interventions is *not appropriate* in the management of hyperkalemia?
   1. Kayexalate 45 g PO (oral) or rectally.
   2. Calcium gluconate 8 mEq IV push.
   3. Aluminum hydroxide antacids.
   4. Hemodialysis or peritoneal dialysis.

10. Appropriate nursing interventions for the patient with acute glomerulonephritis includes
    1. Instructing regarding a permanent need for low-protein, low-sodium diet.
    2. Encouraging activities as tolerated.
    3. Instructing regarding fluid restriction.
    4. Monitoring for fluid volume deficit.

11. John, a 51-year-old man, was admitted with a medical diagnosis of hydronephrosis secondary to renal calculi. Lithotripsy was successful in relieving the obstruction caused by the calculi. Postprocedure, this client must be closely monitored for
    1. Crystalluria and hypertension.
    2. Fluid volume deficit and hypernatremia.
    3. Increased urine specific gravity and hypokalemia.
    4. Inability to void and reflex diuresis.

12. Bladder cancer is the most common neoplasm of the urinary tract. The *first* sign of bladder cancer usually is
    1. Dysuria.
    2. Pyuria.
    3. Painless hematuria.
    4. Retention secondary to obstruction.

13. Tom, a 55-year-old man, is being treated for recurrent UTIs secondary to BPH. This patient should be instructed to avoid
    1. Alcohol consumption.
    2. Hot tub baths.
    3. Sexual intercourse.
    4. Foods that increase urine acidity.

14. Ray, a 25-year-old man, is admitted for diagnostic studies. His symptoms include flank pain, cloudy urine, and

persistent fatigue. Acute glomerulonephritis is suspected. The data about Ray that would have the greatest significance are

1. Temperature 103°F, polyuria, and tachycardia.
2. Pulse 92, temperature 102°F, and hematuria.
3. Respirations 22, decreased urine specific gravity, and anuria.
4. Blood pressure 152/96, increased urine specific gravity, and proteinuria.

15. Which of the following is the pathologic alteration that occurs with acute glomerulonephritis?

1. Crystallization in the distal tubules of the kidney due to an untoward effect of antipyretic medication.
2. Destruction of glomeruli due to the trapping of circulating antigen–antibody complexes.
3. Inhibition of antibodies resulting from an excess of leukocytes.
4. Sensitivity of toxins resulting from an invading microorganism.

16. The type of prostatectomy most likely to result in impotence is

1. Transurethral.
2. Retropubic.
3. Perineal.
4. Suprapubic.

17. To prevent the *most common* type of urinary calculi from precipitating out in the urine, the treatment most appropriate would be

1. Low-sodium diet and increased hydration.
2. Acid-ash diet and increased hydration.
3. Alkaline-ash diet and allopurinol.
4. Increased fiber in diet.

18. Joel, a 32-year-old man, is admitted with a diagnosis of renal calculus. On admission to the unit, the most nursing priority for this client is to

1. Restrict fluids until the type of stone is diagnosed.
2. Relieve pain until the stone can be removed.
3. Monitor urinary output.
4. Prepare the client for diagnostic studies.

19. Which of the following is a risk factor for developing uric acid kidney stones?

1. Gout.
2. Primary aldosteronism.
3. Large intake of dairy products.
4. Recurrent UTIs.

20. Which of the following may contribute to the formation of urinary calculi?

1. Urinary stasis.
2. An increase in BUN level.
3. Elevated serum creatinine levels.
4. Increased fluid intake.

21. Robert, a 62-year-old man with invasive bladder cancer, is scheduled for a total cystectomy and Kock's pouch. Kock's pouch

1. Is a large segment of ileum that is formed into a bladder, with urine entering via the ureters and exiting via the urethra.
2. Results in continuous flow of urine from an abdominal stoma.
3. Is preferred over an ileal conduit because it eliminates the need for an external collection bag and lessens the potential for skin impairment.
4. Is a temporary reservoir for the collection of urine during treatment of bladder cancer.

22. Following an ureterolithotomy, Thomas has a Foley catheter, a ureteral stent, and a Penrose drain. His I&O are closely monitored. If his urinary output decreases, the RN should *first*

1. Notify the surgeon if the change in urinary output occurs suddenly.
2. Reposition the client onto his side to facilitate drainage of the catheter and stent.
3. Gently irrigate the ureteral stent with 30-cc sterile normal saline.
4. Check tube patency for possible kinks.

23. In which kidney structure does filtration occur?

1. Loop of Henle.
2. Bowman's capsule.
3. Glomerulus.
4. Distal convoluted tubule.

24. Calcium imbalance is commonly seen in patients with renal failure. Appropriate treatment includes

1. Calcium- and phosphorus-restricted diet.
2. High-fiber diet.
3. Aluminum hydroxide (Amphojel) 15 mL qid with meals.
4. Calcitonin (Cibacalcin) 0.5 mg SC daily.

25. The most common complication of peritoneal dialysis is

1. Bowel or bladder perforation.
2. Peritonitis.
3. Hypovolemia.
4. Disequilibrium syndrome.

26. Arthur, a 19-year-old man, is diagnosed with acute glomerulonephritis. The nurse should expect the laboratory results of this patient's urinalysis to show

1. Alkaline pH and specific gravity of 1.008.
2. Albumin 3+ and presence of red blood cells.

3. Clear amber color and small amount of sediment.

4. Decreased uric acid and presence of casts.

27. The type of vascular access for hemodialysis that is least likely to become infected is the
   1. Femoral vein catheter.
   2. Subclavian vein catheter.
   3. External shunt.
   4. Arteriovenous fistula.

28. Infection is a common complication associated with chronic hemodialysis. The most common infecting organism is
   1. *Staphylococcus aureus*.
   2. *Escherichia coli*.
   3. Hepatitis B.
   4. *Pseudomonas*.

29. Ruth is to have a 24-h urine specimen from 10 AM Wednesday until 10 AM Thursday. The nurse should instruct the patient to
   1. Discard urine voided at 10 AM on Wednesday and begin the specimen collection after that, ending at 10 AM Thursday.
   2. Begin the collection with urine voided at 10 AM on Wednesday and end at 10 AM Thursday.
   3. Discard urine voided at 10 AM on Thursday and consider the specimen completed.
   4. Discard only the urine voided on arising Thursday morning, during the 24-h period.

30. The physician ordered Peggy to be catheterized for residual urine. If the urine stops flowing while the patient is being catheterized, the nurse should
   1. Slowly remove the catheter to drain urine that may be near the exit of the bladder.
   2. Quickly remove the catheter because the bladder is considered empty when the urine flow stops.
   3. Carefully move the catheter in and out of the bladder approximately 1 inch to drain urine pooled at any location in the bladder.
   4. Gently push the catheter into the bladder further to drain urine that may have pooled in the upper part of the bladder.

31. Fred comes to the office to have his retention catheter changed. He complains of pain while the nurse is inflating the balloon after the new catheter is in place. The *most likely* cause of discomfort is that the balloon is
   1. In the urethra.
   2. Near the urethral orifice.
   3. Located too low inside the bladder.
   4. Overdistended in the bladder.

32. When a retention catheter is in place, the preferred method of obtaining urine for culture and sensitivity is to
   1. Use a bulb syringe to withdraw urine from the catheter.
   2. Use a sterile syringe and needle to withdraw urine from the catheter port.
   3. Disconnect the tubing and drain the tube between the catheter and drainage bag, using sterile technique.
   4. Using sterile technique, drain 30 mL of urine from the catheter collection bag.

33. David is a 50-year-old man with newly diagnosed end-stage renal disease that resulted from long-term overuse of salicylates. He is admitted to the hospital for construction and maturation of an arteriovenous fistula. Of the following assessment findings, which are consistent with this patient's diagnosis?
   1. Sudden decrease in serum creatinine level and proportional rise in BUN level, loss of skin turgor, and hypokalemia.
   2. Slow decrease in glomerular filtration rate as measured by below-normal creatinine clearance, generalized edema, and hypercalcemia.
   3. Slowly rising serum creatinine level with small contracted kidneys and anemia.
   4. Rapidly rising serum creatinine, polycythemia, and anuria.

34. Mary will receive her first hemodialysis treatment this morning. The nurse plans to withhold breakfast and the AM doses of methyldopa (Aldomet) and hydralazine (Apresoline). The primary reason for withholding these medications is
   1. To prevent nausea and vomiting, as the client will not be given breakfast.
   2. The dosage and patient response would be unpredictable, because the medications would be dialyzed off during the treatment.
   3. Ultrafiltration during dialysis will act as a substitute for the medication.
   4. The medications could cause severe hypotension during dialysis.

35. The best rationale for using a warm dialyzing solution for peritoneal dialysis is that it helps
   1. Promote relaxation of abdominal muscles.
   2. Decrease the risk of peritoneal infection.
   3. Constrict the blood vessels in the peritoneum.
   4. Prevent the body temperature from falling precipitously.

36. Ben, a 52-year-old man, received a kidney transplant. The nurse should implement which of the following measures to avoid a common complication of transplants?
   1. Reverse isolation precautions.
   2. Assessment of clotting time twice daily.

3. Allow the client only limited rest periods.

4. Increase fluid intake to 2500 mL daily.

37. Which of the following criteria must a potential cadaver kidney donor meet?

1. Age below 40 years.

2. No significant illness within last 30 days.

3. No significant hypertension.

4. No significant damage to central nervous system.

38. Stella, a 35-year-old woman, is admitted to the hospital for hypertension. Her blood pressure is 175/96 and pulse rate is 86. Her physician orders a renal arteriogram and an IV of D_5 $1/2$NS to run at 125 mL/h. The reason for ordering the IV to run at this rate prior to the procedure is to

1. Reduce the chances that the dye used in the procedure will damage the kidneys.

2. Allow for better visualization of the kidneys.

3. Reduce chances of an allergic reaction to the dye.

4. Prevent thirst, as the client must be NPO.

39. Which of the following interventions is appropriate when preparing a client for an IVP?

1. Maintain NPO status as ordered for 6 to 8 h prior to procedure and prep bowel as ordered.

2. Maintain IV flow rate at 150 mL/h and encourage PO fluids.

3. Encourage increased fluid intake and check for iodine sensitivity.

4. Advise the patient that the procedure will be done under general anesthesia and obtain a signed consent form.

40. The test for BUN measures the nitrogen portion of urea in the blood. This test is used as a gross index of glomerular function and excretion of urea. The BUN level is increased in

1. Impaired liver function and celiac disease.

2. Overhydration and liver failure.

3. Decreased protein intake and liver failure.

4. Impaired renal function and dehydration.

41. The correct procedure for obtaining specimens to measure creatinine clearance is to

1. Obtain a venous blood sample of 5 mL prior to breakfast.

2. Collect a 24-h urine specimen.

3. Collect a series of venous blood samples: 5 mL every 30 min for a 2-h period.

4. Collect an early-morning clean-catch midstream urine specimen.

42. Judy returns from surgery following a cystectomy and ileal conduit. After surgery, the nurse would anticipate that the physician's orders would include

1. A clear liquid diet.

2. Notifying the physician if mucus or blood is noted in urinary drainage.

3. Hourly measurement of urine output.

4. Catheterization for residual urine after first voiding.

43. In assessing the following renal function test results, the nurse should recognize which values as *abnormal*?

1. Urine specific gravity 1.025, BUN 12 mg/dL.

2. Serum creatinine 0.8 mg/dL, BUN 8 mg/L.

3. Creatinine clearance 120 mL/min, urine specific gravity 1.005.

4. BUN 25 mg/dL, serum creatinine 12 mg/dL.

44. Dennis is scheduled for ESWL. The teaching plan should describe this procedure as

1. Surgical removal of kidney stones.

2. Capture of stones via a cystoscopy.

3. Fragmenting of stones by vibration.

4. Dissolution of stones through medication.

45. Which of the following medications will change the color of urine to red or orange?

1. Amitriptyline (Elavil) and chloroquine (Aralen).

2. Phenytoin (Dilantin) and phenazopyridine (Pyridium).

3. Multiple vitamins and chlorzoxazone (Paraflex).

4. Rifadin (Rifampin) and sulfasalazine (Azulfidine).

46. Which of the following may increase the BUN level?

1. Severe dehydration.

2. Hypervolemia.

3. Long-term use of loop diuretics.

4. Hypernatremia.

47. Nursing care for a patient in the oliguric phase of renal failure would include

1. Encouraging activity and frequent ambulation.

2. Restricting fluid and protein intake.

3. Encouraging fluid intake to 2 to 3 L/24 h.

4. Providing a high-carbohydrate, high-protein diet.

48. The major effects of acute renal failure include all of the following *except*

1. Fluid overload.

2. Alkalosis.

3. Platelet dysfunction.

4. Anorexia.

49. Peritoneal dialysis has been initiated. When the outflow tubing is unclamped to allow the fluid to drain from the peritoneal cavity, no drainage occurs. The priority nursing intervention would be to

1. Connect the tubing to suction.

2. Notify the physician immediately.

3. Change the peritoneal catheter.

4. Turn the client from side to side.

50. Jim underwent surgery to remove his bladder and create an ileal conduit. Which of the following complications is this patient at increased risk for developing compared with other clients undergoing major surgery?

1. Atelectasis.

2. Hemorrhage.

3. Sepsis.

4. Thrombophlebitis.

51. When teaching patients with an ileal conduit how to care for the skin surrounding the stoma, the nurse should advise them to use which of the following?

1. Stomahesive.

2. Karaya.

3. Bacitracin.

4. Denatured alcohol.

52. Which of the following symptoms would the patient with cystitis most likely report?

1. Abdominal pain and dark urine.

2. Dysuria and frequency.

3. Frequent voiding of large amounts of urine and general malaise.

4. Flank pain and fever.

53. The organism most often responsible for a UTI is

1. *Staphylococcus aureus*.

2. *Streptococcus*.

3. *Pseudomonas*.

4. *Escherichia coli*.

54. Peritonitis is a potential complication for the patient receiving peritoneal dialysis. Which of the following findings is most suggestive of this complication?

1. Cloudy return dialysate.

2. Blood-tinged return dialysate.

3. Abdominal pain associated with the dialysis treatment.

4. Difficulty instilling the dialysate into the abdomen.

55. John has a 5-year history of chronic renal failure and is maintained on hemodialysis three times weekly. He has recently developed symptoms of gastritis and tells the nurse that antacids seem to help. Which of following information must the nurse provide for this patient?

1. Be sure to take the antacid after meals to enhance its effect.

2. Avoid antacids containing magnesium.

3. Discontinue the use of antacids and change to a bland diet.

4. Use milk and dairy products instead of antacids to soothe the stomach irritation.

56. Calcium gluconate may be ordered to be given intravenously to a patient with severe hyperkalemia to

1. Decrease the potassium level by active transport.

2. Antagonize the action of potassium on the heart.

3. Prevent acute renal failure.

4. Treat the muscle weakness.

57. James, a 72-year-old man, is admitted with CHF and extracellular fluid volume excess. During the initial assessment of this patient, the nurse should expect to find

1. Absence of breath sounds in the lower lobes of the lungs.

2. Postural decrease in central venous pressure.

3. Moist rales (crackles).

4. Hyperactive reflexes.

58. James is placed on a 2-g sodium diet. The nurse asks him to select foods that best meet his diet prescription. This patient's knowledge of foods lowest in sodium would be accurate if he selected which of the following menus?

1. Tossed salad with blue cheese dressing, canned tuna, and vanilla cookies.

2. Split pea soup, cheese sandwich, and a banana.

3. Baked chicken, lettuce with sliced tomatoes.

4. Beans and frankfurters, carrot and celery sticks, and a plain cupcake.

59. Jill had an appendectomy yesterday. She has a nasogastric tube to low intermittent suction. She is NPO with only ice chips allowed. During her morning bath, Jill complains of a headache and of being more anxious than usual. She is confused. The nurse should recognize these symptoms probably are resulting from

1. Hyponatremia.

2. Hypocalcemia.

3. Hypokalemia.

4. Hyperkalemia.

60. Jane, a 23-year-old woman, is admitted with a diagnosis of dehydration secondary to vomiting for 3 days. Which acid–base imbalance is Jane most likely suffering from?

1. Respiratory acidosis.

2. Respiratory alkalosis.

3. Metabolic acidosis.

4. Metabolic alkalosis.

61. Lillian, age 74 years, develops signs of circulatory overload. She has an IV of D_5 $1/2$NS infusing at 125 mL/h. Which of the following nursing interventions should be included in her plan of care?

1. Consult with physician for IV rate change.

2. Monitor for oliguria.

3. Provide frequent oral care.

4. Assess for diminished breath sounds.

62. Elliott, a 66-year-old man, has been placed on furosemide (Lasix) 40 mg daily. For which one of the following electrolyte imbalances is this patient at risk?
    1. Hypocalcemia.
    2. Hypokalemia.
    3. Hypermagnesemia.
    4. Bicarbonate deficit.

63. Donald's laboratory results indicate that he is in metabolic acidosis. The nurse would be alert to which of the following signs of metabolic acidosis?
    1. Hyperreflexia, paresthesias, and tetany.
    2. Giddiness, irregular respiratory pattern, and moist cool skin.
    3. Muscle weakness and numbness and tingling in the extremities.
    4. Lethargy, disorientation, and tachypnea.

64. As a result of the metabolic acidosis, Donald must be closely monitored for which of the following electrolyte imbalances?
    1. Hypokalemia.
    2. Hyperkalemia.
    3. Hyponatremia.
    4. Hypernatremia.

65. Which of the following is an indication of extracellular fluid volume excess?
    1. Hypernatremia.
    2. Increased hematocrit.
    3. Rapid, thready pulse.
    4. Rapid weight gain.

66. A specific nursing intervention for the patient with *suspected* insufficient ADH would be
    1. Checking vital signs every 4 h.
    2. Restricting fluids.
    3. Checking the urine specific gravity.
    4. Lowering the head of the bed.

67. A patient with chronic obstructive pulmonary disease is admitted with severe dyspnea and copious respiratory secretions. From which of the following acid–base imbalances is this patient most likely suffering?
    1. Metabolic acidosis.
    2. Metabolic alkalosis.
    3. Respiratory acidosis.
    4. Respiratory alkalosis.

68. Judy, a 54-year-old woman, has just returned from the recovery room to the surgical unit following a thyroidectomy. During the next 24 to 48 h, the nurse will periodically assess this patient for a positive Chvostek's sign, which would indicate the patient is developing

    1. Respiratory stridor.
    2. A low hematocrit.
    3. A fluid volume deficit.
    4. A calcium deficit.

69. Sam, a 68-year-old man, periodically develops hypokalemia as a side effect of his medications. Which of the following foods would be helpful for him to include in his diet?
    1. Peanut butter and milk.
    2. Pork and squash.
    3. Yogurt and cheese.
    4. Bananas and cantaloupe.

70. Which of the following electrolyte imbalances predisposes to the development of digitalis toxicity?
    1. Hyponatremia.
    2. Hypokalemia.
    3. Hypocalcemia.
    4. Hyperkalemia.

71. Betty has an elevated blood pressure, neck vein distention, an increased central venous pressure, and a weight gain of 4 pounds in the past 24 h. The nurse should question which of the following physician's orders?
    1. 2-g sodium diet.
    2. 1000 mL normal saline IV at 125 mL/h.
    3. Furosemide (Lasix) 40 mg bid.
    4. High Fowler's position.

72. Which of the following arterial blood gas findings is characteristic of metabolic acidosis?
    1. Increased bicarbonate content.
    2. Decreased bicarbonate content.
    3. Increased carbon dioxide content.
    4. Decreased carbon dioxide content.

73. Joan, a 35-year-old housewife, was admitted to the hospital with nausea, vomiting, and diarrhea for several days. Nursing assessment of this patient would likely reveal
    1. Puffy eyelids, moist rales, and shortness of breath.
    2. Polyuria, decreased body temperature, and hypertension.
    3. Exaggerated reflexes, acute weight gain, and dyspnea.
    4. Oliguria, tachycardia, and fever.

74. Potassium imbalance in the body will result in signs and symptoms that relate to this electrolyte's effect on
    1. Cardiac and skeletal muscle.
    2. Fluid shifts between the extracellular and intracellular compartments.
    3. The formation of clotting factors.
    4. Deep tendon reflexes.

75. Kathy's laboratory results are as follows: sodium = 155 mEq/L and potassium = 4.5 mEq/L. The nurse should recognize that this client is experiencing
   1. Hyponatremia.
   2. Hypernatremia.
   3. Hypokalemia.
   4. Hyperkalemia.

76. Sally is experiencing numbness and tingling of her fingers, toes, and circumoral area. This patient may be exhibiting symptoms of
   1. Sodium excess.
   2. Calcium deficit.
   3. Magnesium excess.
   4. Potassium deficit.

77. Brandon has a vitamin D deficiency. This may result in
   1. Hypokalemia.
   2. Hypocalcemia.
   3. Hyponatremia.
   4. Hypomagnesemia.

78. Severe prolonged diarrhea may result in which of the following acid–base imbalances?
   1. Metabolic acidosis.
   2. Metabolic alkalosis.
   3. Respiratory acidosis.
   4. Respiratory alkalosis.

79. Which of the following patients is at risk for developing metabolic alkalosis?
   1. A gunshot victim who is going into shock.
   2. A diabetic who has omitted several doses of insulin.
   3. A depressed patient who has overdosed on aspirin.
   4. A patient with prolonged nausea and vomiting.

80. Which of the following physician's orders should the nurse expect for a client with severe metabolic acidosis?
   1. Oxygen at 2 L per nasal cannula.
   2. Sodium bicarbonate 7.5% IV push.
   3. Potassium chloride 40 mEq IV push.
   4. Magnesium sulfate 1 mEq/kg body weight IV push.

81. Infants and young children do not tolerate fluid imbalances as well as adults do because their body fluids
   1. Are less concentrated.
   2. Are more concentrated.
   3. Account for a lower percentage of the total body weight.
   4. Account for a high percentage of the total body weight.

82. John is suffering from end-stage renal disease. The nurse should question which of the following physician's orders for this patient?

   1. Restrict oral fluid intake to 800 mL/24 h.
   2. Institute low-protein diet.
   3. Administer milk of magnesia 30 mL PO PRN.
   4. Place on cardiac monitor telemetry.

83. Which of the following would be used to correct edema associated with hypoproteinemia?
   1. Dextran.
   2. Salt-poor albumin.
   3. Isotonic IV fluids (e.g., Ringer's lactate).
   4. Hypotonic IV fluids (e.g., 5% dextrose in water).

84. Which of the following is the *best* indicator of a patient's fluid status?
   1. Skin turgor.
   2. Urinary output.
   3. Amount of edema present.
   4. Condition of mucous membranes.

85. Abby, a 68-year-old woman, has a history of hypertension for which she has been taking a thiazide diuretic. Her plasma potassium is 3.0 mEq/L. Nursing interventions for this patient should include which of the following?
   1. Monitor for muscle weakness and fatigue.
   2. Assess for positive Chvostek's sign.
   3. Administer Kayexalate enema as ordered.
   4. Observe cardiac monitor pattern for elevation of T wave.

86. Which of the following patients would be predisposed to the development of hypomagnesemia?
   1. Patient with chronic alcoholism.
   2. Patient with renal insufficiency.
   3. Patient taking antacids for chronic gastritis.
   4. Patient on a high-protein diet.

87. During a difficult procedure Jack begins to hyperventilate. The nurse understands that this can lead to
   1. Respiratory acidosis.
   2. Respiratory alkalosis.
   3. Hyponatremia.
   4. Hypernatremia.

88. Which of the following signs and symptoms are indicative of metabolic acidosis?
   1. Lethargy, disorientation, and tachypnea.
   2. Tetany, tachycardia, and respiratory depression.
   3. Circumoral tingling, muscle weakness, and bradypnea.
   4. Muscle twitching, anxiety, and disorientation.

89. Which of the following occurs as a compensatory mechanism when metabolic acidosis develops?
   1. Body temperature rises.
   2. Heart rate slows.

3. Respiratory rate increases.

4. Urinary output decreases.

90. John, a 68-year-old man, reports taking large amounts of antacids for the relief of "heartburn." The nurse explains to him that this practice may result in

1. Hyperkalemia.

2. Hyponatremia.

3. Metabolic alkalosis.

4. Metabolic acidosis.

91. A patient is admitted to the hospital with pneumonia. The nurse notes that moist crackles are present and the patient is experiencing shortness of breath. This patient is most likely suffering from the following acid–base imbalance:

1. Respiratory acidosis: pH 7.25, pCO_2 60, HCO_3 26.

2. Metabolic acidosis: pH 7.29, pCO_2 32, HCO_3 15.

3. Metabolic alkalosis: pH 7.40, pCO_2 30, HCO_3 20.

4. Respiratory alkalosis: pH 7.60, pCO_2 25, HCO_3 24.

92. Which arterial blood gas finding is characteristic of a compensatory action in metabolic acidosis?

1. Increased bicarbonate content.

2. Decreased bicarbonate content.

3. Increased carbon dioxide content.

4. Decreased carbon dioxide content.

93. The most appropriate nursing intervention when a patient's serum sodium level is 140 mEq/L is

1. Advising the patient to avoid canned soups and vegetables, processed meats, and added table salt.

2. Carefully monitoring ECG pattern for dysrhythmias.

3. Notifying the physician.

4. Continuing to monitor electrolyte values.

94. An excess of extracellular sodium causes

1. An increase in aldosterone production.

2. Fluid to leak out of the cells.

3. Cell size to increase.

4. Transient pain.

95. A patient with diarrhea should be observed for hyponatremia because

1. Sodium is concentrated in gastrointestinal fluid.

2. Water lost in diarrhea causes an increase in sodium concentration.

3. Diarrhea triggers renal mechanisms to waste sodium.

4. Hyponatremia occurs as a result of treatment for diarrhea.

96. The patient with a nasogastric tube to suction should be observed for

1. Metabolic alkalosis.

2. Muscle flaccidity.

3. Tachypnea.

4. Skin discoloration.

97. While Mr. Williams is using the mechanical ventilator, some of his arterial blood gas findings are as follows: pH 7.48, pCO_2 30, pO_2 88, HCO_3 25. These findings indicate that this patient is experiencing which type of acid–base abnormality?

1. Metabolic acidosis.

2. Metabolic alkalosis.

3. Respiratory acidosis.

4. Respiratory alkalosis.

98. Joel, a 47-year-old man, has been experiencing symptoms of fluid retention. His physician prescribed spironolactone (Aldactone). Nursing intervention related to this medication includes

1. Watching for muscle weakness and giving diluted potassium chloride (KCl) supplement as ordered.

2. Monitoring urine for changes in sugar and acetone.

3. Not giving medication at bedtime and observing for digitalis toxicity.

4. Not giving supplemental KCl and monitoring for signs of electrolyte imbalance.

99. The nurse is directed to administer a hypotonic IV solution. Looking at the following labeled solutions, she should choose

1. 0.45% sodium chloride.

2. 0.9% sodium chloride.

3. 5% dextrose in water.

4. 5% dextrose in normal saline.

100. IV therapy is started to help correct electrolyte imbalances that Julie demonstrates. If this patient receives IV fluid too rapidly and the nurse assesses her peripheral veins, the nurse should expect to find veins that are

1. Tortuous.

2. Collapsed.

3. Inflamed.

4. Distended.

ANSWERS AND RATIONALES

1. ❶ Nephrotic syndrome is thought to be an antigen–antibody reaction that causes the glomerular membrane to become permeable to large protein molecules (albumin), resulting in proteinuria and hypoalbuminemia. When the serum protein level drops, the colloid osmotic pressure drops, allowing fluid to flow through the capillaries into the extracellular space, producing edema.

(2) Cystinuria results from a metabolic disturbance and has no relationship to proteinuria, hypoalbuminemia, or edema.

(3) Renal tubular acidosis is a disorder in which the distal tubule cannot excrete hydrogen ions; as a result there is increased loss of potassium and bicarbonate in the urine, and systemic acidosis develops.

2. **②** Azotemia (uremia frost) is the presence of urea and nitrogenous bodies in the blood, which is seen in patients experiencing renal failure.

(1) The glomerular filtration rate is decreased with azotemia.

(3) The BUN level rises with azotemia.

(4) Edema is present in the patient with azotemia; however, it usually develops gradually. Rapid development of edema does not result in azotemia.

3. **②** A patient with a high BUN level will display symptoms of confusion and disorientation because of the effect of urea nitrogen on the brain.

(1) Hematuria and dysuria are indicative of calculi or an inflammatory process in the urinary tract. An elevated BUN level indicates declining function of the kidney nephron unit.

(3) A patient with a high BUN level may have oliguria, but there is no reason for increased respiratory rate.

(4) A fruity odor of breath is caused by the breakdown of fat into ketone bodies. This occurs in patients with diabetes mellitus or chronic malnutrition and has no relationship to the BUN level.

4. **①** In response to hypotension, renin is secreted by the kidney to cause vasoconstriction. Aldosterone is released from the adrenal cortex to cause the kidneys to retain sodium and water, in an effort to increase the total blood volume and blood pressure.

(2) Angiotensin is a part of the renin chain. Sodium is retained, not secreted, by the kidneys.

(3) Renin is correct; however, parathormone is a substance secreted by the parathyroid glands to increase the serum calcium level, which has no relationship to the physiologic response to shock.

(4) ADH is secreted by the posterior pituitary to cause fluid retention and thereby increase the blood pressure; however, corticosteroids are not a part of the body's physiologic response to shock.

5. **③** Damaged glomeruli will decrease the ability of the glomeruli to filter selectively. Permeability is increased; therefore, protein molecules and red blood cells are filtered from the plasma into the urine.

(1, 2, 4) These structures are not affected by this process.

6. **①** The most common etiologic factor for acute glomerulonephritis is group B hemolytic streptococci. Often streptococcal infection of the throat precedes the onset of glomerulonephritis.

(2, 3, 4) These usually are associated with the development of glomerulonephritis.

7. **②** Protein restriction is used (when BUN level is elevated) to rest the kidneys and to decrease nitrogenous substances in the blood.

(1) Protein does not act as an antidiuretic.

(3) Protein intake does not affect the antigen–antibody reaction.

(4) Protein increases osmotic pressure in the vascular system, not in the renal system.

8. **③** In acute renal failure, the patient passes through oliguria and then diuresis before renal function returns to normal or near normal.

(1, 2, 4) These options are incorrect as seen in rationale (3).

9. **③** Aluminum hydroxide antacids are not effective in decreasing the potassium in the blood. They have no systemic effect.

(1) Kayexalate aids in eliminating excess potassium by exchanging sodium ions for potassium ions in the gastrointestinal tract. Potassium is then excreted in the stool.

(2) Calcium salts are given to antagonize the action of the hyperkalemia on cardiac muscle, until the Kayexalate and/or dialysis removes the excess potassium from the blood.

(4) Hemodialysis or peritoneal dialysis will eliminate excess potassium from the blood.

10. **③** Instructing a patient regarding fluid restriction is necessary to help prevent fluid overload because the poorly functioning kidney cannot eliminate large amounts of fluid.

(1) The acute phase of an illness is not the appropriate time to work on long-term goals. The need for a permanent low-protein or low-sodium diet will depend on the kidney damage; 60 to 70 percent of adult patients recover completely.

(2) Bed rest, not activity, is prescribed to rest the kidney until edema and elevated blood pressure are under control.

(4) The patient with acute glomerulonephritis develops a fluid volume excess, not a fluid volume deficit.

11. **④** Kidney stones that obstruct a ureter cause backflow of urine into the kidney pelvis. This dilates the kidney (hydronephrosis) and eventually results in nephron destruction. After the stone is removed, the patient may develop reflex diuresis, which is caused by a decrease in ADH secretion. If not closely monitored and given appropriate fluid replacement, the patient can rapidly dehydrate. This patient must be closely monitored for an inability to void, which can develop due to obstruction of urine flow by the stone fragments remaining in the urinary tract.

(1, 2, 3) These options are incorrect as seen in rationale (4).

12. **③** Painless hematuria is the initial symptom in 75 percent of cases of bladder and renal cancer.

(1, 2, 4) Dysuria, pyuria, and obstruction may develop in a patient with bladder cancer, but not until the late stages.

13. **①** Alcohol intake is the most common precipitating factor for acute urinary retention in a patient with prostatic enlargement.

(2) A hot tub bath would cause relaxation of the urethra and may facilitate urination.

(3) Sexual intercourse with ejaculation may relieve some congestion and actually facilitate urination.

(4) Foods that increase urine acidity should be encouraged in a patient with prostatic hypertrophy to discourage bacterial growth in urine retained within the bladder.

14. ❹ Clinical manifestations of acute glomerulonephritis include hypertension, hematuria, proteinuria, increased urine specific gravity, headache, edema, elevated serum creatinine and BUN levels.

(1) The temperature would not be significantly elevated, as glomerulonephritis is an inflammatory response rather than an acute infection. This patient would have oliguria, not polyuria, and there would be no reason for tachycardia to occur.

(2) This option is incorrect as explained in rationale (1).

(3) There would be no reason for tachypnea to occur. The urine specific gravity would be elevated due to protein and red blood cells in the urine.

15. ❷ Antigen–antibody complexes are trapped in the glomeruli, causing glomerular damage.

(1, 3, 4) These options are incorrect as seen in rationale (2).

16. ❸ In perineal prostatectomy, an incision is made in the perineum, between the scrotum and anus. Nerve pathways can easily be destroyed, resulting in sexual dysfunction (impotence).

(1, 2, 4) These surgical approaches do not involve the perineal area and therefore are less likely to result in impotence.

17. ❷ Eighty percent of all urinary stones contain calcium. An acid-ash diet is helpful in preventing calcium ions from precipitating out of the urine and forming crystals and stones. Increased hydration also helps prevent precipitation of calcium out of the urine.

(1, 3, 4) These diets will not aid in preventing calcium stone formation.

18. ❷ Pain from renal calculi is excruciating and must be controlled with narcotic analgesics as a first priority, after which urinary output can be monitored and the patient can be prepared for diagnostic studies.

(1) Fluids are increased, not restricted, to aid in the "flushing" of stones and stone fragments out of the urinary tract.

(3) Urinary output must be monitored because of the possibility of developing an obstruction to urine flow; however, administration of pain medication must be the nurse's first priority in this case.

(4) Diagnostic studies will be ordered but are not the first priority.

19. ❶ Gout is a metabolic disease characterized by urate deposits, which cause painful arthritic joints. It strikes mainly the feet and legs and especially the great toe. As the disease progresses, it may cause nephrolithiasis, as uric acid precipitates out of the urine into crystals and stones.

(2) Primary aldosteronism results in hypernatremia and has no relationship to uric acid calculi.

(3) Large intake of dairy products may result in development of renal calculi, but the composition would be calcium instead of uric acid.

(4) Recurrent UTIs are associated with renal calculi but are not a risk factor for uric acid stones.

20. ❶ Risks factors for urinary calculi include anything that causes either urinary stasis or supersaturation of the urine with particles. This includes dehydration, immobility, and increased calcium or other ions in the urine.

(2, 3, 4) These are incorrect options as seen in rationale (1).

21. ❸ A continent urostomy (or Kock's pouch) differs from an ileal conduit because it has a nipple valve beneath the stoma that prevents urine from flowing through the stoma and, therefore, prevents excoriation of the surrounding skin. The client must catheterize the stoma at least every 6 h to empty the "pouch."

(1) A large segment of ileum is used to form the "pouch," but urine does not exit via the urethra. It exits via an abdominal stoma.

(2) This option is incorrect as seen in rationale (3).

(4) Kock's pouch is not temporary; it is a permanent replacement for the bladder.

22. ❹ If urinary output decreases, the first action by the nurse is to check the Foley catheter tube for kinks.

(1) When notified, the physician will want to know if the patency of the tube has been checked.

(2) Repositioning a patient on his or her side does not facilitate drainage from the catheter or the stent.

(3) A physician's order is needed to irrigate the stent, and no more than 5 cc should be instilled into a stent via gravity (never force it) at one time.

23. ❸ Glomerular filtration occurs in the glomerulus. It is the process of filtering the blood as it flows through the kidney.

(1, 2, 4) These options are incorrect as seen in rationale (3).

24. ❸ In chronic renal failure, the serum phosphorus level is elevated. There is an inverse relationship between phosphorus and calcium in the blood; therefore, whenever one of these ions is elevated (phosphorus), the other (calcium) is below normal. To correct the hypocalcemia, aluminum hydroxide (Amphojel) is given. It acts by binding with phosphorus in the gastrointestinal tract and preventing absorption, thereby decreasing the serum phosphorus level and allowing the serum calcium to rise.

(1) The patient in chronic renal failure should be encouraged to include foods rich in calcium in the diet.

(2) A high-fiber diet is appropriate for the patient in renal failure, to prevent constipation resulting from the significant fluid restriction; however, this would have no impact on the patient's hypocalcemia.

(4) Calcitonin (Cibacalcin) inhibits bone resorption of calcium, lowering the serum calcium level. The patient in chronic renal failure has hypocalcemia.

25. ❷ Peritonitis is the main complication of peritoneal dialysis. The delivery of dialysate into the peritoneal cavity and its removal after a set period can result in introduction of a pathogen into the peritoneal cavity, causing peritonitis.

(1) Perforation of the bowel or bladder may occur when the catheter initially is inserted, but it is not a common problem.

(3) Hypovolemia is not a problem for patients requiring dialysis. They have a fluid volume excess.

(4) Disequilibrium syndrome usually is not a problem in peritoneal dialysis. It is more likely to occur with hemodialysis as a result of rapid change in the composition of the extracellular fluid. Solutes are removed more rapidly from the blood than from the cerebrospinal fluid and brain. The higher osmotic gradient in the brain cells allows fluid to pass into these cells, causing cerebral edema.

26. ❷ In glomerulonephritis, the glomerular membrane becomes permeable to large molecules including protein (albumin) and red blood cells as well.

(1) There is no reason for the urine to become alkaline, and, because of increased amount of solute in the urine, the specific gravity will be significantly elevated rather than within normal limits.

(3) The urine will appear smoky in color (indicating bleeding at the kidney level) as a result of the red blood cells that pass across the glomerular membrane.

(4) These are not findings in the urine of a patient with glomerulonephritis.

27. ❹ The type of vascular access for hemodialysis that is least likely to become infected is the arteriovenous fistula; it is beneath the skin and exposed to pathogens only during the actual dialysis procedure.

(1, 2, 3) The femoral, subclavian, and external shunts protrude through the skin and therefore are more likely to become infected than the fistula. Between dialysis treatments, these shunts are injected with a heparinized normal saline solution, then capped and covered with an occlusive dressing.

28. ❸ Hepatitis B virus is the most common infectious organism associated with hemodialysis. This virus is transmitted via the blood.

(1, 2, 4) These options are incorrect as seen in rationale (3).

29. ❶ If the 24-h urine specimen begins at 10 AM, the urine voided at that time is discarded. Then all urine voided for the next 24 h is collected and maintained on ice until 10 AM the following day, at which time the patient is asked to void and that urine is included in the specimen.

(2, 3, 4) These options are incorrect as seen in rationale (1).

30. ❶ Slowly removing the catheter allows drainage of urine near the exit of the bladder. The total amount of urine obtained is the amount of urine the patient failed to void (residual urine), and it is important to collect all of the urine.

(2) This option is incorrect as seen in rationale (1).

(3) Once the catheter is pulled out of the bladder (even 1 inch), it should never be reinserted, because this may drag bacteria up the urethra toward the bladder and result in a bladder infection. In addition, this action would be very uncomfortable for the patient.

(4) Urine would not have pooled in the upper part of the bladder.

31. ❶ If the balloon is inflated in the urethra, the patient will complain of pain because the balloon is pushing against the side of the small lumen of the urethra.

(2) There is more room for the balloon to be inflated near the opening of the urethra.

(3) The balloon should be inflated low inside the bladder. This should not be the cause of pain.

(4) The balloon can be totally enlarged in the bladder without overdistention of the bladder.

32. ❷ A sterile syringe and needle must be used; urine should be drawn from the catheter port.

(1) A needle and syringe with plunger are necessary to obtain a sterile specimen from the catheter port.

(3) It is never advisable to disconnect the catheter from the drainage tubing to collect a urine specimen because this increases the risk of introducing pathogens.

(4) The urine in the collection bag may have been there for many hours and therefore is not appropriate for a urine specimen.

33. ❸ End-stage renal disease involves progressive, irreversible destruction of both kidneys resulting in their contraction. The serum creatinine level is high and remains relatively stable or continues to rise slowly. Anemia develops because of the inability of the diseased kidneys to produce erythropoietin.

(1) There is an increase, not a decrease, in serum creatinine levels. There is no reason for loss of skin turgor (usually observed with fluid volume deficit or aging), as this patient suffers from a fluid volume excess. The electrolyte imbalance will be hyperkalemia, not hypokalemia.

(2) The glomerular filtration rate decreases, as does the rate of creatinine clearance. This patient suffers from generalized edema, but the calcium level is low (hypocalcemia).

(4) The serum creatinine level gradually rises. The patient develops anemia, as explained in rationale (3), and becomes oliguric and then anuric.

34. ❷ All medications are withheld on the morning of dialysis because they will be removed from the blood during the dialysis. Therefore, the amount of medication available for use by the body prior to hemodialysis and the patient's response would be unpredictable. Medications are given after the dialysis treatment is complete.

(1, 3, 4) These options are incorrect as seen in rationale (2).

35. ❹ Warm dialyzing solution is used to help prevent body temperature from falling precipitously.

(1) Relaxation of the abdominal muscles would be of no benefit to peritoneal dialysis.

(2) Warm dialyzing solution increases the risk of peritoneal infection because pathogens thrive in warm moist environments.

(3) Blood vessels will not constrict as a result of warm dialyzing solution; they may dilate, which would increase the efficiency of the treatment.

36. ❶ One of the common complications associated with kidney transplants is infection, which can cause rejection; reverse isolation helps to prevent infection. Remember that these patients are receiving immunosuppressant medications to decrease the risk of organ rejection. This places them at an increased risk of developing infections.

(2) Assessment of clotting time is the responsibility of the physician; clotting abnormalities are not a common complication associated with a kidney transplant.

(3) Allowing only limited rest would increase the likelihood of this patient's rejecting the kidney. Rest is imperative to restore the body's equilibrium.

(4) It is the physician's responsibility to increase fluid intake. Increasing fluid intake to 2500 mL daily likely would result in a fluid volume overload in a patient with a renal transplant. A common order for fluid replacement is 30 mL/h, or 720 mL/24 h, or an amount that closely approximates the initial urine output.

37. ❸ A potential cadaver kidney donor must meet the following criteria: criteria for brain death, age younger than 60 years, normal renal function, no malignant disease, no generalized infection, no significant hypertension (which would indicate probable kidney damage that otherwise may be indiscernible at that time), no abdominal or renal trauma, negative hepatitis B antigen and HIV antibody, and continuous ventilation and heartbeat until the kidneys are surgically removed from the body.

(1, 2, 4) These options are incorrect as seen in rationale (3).

38. ❶ IV fluids are run at approximately 125 mL/h for 8 h before a renal arteriogram (procedure used to permit visualization of the renal vasculature) to reduce the chance that the dye used in this procedure will damage the kidney. The medium used can be nephrotic.

(2) Increased fluid in the vascular system will not increase visualization of the kidney.

(3) Increased fluid in the vascular system will not reduce the chances of an allergic reaction. If the patient is allergic to the dye, she or he will have an allergic reaction regardless of the amount of hydration. If there is any indication that the patient is allergic to iodine, the renal arteriogram should not be done.

(4) Although the patient may complain of thirst as a result of being NPO, this is not the rationale for the IV flow rate.

39. ❶ In preparation for an IVP, a client is NPO for two reasons. The first is to cause a relative fluid depletion so that the radiopaque contrast medium will be more concentrated when it passes through the kidneys and the x-ray films will be clearer. The second reason is to keep the gastrointestinal tract empty so that the kidneys, which are behind the bowel, will be better visualized. This is also why the bowel prep may be ordered.

(2, 3) These options are incorrect as seen in rationale (1).

(4) The IVP will not be performed under general anesthesia. A consent form should be signed prior to the procedure.

40. ❹ BUN measures the amount of urea nitrogen (the end-product of protein metabolism normally excreted by the kid-

neys) in the blood. Any renal function impairment causes an increase in BUN level. Other factors that also may result in an increased BUN level include hypovolemia (dehydration), excessive protein intake (high-protein diets), starvation (which results in breakdown of the body's protein stores for energy), and gastrointestinal bleeding (which contains a large amount of plasma proteins).

(1) Impaired liver function would result in a decreased BUN level. Celiac disease (which results in abnormal fat absorption from the gastrointestinal tract) has no impact on the BUN level.

(2) Overhydration and liver failure would result in a low BUN level.

(3) Decreased protein intake and liver failure would result in a low BUN level.

41. ❷ The correct procedure used to assess creatinine clearance is a 24-h urine specimen, collected and maintained in a container on ice. Exact start time and date are recorded on the container and on the patient's record.

(1, 3, 4) These options are incorrect as seen in rationale (2).

42. ❸ Urine output must be closely monitored to ensure patency of the ureters at the junction with the conduit and unobstructed flow through the stoma.

(1) The patient will be NPO until bowel sounds return. A small portion of the small intestine has been resected; therefore, gastrointestinal function will be altered for 2 to 3 days after surgery, during which time the patient will be unable to tolerate oral feedings.

(2) Some blood is expected in the urine initially. The amount should be small and should gradually disappear over the first 24 h. Mucus in the urine is expected, as the small bowel secretes mucus and a portion of the small bowel is now being used as a bladder.

(4) The ileal conduit should be draining continuously. The patient is unable to "void."

43. ❹ Normal BUN level is 11 to 20 mg/dL in adults and normal creatinine level is 0.6 to 1.2 mg/dL; so a BUN level of 25 mg/dl and serum creatinine level of 12 mg/dL are abnormal values (see Appendix 2).

(1, 2, 3) These options are all normal values.

44. ❸ In ESWL, a noninvasive procedure, the patient is anesthetized (spinal or general) and placed in a water bath. Electrically generated shock waves are directed toward the kidney to fracture the stones. The procedure usually lasts from 30 to 45 min, and immobility is essential. Early ambulation and adequate fluid intake are important to fully "wash out" the stone fragments.

(1, 2, 4) These are procedures to remove stones, but they are not lithotripsy.

45. ❷ Phenytoin (Dilantin), an anticonvulsant drug, will color the urine red. Phenazopyridine (Pyridium), a urinary antiseptic and analgesic, will color the urine orange.

(1, 3, 4) These medications will not color the urine red or orange.

46. **❶** Severe dehydration increases the BUN level by increasing the concentration of urea nitrogen per volume of blood.

(2, 3, 4) None of these results in an increased BUN level.

47. **❷** Nursing care for a patient in the oliguric phase (urine output <400 mL/d) includes restricting fluid to prevent a fluid volume excess. Protein intake is reduced to decrease the workload of the kidney in eliminating the urea nitrogen end-product of protein metabolism.

(1) Patients in the oliguric phase of renal failure require rest.

(3) Encouraging fluid intake during the oliguric phase will result in a fluid volume excess.

(4) The diet should be low protein as explained in rationale (2). Most of the caloric intake is supplied by carbohydrates.

48. **❷** The patient in acute renal failure goes into metabolic acidosis, not alkalosis, because the kidney becomes unable to eliminate excess hydrogen ions or to conserve bicarbonate.

(1, 3, 4) All of these do occur in the patient in renal failure.

49. **❹** Turning the patient from side to side will increase the outflow of the dialysate fluid.

(1) The dialysate solution must run out by gravity. Suction would remove it too rapidly, not allowing adequate dwell time for the waste products to move across the peritoneum into the dialysate to be removed.

(2) There is no reason to call the physician. The nurse needs only to turn the patient from side to side to facilitate drainage.

(3) The peritoneal catheter is tunneled through the subcutaneous tissue into the abdomen. It is the physician's responsibility to determine when the catheter requires replacement and to perform that procedure. It is a nursing responsibility to assess for indications of blockage, kinks, or infection.

50. **❹** Patients undergoing surgical procedures involving the pelvic region are at increased risk for developing thrombophlebitis. The edema in that area slows the venous return, encouraging clot formation.

(1, 2, 3) The risk of developing atelectasis, hemorrhage, or sepsis is no greater for this patient than for patients undergoing other major surgeries.

51. **❶** Stomahesive is used to increase adherence of the ostomy appliance to the skin.

(2) Karaya, which is used with ileostomies and colostomies, cannot be used for ileal conduits, because urine will deteriorate Karaya.

(3) Bacitracin is not necessary. The skin should be cleansed with mild soap and water and gently patted dry. An emollient skin lotion or cream may be applied around the appliance face plate to protect against skin contact with any urine leak.

(4) Denatured alcohol will dry out the skin, making it more prone to cracking and breakdown.

52. **❷** The patient with cystitis presents with dysuria, frequency (frequent voiding of small amounts), urgency, abdominal pain, fever, general malaise, and cloudy urine.

(1, 3, 4) These options are not correct as seen in rationale (2).

53. **❹** The organism most often responsible for UTI is *Escherichia coli*, which is a normal flora in the intestines.

(1, 2, 3) These options are incorrect as seen in rationale (4).

54. **❶** The finding most suggestive of peritonitis in the patient receiving peritoneal dialysis is cloudy return dialysate.

(2) Blood-tinged return dialysate is not expected unless the catheter has just been inserted. This is not indicative of peritonitis.

(3) Abdominal pain during the dialysis treatment may result from very rapid instillation of the solution. This is not indicative of peritonitis.

(4) If the dialysate is difficult to instill, the most likely cause is obstruction of the catheter.

55. **❷** The patient in chronic renal failure must be warned against taking over-the-counter medications that contain magnesium. Without the kidney's ability to excrete excess magnesium in the urine, this patient will develop hypermagnesemia.

(1, 3, 4) These options are incorrect as seen in rationale (2).

56. **❷** Calcium gluconate is given to the patient with hyperkalemia to counteract the effect of the potassium on the cardiac muscle until other measures can be implemented to remove the excess potassium from the blood.

(1, 3, 4) These options are incorrect as seen in rationale (2).

57. **❸** Because of the pump's failure, the pressure in the pulmonary circulation is increased, which results in an increased fluid shift from the vasculature into the lung tissue. The moist crackles result from the movement of air past the fluid.

(1) Absence of breath sounds would be more indicative of atelectasis.

(2) Central venous pressure would be increased because of the fluid excess and the heart's inability to pump the blood.

(4) Hyperactive reflexes are not associated with this clinical picture.

58. **❸** Baked chicken, lettuce, and sliced tomatoes are all low in sodium.

(1, 2, 4) Salad dressings, canned vegetables and soups, and processed meats (frankfurters) are all high in sodium.

59. **❶** Giving ice chips indiscriminately to patients with a nasogastric tube to suction may result in loss of electrolytes found in the stomach (sodium, chloride, and potassium). This patient is most likely suffering from hyponatremia (low sodium level), because her symptoms are neurologic in nature. A low sodium level results in a fluid shift from the extracellular space into the intracellular space (cells swell), which has the greatest impact on the brain cells.

(2, 3, 4) These options are incorrect as seen in rationale (1).

60. **❹** The contents of the stomach are acidic. Vomiting results in the loss of acid from the body, leaving the patient in an alkalotic state. This acid–base imbalance was not caused by a problem with the respiratory system; therefore, it must be a metabolic alkalosis.

(1, 2, 3) These options are incorrect as seen in rationale (4).

61. ① If this patient is in circulatory overload, the IV rate must be decreased. This requires a physician's order; therefore, it is necessary to notify the physician of the patient's status and get an IV order. Other nursing interventions include placing the patient in Fowler's position, monitoring breath sounds for moist crackles, and administering diuretics as ordered.

(2, 3, 4) These options are incorrect as seen in rationale (1).

62. ② Furosemide (Lasix) is a loop diuretic with the side effect of hypokalemia. It may also result in hyponatremia and hypochloremic alkalosis.

(1, 3, 4) These options are incorrect as seen in rationale (2).

63. ④ Clinical manifestations of metabolic acidosis include drowsiness, confusion, coma, headache, and compensatory hyperventilation (tachypnea).

(1, 2, 3) These options are incorrect as seen in rationale (4).

64. ② When acidosis develops, a cellular buffer system causes hydrogen ions from the blood to be exchanged for potassium ions from the cells. This results in a decrease in acidity (hydrogen ions) in the blood and an increase in the serum potassium level (hyperkalemia).

(1, 3, 4) These options are incorrect as seen in rationale (2).

65. ④ A rapid weight gain is indicative of fluid retention or fluid volume excess.

(1) There would be no reason for the sodium level to be high; however, if the fluid overload is caused by hypotonic solution, the sodium level would be low.

(2) When the fluid volume of the blood increases, the hematocrit (packed cell volume) decreases as a result of dilution.

(3) The pulse would be bounding as a result of the increased volume of the blood.

66. ③ Insufficient ADH results in large volumes of very dilute urine output, the specific gravity of which is very low.

(1) Checking vital signs every 4 h is not indicated unless the patient is allowed to dehydrate.

(2) Fluids must be encouraged if the client has insufficient ADH.

(4) This option has no relationship to this patient's situation.

67. ③ Any process that interferes with adequate ventilation (exchange of oxygen and carbon dioxide) will result in respiratory acidosis. The carbon dioxide is converted to carbonic acid.

(1, 2, 4) These options are incorrect as seen in rationale (3).

68. ④ Chvostek's sign is elicited by tapping on the facial nerve in front of the ear. It is positive if the tapping results in facial twitching. Muscle twitching progressing to tetany is a symptom of hypocalcemia. When the thyroid gland is removed, the parathyroid tissue is sometimes inadvertently removed or damaged, which results in decreased parathyroid hormone and a low serum calcium level.

(1, 2, 3) These options are incorrect as seen in rationale (4).

69. ④ Bananas and cantaloupe are high in potassium. Other foods rich in potassium include apricots, oranges, strawberries, tomatoes, and leafy green vegetables.

(1, 2, 3) These options are incorrect as seen in rationale (4).

70. ② Hypokalemia, hypercalcemia, and hypomagnesia predispose patients to develop digitalis toxicity. Manifestations of toxicity include green or yellow vision, halo vision, nausea, vomiting, abdominal cramps, bradycardia, tachycardia, and dysrhythmias.

(1, 3, 4) These options are incorrect as seen in rationale (2).

71. ② This patient has clinical manifestations of fluid volume excess; therefore, fluids should be restricted, not administered IV at 125 mL/h.

(1) Sodium restriction is appropriate for the patient with fluid volume excess. As water follows sodium in the fluid compartments of the body, if the serum sodium level decreases, the amount (volume) of water in the blood will also decrease.

(3) Furosemide (Lasix) is a loop diuretic frequently used to correct a fluid volume excess.

(4) The patient with a fluid volume excess develops edema from fluid being stored in the interstitial spaces. When this occurs in the lungs, the alveoli begin to fill up with fluid (pulmonary edema) and gas exchange across the alveolar membrane is diminished. Placing the patient in Fowler's position allows for maximum ventilation of the compromised lung.

72. ② In metabolic acidosis, there is a relative decrease in the bicarbonate content of the blood. This occurs as hydrogen ions (acid) are "dumped" into the blood and the bicarbonate is "used up" while acting as a buffer for the acid.

(1) This option is incorrect as seen in rationale (2).

(3, 4) Changes in the carbon dioxide content are related to the respiratory system and result in either respiratory acidosis or respiratory alkalosis.

73. ④ The patient experiencing vomiting and diarrhea for several days is likely to have a fluid volume deficit (dehydration), symptoms of which are oliguria, tachycardia, hypotension, acute weight loss, loss of skin turgor, dry mucous membranes, furrowed tongue, and fever.

(1, 2, 3) These options are incorrect as seen in rationale (4).

74. ① Clinical manifestations of potassium imbalance are related to the role this electrolyte plays in repolarization of nerve and muscle fibers and include skeletal muscle weakness and cardiac dysrhythmias.

(2) Fluid shifts between intracellular and extracellular compartments are determined by the sodium content, not potassium content.

(3) This option is incorrect as seen in rationale (1).

(4) Deep tendon reflexes are affected by serum calcium and magnesium levels.

75. ② The normal serum sodium level is 135 to 145 mEq/L. The normal serum potassium level is 3.5 to 5 mEq/L.

(1, 3, 4) These options are incorrect as seen in rationale (2).

76. ② Clinical manifestations of hypocalcemia are those of increased neuromuscular irritability and include numbness and tingling (especially of fingers and circumoral area), muscle spasms, tetany, cramps, convulsions, positive Trousseau's sign, positive Chvostek's sign, and laryngospasm.

(1, 3, 4) These options are not manifestations of a sodium excess, magnesium excess, or potassium deficit.

77. ❷ Vitamin D is necessary for the absorption of calcium from the diet. Therefore a vitamin D deficiency will result in hypocalcemia.

(1, 3, 4) These options are incorrect as seen in rationale (2).

78. ❶ The contents of the lower gastrointestinal tract are alkaline. Therefore, a patient who has prolonged loss of these contents enters into an acidotic state. This process has nothing to do with the respiratory tract and therefore must be a metabolic imbalance.

(2, 3, 4) These options are incorrect as seen in rationale (1).

79. ❹ The contents of the upper gastrointestinal tract are acid. Therefore, a patient who has prolonged loss of these contents through vomiting or gastric suction enters into an alkalotic state.

(1) The patient who is going into shock suffers from hypoxia at the cellular level. The cells go into an anaerobic cycle, the end-product of which is lactic acid, which results in metabolic acidosis.

(2) The diabetic patient who has inadequate insulin is unable to use glucose to meet energy requirements. Therefore, the body begins breaking down fat for energy, which results in ketones (acid by-products) and ketoacidosis (a metabolic acidosis).

(3) An overdose of aspirin (salicylic acid) results in metabolic acidosis.

80. ❷ Sodium bicarbonate is ordered to buffer the excess acid in the patient with metabolic acidosis.

(1) Oxygen may be prescribed for the patient with respiratory acidosis but will not help correct a metabolic problem.

(3) When acidosis occurs, some of the potassium ions inside the cells go out into the blood in exchange for hydrogen ions going out of the blood and into the cells. This is a cellular buffer system. It results in hyperkalemia until the acidosis is otherwise corrected. Therefore, the nurse would not expect an order to administer potassium to this patient.

(4) There is no reason to expect an order for magnesium sulfate for this patient.

81. ❹ Total body water in an infant is approximately 77 percent in relation to weight. Total body water in an adult is 45 to 60 percent weight, decreasing with age.

(1, 2) Body fluids have the same concentration in infants and children and in adults.

(3) This option is incorrect as seen in rationale (4).

82. ❸ Any medication containing magnesium is contraindicated for the patient with renal failure because the only route for excretion is the kidneys.

(1) Oral fluids are restricted in the patient with renal failure, to prevent fluid overload.

(2) A low-protein diet is prescribed for the patient with renal failure to decrease the urea nitrogen in the blood.

(4) The patient with renal failure may be monitored with cardiac telemetry to observe for dysrhythmias due to hyperkalemia.

83. ❷ Salt-poor albumin replaces the lost serum protein and restores the colloid osmotic pressure, causing the interstitial fluid (edema) to return to the vascular compartment.

(1) Dextran is a plasma volume expander that works by increasing the colloid osmotic pressure and drawing fluid from the interstitial spaces (edema) back into the vascular compartment; however, it does not replace the serum proteins. Dextran is used primarily to restore blood volume for the patient in shock.

(3, 4) These IV solutions would not correct the hypoproteinemia. They would simply provide additional fluid volume.

84. ❷ The best indicator of a patient's fluid status is urinary output.

(1, 3, 4) These options are incorrect as seen in rationale (2).

85. ❶ Muscle weakness and fatigue are symptoms of hypokalemia that should be monitored for in a patient receiving a thiazide diuretic.

(2) A positive Chvostek's sign is seen in patients with hypocalcemia, not hypokalemia.

(3) A Kayexalate enema will further decrease this patient's potassium level, which already is below normal.

(4) This patient's cardiac pattern should be monitored; however, the T wave will be depressed, not elevated, as a result of hypokalemia.

86. ❶ Patients who are at increased risk for developing hypomagnesemia include those with severe malnutrition, alcoholism (due to inadequate diet), and prolonged IV or total parenteral nutrition without magnesium replacement.

(2) The patient with renal insufficiency is prone to hypermagnesemia, not hypomagnesemia, because the kidneys are the primary route for excretion of this electrolyte.

(3) The patient taking antacids is prone to hypermagnesemia, not hypomagnesemia, if the antacid contains magnesium.

(4) A high-protein diet should not be deficient in magnesium and therefore would not result in hypomagnesemia.

87. ❷ Hyperventilation results in excessive loss or "blowing off" of carbon dioxide, which causes alkalosis. As the respiratory system is at fault, it would be respiratory alkalosis.

(1) This option is incorrect as seen in rationale (2).

(3, 4) Hyperventilation alone should have no substantial effect on the serum sodium level.

88. ❶ Clinical manifestations of metabolic acidosis include drowsiness, confusion, coma, headache, increased respiratory rate (tachypnea), arterial pH <7.35, bicarbonate <22 mm Hg, and pCO_2 normal or slightly decreased (compensatory).

(2, 3, 4) These options are incorrect as seen in rationale (1).

89. ❸ When metabolic acidosis develops, the body increases its respiratory rate and depth to "blow off" carbon dioxide (which combines with water to form carbonic acid) and thereby decrease the acid level (compensate).

(1) The body temperature does not increase in response to metabolic acidosis.

(2) The heart rate actually increases, rather than slows, in response to increased respirations.

(4) Metabolic acidosis does not result in decreased urinary output.

90. ❸ Taking large amounts of antacids, particularly baking soda, may result in metabolic alkalosis.

(1) Taking large amounts of antacids does not result in hyperkalemia. If the antacids are absorbed systemically and result in metabolic alkalosis, the serum potassium level would actually decrease.

(2) Taking large amounts of antacids may result in hypernatremia, not hyponatremia, if the antacids contain sodium.

(4) Antacids cannot cause metabolic acidosis.

91. ❶ The patient with moist rales and shortness of breath is not ventilating adequately. This results in a decreased pO_2 (<80 mm Hg), an increased pCO_2 (>45 mm Hg), and respiratory acidosis (pH <7.35). The bicarbonate level would be normal or above normal (>26 mm Hg) once compensation occurs.

(2, 3, 4) These options are incorrect as seen in rationale (1).

92. ❹ When metabolic acidosis occurs, the respiratory system attempts to correct the pH imbalance by "blowing off" (rapid, deep breathing) carbon dioxide. This results in an arterial pCO_2 <35 mm Hg.

(1, 2) In metabolic acidosis, the bicarbonate content is decreased. This is the initial problem, not a compensatory effort.

(3) If the carbon dioxide content is increased, respiratory acidosis would result. This certainly would not compensate for metabolic acidosis; instead it would compound the problem.

93. ❹ A serum sodium level of 140 mEq/L is within the normal range of 135 to 145 mEq/L; therefore, there is no need for a nursing intervention other than to continue monitoring.

(1, 2, 3) These options are incorrect as seen in rationale (4).

94. ❷ When the extracellular sodium content is increased, water from the cells moves out from the area of lower concentration to the area of higher concentration (osmosis).

(1) A decrease, not an increase, in extracellular sodium results in stimulation of the renin-angiotensin response, which results in an increase in aldosterone.

(3, 4) This option is incorrect as seen in rationale (2).

95. ❶ Gastrointestinal contents have a high sodium content; therefore, loss of fluid from this area can result in hyponatremia.

(2, 3, 4) These options are incorrect as seen in rationale (1).

96. ❶ The contents of the stomach are acidic. When these contents are removed from the body via suction, the result is a net loss of acid and gain of alkali. The patient must be monitored for metabolic alkalosis.

(2, 4) There is no reason to assess this patient for muscle flaccidity or skin discoloration.

(3) When a patient develops metabolic alkalosis, the respiratory system attempts to compensate by retaining carbon dioxide. Therefore, the respiratory rate is decreased (bradypnea).

97. ❹ This patient has respiratory alkalosis as a result of hyperventilation. Arterial blood gas findings in respiratory alkalosis are pH normal or >7.45, and pCO_2 and bicarbonate normal (21–28 mEq/L).

(1, 2, 3) These options are incorrect as seen in rationale (4).

98. ❹ Spironolactone (Aldactone) is a potassium-sparing diuretic; therefore, potassium supplements are not appropriate. Electrolyte imbalances can occur with the use of any diuretic.

(1) This option is incorrect as seen in rationale (4).

(2) There should be no changes in the presence or absence of sugar and acetone in the urine as a result of this medication.

(3) All diuretics should be given in the morning to lessen nocturia. Patients receiving diuretics that are not potassium-sparing must be monitored for digitalis toxicity because hypokalemia predisposes to this condition. However, spironolactone (Aldactone) is potassium-sparing.

99. ❶ Sodium chloride 0.45% is hypotonic compared with normal physiologic saline (0.9%).

(2) Sodium chloride 0.9% is isotonic (the same as normal saline).

(3) Dextrose 5% in water has the same osmolality as normal saline and therefore is isotonic; however, once administered it becomes hypotonic as the body metabolizes the dextrose, leaving only water behind.

(4) Dextrose 5% in normal saline is hypertonic.

100. ❹ Administration of IV fluids at a rapid rate would cause distended veins because the fluid is entering the veins more rapidly than the veins can disseminate it.

(1, 2, 3) Very rapid infusion of IV fluid would not cause tortuous, collapsed, or inflamed veins.

Gastrointestinal, Accessory Organ, and Nutritional Anemia Disorders

TOPICAL OUTLINE

I. INFLAMMATORY DISORDERS OF THE ORAL CAVITY

A. Stomatitis

1. Etiology

Stomatitis is an inflammation of the oral cavity with numerous causes, such as bacteria, viruses, nutritional deficiencies, irritants, mechanical trauma, periodontal disease, and systemic infections.

2. Signs and Symptoms

Pain, increased flow of saliva, halitosis, inflammation, ulcers, fever blisters, and tendency to bleed.

3. Treatment

a. Clean mouth thoroughly as needed.

b. Toothbrush should be small enough to reach all teeth. The bristles should be firm enough to clean but not so firm that they are likely to injure tooth enamel and gum tissue. When cleaning dentures, the nurse should hold them over a soft towel so that if they slip from the nurse's grasp, they will not fall on a hard surface and break. Use of a brush and a nonabrasive powder or paste is recommended. The dentures are rinsed well in warm water after cleaning. Water spray units are available to assist with oral hygiene. Flossing at least once per day is recommended. Commercial mouthwashes may be helpful, and many clients enjoy the fresh aftertaste. Steroids (topical or systemic) may be ordered by the physician. Avoidance of smoking and alcoholic beverages is recommended.

c. For local symptoms, supportive measures include warm mouth rinses and topical antihistamines, antacids, or corticosteroids.

II. TYPES OF STOMATITIS

A. Gingivitis (Trench Mouth)

1. Etiology

Gingivitis is inflammation of the gingivae (gums). It may be caused by improper dental or oral hygiene, poorly fitting dentures, or tobacco. It may be a side effect of Dilantin.

2. Signs and Symptoms

Inflamed gingivae, tendency to bleed, redness, swelling, development of gum pus, and abscess formation with loss of teeth.

3. Treatment

Focus on prevention by providing excellent mouth care, which includes gum massage, professional teeth cleaning, health teaching, and conscientious brushing habits. Physician may order application of antibiotics and mouth irrigations.

B. Leukoplakia ("Smoker's Patch")

1. Etiology

Leukoplakia is the formation of white spots or patches on the mucous membrane of the tongue or cheek. The etiology includes tobacco: pipes, cigars, cigarettes, and chewed or "dipped." Other factors are alcohol, iron deficiency, and vitamin deficiencies.

2. Signs and Symptoms

White patches on the oral mucosa that cannot be rubbed off. Leukoplakia is the most common form of precancerous lesions in the oral cavity.

3. Treatment

Benign leukoplakia usually resolves on cessation of tobacco (e.g., of pipe smoking). Removal of irritant leads to healing in 2 to 4 weeks.

C. Herpes Simplex (Cold Sore, Fever Blister)

1. Etiology

Herpes simplex virus type I. The etiology includes upper respiratory infections, excessive exposure to sunlight, food allergies, emotional tension, and onset of menstruation.

2. Signs and Symptoms

Lip lesions, mouth lesions, vesicle formation (single or clustered), and painful ulcers.

3. Treatment

Spirit of camphor, mild antiseptic mouthwash (without alcohol), viscous lidocaine (to alleviate pain), removal of predisposing factors. Physician may order antiviral agents or steroids (topical or systemic).

4. Nursing Implications

a. Assess patient for signs and symptoms of inflammation of the oral cavity.

b. Assess gums for inflammation and bleeding.

c. Assist patient if necessary to clean mouth as needed.

d. Clean dentures over a soft towel, using a brush and a nonabrasive powder or paste. Rinse the dentures well with warm water after cleaning. Dentures should fit properly or they can become a source of irritation.

e. Administer medications as ordered by the physician.

f. Prevent or cure oral cavity inflammation by educating the patient about good oral hygiene and the need to eliminate the use of alcohol and tobacco.

III. ESOPHAGEAL DISORDERS

A. Esophageal Achalasia

1. Etiology

a. The cause is unknown, but the disorder is a direct result of disruptions of the normal neuromuscular mechanism of the esophagus. In achalasia there is decreased motility of the lower two thirds of the esophagus with the absence of effective coordinated peristalsis.

b. The lower esophageal sphincter does not relax normally with swallowing, and obstruction of the esophagus at or near the diaphragm occurs.

c. Food and fluid accumulate in the lower esophagus. Altered peristalsis due to impairment of the esophagus affects all ages and both sexes. The course of the disease is chronic.

2. Signs and Symptoms

a. Dysphagia is the most common symptoms and occurs most frequently with both liquids and solids.

b. Halitosis and regurgitation of sour-tasting liquids are common symptoms if diverticula are present.

c. Loss of weight.

3. Treatment

a. The aim of medical management is to relieve symptoms. Symptomatic treatment consists of sedatives, a semisoft bland diet, eating slowly, drinking fluids with meals, sleeping with the head of the bed elevated, H_2 histamine receptor antagonists such as ranitidine (Zantac), and cholinergic gastrointestinal (GI) agents such as cisapride.

b. The most successful treatment for relieving symptoms is forceful dilation of the entrance into the stomach.

c. Surgical intervention may become necessary. An esophagomyotomy may be done, in which the muscle fibers that enclose the narrowed area of the esophagus are divided.

B. Esophagitis

1. Etiology

a. Esophagitis (inflammation of the esophagus) is very common and may occur as a result of excessive alcohol intake, excessive use of tobacco, chemical irritation, and ingestion of lye or dust. Esophagitis may be caused by gastroesophageal reflux disease (GERD). Causes of GERD include an idiopathic incompetent lower esophageal sphincter, pregnancy, obesity, ascites, hiatal hernia, and postoperative resection of the lower esophagus (sliding hiatal hernia).

b. Reflux esophagitis is very common. It is due to the reflux of gastric contents into the esophagus.

c. A sliding hiatal hernia is a common cause of reflux esophagitis. Gastric secretions cause inflammation of the esophagus. Reflux is due to an incompetent lower esophageal sphincter.

2. Signs and Symptoms

a. Pain in the esophageal and epigastric areas

b. Reflux of gastric contents into mouth, causing a sour, bitter taste

3. Treatment

a. Treatment of esophagitis depends on the cause. If strong acid causes acute esophagitis, prompt and vigorous treatment is necessary to stop the acid from eroding through the esophagus.

b. Treatment of chronic esophagitis includes oral antacids, bland diet, and sleeping with the head of the bed elevated. The physician may prescribe gastric pump inhibitors (e.g., Prilosec, Prevacid, or Nexium). See *Handbook of Medications for the NCLEX-RN Review,* Chapter 10, for more information on drug therapy.

C. Hiatal Hernia

1. Etiology

   a. A hiatal hernia is a protrusion of part of the stomach into the thoracic cavity through the opening in the diaphragm through which the esophagus passes.

   b. It occurs more often in women (ages 40–70 years) than in men and is the most common upper GI pathologic condition of the upper GI tract.

   c. The etiology is a weakening of the diaphragmatic muscle. It may be congenital, with symptoms occurring later in life, or it may result from aging.

   d. The major factor contributing to the development of hiatal hernia is increased intraabdominal pressure. This can result from lifting heavy objects, coughing, vomiting, obesity, and pregnancy.

2. Signs and Symptoms

   a. No symptoms occur until the lower esophageal sphincter becomes incompetent.

   b. The lower esophageal sphincter refers to the muscle at the point of the junction of the esophagus and stomach.

   c. It encircles the esophagus and usually is contracted. This prevents gastric reflux. When the sphincter develops less pressure and tone, the contraction of the esophagus is not complete.

   d. This permits gastric reflux to occur. Regurgitation (effortless return of gastric contents into esophagus or mouth) is a fairly common manifestation of hiatal hernia.

   e. It often is described as bitter, hot, or sour liquid coming into the throat or mouth.

   f. Other symptoms of hiatal hernia include feelings of a lump in the throat or of food stopping, dysphagia (difficulty swallowing), and painful swallowing. Some patients with hiatal hernia are asymptomatic. Some patients have pain that they believe may be cardiac in nature, and they may seek assistance in an emergency room.

3. Diagnosis

   a. The latest diagnostic test for GERD involves inserting into the esophagus a wireless transmitter called a Bravo, which is approximately 1 inch long and as wide as a pencil. It is a major improvement over the standard nasal catheter inserted through the nose and down the throat for 24 h.

   b. The Bravo, which wirelessly transmits data to a small receiver worn by the patient for 48 h, detaches within a few days and then passes through the body's digestive tract.

   c. Once hiatal hernia is diagnosed, treatment can begin. Untreated, it can lead to respiratory problems, noncardiac chest pain, or even a precancerous condition.

4. Treatment

   a. Medical treatment consists mainly of various measures to prevent gastric reflux and medications to relieve symptoms.

   b. Administration of gastric pump inhibitors (e.g., Prilosec, Prevacid, or Nexium), elimination of alcohol and tobacco, avoidance of lifting and straining, and elevation of the head of the bed all help to relieve symptoms. The patient is instructed to remain in an upright position after eating instead of reclining.

   c. The obese patient is encouraged to lose weight.

   d. Surgical intervention for hiatal hernia is indicated when medical therapy fails or for complications such as stenosis, strangulation, and bleeding.

   e. The object of surgery is to restore gastroesophageal integrity and prevent gastric reflux by reinforcing the sphincter muscle.

IV. DISORDERS OF THE STOMACH, WITH DIAGNOSTIC PROCEDURE

A. Gastritis

1. Etiology

   a. Gastritis refers to any diffuse lesion in the gastric mucosa that can be identified histologically as inflamed.

   b. Gastritis may occur as an acute or chronic disorder and is more common in the elderly population.

   c. Acute gastritis is a short-lived inflammatory process affecting the mucosa of the stomach. It involves erosion of the mucosa.

   d. A number of drugs, stimuli, and circumstances are associated with acute gastritis, including ingestion of aspirin, antiinflammatory agents, corticosteroids, alcohol, major physiologic stress, and intense emotional reactions.

   e. The most common cause of acute superficial gastritis is alcohol.

   f. Stress ulcers are a form of acute gastritis. They occur frequently after burns or other major physiologic stressors.

   g. Chronic gastritis often is referred to as *nonerosive* and is differentiated by the histologic appearance of the gastric mucosa. The gastric mucosa is thin with decreased hydrochloric acid secretion. With loss of intrinsic factor, the patient develops pernicious anemia and experiences fatigue and neurologic problems due to decreased vitamin B_{12} production. Several etiologic mechanisms may be involved in the production of chronic gastritis. It may be the result of an autoimmune disorder. Antibodies directed against the parietal cells have been isolated from patients with chronic gastritis.

2. Signs and Symptoms

   a. The symptoms of chronic gastritis depend on the etiologic factors and the extent of inflammation. Patients with chronic gastritis may be asymptomatic until damage is sufficient to produce symptoms.

b. The patients with gastritis as a result of hypersecretion of acid will experience symptoms similar to those of peptic ulcer disease.

c. Assessment may reveal anorexia, a feeling of fullness, belching, vague epigastric pain, nausea, vomiting, and intolerance of spicy or fatty food.

3. Treatment

a. Treatment of gastritis is dictated by the etiologic factors. The aim of medical therapies is to alleviate symptoms.

b. The patient with acute pain may need a topical anesthetic such as benzocaine (used as a gastric mucosal anesthetic and antacid).

c. Discomfort may be lessened with a bland diet, small frequent meals, antacids, antihistamine H_2 antagonist, and avoidance of foods that cause symptoms.

4. Nursing Implications

a. Assess patient for symptoms of gastritis.

b. Administer medications (e.g., gastric pump inhibitors [Prilosec, Prevacid, and Nexium]). Bacterial gastritis is treated with antibiotics (e.g., Flagyl or tetracycline)

c. Instruct the patient to chew food thoroughly, to avoid medications that can irritate the gastric mucosa, such as salicylates, and avoid use of steroids on an empty stomach.

d. Administer vitamin B_{12} by intramuscular (IM) injection if the patient has pernicious anemia.

5. Diagnostic Procedures

a. Gastric analysis

◆ In this procedure, the contents of the stomach are examined to determine whether hydrochloric acid is present and in what amount.

(1) It is useful in the diagnosis of ulcer disease, which is characterized by high gastric acidity, and of pernicious anemia, in which gastric acid is absent.

(2) The evening before gastric analysis, the patient is NPO after midnight and is not allowed to smoke the morning of the test because smoking can stimulate the production of gastric acid and affect test results.

(3) A nasogastric tube is inserted through the nose or mouth into the stomach and is taped in place. Gastric contents are withdrawn using a syringe and gentle suction at 15- to 20-min intervals for 1 to 3 h.

(4) A stimulus in the form of caffeine, alcohol, or injection of histamine may be given to stimulate gastric secretion.

b. Barium swallow (fluoroscopy), an upper GI procedure

(1) This is an x-ray examination of the esophagus, stomach, and duodenum.

(2) The procedure is used to detect esophageal tumors, esophageal varices, gastric ulcers, and gastritis.

(3) Barium sulfate, a white, chalky radiopaque substance, is swallowed to allow x-ray visualization of the structures.

(4) Basic preparation for an upper GI series may be done at home. The patient is on a low residual diet for 2 days and clear liquid diet the day before the procedure. The patient remains on NPO status after midnight and on the morning of the examination.

c. Barium enema, a lower GI procedure

(1) This procedure is used to diagnose problems of the large intestine, such as polyps, diverticula, tumors, Crohn's disease, and ulcerative colitis. Crohn's disease, also known as *regional enteritis,* is an inflammation of any part of the GI tract (usually the proximal portion of the colon or, less often, the terminal ilium) that extends through all layers of the intestinal wall.

(2) A bowel preparation is done prior to the procedure to adequately cleanse the bowel of feces, which would interfere with the test and produce inaccurate results. The patent may receive a mild sedative before the procedure.

(3) If the procedure is done in the hospital or outpatient clinic, four or more enemas are given until clear, and an oral cathartic is administered the evening before the examination.

(4) Alternative bowel preparation, used for outpatients, consists of a Fleet enema and GoLYTELY (an osmotic solution taken orally to induce diarrhea), which is consumed every 10 to 15 min. No food or fluid is taken after midnight or on the morning of the examination. Enemas and strong irritants usually are not administered to the elderly or severely ill patients. These patients usually are given Fleet's Phosphate of Soda enemas the evening prior to the GI procedure and a low volume of enema the morning of the procedure.

(5) A barium enema is administered, and the progress of the barium enema is followed on a fluoroscopy screen. X-ray films are taken with the patient in different positions. Different positions allow for visualization of all areas of the large bowel.

(6) When the procedure is completed, the patient is allowed to expel the barium, and additional films are taken of the entire lower GI tract.

d. Consideration of upper and lower GI procedures

(1) The major complications of an upper or lower barium enema are severe constipation and impaction of barium in the bowel.

(2) A barium study of the upper or lower GI tract is contraindicated in patients with megacolon, perforation, or obstruction of the GI tract.

(3) A pregnant woman should not undergo this procedure done except in emergency situations because the x-rays might damage the fetus.

(4) If upper and lower GI procedures are scheduled, the lower GI procedure must be done first because several days are required for swallowed barium to pass completely out of the GI tract. The residual barium can distort the results of the lower GI procedure.

(5) Because barium sulfate is a constipating substance that can cause obstruction of the GI tract if not eliminated, cathartics must be given after the procedure is completed.

e. Endoscopic retrograde cholangiopancreatography (ERCP), a nonsurgical procedure

(1) This procedure allows for visualization of the pancreas, gallbladder, and biliary tree—the system of ducts that carries bile and pancreatic juices from the liver and the gallbladder into the first section of the intestine.

(2) The physician injects x-ray contrast (dye) into the bile ducts so that stones will show up clearly. The physician passes an endoscope into the stomach and places a mouthpiece in the patient's mouth to hold the teeth apart and the mouth open. A nurse suctions fluid from the patient's mouth as necessary.

(3) If a stone is present in the common bile duct, an endoscopic papillotomy (EPT) can be performed. The cannula of the endoscope is replaced with an electric surgical cutter. The sphincter of Oddi is enlarged by cutting it open (sphincterotomy). A basket is passed through the endoscope to retrieve the stone. The stone can be placed in the duodenum and passed naturally in the stool or removed in the basket. The opening of the bile duct will retain its new width, allowing same-size or smaller stones to pass through it should they recur. Patients may go home several hours after the procedure. They are instructed to drink no alcoholic beverages for the next 24 h. They cannot drive a car or operate any hazardous machinery for the next 12 h. Complications of this procedure can occur but are uncommon. One possible complication is pancreatitis due to irritation of the pancreatic duct.

B. Peptic Ulcer

1. Etiology

a. Development of peptic ulceration depends on the defensive resistance of the mucosa, relative to the volume of hydrochloric acid. Ulceration occurs when aggressive factors exceed defensive factors.

b. Emotional stress can cause an increase in gastric motility via thalamus stimulation to the vagal nerves.

c. When patients undergo stress reactions, the sympathetic nervous system causes the blood vessels in the duodenum to constrict, which makes the mucosa more vulnerable to trauma from gastric acid and pepsin secretion. Prolonged stress from burns and severe trauma can produce stress ulcers (also known as *Curling's ulcers*) within the GI tract.

d. Certain medications may contribute to gastroduodenal ulcerations by altering gastric secretion, producing local damage to mucosa. Antiinflammatory agents such as phenylbutazone (Butazolidin) and indomethacin (Indocin) decrease mucosal resistance and should be used with caution. Reserpine (Tensin), alcohol, and caffeine stimulate acid production. Aspirin ingestion is frequently related to mucosal damage and suppressed mucus secretion.

e. *Helicobacter pylori* is a gram-negative bacteria that can colonize in the stomach and duodenum. By taking up residence between epithelial cells and the mucous barrier that protects them, this organism manages to escape destruction by acid and pepsin.

(1) There is a strong association between *H. pylori* infection and peptic ulcer.

(2) *H. pylori* is present in 95 percent of patients with duodenal ulcers and 75 percent of patients with gastric ulcers. Eradication of the bacteria promotes ulcer healing and minimizes recurrence.

(3) Although the mechanism by which *H. pylori* promotes ulcers is not firmly established, research has shown a definite association.

(4) Antibiotics (e.g., Flagyl) are used to eradicate *H. pylori*.

2. Signs and Symptoms

a. The principal symptom experienced by the patient with stomach ulcers and duodenal ulcers is an aching, burning, cramplike, gnawing epigastric pain. The pain has a definite relationship to eating, and pain may be relieved by food or antacids. If the ulcer is located in the stomach, symptoms will occur on an empty stomach. With duodenal ulcers, symptoms may occur after eating.

b. Clients have a normal appetite unless pyloric obstruction is present. Carcinoma or gastritis may be associated with anorexia, weight loss, and dysphagia.

c. Vomiting usually results from gastric stasis or pyloric obstruction.

V. MAJOR COMPLICATIONS OF ULCERS

A. Hemorrhage

Occurs when ulcers perforate blood vessels. Hemorrhage varies from minimal bleeding, manifested by occult blood in the stool (melena), to massive bleeding, in which the patient vomits bright red blood (hematemesis).

1. Signs and Symptoms

The usual symptoms of GI bleeding are either vomiting of coffee ground-colored material or passing of tarry stools. Symptoms of severe blood loss of more than 1 L in 24 h may cause the manifestations of shock, such as hypotension, weak thready pulse, palpitations, diaphoresis, and chills.

2. Interventions

a. Monitor vital signs every 15 to 30 min. Early recognition of changes in vital signs and an increase in the amount and redness (blood) of nasogastric drainage often signal massive upper GI bleeding.

b. It is important to maintain the patency of the nasogastric tube so that blood clots do not obstruct the tube. The patient should be observed closely for bleeding.

c. Monitor the results of hemoglobin and hematocrit laboratory values.

d. Assess the patient's level of consciousness, vital signs, skin color, and capillary refill.

e. Check the abdomen for distention, guarding (client does not want abdomen touched), peristalsis, and the presence of a boardlike rigid abdomen.

f. Signs and symptoms of shock include low blood pressure (BP); rapid, weak pulse; increased thirst; cold, clammy skin; and restlessness.

g. When a patient has a base systolic pressure of 130 mm Hg that drops to less than 104 mm Hg, the drop suggests a blood loss of more than 20 percent. Check the BP several times before calling the physician.

h. Use of cool (not ice) lavages with saline is a standard treatment modality for upper GI bleeding, and vasopressin is used to constrict bleeding blood vessels.

i. Approach the patient in a calm and assured manner to help decrease the level of anxiety.

j. Measure urine output hourly. A rate of at least 30 mL/h indicates minimum renal perfusion. Lesser amounts may indicate renal ischemia, secondary to loss of blood volume.

k. Measure urine specific gravity because it will provide additional information regarding the patient's hydration status. Consistent readings greater than 1.025 (normal = 1.005–1.025) indicate the urine is very concentrated and that there is probably a low blood volume.

l. If the patient has a central venous pressure (CVP) line in place, record readings every 1 to 2 h (normal CVP = 3–12 cm H_2O or 2 to 6 mm Hg).

m. Administer antihypotensive agents such as dopamine as ordered.

B. Perforation

This usually is a surgical emergency.

1. Etiology

The ulcer perforates the stomach and gastroduodenal contents enter the peritoneal cavity, causing chemical peritonitis, bacterial septicemia, and hypovolemic shock.

2. Signs and Symptoms

a. Sudden, sharp, severe pain beginning in the midepigastrium.

b. Diminished peristalsis or ileus may develop.

3. Treatment

a. Immediate replacement of fluid, blood, and electrolytes and administration of antibiotics in preparation for surgery.

b. Nasogastric suction to drain gastric secretions and prevent further gastric spillage in preparation for surgery.

4. Nursing Implications

a. Aim interventions at controlling hypovolemic shock by preventing dehydration and electrolyte imbalance and stopping bleeding.

b. Insert a nasogastric tube (with physician's order) to assess rate of bleeding and to administer cool saline lavage. The cool saline will constrict blood vessels in the stomach and slow bleeding. Iced saline usually is not used because it may cause more mucosal damage by decreasing perfusion of the gastric mucosa, and it may cause a vagal response that could result in cardiac asystole.

c. Maintain patient on bed rest for several days after bleeding has subsided. Rest decreases BP and GI activity.

C. Types of Gastric Surgery

In a *total gastrectomy*, the entire stomach is removed. This radical surgery is performed infrequently to treat stomach cancer. A *subtotal gastrectomy*, a generic term referring to any surgery that involves partial removal of the stomach, may be performed by either a Billroth I or a Billroth II procedure. In *Billroth I*, or *gastroduodenostomy*, part of the stomach is removed and the remainder is anastomosed to the duodenum. In *Billroth II*, or *gastrojejunostomy*, the lower part of the stomach is removed and the remaining stomach is anastomosed to the jejunum. In *Billroth III*, all of the stomach is removed and the esophagus is anastomosed to jejunum. This is the same as a total gastrectomy.

1. Pernicious Anemia after Total Gastrectomy

a. The patient is unable to absorb vitamin B_{12} because the intrinsic factor necessary for the absorption of vitamin B_{12} has been removed.

b. When vitamin B_{12} is not absorbed, pernicious anemia develops. The patient must receive IM vitamin B_{12} injections lifelong.

c. Signs and symptoms include weakness, numbness, and tingling in extremities.

2. Dumping Syndrome after Gastrectomy

a. Dumping syndrome may occur because ingested food enters the jejunum too rapidly.

b. Early manifestations occur 5 to 30 min after eating and include sweating, pallor, diarrhea, palpitations, and nausea.

c. Late manifestations occur 2 to 3 h after eating and are caused by the rapid entry of high-carbohydrate food into the jejunum. This increases the blood sugar level and causes excessive production of insulin. This, in return, results in symptoms of hypoglycemia.

3. Nursing Implications after Gastrectomy

a. After surgery check vital signs, dressing for drainage, suture line for signs of infection and dehiscence, patency of nasogastric tube, and character of nasogastric drainage (normally bloody for 12–24 h, then brown-tinged, and finally light yellow or clear).

b. The amount of nasogastric drainage decreases as peristalsis returns.

c. Assess for passage bowel sounds and the passage of flatus.

d. Monitor for nausea and vomiting.

e. Assess tolerance to food and fluid when oral intake is resumed.

f. Have the patient turn, cough, and deep breathe every 2 h while on bed rest and ambulate as ordered. Keep the head of the bed slightly elevated to decrease pull on incision. Splint incisions with pillow when coughing, deep breathing, or turning.

g. Check patency of nasogastric tubing when patient complains of nausea or vomits. Administer antiemetic such as promethazine hydrochloride (Phenergan), as ordered.

h. Administer intravenous (IV) fluid to replace nasogastric drainage, as ordered.

i. Administer vitamin B$_{12}$ IM for pernicious anemia.

j. Combat dumping syndrome by instructing patient to avoid fluid with meals; assume low Fowler's position during and after meals for 1 h; and avoid high-carbohydrate foods. Administer antispasmodics such as belladonna (Donnatal) as ordered to help delay gastric emptying.

VI. DISORDERS OF THE INTESTINES AND SURGICAL MANAGEMENT

A. Diverticular Disease

Diverticula are outpouchings of the intestine. When diverticula are not inflamed, the condition is called *diverticulosis,* and the patient may be asymptomatic. When inflammation is present, the condition is referred to as *diverticulitis.*

1. Incidence
Diverticular disease is most prevalent in men older than 40 years.

2. Etiology

a. Diet may be a contributing factor as lack of roughage reduces fecal residue, narrows the bowel lumen, and leads to higher intraabdominal pressure during defecation.

b. The fact that diverticulosis is most prevalent in western industrialized nations, where processing removes much of the roughage from foods, supports this theory.

c. Diverticulosis is less common in nations where the diet contains more natural bulk and fiber.

3. Signs and Symptoms
Diverticulitis causes spasms and constipation alternating with diarrhea, blood in stool, severe abdominal pain, fever, nausea, and vomiting.

4. Nursing Assessment

a. Assess for abdominal pain (onset, type, location, and intensity), abdominal distention, and fever.

b. Assess elimination pattern, frequency, consistency of stool, and time and ease of defecation. Observe for melena. Assess use of laxatives.

c. Review dietary pattern including type and amount of food ingested.

d. Assess for abdominal rigidity (boardlike), tenderness, tachycardia, and hypotension, which can indicate perforation of the intestine.

5. Nursing Interventions

a. Instruct patient with diverticulosis to eat high-fiber foods such as fresh fruits with skin, whole-wheat bread and cereal, and raw vegetables such as lettuce, carrots, and cauliflower. These high-fiber foods add bulk to stool and speed its passage through the bowel.

b. Instruct patient to add bran to food on a daily basis. Begin with 1 teaspoon per day and gradually progress to 2 to 4 teaspoons per day.

c. Instruct patient to drink 8 to 10 glasses of water per day (unless otherwise contradicted) because fiber retains water and decreases its absorption.

d. Instruct patient to avoid strong enemas and laxatives and to use hydrophilic colloid laxatives (Metamucil) and stool softeners.

e. Caution patient against overuse of enemas, laxatives, stool softeners, and an extremely high-fiber diet. Excessive bulk in diet may damage the lining of the intestines.

f. The patient with diverticulitis may be NPO during the severe inflammatory stage. Administer IV fluids as ordered; monitor nasogastric suctioning; and administer antispasmodics (e.g., Donnatal), analgesics, steroids, and antibiotics, as ordered.

g. Maintain patient on bed rest during acute phase of diverticulitis to decrease GI activity.

h. Monitor for hemorrhage, bowel obstruction, and intestinal perforation.

B. Ulcerative Colitis Disease

1. Etiology and Incidence
Causes of ulcerative colitis are unknown, although it is related to abnormal immune response in the GI tract, possibly associated with food or bacteria such as *Escherichia coli.* Ulcerative colitis occurs primarily in young adults, especially women. It is prevalent among those of Jewish ancestry, indicating a possible familiar tendency.

2. Signs and Symptoms

a. Onset of signs and symptoms occur between the ages of 15 and 35 years, but it has been reported in every decade of life.

b. The patient with severe ulcerative colitis may have frequent liquid stools (10–20 liquid stools per day) containing blood and pus. The patient may complain of severe cramps and demonstrate signs and symptoms of dehydration, fever, weight loss, electrolyte abnormalities, especially hypokalemia, anorexia, nausea, and vomiting.

c. Ulcerative colitis may lead to complications, such as hemorrhage, stricture, or perforation of the colon.

3. Pathology

a. In ulcerative colitis, there is an inflammatory, usually chronic, disease that affects the mucosa of the colon. When there is involvement of the entire colon, there may be minimal involvement of a few centimeters of the terminal ileum.

b. Severity ranges from a mild, localized disorder to a fulminant disease that may cause a perforating colon, progressing to potentially fatal peritonitis and toxemia.

c. A striking feature of the inflammation is that it is uniform and continuous with no intervening areas of normal mucosa.

◆ The aim of therapy is to control the inflammatory process and to replace nutritional losses.

4. Treatment

a. In the severely ill patient, even clear liquids taken orally may stimulate colonic activity; therefore, the patient should receive nothing by mouth.

b. Total parenteral nutrition (TPN) administered IV; is used to rest the intestinal tract and decrease stool volume. Blood transfusions or iron supplements may be needed to correct anemia.

5. Nursing Interventions

a. Monitor intake and output.

b. Replace fluid, nutritional, and electrolyte losses with IV fluids. TPN may be ordered.

C. Crohn's Disease

1. Etiology

a. Although the exact cause of Crohn's disease is unknown, autoimmune and genetic factors are thought to play a role. Up to 5 percent of those affected have one relative with the disease. Jewish ancestry is a risk factor.

b. The incidences of Crohn's disease have risen steadily over the past 50 years. It now affects 7 of every 100,000 people. Crohn's disease is most prevalent in adults ages 20 to 40 years. It is two to three times more common in those of Jewish ancestry and least common in blacks.

2. Signs and Symptoms

a. Clinical effects initially may be mild and nonspecific. They vary according to the location and extent of the lesion.

b. Acute inflammatory signs mimic appendicitis and include steady, colicky pain in the right lower quadrant, cramping, tenderness, flatulence, nausea, fever, and diarrhea. Bleeding may occur and, although usually mild, may be massive. Blood in stools may occur. Chronic symptoms, which

are more typical of the disease, are more persistent and less severe. They include diarrhea (4–6 stools per day) with pain in the right lower abdominal quadrant, steatorrhea fat in feces), and marked weight loss.

3. Treatment

a. The principal drugs used for therapy are the antiinflammatory agents sulfasalazine (Azulfidine), steroids, and Donnatal to reduce intestinal spasms. Agents to control diarrhea include Atropine, Lomotil, and codeine. Lomotil is the drug used most often.

b. There may be iron deficiency anemia, which reflects chronic disease from chronic blood loss and poor iron absorption.

4. Pathology

In Crohn's disease, the inflammation often is discontinuous. Severely involved segments of bowel are separated from each other by "skip areas" of apparently normal bowel. In 50 percent of patients with Crohn's disease of the colon, the rectum is spared. In contrast to ulcerative colitis, Crohn's disease is characterized by chronic inflammation extending through all layers of the intestinal wall.

5. Nursing Assessment

a. Assess for abdominal cramps, intestinal spasms, and abdominal distention.

b. Assess for signs of dehydration, fever, frequency and consistency of stools, and weight loss.

c. Assess for electrolyte abnormalities, anemia, and blood in stool.

VII. CORRECTIVE SURGERY

A. Surgical Management of Crohn's Disease and Ulcerative Colitis

1. Medical Treatment

a. The majority of patients with Crohn's disease eventually require surgery at least once during the course of their disease.

b. This in contrast to ulcerative colitis, where colectomy is curative. In Crohn's disease, surgical resection of the small or large intestine is followed by a high rate of recurrence.

c. Temporary colostomy may be used to rest and heal the colon in clients with ulcerative colitis.

d. Faced with the possibility of recurrent disease, many physicians are reluctant to advise surgery for Crohn's disease, except for the following complications: fixed bowel narrowing or obstruction, persistent fistulas, massive hemorrhage, perforation, and severe anorectal disease.

e. Approximately 85 percent of patients with ulcerative colitis go into remission with medical management. Surgery is indicated for the same reasons given for Crohn's disease.

2. Types of Surgical Procedures

a. Proctocolectomy

A proctocolectomy results in an external ileostomy. The diseased colon and rectum with the terminal ileum are removed through the abdominal wall.

(1) Drainage into an ileostomy bag is continuous because the bag is the small intestine; water is absorbed in the large bowel.

(2) The ileostomy is not irrigated because stool has liquid consistency.

b. Kock's pouch (continent ileostomy)

A reservoir or pouch is constructed from a loop of the ileum. This reservoir stores fecal content intraabdominally. It is drained several times per day through a nipple valve using a soft rubber catheter.

(1) Advantages

(a) No external pouch

(b) Minimal skin irritation

(2) Cautions

(a) Problems with leakage and frequent revisions have made this procedure less attractive.

(b) Kock's pouch can be used for treatment of ulcerative colitis when a major part or all of the colon must be removed but is not recommended as treatment for Crohn's disease because recurrence of the disease (50 percent incidence) would destroy the pouch.

(c) Fecal content must be drained frequently for the first few weeks after surgery. It takes several weeks for the pouch to enlarge enough to hold normal amounts of fecal drainage.

(d) Liquid fecal content left in pouch 6 to 8 h may become semisolid as a result of water evaporation and absorption. When this occurs, a small amount of fluid is added to allow easy removal of fecal drainage.

c. Ileorectal anastomosis

Can be used when all of the colon is removed but the rectum is only mildly affected. The terminal small bowel is used to create an internal ileal pouch that is anastomosed to the rectal stump, thus preserving rectal function.

(1) There is great enthusiasm for ileorectal anastomosis with an internal ileal pouch created to act as a reservoir.

(2) This often produces a highly satisfactory result, with continence and five to seven stools per day passed through the rectum.

(3) Complications such as pouchitis and the need for surgical revision seem less frequent than with the continent ileostomy (Kock's pouch).

(4) The procedure is an excellent alternative for clients who will not accept an external ileostomy or Kock's pouch.

3. Nursing Care for Ileostomy

Nursing care for a patient with a conventional ileostomy is similar to that for a patient with Kock's pouch and ileorectal anastomosis.

a. Expect the ileorectal anastomosis to be noisy initially as the result of tissue edema; the noise decreases with time.

b. Expect foods such as seeds and kernels to pass through undigested.

c. Give meticulous care to the skin surrounding the stoma of the external ileostomy and the very small stoma of the Kock's pouch.

d. Continuously assess the patient for signs of dehydration, hypokalemia, and hyponatremia.

e. Avoid laxatives.

f. Treat blockage of the conventional ileostomy caused by a mass of undigested high-fiber foods by gently massaging the area below the stoma. Call physician if lumen remains blocked because a lavage by bulb syringe with 30 to 50 mL of normal saline may be required.

VIII. BOWEL DISORDERS

A. Organic (Mechanical)

1. Etiology

Paralytic ileus or mechanical blockage caused by neoplasms, fecal impaction, intussusception, or neurogenic impairment.

2. Signs and Symptoms

a. The clinical manifestations vary depending on the location of the obstruction (small or large intestine) and whether it is partial or complete.

b. Vomiting is common in obstruction in the small intestine and occurs earlier and more profusely the higher in the intestine that the obstruction occurs.

c. If the obstruction is in the large intestine, vomiting usually does not occur because the ileocecal valve prevents backflow from the colon into the ileum.

d. Abdominal distention is a common manifestation of all intestinal obstructions.

3. Treatment

a. Mechanical intestinal obstructions are treated surgically.

b. Prophylactic antibiotics given intramuscularly or intravenously.

c. Surgical intervention consists of resecting the occluded bowel and anastomosing the remaining healthy segments.

d. Treatment of bowel obstruction consists of intestinal intubation and decompression to remove gas and fluid prior to surgery. This procedure relieves vomiting and reduces distention.

e. Enemas are never given to a patient with bowel obstruction because they may cause rupture of the colon.

B. Paralytic Ileus

1. Etiology

   a. A paralytic ileus is the cessation of peristalsis (ileus) as a result of neurogenic impairment.

   b. Paralytic ileus commonly results from direct irritation of the GI tract (occurring during surgery), peritoneal irritation, major trauma, use of large amounts of narcotics, sepsis, and severe electrolyte abnormalities (particularly hypokalemia).

2. Signs and Symptoms

   a. Abdominal distention

   b. Absent or decreased bowel sounds

   c. Vomiting and signs of dehydration

3. Treatment and Nursing Implications

   a. GI intubation with a nasogastric tube until peristalsis resumes.

   b. IV fluids and electrolytes to replace nasogastric drainage.

   c. Gradual resumption of fluids and food when bowel function returns.

   d. Nasogastric drainage is assessed for color, measured, and emptied every shift.

C. Inguinal Hernia

1. Etiology

   A hernia occurs when part of an internal organ protrudes through an abnormal opening in the containing wall of its cavity. Most hernias occur in the abdominal cavity. Although many kinds of abdominal hernias are possible, inguinal hernias are most common. In an inguinal hernia, the large or small intestine protrudes into the inguinal canal. Some hernias can be manipulated back into place. A herniated intestine that becomes twisted or edematous can seriously interfere with normal blood flow and may lead to intestinal obstruction and necrosis.

2. Signs and Symptoms

   Inguinal hernia usually causes a lump to appear over the herniated area when the patient stands or strains. The lump disappears when the patient is supine. Tension on the herniated contents may cause a sharp, steady pain in the groin, which fades when the hernia is reduced. Strangulation produces severe pain and may lead to partial or complete bowel obstruction and even intestinal necrosis. Partial bowel obstruction may cause anorexia, vomiting, pain and tenderness in the groin, an irreducible mass, and diminished bowel sounds. Complete obstruction may cause shock, high fever, absent bowel sounds, and bloody stools. In an infant, an inguinal hernia often coexists with an undescended testicle or hydrocele.

3. Treatment

   a. If the hernia is reducible, the pain may be temporarily relieved by pushing the hernia back into place. A truss may keep the abdominal contents from protruding into the hernial sac, although it will not cure the hernia. This device is especially beneficial for an elderly or debilitated patient because any surgery is potentially hazardous to the patient.

   b. For infants, adults, and otherwise healthy elderly patients, herniorrhaphy is the treatment of choice. Herniorrhaphy replaces the contents of the hernial sac into the abdominal cavity and closes the opening or reenforces the opening with medical mesh.

IX. TUMORS OF THE BOWEL

The most frequent tumors of the bowel are polyps (small tissue that protrudes into the bowel lumen). The two major types of polyps are hyperplastic polyps (not premalignant) and neoplastic polyps (malignant). Malignant tumors of the colon and rectum are among the most commonly occurring malignancies in the United States.

A. Colorectal Cancer

1. Etiology and Incidence

   a. The American Cancer Society estimates an incidence of 87,000 cases of colon and rectal cancer in 1992.

   b. Colorectal cancer is the second most common visceral malignant neoplasm in the United States. Incidence is equally distributed between men and women. It ranks just behind lung cancer as a leading cause of cancer deaths in the United States.

   c. Most tumors are found in the distal portion of the large bowel from the sigmoid colon to the anus.

   d. No cause is known.

   e. Colorectal cancer tends to progress slowly and remains localized for a long time. Consequently, it is potentially curable if early resection is performed before nodal involvement.

2. Risk Factors

   a. Family history of colon cancer

   b. Previous colon cancer

   c. Ulcerative colitis

   d. Familial intestinal and rectal polyps

   e. Low-residue diet that is high in refined foods

   f. Residence in highly industrialized or urban societies

   g. Age over 40 years.

3. Signs and Symptoms

   a. Rectal bleeding, changed bowel habits, and intestinal obstruction

   b. Weight loss, anorexia, nausea and vomiting, anemia, and palpable mass

4. Surgical Treatment of Colon Cancer

   a. Total resection of tumor represents optimal management when a malignant lesion is endoscopically or radiographically detected in the large bowel. Although postoperative radiation therapy has been offered to some patients following such total resection, most authorities favor short-term systemic treatment with combination chemotherapy.

b. Radiation therapy to the pelvis is generally recommended for patients with rectal cancer because of the 30 to 40 percent probability of regional recurrence following complete surgical resection of the tumor.

c. Chemotherapy in patients with advanced colorectal cancer has been found to be of only marginal benefit. Clinical trials have found 5-fluorouracil (5-FU) to be the most effective treatment.

d. If enough colon remains, an end-to-end anastomosis is performed; if not, a permanent colostomy is created. A colostomy is the creation of an opening between the colon and the abdominal wall through which fecal content passes.

e. Temporary colostomy (usually double-barreled) may be used to allow the bowel to rest and heal (e.g., ulcerative colitis).

f. Double-barreled colostomy has proximal and distal stomas. The proximal stoma is irrigated but the distal stoma is not; it is allowed to rest and heal. Liquid antibiotics may be inserted into the distal stoma if needed for infections.

5. Nursing Implications

a. The preoperative period begins when surgery is determined to be the best course of treatment. Diagnostic studies are initiated, body system disorders are stabilized, and consent for surgery is obtained.

b. Obtain history of hospitalization and surgical experience.

c. Determine the patient's knowledge base about planned surgery.

d. Check vital signs as needed.

e. Observe for nonverbal signs of anxiety, such as nervousness, withdrawal, and increasing pulse rate.

f. Ask about significant others, coping mechanisms, and other support systems.

g. Teach the patient about deep breathing and leg exercises and educate about colostomy irrigation before surgery.

h. If colostomy will be permanent, the patient should be allowed to express feelings and have time to discuss treatment and prognosis before surgery.

i. The patient will have a nasogastric tube inserted for suctioning after surgery.

j. Provide opportunities for the patient and significant others to ask questions and express concerns.

k. Provide information without giving false or inappropriate hope.

l. Reinforce explanations given by the physician.

m. Refer questions and concerns that cannot be answered to other members of the health care team.

n. Use the assistance of clergy or other support personnel to counsel the patient.

o. After surgery, dilate colostomy stoma as ordered. Assess for the return of peristalsis and begin colostomy irrigation as ordered. Assess the appearance of the stoma and report any sign of cyanosis.

p. Amount of colostomy irrigation for an adult varies from 500 to 1500 mL of tap water; the amount is determined by the patient's weight. The irrigation usually is three times per week and should be administered at the same time each day.

q. Take special care to keep fecal contents off patient's skin around the stoma; clean with tap water (soap irritates). The digestive enzymes will erode the skin.

r. The patient needs a great deal of support; his or her self-image may be altered. The patient must accept colostomy before accepting the responsibility of colostomy care. It takes from 2 to 3 h to complete a colostomy irrigation and drainage until it is well established. After the colostomy has been used for several months it will then take approximately 45 to 60 min to irrigate the colostomy.

s. If the colostomy continues to drain after irrigation is completed, the amount of irrigation fluid must be increased. Continuous drainage after irrigation is a sign that the feces were not sufficiently removed from the colon.

X. APPENDICITIS

1. Definition and Classification

a. Appendicitis is inflammation of the vermiform appendix. It can be classified as simple, gangrenous, or perforated.

b. *Simple appendicitis* involves an inflamed and intact appendix. In *gangrenous appendicitis,* the appendix may have focal or extensive necrosis with microscopic perforations. *Perforated appendicitis* may allow bacteria into the abdominal cavity, causing chemical peritonitis.

2. Incidence and Epidemiology

a. Appendicitis occurs more commonly in men than in women, with a peak incidence in late teens and early 20s. About 250,000 cases are reported annually.

b. It is a common cause of surgical emergency in children, with 4 appendectomies per 1000 admissions for appendicitis annually in the United States.

c. Appendicitis probably results from an obstruction of the intestinal lumen caused by a fecal mass, structure, barium ingestion, or viral infection. This obstruction sets off an inflammatory process that can lead to infection, thrombosis, necrosis, and perforation.

d. If the appendix ruptures or perforates, the infected contents spill into the abdominal cavity, causing peritonitis, the most common and most serious complication of appendicitis.

3. Signs and Symptoms

a. Typically, appendicitis begins with generalized or localized abdominal pain in the upper right abdomen, followed by anorexia, tachycardia, nausea, and vomiting.

b. Pain eventually localizes in the lower right abdomen (McBurney's point), with increasing tenderness, increasingly severe abdominal spasms, and rebound tenderness.

c. Findings supporting this diagnosis include a temperature of 99°F to 102°F and a moderately elevated white blood cell count (13,000–16,000 mm³).

4. Nursing Implications

a. If appendicitis is suspected or during preparation for appendectomy, never administer cathartics or enemas because they may rupture the appendix.

b. Administer IV fluids to prevent dehydration.

c. The client should have nothing by mouth (NPO).

d. Administer analgesics only after the diagnosis has been made and then give judiciously because they may mask symptoms.

e. To lessen pain, place the patient in Fowler's position. (This also is helpful after surgery.) Fowler's or semi-Fowler's positioning relieves pressure over the appendix.

f. Never apply heat to the lower right abdomen; this may cause the appendix to rupture.

g. After appendectomy, give analgesics as ordered; encourage the patient to cough, deep breathe, and turn frequently to prevent pulmonary complications.

h. Document bowel sounds, passing of flatus, or bowel movement and signs of return of peristalsis.

i. Observe closely for possible surgical complications.

j. Assist the patient to ambulate as soon as possible after surgery, usually within 8 to 12 h.

5. Complications

Peritonitis may be a complication of appendicitis. The most common causes of bacterial peritonitis are appendicitis with perforation and associated with diverticulitis and peptic ulcer.

a. Signs and Symptoms

(1) The cardinal manifestations of peritonitis are acute abdominal pain and tenderness. Rigidity of the abdominal wall is a common finding in peritonitis and may be localized or generalized.

(2) Peristalsis may be present initially but usually disappears as the illness progresses and bowel sounds disappear.

(3) Hypotension, tachycardia, oliguria, and leukocytosis, with white blood cell counts greater than 20,000 common, especially in generalized peritonitis.

6. Nursing Interventions

a. Maintain patient on bed rest in semi-Fowler's position to minimize discomfort and promote localization of infection in abdomen.

b. Use nonpharmacologic measures to promote comfort; analgesics are used sparingly because they can mask symptoms.

c. Administer IV fluids, electrolytes, and antibiotics as ordered.

d. Keep nasogastric tube taped securely to nose and maintain its function.

e. Apply water-soluble lubricant to nose to prevent irritation and discomfort.

f. Apply water-soluble lubricant to lips to prevent drying and cracking.

g. Brush teeth and rinse mouth frequently, avoiding use of lemon and glycerin swabs and alcohol-containing commercial mouthwashes, which are drying.

h. Give clear fluids as ordered when peristalsis returns and progress diet as tolerated.

XI. DISORDERS OF THE LIVER AND THEIR TREATMENT

A. Hepatitis

Acute inflammation of the liver caused by toxin or virus.

1. Viral Hepatitis

A fairly common systemic disease, viral hepatitis is marked by liver cell destruction and necrosis. This disease has four forms: types A, B, D, and C.

a. *Type A:* Hepatitis A virus (HAV), also known as short-incubation hepatitis and infectious hepatitis.

(1) Causes of epidemics include drinking infected water or milk or eating infected food, especially raw or inadequately cooked shellfish from contaminated waters.

(2) Person-to-person spread of HAV is enhanced by poor personal hygiene and overcrowding.

(3) Incidence: In the general population, those younger than 15 years and college students living in close quarters are at most risk.

b. *Type B:* Hepatitis B (HBV), also known as *serum hepatitis,* is spread primarily through contact with infectious blood or blood products.

(1) The virus also may be transmitted by other body fluids, such as saliva and semen, but at lesser concentrations compared with those found in blood.

(2) Accidental needle puncture with HBV-contaminated needles or parenteral inoculation with contaminated blood, plasma, or serum is a common route of entry into the host.

(3) Hepatitis B virus also can be transmitted by shared needles of illicit drug users.

(4) Populations at risk for developing hepatitis B include health care professionals, who are frequently exposed to blood; laboratory personnel; dialysis unit staff members; dentists and dental practitioners; close contacts of clients with a current HBV infection; illicit parenteral drug users; and male homosexuals.

(5) Prevention of hepatitis B by use of hepatitis B vaccine is recommended for hospital personnel who are frequently exposed to blood and blood products.

c. *Type D:* Delta hepatitis appears to coexist with hepatitis B; therefore, the hepatitis B vaccine can also help to prevent hepatitis delta virus (HDV). HDV can either infect a client or superinfect a client already infected with HBV (superinfection). Hepatitis D is responsible for approximately 50 percent of all cases of fulminant hepatitis, which has a high mortality rate. It is confined to people who frequently are exposed blood products, such as IV drug users and patients with hemophilia.

d. *Type C:* Hepatitis C (formerly called non-A, non-B hepatitis): An almost 15-year quest to identify an agent of non-A, non-B viral hepatitis ended in 1988 with the identification of an RNA virus with immunologic specificity for transfusion-associated non-A, non-B hepatitis, now known as hepatitis C virus (HCV). Transmitted by blood or sexual activity and other body fluids.

(1) Alpha-interferon reduces liver swelling and thus reduces cell destruction, but it does not eliminate the virus.

(2) An estimated 150,000 people per year are infected with HCV in the United States.

(3) People with multiple sex partners are encouraged to use condoms to reduce sexual transmission.

(4) Screening of all blood donations for HCV has been required since May 1990.

(5) All clients infected with HCV should be vaccinated against hepatitis B.

(6) Hepatitis C, which kills up to 10,000 Americans each year, is the most common bloodborne infection in the United States and is the leading reason for liver transplants.

(7) Some people overcome the virus without medical help. However, 85 percent develop a chronic, simmering infection that they can spread to others. Most will suffer at least some liver damage, especially if they also drink alcohol, and 15 percent develop severe damage.

(8) Sharing IV drug needles is the chief source of hepatitis C, causing 60 percent of cases. Tattooing is also a contributing factor.

(9) The Centers for Disease Control and Prevention (CDC) in Atlanta, Georgia, recommends testing for all individuals, especially hemophiliacs and anyone who ever injected drugs, even as a teenager.

2. Toxic and Drug-Induced Hepatitis

a. Liver injury may follow the inhalation, ingestion, or parenteral administration of a number of pharmacologic and chemical agents.

b. These agents include industrial toxins (e.g., carbon tetrachloride, trichloroethylene).

c. A more common cause is pharmacologic agents used in medical therapy (e.g., anesthetics, anticonvulsants, antihypertensive agents, anticholesterol drugs, antibiotics, antiinflammatory agents, calcium channel blockers).

d. Treatment of toxic and drug-induced hepatitis is mainly supportive, as in acute viral hepatitis. Withdrawal of the suspected agent is indicated at the first sign of an adverse reaction.

3. Immunization

a. Hepatitis B vaccine (Engerix-B or Recombivax HB) is used to provide active immunization before exposure to HBV; the vaccine is also used to treat HDV.

b. After exposure to HBV, specific hepatitis B immunoglobulin is preferred.

c. Standard immunoglobulin is used to provide active immunization after exposure to HAV.

d. There is no specific vaccine for hepatitis except for hepatitis C or D. Standard immunoglobulin is of questionable value after exposure.

4. Nursing Implications

a. The CDC has developed standard precautions for all health care workers.

b. Under universal precautions, blood and certain body fluids of all patients are considered potentially infectious for human immunodeficiency virus (HIV), the virus that causes acquired immunodeficiency syndrome (AIDS); HBV; and other bloodborne pathogens.

c. Precautions are intended to prevent parenteral, mucous membrane, and nonintact skin exposure of health care workers to bloodborne pathogens.

d. Immunization with HBV vaccine is recommended as an important adjunct to standard precautions for health care workers who have been exposed to blood.

e. Universal precautions also apply to semen and vaginal secretions, tissues, and the following fluids: cerebrospinal, peritoneal, synovial, pleural, saliva, peritoneal, pericardial, and amniotic.

f. Use standard precautions for all patients.

g. Use appropriate barrier precautions routinely when contact with blood or body fluids of any patient is anticipated.

h. Take precautions to prevent injuries caused by needles, scalpels, and other sharp instruments or devices during procedures; when cleaning used instruments; during disposal of used needles; and when handling sharp instruments after procedures.

i. Discard uncapped needle units capped and unbroken after use.

j. Place disposable syringes and needles, scalpel blades, and other sharp items in puncture-resistant containers.

k. Place puncture-resistant containers as near as practical to the area of use.

l. Wear gloves when touching blood or body fluids, mucous membranes, or nonintact skin; when handling items or surfaces soiled with blood or body fluids; and when performing venipuncture, other injections, and other vascular access procedures.

m. Change gloves after each contact with patients. Wear masks, protective eye wear, or face shields during procedures that are likely to generate drops of blood or other body fluids to prevent exposure of mucous membranes of mouth, nose, and eyes.

n. Wash hands and other skin surfaces immediately and thoroughly if contaminated with blood or other body fluids.

o. Wear gowns during procedures that are likely to generate splashes of blood or other body fluids.

p. Handle soiled linen as little as possible and with minimum agitation.

q. Bag all soiled linen at the location where it is used.

r. Place and transport linen soiled with blood or body fluids in bags that prevent leakage.

B. Cirrhosis of the Liver

Disease of the liver marked by progressive destruction of liver cells, accompanied by regeneration of the connective tissue causing widespread fibrosis and module formation.

1. Etiology and Incidence

a. It is twice as common in men as in women. It is especially prevalent among malnourished, chronic alcoholics older than 50 years.

b. The number one cause is alcoholism.

c. Other causes include malnutrition, hepatitis, right-sided heart failure, and biliary tract obstruction.

2. Signs and Symptoms

a. In the early stage of cirrhosis, assessment findings include enlarged liver, vascular changes, and abnormal laboratory test results.

b. In the late stage of cirrhosis, assessment findings include ascites, hepatic encephalopathy, portal hypertension, and rupture of esophageal varices.

c. Late manifestations are due partly to chronic failure of liver function and partly to obstruction of the portal circulation. Practically all blood from the digestive organs is collected in the portal veins and carried to the liver.

d. Because a cirrhotic liver does not allow the blood free passage, the blood is dammed back into the spleen and GI tract. As a result, these organs become congested; they are stagnant with blood and cannot function properly. This causes portal hypertension and esophageal varices.

e. Another late symptom of cirrhosis is retention of aldosterone, which occurs because the failing liver cannot break down aldosterone for excretion, causing sodium and water retention.

f. There are inadequate formation and storage of certain vitamins (notably vitamin A, C, and K). Deficiency of vitamin K may lead to hemorrhage.

g. Chronic gastritis, poor diet, and impaired liver function account for the anemia often associated with the disease.

3. Treatment

a. Management of the patient with cirrhosis usually is based on the presenting symptoms, for example, vitamins and nutritional supplements to treat anemia and promote healing of damaged liver cells.

b. The physician strongly encourages the patient to avoid future alcohol use.

c. Specific treatment is directed at complications such as ascites, esophageal varices, and portal hypertension (see next section).

C. Portal Hypertension

Persistent increase in pressure in the portal venous system.

1. Etiology

Obstruction of blood flow by cirrhosis of the liver forces blood into veins of the abdominal wall and into the esophagogastric veins, causing in esophageal varices, splenomegaly, ascites, and cor pulmonale (right-sided heart failure).

2. Treatment

a. Although treatment usually is directed toward a specific complication of portal hypertension, attempts are sometimes made to reduce the pressure in the portal venous system.

b. Surgical decompression procedures have been used for many years to lower portal pressure in patients with bleeding esophageal varices; however, portal–systemic shunt surgery does not improve survival rates in patients with cirrhosis.

c. Numerous variations of systemic shunt procedures are performed. These procedures reroute most of the portal blood flow past the liver to reduce portal hypertension.

d. These procedures may place the patient at increased risk for hepatic encephalopathy because a large amount of blood is not going to the liver for the breakdown of protein to urea for excretion.

e. Beta-adrenergic blocking agents (e.g., propranolol [Inderal] or nadolol [Corgard]) reduce portal pressure through vasodilatory effects on both the splanchnic arterial bed and the portal venous system in combination with reduced cardiac output.

D. Ascites

Accumulation of fluid in the peritoneal cavity.

1. Etiology

a. Accumulation of ascitic fluid represents a state of total sodium and water excess.

b. Portal hypertension plays an important role in the formation of ascites by raising hydrostatic pressure within the splanchnic capillary bed.

c. Hypoalbuminemia, which results in reduced osmotic pressure in the vascular system, favors the moving of fluid from the vascular system to the peritoneal cavity.

d. Renal factors also play an important role in perpetuating ascites. Patients with ascites fail to excrete fluid in a normal fashion. There is an increase in renal sodium reabsorption of both proximal and distal tubules. Renal vasoconstriction caused by high levels of catecholamines (epinephrine, norepinephrine, dopamine) reduces kidney perfusion. When the kidney is not perfusing, it "thinks" the body needs water and retains it.

2. Treatment

   a. Strict bed rest is often recommended because of improved renal clearance in the supine position.

   b. Salt restriction is the most important cornerstone of therapy. A diet of 800-mg sodium often is adequate to induce a negative sodium balance and permit diuresis.

   c. Conventional diuretics such as spironolactone (Aldactone) and furosemide (Lasix) may be used to initiate diuresis.

   d. In patients with a large accumulation of ascitic fluid, particularly those requiring hospitalization, large-volume paracentesis has proved to be an effective and less costly approach to initial management than prolonged bed rest and conventional diuretic treatment.

E. Esophageal Varices

1. Etiology
   Portal hypertension.

2. Signs and Symptoms

   a. Usually present with painless but massive hematemesis.

   b. Associated signs range from mild tachycardia to profound shock, depending on the extent of blood loss and degree of hypovolemia.

3. Treatment

   a. Varices bleeding is a life-threatening emergency.

   b. Prompt estimation and vigorous replacement of blood losses to maintain intravascular volume are essential.

   c. IV infusion of vasopressins is used for generalized vasoconstriction. This diminishes blood flow in the portal venous system and reduces bleeding.

   d. Balloon tamponade of the bleeding varices may be accomplished with a triple-lumen (Sengstaken-Blakemore) or four-lumen (Minnesota) tube with esophageal and gastric balloons. After the tube is introduced into the stomach, the gastric balloon is inflated and pulled back into the cardiac sphincter muscle of the stomach.

   e. A football helmet is placed on the patient. The tubing comes out of the nose and is attached to the football helmet. It then is pulled tightly after the gastric tube is inflated to maintain the tubing in proper position and prevent it from blocking the airway. Because of the high risk of aspiration, endotracheal intubation should be performed prior to attempts to place one of these tubes.

   f. Endoscopic sclerotherapy intervention should be used as the first line of treatment to control bleeding acutely. The varices are injected with one of several sclerosing agents (e.g., sodium morrhuate) via a needle-type catheter passed through the endoscope.

   g. In addition, repeated sclerotherapy can be performed until obliteration of all varices is accomplished in an effort to prevent recurrent bleeding.

   h. Recently, endoscopic ligation of varices has proved to be equally effective in controlling bleeding with fewer treatment-related complications. In this technique, varices are ligated and strangled with small, elastic O-rings placed endoscopically.

4. Nursing Implications after Surgery

   a. If the patient develops respiratory difficulty, cut the Sengstaken-Blakemore tubing immediately. Pull the deflated tubing out of the esophagus and notify the physician immediately.

   b. Assess and suction the patient as needed to prevent aspiration of secretions.

   c. Assess for signs of bleeding and aspiration.

F. Hepatic Encephalopathy

1. Etiology

   a. Develops when the liver is no longer able to break down ammonia into urea (by-product of protein metabolism). The ammonia will go to the brain and cause encephalopathy.

   b. In patients with severe cirrhosis of the liver, hepatic encephalopathy (coma) can occur from intake of excessive amounts of protein but most often is caused by bleeding from esophageal varices resulting from portal hypertension. The blood from the esophagus enters the stomach and is used as protein.

2. Signs and Symptoms

   a. Decreased level of consciousness.

   b. During the prodromal stage, early signs and symptoms are commonly overlooked because they are subtle. The patient demonstrates personality changes (disorientation, forgetfulness, and confusion, impaired speech) and slight tremors.

   c. During the impending stage, tremor progresses to asterixis (liver flap and flapping tremor), the hallmark of hepatic encephalopathy. Asterixis is characterized by quick, irregular extension and flexion of the wrist and fingers when the wrist are held out straight and the hand flexed upward.

3. Treatment
   Early recognition and prompt treatment of hepatic encephalopathy are essential. Treatment includes the following:

   a. Lowering blood ammonia (and other toxin) levels by decreasing absorption of protein and nitrogenous products from the intestine.

   b. Excluding protein from the diet in acute hepatic encephalopathy and restricting protein in the diet in chronic encephalopathy.

   c. Decreasing ammonia absorption by administering lactulose. Lactulose is an osmotic laxative agent that prevents absorption of ammonia from the colon into the blood and thereby reduces blood ammonia levels. Absorbed lactulose is excreted in urine. Neomycin sulfate is used to reduce ammonia-forming bacteria in the GI tract.

4. Functions of the Liver Inhibited by Cirrhosis

a. Synthesis of albumin, clotting factors (factor VIII, IX and X), and other proteins.

b. Prothrombin formation; liver uses vitamin K (produced by bacteria in intestines).

c. Detoxification of drugs and other substances, breakdown of ammonia to urea for excretion, and blood filtering action.

d. Formation of glycogen from carbohydrate source (gluconeogenesis).

e. Formation of glycogen from noncarbohydrates, such as fat or amino acids from protein.

f. Conversion of glycogen into glucose in body tissue (glycogenolysis).

g. Storage of vitamins (e.g., vitamin K) and minerals (e.g., iron).

5. Liver Diagnostic Tests

a. Liver enzymes reflect liver damage caused by injury or disease. Liver enzymes are released into the bloodstream, resulting in increased enzyme levels. Enzymes that usually are analyzed to evaluate for suspected liver disease are alkaline phosphatase (ALP), alanine aminotransferase (ALT or SGPT), 5'-nucleotidase (5-NT), leucine aminopeptidase (LAP), and gamma-glutamyl transferase (GGT).

b. Albumin level is decreased and gamma-globulin level is elevated in cirrhosis of the liver.

c. Level of ammonia, a by-product of protein metabolism converted to urea by the liver, is elevated in severe liver disease.

d. Prothrombin time (PT) is increased; therefore, bleeding may occur.

e. Serum and urine bilirubin levels are increased. Bilirubin is derived from hemoglobin and results from the breakdown of red blood cells. Bilirubin is responsible for the color of bile. It is sometimes found in urine and may occur in blood and tissue as jaundice.

XII. DISORDERS OF THE GALLBLADDER

A. Function of the Gallbladder

The gallbladder stores bile. When there is fat in the duodenum, the sphincter of Oddi opens to allow bile to pass into the duodenum. Bile is needed for the absorption of the fat-soluble vitamins A, D, E, and K. Bile colors the stool brown; without bile, the stool is clay-colored.

B. Diseases

1. Cholelithiasis (Stones in Gallbladder)

a. Extremely painful.

b. Treatment with analgesic. Analgesics are may be given before diagnosis is made if the patient is having severe pain.

2. Cholecystitis

Inflammation of the gallbladder (usually associated with gallstones). Gallstones usually produce symptoms by causing inflammation or obstruction following their migration into the cystic duct or common bile duct.

a. The most specific and characteristic symptom of gallstone disease is biliary colic.

b. The visceral pain characteristically is a severe steady ache or pressure in the epigastrium or right upper quadrant of the abdomen with frequent radiation to the right shoulder.

c. Biliary colic begins quite suddenly and may persist with severe intensity for 1 to 4 h, subsiding gradually or rapidly.

d. Biliary colic may be precipitated by eating a fatty meal.

C. Gallbladder Diagnostic Tests

1. Plain Abdominal X-Ray Film

Advantage is cost, but stones that are not calcified and stones that are not composed of cholesterol will not be seen.

2. Oral Cholecystography (New Procedures Have Reduced the Use of This Procedure)

X-ray test used to visualize stones and to diagnose inflammatory disease and tumors of the gallbladder. The patient ingests radiopaque iodinated dye tablets the night before the test. The client is NPO, and the dye is concentrated in the gallbladder 12 to 14 h after ingestion. The test should be performed 2 to 4 days after upper GI and small-bowel series, as the barium would hamper visualization.

3. Cholangiography

X-ray examination of the bile ducts using contrast medium either intravenously or percutaneously or through the common bile duct using a T-tube to study the biliary duct for gallstones and tumors or stricture.

4. Ultrasonography

Noninvasive procedure using sound waves that provides accurate visualization of gallbladder, liver, biliary tree, and pancreas. Before the procedure, obtain informed consent and tell patient that although no fasting is required, the gallbladder is more easily visualized after 8 h of fasting.

5. Computed Tomography

Noninvasive yet very accurate x-ray procedure used to diagnosis pathologic conditions such as tumors, cysts, abscesses, inflammation, gallstones, and tumors. The computed tomography (CT) scan results from passage of x-rays through the abdominal organs at many angles. CT cannot be used on patients who are very obese, usually more than 300 lb, or on patients who are claustrophobic. The physician may order a contrast dye for better visualization.

6. Cholescintigraphy (HIDA Scan)

Hydroxy iminodiacetic acid (HIDA) scan is an imaging test used to examine the gallbladder and the ducts leading into and out of the gallbladder. In this test, also referred to as cholescintigraphy, the patient receives an intravenous injection of a radioactive material call hydroxy iminodiacetic acid (HIDA). The HIDA material is taken up by the liver and excreted into the biliary tract. In a healthy person, HIDA will pass into the common bile duct and enter the small intestine, from which it eventually makes its way out of the body into the stool.

HIDA imaging is done by a nuclear scanner, which takes pictures of the patient's biliary tract over the course of about two hours. The images are then examined by a radiologist, who interprets the results. It is generally a very safe test and is well tolerated by most patients.

Valuable in evaluating patients for suspected gallbladder disease. This procedure is superior to oral cholecystography, IV cholangiography, ultrasonography, and CT of the gallbladder in detecting cholecystitis.

7. Endoscopic Retrograde Cholangiopancreatography

Contrast medium (dye) is injected through a fiberoptic endoscope into the duodenal papilla to visualize the biliary tract and determine the cause of obstructive jaundice. Use of ERCP has increased since the development of the fiberoptic endoscope. This test is used when other diagnostic tests fail to determine the cause of jaundice (e.g., stones, tumor).

D. Nursing Implications Related to Diagnostic Tests

1. Nursing Care Prior to Diagnostic Examination

a. Explain procedure to patient.

b. Obtain informed consent if required by the institution.

c. Assess the patient for allergies to iodinated dye or shellfish.

d. Adverse reaction rarely occurs if iodine dye is administered orally.

e. Advise patient that iodinated dye is contraindicated in pregnancy.

f. Instruct patient having a CT scan that he or she will have to lie still in an enclosed area for approximately 30 min; show the patient a picture of a CT machine.

2. Nursing Care after Diagnostic Examination

a. Mild nausea is a common sensation when contrast dye is used.

b. Encourage the patient to drink fluids to promote dye excretion and prevent dye-induced renal failure.

c. Evaluate the patient for delayed reaction to dye (dyspnea, rash, tachycardia, and hives). This reaction may occur 2 to 26 h after the test.

d. Treat with antihistamines and steroids as ordered if reaction occurs.

E. Surgical Management of Gallbladder Disorders

1. Cholecystectomy
Excision of the gallbladder from the posterior wall.

a. The surgeon makes an incision in the upper right quadrant of the abdomen and removes the gallbladder.

b. Common bile duct exploration may also be done through the incision site, if necessary. If stones are suspected in the common duct, an operative cholangiography may be performed.

c. Following exploration of the common duct, the surgeon usually inserts a T-tube to ensure adequate bile drainage during duct healing.

d. The bile drains into an external bag and is emptied and measured by the nurse at the end of each shift. Sterile procedure must be used.

2. Laparoscopic Cholecystectomy

◆ Most cholecystectomies are performed by a laparoscopy procedure when cancer is not present and the patient is not obese.

◆ With the patient under general anesthesia, carbon dioxide is inserted through a needle near the umbilicus; this will lift the abdomen wall off the viscera to give the surgeon room to operate.

a. An endoscope is inserted through a small incision near the umbilicus to view the gallbladder.

b. Three other small incisions are created: one for suction, one for grasping the gallbladder, and another for dissection instruments and applying clips. The patient has a smaller risk of postoperative complications than with traditional cholecystectomy because incision pain is lessened and the suture line is small.

F. Nonsurgical Treatments

1. Percutaneous Cholecystolithotomy
The surgeon extracts gallstones using a cystoscope stone basket, an instrument designed for extracting stones.

a. If stones are too large to be extracted manually, they can be fragmented using a lithotriptor or laser.

b. General anesthesia is not necessary for the procedure. The surgeon passes an endoscope into the esophagus through the duodenum and into the common bile duct and extracts the stones.

c. Currently, percutaneous insertion of a dissolution agent that can dissolve cholesterol gallstones is being studied. Chenodeoxycholic acid has been effective in dissolving approximately 66 percent of radiolucent gallstones composed primarily of cholesterol.

2. Extracorporeal Shock Wave Lithotripsy
This noninvasive procedure uses repeated shock waves aimed directly at the gallstone location in the gallbladder or common bile duct to fragment the stones.

a. The shock waves are timed with an electrocardiogram to reduce the risk of dysrhythmias.

b. After the stones are gradually broken up, the stone fragments pass from the gallbladder or common bile duct spontaneously and are removed by endoscopy, dissolved with oral bile or solvents, or left in the intestine and excreted with feces.

G. Nursing Implications for Surgical Management of Gallbladder Disorders

1. Preoperative Nursing Care

a. Assess for clinical manifestations of cholecystitis: intolerance to fatty foods, nausea with or without vomiting, elevated temperature, right upper quadrant discomfort or pain radiating to right scapula, jaundice, clay-colored stool, and dark-colored urine.

b. Monitor serum PT in patients with obstructive jaundice and administer vitamin K before surgery as ordered.

2. Postoperative Nursing Care

a. Check vital signs and intake and output; auscultate the lung.

b. Observe the amount, color, consistency, and odor of the drainage from the T-tube, Penrose drain, and nasogastric tube if in place. Inspect the suture line for signs of infection.

c. Inspect the sclera for jaundice.

d. Administer small amounts of analgesics every 3 to 4 h for the first 24 to 48 h as ordered to facilitate deep respiratory breathing.

e. Splint the incision site with a pillow while encouraging the patient to cough and breathe deeply every 2 h in the early postoperative period.

f. Cholecystoileostomy by laparoscopic procedure usually allows the patient to be discharged within 24 h.

XIII. DISORDERS OF THE PANCREAS

A. Acute Pancreatitis

Pancreatitis is an inflammatory disorder of the pancreas that can be acute or chronic. Acute pancreatitis can occur as a single episode or as recurrent attacks (recurrent acute episodes). Except in cases of alcohol-induced pancreatitis, the pancreas returns to normal after successful treatment.

1. Incidence and Etiology

a. Numerous factors have been identified as causative agents of acute pancreatitis, including alcoholism, biliary tract disease, viral infections, and intestinal diseases such as regional enteritis.

b. In the United States the most common cause is alcoholism. It is estimated that approximately 6000 new cases of acute pancreatitis are diagnosed each year in the United States.

2. Pathophysiology

a. Although there are many known causes of pancreatitis, the manner in which they cause acute inflammation is unknown.

b. Most authorities believe the pathologic factor leading to acute inflammation is autodigestion.

c. Autodigestion is the process by which proteolytic enzymes, particularly trypsinogen, are activated within the pancreas itself.

(1) The activated proteolytic enzymes digest pancreatic and surrounding tissues.

(2) This autodigestion results in edema, interstitial hemorrhage, and cell necrosis.

(3) The injured cells release histamine and bradykinin, which increase vascular permeability and vasodilation and cause more edema.

(4) The initiation of enzyme activation is thought to result from reflux of bile, obstruction of the pancreatic duct, ampulla, and vapor, or ischemia.

(5) Regardless of the cause, the acute inflammation process and autodigestion result in physiologic alterations that can occur as a mild or acute event.

d. Some of the major complications of acute pancreatitis are (1) hypotension/shock, (2) leukocytosis, (3) disseminated intravascular coagulation, (4) oliguria, (5) hyperglycemia (from decreased insulin), and (6) hypercalcemia.

3. Signs and Symptoms

a. The major symptom of acute pancreatitis is pain. The pain varies from mild to severe and is constant.

b. Pain may be experienced in the epigastric area and may radiate to the back. It usually is more intense when the person is supine.

c. Other common symptoms include nausea, vomiting, and abdominal distention.

d. Signs and symptoms of shock may be present (hypotension, tachycardia).

e. Jaundice may be present from obstruction of the common bile duct.

4. Diagnostic Tests

a. The greatest value in establishing the diagnosis of acute pancreatitis is an increase in the serum amylase level to greater than 300 Somogyi units in the presence of the symptoms.

b. Serum amylase levels usually become elevated within 24 to 48 h of the acute pancreatitis and may range from 300 to 800 U.

c. Serum lipase also rises in pancreatitis and reaches its peak 72 to 96 h after onset of acute pancreatitis.

d. Other laboratory findings include leukocytosis, anemia, increased serum bilirubin level, and hyperglycemia.

e. Elevated levels of the liver enzymes ALT and aspartate aminotransferase (AST) are useful for diagnosis if there is no history of excessive alcohol consumption or other etiologic factors responsible for elevated levels of these enzymes.

5. Treatment

Medical management is directed toward decreasing the secretion of the pancreas cells and resting the pancreas.

a. Replace fluids and electrolytes intravenously.

b. Client is NPO to rest the pancreas. Nasogastric suctioning may also be used to decrease gastric contents, which stimulate gastric secretion.

c. Counsel patient to abstain from alcohol.

d. Antibiotics are used in patients with pancreatic necrosis.

e. Pain is treated with drugs such as meperidine (Demerol), which is given every 3 to 6 h. Morphine is contraindicated because it causes spasms of the sphincter of Oddi, which will further decrease pancreatic flow.

f. Antiemetics are given for nausea and vomiting.

6. Nursing Implications

a. Nursing assessment includes determining the location and perceived intensity of pain.

b. Weight is recorded and compared with previous weights as an indication of nutritional status.

c. The abdomen is gently palpated for rigidity and auscultated for presence of bowel sounds.

d. Vital signs are taken frequently to detect signs of hypotension and impending shock.

e. White blood cell count and lipase, amylase, calcium, and albumin levels are monitored.

B. Chronic Pancreatitis

Incidence, etiology, pathophysiology, and nursing implications are very similar to those of acute pancreatitis.

1. Etiology

a. Chronic pancreatitis refers to the presence of permanent histologic alterations of the pancreas. It is a progressive, destructive disease of the pancreas in which normal tissue is replaced by connective tissue. The end result of chronic pancreatitis is pancreatic insufficiency.

b. Chronic pancreatitis may develop after repeated episodes of acute pancreatitis, resulting from chronic alcohol abuse or chronic obstruction of the common bile duct. However, there are clients with chronic pancreatitis who have a negative history of acute pancreatitis.

c. Chronic pancreatitis is characterized by acute bouts of abdominal pain and pain-free periods.

2. Treatment

Chronic pancreatitis is an irreversible process; as such, there is no curative treatment.

a. Treatment is focused on preventing acute exacerbations of the disease, providing symptomatic relief, and treating pancreatic insufficiency.

b. Pancreatic insufficiency is treated with pancreatic enzyme supplement (see *Handbook of Medications for the NCLEX-RN® Review* Chapter 10, for more information).

c. A low-fat diet is prescribed to reduce discomfort and steatorrhea.

d. Histamine blockers such as cimetidine (Tagamet) and antacids are used to reduce and neutralize gastric secretions and thereby reduce pancreatic workload.

e. Antiemetics are used to reduce nausea and vomiting.

f. Operative procedures can be used in chronic and critically ill patients with acute pancreatitis to relieve pain. These procedures are pancreatic resection of the head, body, and tail or total removal of the pancreas (pancreatotomy). All of these procedures result in compromised pancreatic function.

g. Surgery for pancreatitis is not curative, but removal of cysts may improve pancreatic function.

h. Patients with chronic pancreatitis have a shortened life expectancy.

i. Pancreas transplant is performed on some patients with insulin-dependent diabetes mellitus (IDDM). This procedure is used most often in patients with IDDM who have received a kidney transplant.

(1) This is because the cyclosporine used to prevent transplant rejection can cause diabetes and nephrotoxicity.

(2) The patient's own pancreas is left intact and the new pancreas usually is anastomosed to the iliac artery and vein, where insulin can enter the systemic pathway.

(3) Research is being conducted on the use of transplanted pancreatic islets rather than the entire pancreas.

3. Signs and Symptoms

a. Because chronic pancreatitis is progressive, the patient has intermittent problems with pain, anorexia, nausea, vomiting, hyperglycemia, jaundice, and abnormal levels of pancreatic enzymes.

b. When more than 90 percent of the pancreas no longer functions, malabsorption becomes a primary problem as a result of pancreatic insufficiency. Malabsorption produces diarrhea, steatorrhea, weight loss, and symptoms of fat-soluble vitamin deficiency.

XIV. COMMON DISORDERS ASSOCIATED WITH GASTROINTESTINAL AND ACCESSORY ORGANS

A. Bacillary Dysentery (Shigellosis)

1. Etiology and Incidence

a. Acute intestinal infection caused by *Shigella* bacteria.

b. Bacillary dysentery can occur at any age, in males or females, but is most common in children aged 1 to 4 year. Adults often acquire the illness from children.

2. Signs and Symptoms

a. In children, *Shigella* usually produces high fever, diarrhea, nausea and vomiting, irritability, drowsiness, and abdominal pain and distention. Stools may contain pus and mucus from intestinal ulceration, which is typical of this infection.

b. In adults, *Shigella* produces intense abdominal pain, headache, and stool containing pus, mucus, and blood. Adults usually do not have fever.

3. Treatment

a. Enteric precautions, including low residual diet and, most importantly, replacement of fluids and electrolytes with IV infusion of normal saline solution (with electrolytes) in quantities sufficient to maintain urine output at 40 to 50 L/h.

b. Antibiotics are of questionable value but may be used to eliminate any pathogens. Amoxicillin, tetracycline, or sulfamethoxazole may be used.

c. Lomotil is given to control diarrhea and steroids to reduce inflammation.

B. Botulism

Life-threatening paralytic disease.

1. Etiology and Incidence

a. Caused by the gram-positive, anaerobic *Clostridium botulinum,* botulism food poisoning usually results from ingesting cooked contaminated foods, especially those with low acid content, such as improperly canned foods.

b. Botulism can occur at any age and is a relatively common disease. Approximately 400 cases occur per year in the United States.

2. Signs and Symptoms

a. Symptoms usually appear within 12 to 36 h of ingestion of contaminated food. Severity varies with the amount of toxin ingested.

b. Initial symptoms are vomiting, diarrhea, weakness, dry mouth, and sore throat.

c. If severe, cranial nerve impairment causes ptosis (drooping upper eyelid), diplopia (double vision), and dysarthria (difficult and defective speech as a result of impairment of the tongue or other muscles essential for speech), followed by descending weakness or paralysis of muscles in the extremities or trunk and dyspnea from respiratory muscle paralysis.

d. Such impairment does not affect mental or sensory processes.

3. Treatment

Administration of IV or IM botulinum antitoxin (available through the CDC). Antibiotics should be given prophylactically.

C. Esophageal Cancer

1. Etiology and Incidence

a. The cause is unknown. Predisposing factors are chronic irritation of the esophagus, excessive smoking of tobacco, and achalasia (failure of relaxation of the cardiac sphincter muscle, resulting in difficulty in passage of food to stomach).

b. More than 8000 cases of esophageal cancer are diagnosed annually in the United States. It is most common in Japan, China, Russia, the Middle East, and South Africa.

c. The greatest incidence is in men older than 60 years.

2. Signs and Symptoms

Dysphagia and weight loss followed by pain on swallowing, hoarseness, coughing, regurgitation and, later, inability to swallow liquids.

3. Treatment

Esophagogastrectomy, radiation, chemotherapy, and gastrostomy (Peg tube). Feeding tube for nutrition.

D. Folic Acid Deficiency Anemia

Common, slowly progressive anemia.

1. Etiology and Incidence

a. Alcohol abuse, poor diet, impaired absorption, excessive cooking of foods containing folic acid, limited storage capacity in infants, prolonged drug therapy (anticoagulants, estrogen).

b. Occurs most often in infants, adolescents, pregnant and lactating women, alcoholics, the elderly, and patients with cancer or GI disease.

2. Signs and Symptoms

Progressive fatigue, shortness of breath, palpitations, weakness, glossitis, fainting, pallor, forgetfulness, irritability, slight jaundice, nausea and vomiting.

3. Treatment

Folic acid supplementation and inclusion of folic acid–containing foods at every meal. Advise patient to stop taking supplements when condition improves, per physician's orders.

E. Gastric Carcinoma

1. Etiology and Incidence

a. The cause is unknown. Associated with chronic gastritis. Predisposing factors include cigarette smoking and high alcohol intake.

b. Gastric carcinoma is common throughout the world and affects all races. Mortality is high in Japan, Iceland, China, and Austria. In the United States, the incidence has decreased 50 percent in the past 20 years.

c. The incidence is higher in adult men older than 40 years.

2. Signs and Symptoms

Chronic dyspepsia (painful digestion), epigastric discomfort followed by weight loss, anorexia, anemia, fatigue, and, later, often coffee ground vomitus. Patients may have blood in their stools.

3. Treatment

a. Subtotal or total gastrectomy. Chemotherapy includes 5-FU, doxorubicin, and mitomycin.

b. Antiemetics are used to control nausea, and narcotics are administered for pain. Radiation is more successful when combined with chemotherapy.

c. When patient is losing weight and has anorexia, two nutritional IV solutions can be administered.

(1) The two solutions are:

(a) *TPN* (Total Parenteral Nutrition): Amino acid–dextrose formula; 2 to 3 L of solution, usually given over 24 h, and 500 mL of 10% fat emulsions (Intralipid), usually given over 6 h one to three times per week. Fine bacterial filter used.

(b) *TNA* (Total Nutrient Admixture): Amino acid–dextrose–lipid, "3-in-1" formula; 1 L of solution usually is given over 24 h. No bacterial filter needed.

(2) Method of administration is by a central catheter inserted into subclavian vein. The following three methods are used:

(a) Peripherally inserted catheters (PICs) threaded through basilic or cephalic vein to superior vena cava.

(b) Percutaneous central catheters through subclavian vein

(c) Triple-lumen central catheter often used; distal lumen (16-gauge) used to infuse or draw blood samples, middle lumen (18-gauge) used for TPN infusion, proximal port (18-gauge) used to infuse or draw blood and administer medications

(3) Implementation of TPN and TNA include the following:

(a) Initial rate of infusion 50 mL/h and gradually increased (100–125 mL/h) as patient's fluid and electrolyte tolerance permits

(b) Infuse solution by pump at constant rate to prevent abrupt change in infusion rate

(4) Discontinued

(a) Gradually tapered to allow patient to adjust to decreased levels of glucose

(b) After discontinued, isotonic glucose solution administered to prevent rebound hypoglycemia (weakness, faintness, diaphoresis, shakiness, confusion, tachycardia)

F. Iron Deficiency Anemia

1. Etiology and Incidence

a. Iron deficiency anemia is caused by an inadequate supply of iron, which is necessary for formation of red blood cells. Iron deficiency anemia results from:

(1) Inadequate intake of iron (<1–2 mg/d), as in prolonged unsupplemented breast-fed or bottle-fed infants or during rapid growth in children and adolescents.

(2) Iron malabsorption, as in chronic diarrhea (ulcerative colitis), or total gastrectomy and malabsorption syndrome, such as celiac disease.

(3) Blood loss caused by GI bleeding (varices, ulcers) or heavy menses; hemorrhage from trauma.

(4) Pregnancy in which mother's iron supply is not adequate to meet her and fetus' requirement.

b. Iron deficiency anemia occurs most often in premature or low-birth-weight infants, premenopausal women, children, and adolescent girls.

2. Pathophysiology with Signs and Symptoms

a. Patient usually is asymptomatic until anemia is severe.

b. At advanced stages, decreased hemoglobin and the consequent decrease in the blood's oxygen-carrying capacity cause the patient to develop dyspnea on exertion, fatigue, pallor, inability to concentrate, irritability, headache, and susceptibility to infections.

c. Decreased oxygen perfusion causes the heart to compensate with increased cardiac output (tachycardia).

d. In patients with chronic iron deficiency anemia, nails become brittle.

3. Diagnosis

Blood studies show low levels of hemoglobin, hematocrit, serum iron, and serum ferritin, and low red blood cell count.

4. Treatment

a. The first priority of treatment is determining the underlying cause of anemia.

b. Treatment of choice is an oral preparation of ferrous sulfate. Patient is instructed to take ferrous sulfate after eating because it irritates the GI tract.

c. Patient should be told that stools will be black.

d. When patient cannot tolerate oral preparation of iron, parenteral iron therapy is used.

e. Parenteral therapy is also indicated when the patient is unable to absorb iron properly from the GI tract.

f. Because IV infusion of supplemental iron is painless and requires fewer injections, it usually is preferred to IM administration.

g. Poor diet is rarely the sole cause of iron deficiency anemia, but it may be a contributing factor.

h. Use the Z-track injection method when administering iron intramuscularly into a deep muscle to prevent irritation in the tissue.

G. Pernicious Anemia

Characterized by a decrease in the production of hydrochloric acid and deficiency of intrinsic factor. Intrinsic factor is necessary for absorption of vitamin B_{12}.

1. Etiology and Incidence

a. Incidence is higher in patients with immunologically related diseases (e.g., Graves' disease [hyperthyroidism], thyroiditis, myxedema [hypothyroidism]).

b. An inherited or acquired autoimmune response may cause atrophy of gastric mucosa and, therefore, a deficiency of hydrochloric acid and intrinsic factor.

c. Vitamin B_{12} is necessary for growth of cells, particularly red blood cells; decreased production causes anemia. A deficiency of vitamin B_{12} impairs myelin formation, causing neurologic damage.

d. Rarely occurs in children, African-Americans, and Asians; more common in older adults. Onset is usually between ages 50 and 60 years, with incidence rising with increasing age.

2. Signs and Symptoms

a. Weakness, sore tongue, and numbness and tingling in the extremities. The lips and gums appear inflamed and bloody.

b. Hemolysis may cause slight jaundiced sclera and pale or yellow skin.

c. Patient may become highly susceptible to infection. Nausea and vomiting, anorexia, weight loss, and diarrhea or constipation may occur.

d. Neurologic effects of pernicious anemia may include neuritis, weakness in extremities, peripheral numbness and paresthesia, lack of coordination, blurred vision, irritability, and loss of memory, tachycardia, and eventually congestive heart failure.

3. Treatment

a. IM injections of vitamin B_{12} early in course of disease can reverse (not eliminate) pernicious anemia and may prevent permanent neurologic damage.

b. Because vitamin B_{12} injections cause rapid cell regeneration, increased iron replacement is required to prevent development of iron deficiency anemia.

H. Liver Cancer

1. Etiology and Incidence

a. The cause is unknown. May be congenital in children. The number one cause of liver cancer in adults is chronic hepatitis. Another cause is exposure to environmental carcinogens. Occurs more frequently in persons who have had hepatitis B.

b. Most prevalent in men, particularly those older than 60 years. Rapidly fatal (death usually occurs within 6 months of diagnosis).

2. Signs and Symptoms

a. Mass in the upper right quadrant. Severe pain in the epigastric area or upper right quadrant, weight loss, weakness, anorexia, and fever occur only in the advanced stages of the disease.

3. Treatment

a. Liver cancer often is in advanced stages at diagnosis; therefore, very few of these tumors are resectable.

b. A resectable tumor must be a single tumor located in one lobe, with no cirrhosis, jaundice, or ascites.

c. The liver has low tolerance for radiation; therefore, radiation therapy does not increase survival. Chemotherapeutic agents used are 5-FU, methotrexate, and doxorubicin.

d. As with regional infusion of 5-FU, a catheter is placed directly in the hepatic artery or left brachial artery for continuous infusion of 7 to 21 days.

I. Pancreatic Cancer

1. Etiology and Incidence

a. The cause is unknown. Predisposing factors are ingestion and inhalation of carcinogens.

b. Occurs most often in black men 35 to 70 years old.

2. Signs and Symptoms

Include weight loss, abdominal or low back pain, jaundice, and diarrhea.

3. Treatment

a. Treatment of pancreatic cancer rarely is successful because the disease often is widely metastasized at diagnosis.

b. Therapy consists of surgery, radiation, and chemotherapy. Whipple's operation (pancreatoduodenectomy) is associated with a high mortality rate but can obtain wide lymphatic clearance.

c. If the pancreas is removed, pancreatic enzymes must be replaced orally at meals; Viokase is used. A total pancreatomy may increase survival.

d. Pancreatic cancer responds poorly to chemotherapy, but a combination of 5-FU, streptomycin, mitomycin, and doxorubicin shows a trend toward providing longer survival.

e. Other agents include antibiotics to prevent infections; anticholinergic agents to decrease GI spasms; antacids and nasogastric suctioning to remove secretions; insulin (beta cells are destroyed); narcotic analgesics for pain; and pancreatic enzymes to assist digestion of protein, carbohydrates, and fats.

J. Bariatric Surgery for Obesity

1. Obesity

a. Obesity is a complex disorder with many contributing metabolic, psychological, and genetic factors. The traditional view that obese people gain weight because they eat more and exercise less than people of normal weight is only part of the picture. People have remarkably varied energy requirements; some of us can eat twice as much as others and never gain weight.

b. Recent research indicates that ghrelin, a hormone produced by endocrine cells in the stomach, triggers hunger and that controlling ghrelin may be a key to managing weight.

2. Types of Bariatric Surgery

a. Bariatric surgery falls into two broad categories: (1) gastric restrictive surgery and (2) combined gastric restriction and malabsorption surgery, which include stapling and banding (gastric restriction and malabsorption surgery), also known as gastric bypass or Roux-en-Y gastric bypass.

b. Bariatric surgery, which involves surgically reducing stomach capacity, is indicated for dangerously obese patients who have not been able to reduce weight with medically supervised diets, exercise, and behavior modification. An estimated 150,000 people underwent bariatric surgery in 2005, and that number is expected to grow. Although many bariatric surgeries can be done laparoscopically, bariatric surgery is still major abdominal surgery, with all its associated risks. To justify the risks and enjoy long-term benefits of surgery, the patient must be willing and able to modify his or her postoperative eating behavior and take nutritional supplements to keep the weight off and avoid nutritional deficiencies.

c. When a patient has gastric restriction and malabsorption surgery, which bypasses the stomach and duodenum, they are at risk for late complications such as anemia and calcium and vitamin B$_{12}$ deficiency. These patients will require lifelong nutritional supplementation to prevent these problems.

EXAMINATION

1. Recent laboratory values on a patient with a history of severe cirrhosis of the liver include elevated liver function studies, prolonged PT, and hypokalemia. The patient's BP is 160/110; he has lost weight over the past 8 months, and he noticed that his abdominal girth has increased. The nurse teaches the patient that the pathologic basis for the development of ascites may be the presence of portal hypertension and is the result of

   1. Decreased production of serum albumin, decreased colloid osmotic pressure, and increased pressure in the venous system.
   2. Decreased pressure in the venous system and increased colloid osmotic pressure.
   3. Increased aldosterone excretion, decreased colloid osmotic pressure, and lymphatic obstruction.
   4. Excess serum sodium, increased potassium retention, and increased protein metabolism.

2. The physician places the patient on a low-sodium diet and orders a diuretic. Which one of the following drugs will facilitate sodium excretion while conserving body potassium?

   1. Furosemide (Lasix).
   2. Spironolactone (Aldactone).
   3. Hydrochlorothiazide (HydroDIURIL).
   4. Ethacrynic acid (Edecrin).

3. The patient with cirrhosis of the liver receives 200 mL of 25% serum albumin IV over 4 h. The nurse should monitor for

   1. Increased serum protein level.
   2. Reduce ascites and increased urine output.
   3. Increased potassium excretion and decreased BP.
   4. Reduce BP and increased urine output.

4. The nurse observes a patient with severe cirrhosis of the liver for hepatic encephalopathy. The patient must be assessed carefully for a change in

   1. Respiratory status.
   2. Status of ascites.
   3. Bilirubin output.
   4. Level of consciousness (LOC).

5. A male patient diagnosed with cirrhosis of the liver is admitted to the hospital. His serum ammonia level begins to rise rapidly; the physician orders 40 mL of lactulose (Cephulac). The nurse informs the patient that the desired effect of this medication is to

   1. Improve LOC by eliminating ammonia.
   2. Increase urine output and decrease ascites.
   3. Produce nausea and vomiting to eliminate ammonia.
   4. Decrease intestinal motility and eliminate diarrhea.

6. A client on TPN is experiencing hyperglycemia. How should the nurse plan to treat this complication?

   1. Obtain an order for IV solution of 50% dextrose.
   2. Speed up the rate of the feeding.
   3. Notify the physician and report the increase in blood glucose.
   4. Discontinue TPN and notify physician.

7. A female patient is on a 1-g sodium diet for hypertension. She does not like her diet and calls her daughter to bring some good home-cooked food. Initially, the most effective action by the nurse should be to

   1. Ask the dietitian to discuss the patient's diet with her.
   2. Tell the patient that salt will raise her BP.
   3. Explain the diet problems to the physician.
   4. Discuss the diet limitations with the patient and her daughter.

8. A patient is on a clear liquid diet. Which food would the nurse discourage?

   1. Apple juice.
   2. Skim milk.
   3. Broth.
   4. Tea.

9. A patient is on a full liquid diet. Which of the following foods should the nurse allow the client to consume?

   1. Egg whites.
   2. Oatmeal.
   3. Cream of Wheat.
   4. Cherry nut yogurt.

10. To decrease the chances of aspiration from continuous tube feedings, the nurse should

    1. Place the patient on the right side after feeding.
    2. Elevate the head of the bed 30 to 45 degrees.
    3. Position the patient on the left side after feeding.
    4. Position the patient in the supine position after feeding.

11. A nurse indicates a correct understanding of nasogastric tube feedings by the statement: The most serious problem with this method of delivery is

    1. The formula usually causes diarrhea.
    2. This method may makes the client nauseated.
    3. This method may cause aspiration.
    4. The formula usually causes diarrhea.

12. Nurses are expected to write "outcomes" for all nursing interventions. Outcomes must meet all of the following criteria except that they are

    1. Measurable.
    2. Met within the critical period of 12 to 48 h.

3. Realistic.

4. Written in terms of the patient's behavior.

QUESTIONS 13 TO 19: CASE HISTORY

A 52-year-old woman is admitted to the emergency room (ER); her BP is 115/70, pulse 110, and respirations 22. She has been treated for alcoholism, esophageal varices, hiatal hernia, and peptic ulcers for the past 5 years. She was brought to the hospital where she vomited bright red blood.

13. Mrs. Little's signs and symptoms that would indicate the blood vomited blood originated from bleeding esophageal varices are

1. Sharp midepigastric pain and feeling of fullness in the stomach before vomiting.

2. Difficulty swallowing, cyanosis, and hypertension.

3. Anorexia, vomiting of blood, and chronic cough.

4. Midepigastric pain after eating and vomiting.

14. The physician inserted a Sengstaken-Blakemore tube into Mrs. Little's esophagus. Prior to performing the procedure, the nurse told the patient that the purpose of the tube is to

1. Remove blood from the stomach.

2. Apply mechanical compression on the affected vessels.

3. Remove secretions from the stomach.

4. Irrigate the stomach with cool normal saline.

15. After the Sengstaken-Blakemore tube was removed, it was determined Mrs. Little was also hemorrhaging in the stomach. A nasogastric tube was inserted for the purpose of

1. Removing blood from the gastric area.

2. Gavaging the stomach to monitor bleeding.

3. Lavaging the stomach with cool saline solution to monitor bleeding.

4. Stopping bleeding using pressure.

16. Because Mrs. Little has a severe peptic ulcer, the nurse should knows that it is most important to observe for signs and symptoms of

1. Choking, fever, and decreased BP.

2. Severe epigastric pain, blood, diarrhea, and increased temperature.

3. Peritonitis (rigidity of abdominal muscles and nausea and vomiting).

4. Dehydration, chest pain, and bloody diarrhea.

17. The most appropriate nursing care for the patient with peritonitis is

1. Monitor the patient's temperature and intake and output.

2. Assess vital signs and symptoms frequently.

3. Maintain the patient in the supine position and encourage fluids by mouth.

4. Observe for intestinal obstruction.

18. Symptoms of peritonitis include

1. Diminished or no peristalsis (ileus), severe abdominal pain, rapid weak pulse, and rigid abdominal muscles.

2. Increased peristalsis, rapid strong pulse, and severe lower abdominal pain.

3. Hemorrhage, increased BP, and severe abdominal pain.

4. Dysphasia, hematemesis, and increased pulse rate.

19. Mrs. Little was also diagnosed with cancer of the stomach and underwent a total gastric resection. Problems to be anticipated beginning 1 to 2 weeks after surgery include

1. Peritonitis, hemorrhage, and dumping syndrome.

2. Dumping syndrome and pernicious anemia.

3. Chemical peritonitis and hypertension.

4. Bacterial peritonitis and dumping syndrome.

End of Case

QUESTIONS 20 TO 25: CASE HISTORY

Mr. Roberts, a 65-year-old man, is admitted to the hospital for an acute attack of ulcerative colitis; he has suffered from acute gastritis for the past 21 years. He has TPN infusing at 100 mL/h via a subclavian line.

20. Too rapid administration of TPN causes symptoms of fluid overload as well as complications of

1. Pulmonary embolus and hypertension.

2. Hyposmolar diuresis and hypoglycemia.

3. Hyperosmolar diuresis and hyperglycemia.

4. Hypertension, tachycardia, and diabetes.

21. Mr. Roberts' condition improves and he is no longer in the acute stage. Because of the patient's history, the physician recommends that the patient have a total colectomy and ileostomy. In preparing the patient for surgery, the physician orders all of the following medications. The nurse most certainly should question the order for

1. Castor oil to clean out the intestines before surgery.

2. Vitamin K (AquaMEPHYTON) prophylactically.

3. Neomycin sulfates (Mycifradin Sulfate) prophylactically.

4. Diazepam (Valium) to reduce anxiety.

22. During a team conference, the nurse who has been providing care to Mr. Roberts says, "I've had it with Mr. Roberts. Since his surgery, he's done nothing but complain. I can't seem to do anything right for him." The response by a care giver that would best promote the planning of care for Mr. Roberts is:

1. "Mr. Roberts' behavior is characteristic of patients with ulcerative colitis. We have to be consistent in limiting his demands."

2. "Apparently you find it difficult to tolerate extreme dependency in a patient. We can have Mr. Roberts assigned to someone else."

3. "You've done as much as anyone could do for Mr. Roberts. Don't let him get you down."

4. "Mr. Roberts' behavior can certainly be frustrating. Let's try to figure out what he is telling us."

23. Mr. Roberts most likely has which pattern of bowel elimination through this ileostomy?

1. Alternating constipation and diarrhea.

2. Daily evacuation of foul-smelling, frothy stools.

3. Tarry-looking stools after meals that include beets.

4. Daily liquid stools.

24. To evaluate Mr. Roberts' state of hydration, the most reliable information would be obtained by the assessment of

1. Recent food intake, amount vomited, and BP.

2. Weight, number of liquid stools, and BP.

3. Turgor of skin, weight, and fluid intake.

4. Amount of urine output and hematocrit level.

25. To assist Mr. Roberts in adjusting to his ileostomy, the action by the nurse that would be most helpful is to

1. Arrange for a member of Mr. Roberts' family to learn about the care of his ileostomy and about his diet.

2. Plan with the nutritionist to teach Mr. Roberts which foods will regulate drainage so he will not need to use the ileostomy bag all the time.

3. Inform Mr. Roberts about the assistance available from members of an ileostomy organization.

4. Discuss with Mr. Roberts the possible attitudes that he may encounter among family and friends since he has had an ileostomy.

End of Case

26. A patient has been admitted to the hospital for an acute attack of ulcerative colitis. In caring for this patient, which of the following signs and symptoms should the nurse consider the most important to monitor?

1. Low-grade fever, headache, and hypertension.

2. High fever, hematuria, and abdominal pain.

3. Vomiting, uremia, and weakness.

4. Bloody diarrhea, dehydration, and weight loss.

27. Nursing responsibilities for treatment of the individual with ulcerative colitis include administering or providing

1. Vitamins, mineral supplements, and tranquilizers.

2. High-residue, high-fiber diet, and vitamins.

3. Stool softeners, vitamin B_{12}, and antacids.

4. High-protein, high-fiber diet, and antacids.

28. The nurse explains to the client that the main reason for the cecostomy is to

1. Decompress the colon.

2. Restore and maintain a positive nitrogen balance.

3. Lavage the GI tract, causing decompression.

4. Remove formed stool from the colon, causing bowel decompression.

29. An appendectomy involving an abscess requires drainage. In this type of surgery, the complication the nurse would observe for is

1. Septicemia.

2. Local or general peritonitis.

3. Hypotension.

4. Hypokalemia.

QUESTIONS 30 TO 33

Match the diagnostic test with the most appropriate disease being diagnosed.

30. ___ Schilling test

31. ___ Barium enema

32. ___ Gastroscope

33. ___ Proctoscope

1. Gastritis

2. Diverticulosis

3. Pernicious anemia

4. Colitis

End of Case

34. A licensed practical nurse (LPN) assigned to change a client's dressing informs the registered nurse (RN) that although she learned the procedure, she has never performed it. Which of the following is the best approach for the RN to use in instructing the LPN and for meeting the patient's needs?

1. Explain the steps of the procedure before having the LPN complete the assignment.

2. In the presence of the LPN, perform the procedure for the patient while explaining each step.

3. Assign a second LPN to assist in carrying out the procedure.

4. Have the LPN review the procedure manual to be sure that the procedure will be done accurately.

35. The nurse explains to the patient that medical management of an esophageal hiatal hernia usually includes all of the following *except*

1. Antacids.

2. Antibiotics.

3. A bland diet.

4. Semi-Fowler's position.

36. A patient has just been admitted to the ER with severe pain and is being assessed for possible appendicitis. The nurse should anticipate an order for all of the following *except*

1. White blood cell count.

2. An ice bag to the abdomen.

3. The nurse to continue to assess for tenderness at McBurney's point.

4. The patient to have narcotics to relieve pain every 3 to 4 h.

QUESTIONS 37 TO 42: CASE HISTORY

Mrs. Green, a 75-year-old woman, is admitted to the hospital for diagnostic evaluation and probable surgery for a tumor in the colon. She has been having cramping pains in her lower abdomen and has severe abdominal distention.

37. On her second day of hospitalization, Mrs. Green has symptoms of bowel obstruction. Bowel obstruction can occur from
    1. Colitis, paralytic ileus, gastritis, and diverticulosis.
    2. Paralytic ileus, intestinal tumor, and fecal impaction.
    3. Intestinal inflammation, peptic ulcer, gastritis, and colitis.
    4. Fecal impaction, gastritis, colitis, and barium.

38. Mrs. Green is to have decompression of the large intestine prior to GI surgery. This will be accomplished by
    1. Passing a nasogastric tube in the intestines.
    2. Keeping the client NPO and administering IV fluids.
    3. Passing a Miller-Abbott tube into the intestines.
    4. Offering a low-residue diet for 2 days prior to surgery.

39. The nurse explains to Mrs. Green that neomycin is given before surgery to
    1. Prevent paralytic ileus.
    2. Destroy ammonia-producing microorganisms in the colon.
    3. Control extension of the lesion at the splenic flexure.
    4. Lower the bacterial count in the intestines.

40. On the morning of surgery, Mrs. Green's preoperative medication includes atropine sulfate. The anticholinergic action of atropine will cause
    1. Decreased systolic pressure, decreased pulse, and constricted pupils.
    2. Dryness of the oropharyngeal mucosa, decreased respiratory secretions, and increased pulse rate.
    3. Constricted pupils, slow pulse rate, and increased BP.
    4. Drowsiness, decreased pulse rate, dehydration, dryness of the oral mucosa, and increased BP.

41. Mrs. Green has a resection of a segment of the descending colon with an end-to-end anastomosis. After she recovers from anesthesia, she is returned to her room with an IV line and a nasogastric tube in place. Her nasogastric tube is a double lumen with the gastric port to low suction. While the nasogastric tube is in place, the nurse should
    1. Never instill water into the tube before starting the continuous feeding pump.
    2. Instill 3 mL of air into the tube after each normal saline irrigation to ensure patency.
    3. Instill 60 mL of water into the duodenal port every 4 h and whenever the patient complains of pain.
    4. Instill 30 mL of normal saline into the gastric port every 4 h per physician's orders.

42. After surgery, Mrs. Green receives a transfusion of whole blood. The nurse determines that Mrs. Green is experiencing symptoms of a hemolytic transfusion reaction. In addition to notifying the physician, the nurse should
    1. Remove the transfusion and discard the remaining blood.
    2. Stop the transfusion, start the normal saline, and prepare to obtain blood and urine samples.
    3. Slow the transfusion flow rate, cover the patient with blankets, and reassess her in 15 min.
    4. Continue the transfusion and continue to assess the patient.

End of Case

43. Mrs. Benson returns from the operating room after having undergone a partial colectomy and has a double-barrel colostomy. When the physician gives the order to begin irrigation of the colostomy, the nurse should be aware that the
    1. Proximal stoma is irrigated.
    2. Distal stoma is irrigated.
    3. Distal stoma will drain only when the proximal stoma is irrigated.
    4. Proximal stoma and distal stoma must be irrigated.

44. Mrs. Benson's new colostomy drains 1 h after irrigation. The next step is to
    1. Increase liquid intake and increase fiber in the patient's diet.
    2. Decrease fiber in the patient's diet to decrease peristalsis.
    3. Increase the amount of fluid used to irrigate.
    4. Decrease the amount of fluid used to irrigate.

45. Which statement correctly shows the relationship between gastric secretions lost in gastric suctioning and IV therapy?
    1. IV therapy and gastric suctioning accomplish the same purpose.
    2. Electrolytes lost through drainage must be replaced through IV therapy.
    3. Hydration is best accomplished by the use of IV therapy.
    4. IV therapy has a direct relationship with urinary output.

46. The best approach by the nurse that will assist a patient to adapt to an ostomy is to
    1. Begin instruction on stoma care as soon as possible after surgery.
    2. Provide instruction appropriate to the patient's receptiveness.
    3. Be sure the patient helps in stoma care, starting with first or second irrigation
    4. Leave descriptive pamphlets in the patient's room that will answer his or her questions.

47. A patient has been diagnosed with a hiatal hernia. The most appropriate nursing instructions would be
    1. To remain in a sitting position after eating for at least 30 min.
    2. To bend, especially after eating; it will help to move food out of the stomach.
    3. To sleep lying flat on the back with the foot of the bed raised slightly.
    4. Not to drink fluids with meals; it will cause dumping syndrome.

48. A mother of three children has infectious hepatitis (type A). Her children should be
    1. Admitted to the hospital.
    2. Given gamma-globulin.
    3. Placed on a protein-restricted diet.
    4. Placed on bed rest.

49. The most common cause of type A hepatitis is
    1. Consumption of seafood from polluted water.
    2. Ingestion of contaminated foods.v
    3. Transmission via the parenteral route, especially blood products.
    4. Consumption of inadequately processed foods (especially chicken, eggs, turkey, and duck).

50. Which of the following statements regarding the prevention of hepatitis before exposure to hepatitis B virus is most correct?
    1. No specific treatment exists.
    2. Receive gamma globulin.
    3. Receive standard immunoglobulin.
    4. Receive hepatitis B vaccine (Recombivax B).

QUESTIONS 51 TO 55: CASE HISTORY

Mr. Neighbors, a 31-year-old man, is admitted to the hospital to rule out diagnosis of serum hepatitis (type B). His orders include bed rest and diagnostic studies.

51. The nurse assesses the client for early symptoms of serum hepatitis (type B). These include
    1. Loss of appetite, nausea and vomiting, abdominal pain, pruritus, and flulike symptoms.
    2. Capillary fragility, jaundice, dark urine, and pruritus.
    3. Shortness of breath on exertion, bradycardia, and edema.
    4. Ataxia, headache, tachycardia, and polyuria.

52. When taking Mr. Neighbor's admission history, the nurse knows that the factor in the patient's history most likely to be related to his diagnosis is
    1. Recent recovery from an upper respiratory infection.
    2. Being bitten by an insect.

3. Eating home-canned food.
4. Working in a hemodialysis unit.

53. In assessing Mr. Neighbor's laboratory values, the nurse should know that the tests used to assess liver function are
    1. Liver enzymes (AST, ALT, ALP) and biliary excretion.
    2. Iron transferrin, cystography, and biliary excretion.
    3. Creatinine clearance and fatty casts.
    4. Creatine kinase (CK-MB) and LDH.

54. Which of the following precautionary measures is essential in this patient's care?
    1. Serving food on disposable dishes and diligence in hand washing.
    2. Wearing a face mask and diligence in hand washing.
    3. Wearing gloves when carrying out procedures for decontamination of urine and feces.
    4. Wearing gloves when using syringes and needles.

55. The nurse tells Mr. Neighbor the purpose of bed rest is to
    1. Minimize liver damage.
    2. Decrease the circulatory load and reduce cardiac workload.
    3. Control the spread of disease.
    4. Increase the breakdown of fats so that metabolic needs will be met.

End of Case

56. Which of the following statements is true about hepatic encephalopathy?
    1. GI tract fails to absorb ammonia.
    2. Liver fails to convert urea to ammonia.
    3. Liver fails to convert ammonia to urea.
    4. Liver is overloaded with barbiturates, which it cannot break down.

End of Case

QUESTIONS 57 TO 61: CASE HISTORY

X-ray studies reveal that Mrs. White has cholecystitis and cholelithiasis. She has pain in the upper right quadrant of the abdomen radiating to the back and the right shoulder. The biliary colic is severe.

57. The nurse explains to the patient that, before surgery, a cholecystography will be performed to
    1. Detect obstruction at the ampulla of Vater.
    2. Note whether the gallbladder contained stones.
    3. Observe patency of the common bile duct.
    4. Observe patency of the cystic duct and common bile duct.

58. The nurse tells Mrs. White that her PT is decreased because of
    1. An absence of vitamin B_{12} in the intestines.
    2. Accumulation of cholecystokinin.
    3. Decreased synthesis of vitamin K.
    4. Inadequate intake of prothrombin.

59. During surgery, a cholangiography was performed on Mrs. White. She returns to the unit with an abdominal dressing and a T-tube inserted into the common bile duct. Nursing care of the T-tube should consist of
    1. No nursing care; it is a closed vacuum drainage system.
    2. Reporting immediately any bile in the drainage system.
    3. Periodic emptying and measuring of the bile drainage.
    4. Periodic irrigation of the tube with normal saline.

60. The nurse explains to Mrs. White that the main reason the T-tube is inserted after the exploration of the common bile duct is to
    1. Alleviate pain.
    2. Stimulate secretion of bile.
    3. Maintain patency of the common bile duct.
    4. Divert flow of bile away from the GI tract.

61. During the first few days following a laparoscopic cholecystectomy, which one of the following is most important to maintain?
    1. Good oral care.
    2. Good respiratory care.
    3. Client NPO.
    4. Client on bed rest.

End of Case

QUESTIONS 62 TO 68: CASE HISTORY

Mr. Brown, a 42-year-old man, is admitted to the hospital with jaundice, ascites, and weight loss. The following liver function studies are ordered: serum protein concentrations and serum enzymes. A diagnosis of cirrhosis of the liver is made.

62. Serum protein determination measures the liver's ability to
    1. Maintain the integrity of white blood cells and normal amylase level.
    2. Maintain normal amounts of red blood cells and ammonia.
    3. Manufacture antibodies and aldosterone.
    4. Maintain normal levels of liver enzymes and albumin.

63. Mr. Brown's ascites increases and he becomes increasingly lethargic. The ascites is related to
    1. Decreased serum albumin.
    2. Decreased number of platelets.

3. Increased blood urea nitrogen.
4. Increased serum levels of ammonia.

64. Mr. Brown's lethargy indicates some degree of hepatic encephalopathy. The measure that aids in the management of this complication is to
    1. Limit fluids to 500 mL/day.
    2. Restrict dietary sodium.
    3. Maintain high-protein diet.
    4. Restrict dietary protein.

65. The pathophysiology underlying hepatic encephalopathy can best be explained by which statement?
    1. The ability to hold fluid in the intravascular compartment is decreased, causing fluid to leak into interstitial tissue.
    2. The bile flowing into the intestine is increased; this results in its urine concentration in the blood and the brain, causing cell necrosis.
    3. Blood levels of ammonia increase because the liver can no longer remove it from the blood by converting it to urea.
    4. Virus and lymphocytes leave the liver and enter the central nervous system.

66. The nurse would assess an alcoholic patient for signs of alcohol withdrawal, which include
    1. Decreased level of consciousness, vomiting, headache, and blurred vision.
    2. Hypotension, headache, dizziness, seizures, and diaphoresis.
    3. Signs and symptoms of tremors, anorexia, hallucinations, convulsions, delirium tremens, restlessness, diaphoresis, and elevated BP.
    4. Delirium tremens, seizures, decreased level of consciousness, and blurred vision.

67. Mr. Brown asks the nurse why he has ascites and bleeds so easily. The most accurate reply by the nurse would be:
    1. "No one really knows why people with cirrhosis of the liver have these problems."
    2. "It is caused by drinking too much alcohol and not eating right."
    3. "Your diseased liver cannot synthesize vitamin K, and you have not been eating right."
    4. "Your diseased liver cannot synthesize albumin and clotting factors."

68. The nurse tells the patient his diet must be low in protein and high in carbohydrates during the acute phase of his illness. The nurse should teach the patient that which of the following foods are highest in carbohydrates?
    1. Jelly sandwich and a glass of milk.
    2. Hard-boiled egg and bacon.

3. Raw carrot sticks and a banana.

4. Cottage cheese and a hot dog.

End of Case

69. The nurse should anticipate which one of the following laboratory values to be elevated in pancreatitis?

   1. Unconjugated bilirubin.

   2. Prothrombin time.

   3. Serum amylase.

   4. Red blood cell count.

70. A patient is admitted to rule out diagnosis of pancreatitis. The nurse should assess the patient for

   1. Hypertension, bradycardia, and nausea and vomiting.

   2. Extreme pain, tachycardia, fever, nausea and vomiting.

   3. Nausea vomiting, bradycardia, and malaise.

   4. Elevated red blood cell count, malaise, and hematuria.

71. Which one of the following is most likely to cause pancreatitis?

   1. Gold compounds.

   2. Carbon tetrachloride.

   3. Alcohol.

   4. Thorazine.

72. Repeated water enemas (or enemas until clear) are often administered in preparation for a lower GI series. Which of the following electrolyte problems is most likely to occur?

   1. Sodium deficit only.

   2. Potassium deficit only.

   3. Acidosis and sodium and bicarbonate deficits.

   4. Alkalosis and sodium and potassium deficits.

73. The nurse informs the client that frequent sitz baths may be ordered after anorectal surgery to

   1. Relieve pain and reduce sphincter spasm.

   2. Reduce temperature and soften fecal material.

   3. Prevent hemorrhage and increase healing.

   4. Apply medicine using sitz bath water.

74. In assessing a patient with esophageal achalasia, the nurse should observe for symptoms of

   1. Sensation of food sticking in the lower portion of the esophagus, with regurgitation of food.

   2. Dry mouth, thirst, and esophageal pain.

   3. Vomiting after eating and pain in the epigastric area.

   4. Excessive salivation, esophageal spasm, and vomiting.

75. In assessing a patient for a sliding hiatal hernia, the nurse would observe for symptoms of

   1. Fullness in the lower chest and midepigastric pain.

   2. Fullness and pain in the lower abdomen and hematuria.

   3. Chest pain on exertion and nausea.

   4. Abdominal pain on exertion and hematuria.

76. The nurse informs the patient that following a GI barium study, a laxative or enema will be administered because

   1. When barium is digested, it becomes a chalky white powder that is irritating to the intestinal mucosa.

   2. Barium is not digested; when water is absorbed from barium, it solidifies in the intestines and may later cause an obstruction.

   3. The patient may be allergic to the barium, so the impaction needs to be removed immediately.

   4. The barium tablets that the patient swallowed with water the evening before a GI series do not dissolve readily and may result in impaction.

77. The physician states that he is ordering three different acid pump inhibitors for three different patients. You will anticipate that the order may include which of the following?

   1. Prilosec, Prevacid, and Nexium.

   2. Trimethobenzamide (Tigan), atropine, and Carafate.

   3. Propantheline (Pro-Banthine), Atropine, and misoprostol (Cytotec).

   4. Belladonna (Donnatal), Nizatidine (Axid), and Metronidazole (Flagyl).

78. Medications used to treat spastic colon are

   1. Ranitidine (Zantac) and neostigmine (Prostigmin).

   2. Belladonna (Donnatal).

   3. Atropine and propantheline (Pro-Banthine).

   4. Diphenoxylate with atropine (Lomotil) and opium tincture (Paregoric).

79. Which drug is used to treat bladder distention?

   1. Docusate sodium (Colace).

   2. Trimethobenzamide (Tigan).

   3. Neostigmine (Prostigmin).

   4. Belladonna (Donnatal).

80. The nurse should assess patient a week after Billroth II surgery for which of the following problems?

   1. Pernicious anemia and dumping syndrome.

   2. Diarrhea and anemia.

   3. Hypotension and bradycardia.

   4. Gastric bleeding and hypotension.

81. The nurse should assess a patient with dumping syndrome for which of the following signs and symptoms?

   1. Faintness, tachycardia, diaphoresis, and chest palpitations.

   2. Vomiting, bradycardia, diaphoresis, and hemoptysis.

   3. Diarrhea and poor absorption of nutrients.

   4. Faintness, bradycardia, and hypotension.

82. A patient asks the nurse what is a cholangiography. The nurse's correct response is: A cholangiography allows visualization of the

1. Colon.
2. Liver.
3. Gallbladder.
4. Common bile duct and hepatic duct.

83. A male patient with cancer of the pancreas asks the nurse the name of the surgery used to treat his cancer. The nurse's correct response would be a

1. Billroth I.
2. Billroth II.
3. Total gastric resection.
4. Whipple procedure.

84. A 60-year-old woman is admitted to the hospital with a diagnosis of congestive heart failure and ulcerative colitis. Her medications include furosemide (Lasix), digoxin (Lanoxin), tetracycline, and methylprednisolone (Solu-Medrol). Foods that cannot be included in her diet while taking tetracycline are

1. Coffee, cream, and sugar.
2. Beer, beef, and cheese.
3. Milk, antacid, and cheese.
4. Cola, beer, and wine.

85. Without the presence of bile salts in the intestinal tract, which of the following cannot be absorbed?

1. Vitamins B, C, E, and K.
2. Vitamins A, D, E, and K.
3. Bilirubin, and vitamins D and C.
4. Salt and immunoglobulin (hepatitis B immune globulin [H-BIG]).

86. A male patient, aged 72 years, is admitted with jaundice, abdominal pain, and nausea and vomiting. His physician suspects gallstones and possible pancreatic involvement. Which of the following procedures would allow visualization of the biliary and pancreatic ducts and is associated with the least morbidity?

1. Hepatobiliary and scintigraphy.
2. Cholangiography.
3. Percutaneous transhepatic cholangiography (PTHC).
4. Endoscopic retrograde cholangiopancreatography (ERCP).

87. Anemia caused by folic acid deficiency usually occurs in patients in which of the following situations?

1. Malnutrition and alcohol-induced cirrhosis.
2. Sickle cell disease, pernicious anemia, and rheumatic heart disease.

3. Thrombocytopenia purpura, hemophilia, and disseminated intravascular coagulation.
4. Cystic fibrosis and myasthenia gravis.

88. The nurse in caring for a patient after a cholangiopancreatography should assess for

1. Internal bleeding and peritonitis.
2. Hypotension and allergic reaction to radiographic dye.
3. Tachycardia and dyspnea.
4. Allergic reaction to radiographic dye and dyspnea.

89. The nurse is caring for an elderly patient in a long-term care facility. The nurse would consider which of the following changes in relation to liver function in the elderly?

1. Liver function tests are often abnormal.
2. The liver's ability to detoxify drugs is decreased.
3. Production of cholesterol is increased.
4. Hypertension is common.

90. Which of the following assessments would provide the nurse with the most accurate information regarding GI function in a patient with a paralytic ileus?

1. Palpating the abdomen for tenderness.
2. Auscultation of bowel sounds.
3. Monitoring serum electrolyte levels.
4. Monitoring the white blood cell count.

91. The nurse is caring for a patient with cirrhosis and esophageal varices. Which of the following should be reported to the physician immediately?

1. Anorexia and nausea.
2. Weight gain and decrease in urine output.
3. Hematemesis and melena.
4. Increase in abdominal girth and peripheral edema.

92. The nurse is caring for a patient with bleeding esophageal varices with a Sengstaken-Blakemore tube inserted with both the gastric and esophageal balloons inflated. Which of the following nursing assessments and intervention are most important?

1. Encourage sips of cool, clear fluids, and observe for respiratory distress.
2. Deflate the esophageal balloon for 10 min every 2 h.
3. Reposition the tube if the patient complains of nausea and abdominal distention.
4. If sudden respiratory distress occurs, cut all balloon lumens.

93. A 67-year-old male patient is admitted to the hospital with a diagnosis of cancer of the large intestine. He is scheduled for a large-bowel resection. He tells his physician that if he must have an ileostomy, he wants a continent ileostomy. Which statement describes a continent ileostomy?

1. It will have continuous drainage into an external ileostomy bag that must be emptied at least once daily.

2. The ileostomy drainage will be regulated so that a drainage bag will not have to be used continually on a 24-h basis.

3. This method eliminates the need to wear an external appliance or bag over the stoma. The internal pouch will act as a reservoir and can be drained by inserting a catheter.

4. This internal ileostomy pouch will be irrigated every 3 days, and no external bag will be needed.

94. The nurse is caring for a patient with possible appendicitis. Which of the following should be reported immediately?
    1. Temperature of 38°C (100°F).
    2. Leukocyte level count of 10,000 mm³.
    3. Sudden, severe localized abdominal pain.
    4. Nausea and vomiting.

95. The nurse is admitting a patient with a diagnosis of possible appendicitis. All of the following instructions should be given to the patient *except*
    1. Food and fluids will be restricted.
    2. Analgesics are withheld until a diagnosis is made and surgery is scheduled.
    3. A mild laxative will be administered to prepare the patient for surgery.
    4. An ice pack may be used to reduce abdominal pain.

96. When the nurse is obtaining a history from a patient with Crohn's disease, it would be most important to document
    1. Percentage of meals eaten.
    2. Number and character of stools.
    3. Presence of lesions in the oral cavity.
    4. History of allergies.

97. The nurse is assessing a patient with an ulcerative colitis. It would be most important to monitor the
    1. Serum bicarbonate level.
    2. Platelet count
    3. White blood cell count.
    4. Hemoglobin levels.

98. The nurse is caring for a patient with an acute exacerbation of Crohn's disease. Which of the following nursing interventions is appropriate?
    1. Ambulate patient several times each day to prevent joint complications.
    2. Encourage high-fiber and protein intake.
    3. Administer stool softeners, and encourage ambulation.
    4. Place a deodorizer in the room and maintain patient on bed rest.

99. The nurse is admitting a patient with a diagnosis of ulcerative colitis. Which of the following nursing diagnoses would be most important?
    1. High risk for decreased cardiac output related to GI blood loss.
    2. Pain related to inflammation of the intestinal wall.
    3. Constipation related to paralytic ileus.
    4. High risk for pneumonia related to bed rest.

100. Postural drainage and percussion should be done
    1. Immediately after breakfast.
    2. One hour after eating.
    3. Approximately 3 h after eating
    4. Eight hours before eating.

ANSWERS AND RATIONALES

1. ❶ Decreased albumin production in the liver caused by cirrhosis of the liver results in decreased colloidal osmotic pressure, causing fluid to flow out of the vascular system and into the peritoneal cavity. Decreased removal of aldosterone by the liver results in sodium retention and thus water retention, adding to the fluid in the peritoneal cavity. The liver fails to break down aldosterone, so the kidney cannot excrete it.

(2, 3, 4) These options are incorrect as seen in rationale (1).

2. ❷ Spironolactone (Aldactone), a potassium-sparing diuretic, is used because the client's high aldosterone level causes sodium retention. Potassium is lost when sodium is retained.

(1, 3, 4) These medications, although also diuretics, cause urinary loss of potassium.

3. ❷ Serum albumin will increase osmotic pressure in the vascular system and help prevent leakage of fluid from the vascular system. This decreases ascites and increases fluid so that more fluid is available to perfuse the kidneys; this results in increased urine output.

(1, 3, 4) These options are incorrect as seen in rationale (2).

4. ❹ The client has cirrhosis of the liver and cannot break down ammonia to urea; the ammonia may go to the brain and cause hepatic encephalopathy. One of the first signs of hepatic encephalopathy is a decreased level of consciousness.

(1, 2, 3) These options are incorrect as seen in rationale (4).

5. ❶ Cephulac is a laxative that reduces ammonia levels by binding the ammonia in the GI tract and eliminating it in the stool. If enough ammonia can be removed by this laxative, level of consciousness should improve.

(2, 3, 4) These options are incorrect as seen in rationale (1).

6. ❸ When a patient is experiencing hyperglycemia, the nurse needs a physician's order for insulin to decrease blood glucose. Patients on TPN have their blood sugar monitored closely for hyperglycemia.

(1, 2, 4) These options are incorrect as seen in rationale (3). TPN cannot be suddenly discontinued because the patient would develop hypoglycemia.

7. ❹ Patients must be included in decisions that affect their lives. The nurse or dietitian will not be with the patient when she goes home. By discussing the patient's diet with the patient

and the daughter, the nurse can help them plan an acceptable 1-g sodium diet that the patient can live with.

(1, 2, 3) These options are incorrect as seen in rationale (4).

8. ❷ Skim milk is not allowed on a clear liquid diet.

(1, 3, 4) Apple juice, broth, and tea are liquids that can be seen through and therefore are considered clear liquids.

9. ❸ Cream of Wheat can be given to a client on a full liquid diet. It can be made in a semiliquid form and eaten with a spoon.

(1, 2, 4) Egg whites, oatmeal, and cherry nut yogurt are not allowed on a full liquid diet. They would be allowed on a soft diet.

10. ❷ All clients on continuous tube feeding should have the head of their bed in semi-Fowler's position (35–45 degrees) at all times to prevent regurgitation and aspiration of tube feeding.

(1, 3, 4) Placing the client in any of these positions would allow tube feeding to regurgitate into the esophagus and may cause aspiration.

11. ❸ Regurgitation and aspiration are the most serious complications related to tube feeding.

(1, 2, 4) The formula usually does not cause the patient to be nauseated; it may cause diarrhea but these problems are not as serious as regurgitation and aspiration.

12. ❷ The expected nursing "outcomes" for all nursing interventions do not have to be met within a critical period of 12 to 48 h. The expected nursing "outcomes" may be met in 3 h or in weeks.

(1, 3, 4) All expected nursing "outcomes" must be measurable, realistic, and written in terms of the patient's behavior.

13. ❸ Blood draining from the esophageal varices into the stomach will cause anorexia and vomiting. Blood drainage down the throat will produce a tickling sensation, which will cause a chronic cough. The patient has difficulty breathing because of increased abdominal pressure from ascites and portal hypertension. Remember, blood in the stomach will be used as protein. Rubber band ligation may be used to treat esophageal varices. In this procedure, the surgeon goes through the oral cavity into the esophagus and ties off the bleeding veins by stapling them with rubber bands.

(1, 2, 4) These options are incorrect as seen in rationale (3).

14. ❷ A Sengstaken-Blakemore tube is placed in the esophagus to force blood back into the veins and temporarily stop esophageal bleeding.

(1, 3, 4) These options are incorrect as seen in rationale (2).

15. ❸ Lavaging the stomach with cool saline solution may curtail hemorrhaging by vasoconstricting the blood vessels. Gastric cooling with ice is controversial because it may cause more mucosal damage. For this reason, iced saline solution should not be used.

(1, 2, 4) These options are incorrect as seen in rationale (3). Rationale 2 is incorrect because gavage means to feed.

16. ❸ The ulcer may erode through the stomach's vascular system, causing hemorrhaging, and it may erode through the stomach wall, spilling into the peritoneal cavity, causing peritonitis. Signs and symptoms of peritonitis are rigidity of abdominal muscles, nausea and vomiting, and severe abdominal pain.

(1, 2, 4) These options are incorrect as seen in rationale (3).

17. ❷ Frequent assessment of all vital signs and symptoms by the nurse is crucial for early determination of any problems that need medical or surgical intervention by the physician.

(1) Monitoring the patient's temperature and intake and output (I&O) is only part of the assessment; the option does not state frequency.

(3) Maintaining the patient in the supine position and encouraging fluids would cause the patient to vomit and possibly aspirate. The patient has decreased peristalsis and, therefore, would be NPO.

(4) A patient with peritonitis has decreased peristalsis and may have a paralytic ileus (paralysis of intestinal peristalsis). The bowel is already obstructed and the patient is NPO.

18. ❶ The peritoneum that lines the abdominal and pelvic cavities is well supplied with somatic nerves; therefore, irritation causes severe localized pain. Peristaltic activity of the bowel ceases (paralytic ileus) because of a critical fluid and electrolyte imbalance caused by the infectious process. The inflammatory process increases oxygen requirement at a time when the person has a decreased ability to ventilate. The person has difficulty ventilating because of increased abdominal pressure, which elevates the diaphragm; breathing is painful.

(2, 3, 4) These options are incorrect as seen in rationale (1).

19. ❷ Dumping syndrome occurs after partial and total gastrectomy. Because of gravity, ingested food rapidly enters the jejunum without proper mixing with the normal duodenal digestive processing. Approximately 30 min after eating, the person experiences vertigo, tachycardia, syncope, sweating, pallor, palpitation, diarrhea, and nausea. These symptoms are greatly increased if the patient drinks fluids with meals because the fluid flushes the food rapidly down the intestine. Pernicious anemia is caused by the removal of a portion of the stomach that contains intrinsic factor, which is necessary for absorption of vitamin B_{12}.

(1, 3, 4) These options are incorrect as seen in rationale (2).

20. ❸ Hyperglycemia develops when the pancreas cannot secrete sufficient insulin to meet the body's needs. Glucose is "locked" outside the cells without the available insulin to transport it into cells, and it accumulates and raises the blood glucose level (hyperglycemia). The elevated glucose level exerts a strong osmotic force and pulls intracellular fluid out and into the blood, which increases the blood glucose level. The osmotic load of glucose in the urine prevents the reabsorption of water by the kidney tubules, causing hyperosmolar diuresis. When the blood glucose level rises above 140 (normal blood glucose is 75–120), it exceeds the renal threshold and glucose spills into the urine, causing glycosuria. The osmotic load of glucose in the urine prevents the reabsorption of water into the kidney tubules.

This pathologic development results in the three cardinal symptoms of diabetes—polyuria, polydipsia, polyphagia (the three P's)—and weight loss. In addition to the three cardinal symptoms, people with diabetes may develop ketoacidosis, a form of metabolic acidosis, one of the most severe complications of diabetes. Ketoacidosis may arise when hyperglycemia is not controlled by insulin and diet.

(1, 2, 4) These options are incorrect as seen in rationale (3).

21. **①** Ulcerative colitis is an inflammation of the colon causing increased peristalsis; castor oil would exacerbate this problem by increasing peristalsis.

(2) With ulcerative colitis there is gross inflammation of the colon, resulting in bleeding in the colon. Vitamin K is necessary for the synthesis of prothrombin, necessary for clot formation; there would be no reason to question this order.

(3) Neomycin is used to prepare the GI tract for surgery by decreasing the bacteria in the GI tract. Therefore, the use of neomycin would not be contraindicated for a patient with ulcerative colitis.

(4) Diazepam (Valium) is a muscle relaxant used in the management of anxiety and, therefore, can be given to this patient.

22. **④** "Mr. Roberts' behavior can certainly be frustrating. Let's try to figure out what he is telling us." This statement acknowledges that working with this patient can be frustrating, and it encourages the team to discuss the problem.

(1) This is labeling and stereotyping the patient. Setting limits may increase the patient's need to complain because he will not be able to express his feelings.

(2) It is never appropriate to tell another person how he or she feels; it only causes inappropriate feelings and does not solve problems. A nurse needs to learn to work with all patients, so assigning the patient to another nurse is not an option.

(3) This statement is incorrect; there is always room for improvement. This statement does not help solve the problem.

23. **④** Before surgery, a patient with ulcerative colitis has inflammation and hypertrophy of the intestine, and may have 10 to 20 bowel movements per day consisting of blood, mucus, and diarrhea. After a total colectomy and a ileostomy, the patient will have liquid stools through the ileostomy every day because the large bowel, which absorbs water, has been removed.

(1, 2, 3) These options are incorrect as seen in rationale (4).

24. **④** When renal function is normal, urine output is a good measure of hydration; if a patient is adequately hydrated, he will have adequate urine output. If he is dehydrated, he will have a low urine output; the urine will be a dark, yellow-green color, and the specific gravity will be high. The hematocrit is the volume of red blood cells in 100 mL of blood. Hematocrit will be elevated if the patient is dehydrated.

(1) Food intake is not related to hydration; the amount vomited may not dehydrate the patient if the patient was well hydrated before vomiting or if the patient has an IV line infusing at a rate of 125 mL/h. BP is influenced by many factors and is not a good indicator of hydration.

(2) A patient may gain weight from fluid outside the vascular system (edema) and may be dehydrated; therefore, weight is not always a good indicator of hydration. A person who eats too much can gain weight.

(3) Poor skin turgor can be used as an indicator of hydration, but not in the elderly (their skin may normally have poor skin turgor because of loss of elasticity). Weight is discussed in rationale 2. The patient may be taking in small or large amounts of fluids; this is not a good indicator.

25. **③** Organizations with support groups for people who have had an ileostomy can assist patients with information about the care of the ileostomy and can show them different types of ileostomy bags and stoma guard skin barrier preparation. These organizations have members who have had an ileostomy and who will talk with patients about their own experiences after an ileostomy.

(1) Mr. Roberts is able to care for his own ileostomy and does not need a family member to learn about his care. Another member of the family would not help the patient to adjust to the stoma.

(2) Ileostomy drains all of the time and cannot be regulated because an ileostomy is in the small bowel where the bowel content is always liquid. The small bowel absorbs food; the large intestine absorbs water.

(4) Many of Mr. Roberts' family and friends will not know he has had an ileostomy; their attitude is not important, but the patient's attitude is important.

26. **④** Bloody diarrhea results from constant inflammation and irritation of the colon; dehydration occurs because of diarrhea. Weight loss results from liquid loss and poor food absorption because the bowel is hypertrophied from continual inflammation and diarrhea. The patient may also have anorexia caused by the constant inflammation and diarrhea.

(1) The patient may have a low-grade fever because of inflammation in the large intestine. A headache is not associated with ulcerative colitis, and hypertension is not a symptom of ulcerative colitis. Low-grade fever is the only symptom the patient may have but is not as important to monitor as are bloody diarrhea, dehydration, and weakness. If these signs and symptoms are not treated, the patient could die.

(2) A patient with ulcerative colitis will not have a high fever or hematuria (blood in urine). The patient will have abdominal cramping and pain, but none of these signs and symptoms is as life threatening as the signs and symptoms in rationale 4.

(3) Vomiting is not a sign of ulcerative colitis. Uremia is a toxic condition associated with renal insufficiency produced by an excess of urea and other nitrogenous substances in the blood. Weakness may be a sign of ulcerative colitis.

27. **①** Ulcerative colitis is an inflammatory, often chronic, disease that affects the mucosa of the colon and often extends upward into the entire colon. Ulcerative colitis produces mucosal congestion and ulcerations. The major symptom is recurrent bloody, mucous, pus-filled diarrhea causing a loss of nutrients, including vitamins and minerals; therefore, these must be replaced. Although the etiology of ulcerative colitis is unknown, it is thought to be related to abnormal immune response in the GI tract, possibly associated with food or bacteria. Stress once was thought to be a cause of ulcerative colitis; however, research now shows that it is not a cause but that it does increase the severity of the attack. Stress increases an individual's anxiety; therefore, tranquilizers are used to relax the individual with ulcerative colitis.

(2) A high-residue, high-fiber diet will increase peristalsis, inflammation, diarrhea, mucus, and pus in a patient with ulcerative colitis.

(3) A patient with diarrhea does not need a stool softener. Vitamin B_{12} would be helpful to replace vitamins lost. Antacids are used to neutralize acid in the stomach, but there is no acid in the large bowel.

(4) See rationales 2 and 3.

28. ❶ A cecostomy is used to drain fluid from the lower bowel by inserting a tube through the abdominal wall into the colon when there is a higher intestinal obstruction that prevents passage of a Miller-Abbott tube through the nose and down deep into the intestines. A Miller-Abbott tube is inserted through the nose and into the patient's intestine for bowel decompression. These procedures are done before surgery to decompress the bowel so that bowel contents will not leak into the peritoneum when the bowel is opened during surgery to take out the obstruction.

(2) Adequate intake of protein is needed to maintain a positive nitrogen balance, necessary for healing. It has no relationship to a cecostomy.

(3) Lavage means to wash out the GI tract with water, usually after someone has ingested poison (no relationship to a cecostomy).

(4) A colostomy is used to remove formed stool from the bowel; it does not decompress the bowel.

29. ❷ The major complication of an appendectomy is the potential for leakage of contents from the abscessed appendix into the peritoneum, causing local or generalized peritonitis.

(1) Septicemia is the presence of pathogenic bacteria in the blood and is sometimes confused with uremia. Uremia is a toxic condition associated with renal failure, resulting in the retention of nitrogenous substances that are normally secreted by the kidney (causing azotemia and coma).

(3, 4) These options are incorrect as seen in rationale (2).

30. ❸ A Schilling test is performed to detect vitamin B_{12} absorption. Normally, ingested vitamin B_{12} combines with intrinsic factor, which is produced in the stomach. If intrinsic factor is not present in the stomach, vitamin B_{12} is not absorbed, resulting in pernicious anemia. Vitamin B_{12} is necessary for the production of red blood cells.

(1, 2, 4) These options are incorrect as seen in rationale (3).

31. ❷ A barium enema is administered to determine the presence of diverticulosis. A diverticulum is a blind outpouching of the intestinal mucosa in the large intestine. Barium is administered by enema, and x-ray films are taken to observe the flow of barium in the large bowel to detect diverticula.

(1, 3, 4) These options are incorrect as seen in rationale (2).

32. ❶ A gastroscope is passed down through the nose or mouth and into the stomach where the physician can look at the stomach lining and determine if there is inflammation (gastritis).

(2, 3, 4) These options are incorrect as seen in rationale (1).

33. ❹ A proctoscope is passed up the rectum and into the large bowel where the physician can look at the lining of the colon to see if there is inflammation (colitis) of the colon.

(1, 2, 3) These options are incorrect as seen in rationale (4).

34. ❷ The safety of the patient is always the first priority, so the RN should perform the procedure for the patient in the presence of the LPN.

(1, 3, 4) These options are incorrect as seen in rationale (2).

35. ❷ Antibiotics are not used for a hiatal hernia because there is no infection. A hiatal hernia is an enlargement of the cardiac sphincter muscle. This enlargement allows food and gastric juices to flow back into the esophagus, especially when the patient lies down or bends over.

(1) Antacids are used to neutralize the acid in the stomach so that when gastric juices (especially hydrochloric acid flow up into the esophagus, the chance of esophageal ulcers is reduced.

(3) A bland diet is used to reduce the workload of the stomach and thus reduce gastric secretions, especially hydrochloric acid during an acute phase.

(4) Elevating the head of the bed helps to reduce flow of food and gastric juices into the esophagus.

36. ❹ The use of analgesic to relieve pain would interfere with the diagnosis by reducing or removing the pain. The area and intensity of pain help the physician to make an accurate and immediate diagnosis. Remember, this question asked what the nurse would not anticipate.

(1) An elevated white blood cell count would indicate an infection and possible appendicitis.

(2) An ice bag may be ordered for comfort because pain medication cannot be given before a diagnosis is made.

(3) Tenderness at McBurney's point would indicate possible appendicitis. McBurney's point is a point of tenderness in acute appendicitis. It is situated on a line between the umbilicus and the right anterosuperior iliac spine; the latter is an area of the right lower quadrant of the abdomen.

37. ❷ Paralytic ileus is a lack of intestinal peristalsis. With no movement of fecal material in the GI tract, obstruction can easily occur. Intestinal tumor and fecal impaction will obstruct movement of fecal material through the intestine and result in an obstruction.

(1) With colitis, there is increased peristalsis and inflammation of the bowel. Gastritis (inflammation of the stomach) will not cause bowel obstruction. Paralytic ileus can cause bowel obstruction, so this answer is only partially correct. Diverticulosis is pouches in the wall of the intestine. Food falls into pits in the intestines, causing spasms and intestinal inflammation.

(3) An intestinal inflammation will not cause a bowel obstruction. A peptic ulcer and gastritis are located in the stomach, so they cannot cause a bowel obstruction. Colitis is inflammation of the colon; inflammation does not cause obstruction.

(4) Fecal impaction may cause bowel obstruction, but gastritis, colitis, and barium will not. A barium enema causes an obstruction only if barium remains in the intestines after the procedure is completed. See rationale 3 for gastritis and colitis. Remember, the entire option must be correct for the option to be the correct answer.

38. ❸ A Miller-Abbott tube is passed through the nose into the colon to remove fluid before surgery for intestinal obstruction.

(1) A nasogastric tube usually is not long enough to reach the large intestine, so it cannot be used to decompress the large bowel, but it may be used to decompress the small intestine to remove fluid above the obstruction. As you probably know, the word *nasogastric* suggests that it is from the nose to the stomach. It will help you to answer the question if you take time to dissect the meaning of words when answering the question.

(2) Keeping a client NPO or administering IV fluids will not decompress the bowel, but these procedures are performed when the patient has a bowel obstruction.

(4) The client is NPO with bowel obstruction.

39. ❹ Neomycin is given before surgery to lower the bacterial count in the intestine, which helps prevent peritonitis after surgery.

(1, 2, 3) These options are incorrect as seen in rationale (4).

40. ❷ Atropine is an anticholinergic drug that decreases oral and respiratory secretion, helping to prevent aspiration during surgery. The patient will also have an increased pulse rate.

(1) Atropine increases heart rate; it does not decrease systolic BP or slow the pulse rate. It causes mydriasis (pupillary dilation).

(3) Atropine increases the pulse rate and causes pupillary dilation.

(4) Atropine does not cause drowsiness; it increases the pulse rate. It does not cause dehydration but does cause dryness of the mouth.

41. ❹ The nurse usually will have a physician order or an agency with an ongoing policy for instillation of 30 mL of normal saline into the nasogastric tube every 4 h; when gastric drainage slows, this instillation helps ensure patency of the tube.

(1) The client has a nasogastric tube in her esophagus, and the tubing is hooked to low Gomco suctioning or wall suction. It would be very difficult to check for a gag reflex (there is no reason to check).

(2) Instilling 3 mL of air into the tube after each irrigation would not ensure patency but would cause the patient to feel bloated from the air pushed into the stomach.

(3) Instilling 60 mL of water into the duodenal port every 4 h is incorrect; there is no duodenal port. Normal saline, not water, must be used to maintain electrolyte balance.

42. ❷ When a patient demonstrates signs of a hemolytic transfusion reaction, the nurse must stop the infusion and start the normal saline that is always hung with the blood. The nurse must notify the physician and be prepared to obtain blood and urine samples because the physician will use these to diagnose whether the patient is having a hemolytic transfusion reaction and the degree of the reaction.

(1) The nurse would not remove the transfusion without the physician's order.

(3) Slowing the transfusion rate is very dangerous when a hemolytic transfusion reaction is suspected because allowing the blood to run even slowly could be fatal.

(4) Insulin would not be ordered for a hemolytic transfusion reaction. An antihypertensive drug may be ordered to combat shock. Remember that when a patient is in shock, regardless of the cause, the patient's BP will be very low and the patient will have a weak thready pulse.

43. ❶ A proximal stoma is irrigated because it is the part of the intestine connected to the stomach. Fecal material will be formed from food and must be excreted through the proximal stoma. A distal stoma is connected to the part of intestine that is not connected to the stomach and is being allowed to rest and heal from an inflammation, such as colitis.

(2, 3, 4) These options are incorrect as seen in rationale (1).

44. ❸ If a patient with a colostomy is incontinent 1 h after irrigation, this is a sign that the bowel has not been sufficiently cleaned and more irrigation fluid is needed to increase fecal excretion.

(1, 2, 4) These options are incorrect as seen in rationale (3).

45. ❷ Electrolytes are lost in gastric suctioning and must be replaced by IV therapy. The physician monitors the patient's blood chemistry to determine the electrolyte solution needed for therapy for this patient.

(1, 3, 4) These options are incorrect as seen in rationale (2).

46. ❷ The patient will not hear what the nurse is teaching until she or he is ready to listen.

(1) The patient may not be receptive to learning about ostomy care for the first few days after surgery because she or he has other problems to cope with (e.g., pain and self-image). During this early stage, the nurse dilates the stoma using two fingers to keep it patent.

(3) The patient may not be ready to participate in stoma care during the first irrigation and, therefore, will not follow the nurse's instructions. The stoma is not used for irrigation until approximately 4 to 5 days after surgery.

(4) Leaving descriptive pamphlets is a very impersonal approach and would not be helpful at this early stage of her learning.

47. ❶ Clients with a hiatal hernia should remain in a sitting position to help prevent the reflux of food and gastric fluid into the esophagus causing ulcers in the esophagus. Gastric contents would have to move upward against gravity.

(2) Bending after eating may cause vomiting because the gastric contents will move into the esophagus.

(3) Sleeping flat allows the gastric contents to move through the cardiac sphincter muscle and into the esophagus. A

hiatal hernia is caused by incomplete closure of the sphincter muscle.

(4) Dumping syndrome is not associated with hiatal hernia. Drinking fluid with meals is allowed with hiatal hernia. Drinking fluid after a partial or total gastrectomy will cause dumping syndrome because the water flushes the fluid rapidly from the stomach into the intestine.

48. ❷ Hepatitis type A, also known as short-incubation hepatitis or infectious hepatitis, is caused by a virus. If given early, standard immunoglobulin (gamma-globulin) vaccine can prevent hepatitis A or decrease the severity of symptoms.

(1) Patients with hepatitis A usually are not admitted to the hospital because the virus does not remain in the blood for a long time. People who are otherwise healthy usually recover from hepatitis A without major problems.

(3) There is no reason for a protein-restricted diet because the liver usually is not damaged with hepatitis A.

(4) The patient usually is not extremely ill but will need some rest, but not bed rest. The disease is short-lived.

49. ❶ Hepatitis type A is highly contagious and spreads from person to person by close contact or by handling of feces-contaminated articles containing hepatitis A. Feces is piped into rivers and streams, and fish eat feces from polluted water.

(2, 3) These options are incorrect as seen in rationale (1).

(4) Ingestion of inadequately processed foods, especially chicken, egg, duck, and turkey, may cause salmonellosis, not hepatitis type A.

50. ❹ Hepatitis B virus vaccine (Recombivax HB) is used to provide active immunization before exposure. Hepatitis B virus is transmitted parenterally through blood and by contact with blood or other body fluids.

(1) The specific treatment for prevention of hepatitis B is Recombivax HB.

(2, 3) Standard immunoglobulin (gamma-globulin) contains antibodies against hepatitis B. However, hepatitis B immunoglobulin (H-BIG) contains much higher levels of antibody. Gamma-globulin is used after a person has come in contact with a person who has hepatitis B. Those who have received Recombivax before coming in contact with someone with hepatitis B do not need immunoglobulin.

51. ❶ Early symptoms of hepatitis include anorexia, nausea, pruritus, vomiting, abdominal pain, diarrhea or constipation, and flulike symptoms. Later symptoms are pruritus (itching), which typically is mild and transient; jaundice, which is first seen in the eyes and mucous membranes; dark urine and clay-colored stools a few days prior to jaundice; and bleeding tendencies related to reduced prothrombin synthesis by the injured hepatic cells. With hepatitis, the liver is larger than normal and is tender on palpation. If damage to the liver is significant, the patient may develop hepatic encephalopathy. Symptoms are irritability and severe drowsiness and then coma. Encephalopathy is caused by failure of the liver to break down ammonia to urea for excretion; ammonia goes to the brain and causes encephalopathy.

(2) Capillary fragility may be a later symptom related to reduced prothrombin. Jaundice, dark urine, and pruritus are late signs of hepatitis.

(3, 4) These options are not related to hepatitis A or B.

52. ❹ The patient would have been exposed to blood and body fluids on a daily basis while working in a hemodialysis unit.

(1) Upper respiratory infections are not related to hepatitis type A or B.

(2) Insect bites are not related to hepatitis A or B.

(3) Eating home-canned foods, even if contaminated, is not related to hepatitis type A or B. Contaminated canned food can cause botulism if it contains the bacteria *Clostridium botulinum*.

53. ❶ Liver enzymes elevated in liver disease include aspartate aminotransferase (AST), formerly known as serum glutamic oxaloacetic transaminase (SGOT); and alanine aminotransferase (ALT), formerly known as serum glutamic pyruvic transaminase (SGPT). Lactate dehydrogenase (LDH) is elevated in liver disease but is also elevated in heart, lung, and kidney disease. Gamma-glutamyl transpeptidase (GGTP) is an enzyme located in the liver and kidney. Elevation of this enzyme along with alkaline phosphatase (ALP) indicates a liver disorder. The enzyme that is located mainly in the liver and confirms liver disease is ALT. A protein metabolism study evaluates total protein, serum albumin, and blood ammonia.

(2) Iron is coupled with the iron-transporting protein transferrin, which is responsible for transporting iron to the lungs for the purpose of hemoglobin synthesis. Therefore, decreased iron will cause iron deficiency anemia. A cystography using injection of radiopaque dye is used to examine the bladder through roentgenography.

(3) Creatinine clearance is a reliable test for estimating glomerular filtration rate (GFR). In renal insufficiency, GFR is decreased, and serum creatinine is increased. As people age, GFR decreases. A fatty cast study is performed to diagnose nephrotic syndrome.

(4) CK-MB and LDH are elevated after a myocardial infarction.

54. ❹ When working with a client who has hepatitis B, it is important to wear gloves when exposed to the patient's blood. Blood is the major mode of transmission.

(1) Serving food on disposable dishes is not necessary; hepatitis B is not transmitted in this manner. Good hand-washing care is always important.

(2) Wearing a face mask is not necessary; hepatitis B is not transmitted by the respiratory route.

(3) Hepatitis A, not hepatitis B, is transmitted by the fecal–oral route.

55. ❶ Bed rest reduces metabolism, reducing the workload on the liver and allowing it to heal, thereby minimizing liver damage.

(2) The heart is not damaged; the liver needs rest.

(3) Bed rest does not control the spread of the disease.

(4) Bed rest does not increase the breakdown of fats.

56. ❸ When the liver is damaged and is unable to convert ammonia (a by-product of protein) to urea, the ammonia goes to the brain and causes hepatic encephalopathy. The first sign of this may be reduced level of consciousness.

(1) The GI tract does not absorb ammonia.

(2) The liver needs to convert ammonia to urea so that it can be excreted by the urine; it does not convert urea to ammonia. If the liver is damaged, it fails to convert ammonia to urea.

(4) If the liver was overloaded with barbiturates, then the liver could not break down any drug. This problem is not related to an overdose of barbiturates. Kidney failure and need for dialysis would be some of the problems.

57. ❷ Cholecystography is performed to detect whether the gallbladder contains stones.

(1) The ampulla of Vater is an opening at the end of the common bile duct in the duodenum.

(3, 4) A cholangiography, not a cholecystography, is used to visualize the common bile duct and cystic duct.

58. ❸ Vitamin K is a fat-soluble vitamin synthesized in the large bowel and is necessary for synthesis of prothrombin in the liver. When bile is not present in the large intestine, fat-soluble vitamins, including vitamin K, are not absorbed.

(1) The intrinsic factor must be present in the stomach for absorption of the vitamin B_{12} necessary for production of red blood cells.

(2) Cholecystokinin is a hormone secreted into the blood by the mucosa of the small intestine.

(4) Prothrombin is a chemical substance that interacts with calcium salts in the liver to produce thrombin. Thrombin is an enzyme necessary for blood clotting.

59. ❸ The T-tube drainage must be measured, emptied, and recorded at the end of each shift. This is a sterile procedure.

(1) A T-tube is not a closed vacuum drainage system. It is a tube that is placed into the common bile duct after a cholangiogram to ensure patency of the common bile duct. The tube exits the patient's abdomen and drains into a small bag.

(2) Bile drainage is expected for 1 to 2 days to 2 to 3 weeks after surgery; the physician will then remove the T-tube.

(4) The T-tube is never irrigated by the nurse.

60. ❸ When the common bile duct is explored, swelling in the duct may cause obstruction; a T-tube is inserted to maintain patency.

(1, 2, 4) These options are incorrect as seen in rationale (3).

61. ❷ Good respiratory care (turn, cough, and deep breath) is very important after a cholecystectomy because the client may breathe very shallowly to decrease incisional pain. Turn, cough, and deep breath prevents stasis of fluid in the lung and allows the patient to cough up sputum.

(1) Good oral care is not a priority after this surgery but is a priority after oral surgery or when the patient has a nasogastric tube in place.

(3) Client is NPO after a laparoscopy for a maximum of 24 h.

(4) After any surgery, a patient is out of bed and ambulating as soon as possible to prevent pneumonia, blood clot formation, and other complications caused by bed rest.

62. ❹ Serum proteins consists of albumin and globulins. Albumin constitutes the largest percentage of total protein value, and a change in the albumin level affects the total protein value. Albumin plays an important role in maintaining serum colloid osmotic pressure within the vascular system. If serum protein is low, fluid will leak out of the vascular system and cause edema (third spacing of fluids). Inability to maintain normal levels of serum albumin is a sign of liver damage.

(1, 2, 3) These options are incorrect as seen in rationale (4).

63. ❶ Ascites is due to a decrease in serum albumin; the osmotic pressure is low, and fluid leaks out of the vascular system and into the peritoneum.

(2, 3, 4) These options are incorrect as seen in rationale (1).

64. ❹ Protein must be restricted because the liver cannot break down ammonia (a by-product of protein) to urea. Ammonia can go to the brain and cause encephalopathy. Protein is broken down to ammonia in the GI tract by bacterial action.

(1, 2, 3) These options are incorrect as seen in rationale (4).

65. ❸ Blood levels of ammonia increase because the liver can no longer remove ammonia from the blood by converting it to urea, which will then be excreted by the kidneys.

(1, 2, 4) These options are incorrect as seen in rationale (3).

66. ❸ The alcohol withdrawal syndrome includes tremors, anorexia, hallucinations, convulsions, delirium tremens, restlessness, diaphoresis, and elevated BP.

(1, 2, 4) These options are incorrect as seen in rationale (3). A patient with alcohol withdrawal would not have seizures, decreased level of consciousness, or blurred vision. It would depend on patient's past history.

67. ❹ Human survival depends on the liver's role in protein metabolism. The primary function of the liver is protein metabolism. Protein is synthesized into urea by the liver and is excreted by the kidney. In severe liver disease, the liver cannot break down ammonia to urea. The ammonia accumulates and goes to the brain, causing hepatic encephalopathy. The liver also synthesizes plasma proteins, such as albumin, prothrombin, fibrinogen, and clotting proteins (factors V, VI, VII, IX, and X). The severely damaged liver fails to adequately synthesize plasma proteins (albumin). Inadequate amounts of albumin result in reduced intravascular osmotic pressure; fluid leaks out of the vascular system and ascites builds up. A severely damaged liver fails to produce adequate clotting factors, which results in bleeding.

(1, 2, 3) These options are incorrect as seen in rationale (4).

68. ❶ A jelly sandwich and a glass of milk have a higher carbohydrate content than the other options.

(2) Eggs and bacon are high in protein.

(3) Raw carrot sticks and a banana are lower in carbohydrates than option 1.

(4) Cottage cheese and a hot dog are high in protein.

69. ❸ Amylase is a pancreatic enzyme that changes starch to sugar. When serum amylase is slightly or moderately elevated, pancreatitis is suspected.

(1) Unconjugated bilirubin, or indirect bilirubin, is related to increased destruction of red blood cells and not to pancreatitis.

(2) Prothrombin is synthesized by the liver. Prothrombin is converted thrombin, which is needed to form blood clots. Prothrombin is not elevated in pancreatitis. (PT measures clotting ability. If PT is prolonged, bleeding occurs.)

(4) The red blood cell count is not elevated in pancreatitis.

70. ❷ Pancreatitis, or inflammation of the pancreas, may be acute or chronic. Men are more often afflicted with acute pancreatitis than are women, possibly because pancreatitis is strongly linked with alcohol use. Assessment reveals severe pain in the upper left quadrant and the epigastric area, with the pain radiating through to the back. Fever, nausea and vomiting, and tachycardia occur. Pancreatitis can be diagnosed by laboratory testing of serum amylase level, which is elevated in pancreatitis. Tachycardia occurs and is caused by pain, fever, and shock.

(1) With acute pancreatitis, the patient may have hypotension. The patient who goes into shock does not have hypertension. The patient does not have bradycardia, but has tachycardia and nausea and vomiting.

(3) Nausea and vomiting may occur with pancreatitis but are not the major problems. Nausea and vomiting occur for many reasons. Bradycardia does not occur; extreme malaise may occur.

(4) The red blood cell count is not elevated, but the white blood cell count is elevated. Malaise occurs in pancreatitis, but hematuria (blood in the urine) does not.

71. ❸ Alcohol is one of the most common causative factors of pancreatitis.

(1, 2, 4) Gold compounds, carbon tetrachloride, and Thorazine do not cause pancreatitis. Other common causes of pancreatitis are cholecystitis with stones, surgery of the biliary tract, viral hepatitis, and ERCP, a diagnostic procedure. Medications, including thiazide diuretics, furosemide, estrogen, tetracycline, and glucocorticoids, can cause pancreatitis.

72. ❸ Repeated water enemas may cause electrolyte problems of bicarbonate and sodium and potassium deficiencies.

(1) Sodium deficit occurs, but it is not the only deficit. The word "only" should alert you that the answer probably is wrong.

(2) Potassium deficit does not usually occur because very little potassium is present in the GI tract and the kidney is the main regulator of potassium. Remember, if there is kidney failure there is hyperkalemia.

(4) Alkalosis results from nasogastric suctioning because hydrochloric acid is being pulled off, not from water enemas. Calcium and folic acid would not be deficient, so the option is incorrect.

73. ❶ A warm water sitz bath increases blood circulation to the anorectal area, relieves pain, and reduces sphincter spasms.

(2, 3, 4) These options are incorrect as seen in rationale (1).

74. ❶ Esophageal achalasia is caused by neuromotor dysfunction of the lower two thirds of the esophagus, causing the sensation of food sticking in the lower portion of the esophagus (called dysphagia) with regurgitation of food.

(2, 3, 4) These options are incorrect as seen in rationale (1).

75. ❶ One of the major symptoms of a hiatal hernia is the feeling of fullness in the lower chest area. A major problem is gastric reflux. Gastric reflux may cause an ulcer in the lower esophagus, which will cause epigastric pain. A hiatal hernia occurs when the esophageal sphincter is enlarged. This enlargement allows regurgitation of small amounts of chyme or gastric juice into the esophagus. Because gastric juice has a high acid content, esophageal ulcers are a common problem. Patients with hiatal hernias must sleep with the head of the bed slightly elevated to prevent regurgitation and vomiting.

(2) There is no feeling of fullness or pain in the lower abdomen or hematuria.

(3) There is no chest pain on exertion or nausea.

(4) There is no abdominal pain on exertion or hematuria.

76. ❷ Barium is not digested. When the water is absorbed, barium solidifies and causes bowel obstruction; therefore, it is important that the patient receive a laxative and cleansing enema after the diagnostic test is completed. It is the nurse's responsibility to see that these orders by the physician are carried out.

(1) Barium is not irritating to the intestinal mucosa.

(3) A client being allergic to barium and barium impaction are not related.

(4) Barium is not given in tablet form the night before; it is given in liquid form during the procedure.

77. ❶ Prilosec, Prevacid, and Nexium all are gastric pump inhibitors that decrease the production of hydrochloric acid in the stomach.

(2) Trimethobenzamide (Tigan) decreases nausea and vomiting. Atropine competitively blocks the effect of acetylcholine at muscarinic cholinergic receptors that mediate the effects of parasympathetic postganglionic impulses, depressing salivary and bronchial secretions, dilating the bronchi, inhibiting vagal influences on the heart, relaxing the GI and genitourinary tracts, inhibiting gastric secretions (high doses), and relaxing the pupil of the eye (mydriatic effect). Carafate is an antiulcer drug that forms an ulcer-adherent complex at duodenal ulcer sites, protecting the ulcer against acid, pepsin, and bile salts, thereby promoting ulcer healing; it also inhibits pepsin activity in gastric juices.

(3) Propantheline (Pro-Banthine), an anticholinergic medication, inhibits gastric acid secretion by blocking the effects of acetylcholine at muscarinic cholinergic receptors that mediate the effects of parasympathetic postganglionic impulses, thus reducing the signs and symptoms of peptic ulcer disease. For information on atropine see rationale 2. Misoprostol (Cytotec) inhibits gastric secretion and increases bicarbonate and mucus production, protecting the lining of the stomach.

(4) Belladonna tincture (Donnatal) is used for spastic colon. It is the drug of choice for diverticulosis. It provides peripheral

anticholinergic/antispasmodic action and mild sedation. Niza-tidine (Axid) inhibits the action of histamine at the histamine H_2 receptors of the parietal cells of the stomach, inhibiting basal gastric acid secretion and gastric acid secretion that is stimulated by food, caffeine, insuline, histamine. Total pepsin output is reduced. Metronidazole (Flagyl) is an antibiotic that inhibits DNA synthesis in specific (obligate) anaerobes, causing cell death. It is used to treat infection with susceptible anaerobic bacteria. It also is used to eradicate *Helicobacter pylori,* a gram-negative bacteria that can colonize in the stomach and duodenum by taking up residence between epithelial cells and mucus barrier that protects the stomach; this organism escapes destruction by acid and pepsin.

78. ❷ Belladonna (Donnatal) is used to treat spastic colon in diseases such as diverticulosis and colitis.

(1) Ranitidine (Zantac) reduces the production of hydrochloric acid in the stomach. Neostigmine (Prostigmin) is a cholinergic anticholinesterase medication used to increase muscle strength in symptomatic treatment of myasthenia gravis; it also is used for the prevention and treatment of postoperative bladder distention and urinary retention or ileus.

(3) Atropine is an anticholinergic drug used to reduce GI and respiratory secretions. Atropine also increases heart rate. For a discussion of propantheline (Pro-Banthine), see answer 77, rationale (3).

(4) Diphenoxylate with atropine (Lomotil) is an antidiarrheal medication.

79. ❸ Neostigmine (Prostigmin) is a cholinergic agent used to increase muscle strength in symptomatic treatment of myasthenia gravis and in prevention and treatment of postoperative bladder distention and urinary retention.

(1) Docusate sodium (Colace) is the laxative stool softener used to prevent constipation in patients who must avoid straining, for example, after myocardial infarction or rectal surgery.

(2) Trimethobenzamide (Tigan) is an antiemetic used in the management of mild to moderate nausea and vomiting.

(3) See answer 78, rationale (1) for a discussion of neostigmine (Prostigmin).

(4) See answer 77, rationale (4) for a discussion of belladonna (Donnatal).

80. ❶ Pernicious anemia may occur when Billroth II surgery is performed because half of the stomach is removed; therefore, most of the intrinsic factor necessary for the absorption of vitamin B_{12} is removed. Vitamin B_{12} is necessary for the production of red blood cells. Dumping syndrome occurs after Billroth II surgery when the patient begins to ingest food and ingested food rapidly enters into the intestines. The food leaves the stomach faster after a partial gastrectomy because the stomach is much smaller and gravity pulls food down into intestine. Fluid should not be ingested with meals because it flushes the food quickly into the intestines, causing dumping syndrome.

(2) The patient may develop diarrhea if dumping syndrome is severe. The patient may develop pernicious anemia; see rationale (1). Anemia is not specific enough to be a correct answer.

(3) Hypotension and bradycardia are not expected problems following Billroth II surgery. Hypotension may occur as a result of dumping syndrome.

(4) Gastric bleeding and hypotension are not expected complications of Billroth II surgery 1 week after surgery. Bleeding after surgery usually is not the right answer. Bleeding seldom occurs after surgery. However, the nurse should always monitor for bleeding after surgery, especially vascular surgery, because bleeding is life threatening when it occurs.

81. ❶ Signs and symptoms of dumping syndrome are faintness, tachycardia, diaphoresis (sweating), and chest palpitations. These signs and symptoms occur after gastric resection because gastric contents empty rapidly into the small intestine, causing hyperglycemia due to the sudden dumping of carbohydrates into the intestine. This sudden dumping of food also causes a shock to the sympathetic nervous system. The patient is advised not to drink fluids with meals because water increases the dumping of food.

(2, 3, 4) These options are incorrect as seen in rationale (1).

82. ❹ Cholangiography allows visualization of the hepatic common bile ducts. Before IV radiographic dye is administered, the patient should be assessed for allergies, especially to iodine. X-ray filming begins a few minutes after the radiographic dye is inserted.

(1) An endoscopy is used to visualize the colon. Enemas until clear are given the evening before this procedure.

(2) Liver scanning is a radionuclide procedure used to outline and detect structural changes of the liver. No fasting or premedication is required for this procedure. The patient is exposed to small amounts of radiation, as only a tracer dose of isotope is used.

(3) Oral cholecystography is used to visualize stones in the gallbladder or cystic duct. The evening before examination, the patient ingests a radiopaque dye that contains iodine. The patient must be assessed for iodine allergies before and during the procedure. This procedure is seldom used anymore because more effective diagnostic procedures are available (e.g., ultrasonography).

83. ❹ The Whipple procedure, or pancreaticoduodenectomy, is used to treat pancreatic cancer. It involves resection of the pancreatic head, duodenum, distal stomach, and distal part of the common bile duct.

(1) Billroth I surgery removes a portion of the stomach that contains acid-secreting cells and is anastomosed to the duodenum.

(2) Billroth II removes a portion of the stomach containing hydrochloric acid-secreting cells; the remaining portion of the stomach is anastomosed to the jejunum.

(3) Total gastric resection, removal of the entire stomach, is also called a Billroth III.

84. ❸ Milk, antacids, and cheese cannot be included in the diet of a patient taking tetracycline; these foods interfere with absorption of tetracycline. Tetracycline is given to eliminate any pathogenic organism that might be associated with ulcerative colitis.

(1, 2, 4) These options are incorrect as seen in rationale (3).

85. **②** Fat-soluble vitamins A, D, E, and K are not absorbed without bile. Bile is needed for the breakdown of fats, and fat is necessary for the absorption of fat-soluble vitamins.

(1, 3, 4) These options are incorrect as seen in rationale (2).

86. **④** ERCP is a procedure that uses a fiberoptic endoscope for radiographic visualization of the bile and pancreatic ducts. This is especially useful in jaundiced patients. Stones, cysts, ampullary stenosis, and malignant tumors can be identified. Only ERCP and percutaneous transhepatic cholangiography (PTHC) can provide direct visualization of the biliary and pancreatic ducts. PTHC is an invasive procedure with significant potential for complications (disease). ERCP, on the other hand, is associated with much fewer complications but must be performed by an experienced endoscopist. ERCP is performed using a fiberoptic endoscope passed down through the esophagus into the duodenum and then into the ducts. In PTHC, a needle is passed through the liver and into an intrahepatic bile duct. The biliary system can be directly injected with iodinated x-ray contrast dye (radiopaque). The biliary ducts and the gallbladder can be visualized and studied for obstruction by stones, structures, and malignant tumors.

(1) Hepatobiliary scintigraphy is a nuclear scan used for evaluating patients suspected of having gallbladder disease. It does not visualize the pancreatic duct.

(2) Cholangiography, an x-ray procedure using contrast dye, provides visualization of the hepatic duct and common bile duct; it does not visualize the pancreatic duct.

(3) PTHC is explained in rationale (4).

87. **①** Anemia caused by folic acid deficiency usually occurs as the result of malnutrition and alcoholism-induced cirrhosis. Alcohol inhibits folic acid metabolism; malnutrition may also result from lack of folic acid intake. Foods high in folic acid include liver, soybeans, asparagus, green beans, brussel sprouts, and cabbage.

(2) Sickle cell disease is a congenital hemolytic anemia that occurs primarily in African-Americans. Sickle cell anemia results from defective hemoglobin molecules (hemoglobin S) that cause red blood cells to become sickle shaped. Such cells have impaired oxygen-carrying capacity and cell lysis (cell destruction), resulting in chronic ill health (fatigue, dyspnea on exertion, swollen joints), long-term complications, and premature death. Fifty percent of patients with sickle cell disease die by their early 20s; few live to middle age. Pernicious anemia is discussed in answer 80, rationale (1). Rheumatic heart disease is a systemic inflammatory disease of childhood, often recurrent, that follows a group A beta-hemolytic streptococcal infection. Rheumatic heart disease refers to the cardiac manifestation of rheumatic fever, and includes myocarditis, pericarditis, and endocarditis during the early acute phase and later chronic valvular disease. Most clients complain of joint pain, accompanied with swelling and redness; joints commonly affected are knees, ankles, elbows,

and hips. Long-term antibiotic therapy can minimize the recurrence of rheumatic fever, reducing severe valvular deformity.

(3) Idiopathic thrombocytopenia purpura is an autoimmune disorder. Thrombocytopenia is characterized by platelet destruction and may be acute or chronic. Because platelets play a vital role in coagulation, this disease poses a serious threat to hemostasis. Disseminated intravascular coagulation (DIC) occurs as a complication of disease and conditions that accelerate clotting, causing small blood vessel occlusion, organ necrosis, and depletion of circulating clotting factors and platelets. DIC results from infection such as septicemia, obstetric complications, extensive burns, trauma, and surgery. It is not clear why such disorders lead to DIC. See Chapter 3.

(4) Cystic fibrosis is a generalized dysfunction of the exocrine glands affecting multiple organ systems in varying degrees of severity. It is the most common fatal genetic disease of Caucasian children. See Chapter 9.

88. **①** The hazards of a cholangiopancreatography may include bile leakage leading to peritonitis and bleeding caused by accidental rupture of a blood vessel. Although these problems seldom occur, assessment for them must be a priority.

(2, 3, 4) If bleeding occurs, the patient would develop tachycardia as a compensatory mechanism for hypotension, but it is only part of the assessment. Always look for the most global answer. Allergic reaction to the dye usually occurs during administration of the dye.

89. **②** The most consistent finding associated with the aging process is a decrease in liver enzymes needed for drug metabolism and detoxification. Smaller doses of all drugs are recommended for elderly patients. Drug interactions and cumulative drug effects occur with higher frequency in the elderly.

(1) An abnormal liver function test is not associated with aging.

(3) Cholesterol production may decrease with aging, as do almost all functions of the body.

(4) Hypotension, not hypertension, usually is associated with aging. The heart becomes smaller and the force of cardiac muscle contraction is reduced.

90. **②** The major symptoms of paralytic ileus are decreased or absent bowel sounds (due to decreased peristalsis), abdominal distention, vomiting, or increased nasogastric drainage if a nasogastric tube is in the stomach.

(1, 3, 4) These options are not related to a paralytic ileus.

91. **③** Bleeding from esophageal varices is a major, life-threatening complication of portal hypertension. The most common manifestation of ruptured esophageal varices is hematemesis, with rapid development of hemorrhagic shock and severely compromised blood flow to vital organs. The patient has tachycardia, severe hypotension, and melena (black, tarry feces).

(1) Anorexia and nausea can indicate a variety of disorders.

(2) Weight gain is not specific; it could be 1 lb. A decrease in urine output is not specific; it may be a decrease of only 100 mL over 12 h.

(4) An increase in abdominal girth may indicate ascites or abdominal distention. It is not related to esophageal bleeding.

92. ❹ Observe the patient for sudden respiratory distress, which occurs if the gastric balloon ruptures and the entire tube moves upward. Gasping, dyspnea, and cyanosis will be evident. If this occurs, immediately cut all balloon lumens. A pair of scissors must be kept at the patient's bedside at all times.

(1) The patient cannot and should not drink fluid if the balloon is in the esophagus.

(2) Balloons are not deflated until the physician is ready to take the Sengstaken-Blakemore tube out of the patient's esophagus.

(3) The tube cannot be repositioned with balloons inflated.

93. ❸ A continent ileostomy (Kock's pouch) is an intraabdominal reservoir made from the terminal ileum, which stores the ileal contents until the pouch is drained. The stoma site is usually the right lower quadrant above the pubic line. Because the pouch is continent (inside the abdomen), no external appliance has to be worn. The pouch gradually expands until it can hold 8 to 12 h of accumulated fecal material. This helps improve the patient's quality of life and allows emptying of the pouch when convenient, thus offering more control. This pouch cannot be used in patients with Crohn's disease because the disease destroys the pouch.

(1, 2, 4) These options are incorrect as seen in rationale (3).

94. ❸ Appendixes can rupture and cause peritonitis. When peritonitis is a potential problem, monitor the patient's pain. Report severe, well-localized abdominal pain, especially if it is experienced as a sudden change from the previous pain pattern. Signs and symptoms of peritonitis must be reported to the physician immediately.

(1) A temperature of 100°F is not unusual with appendicitis.

(2) A white blood cell count of 10,000/mm^3 is a normal leukocyte level.

(4) Nausea and vomiting are not unusual with appendicitis.

95. ❸ No cathartics or enemas are given because the resultant stimulation of peristalsis irritates the already inflamed area and can precipitate perforation. Normally before intestinal surgery, the intestine is cleaned out with cathartics and enemas; in this case, however, the danger of perforation of appendicitis outweighs the benefits of a clean intestine.

(1) Client is kept NPO because surgery will be performed immediately if a diagnosis of appendicitis is made.

(2) Analgesics are not given until the decision to operate is made because they may mask symptoms needed for differential diagnosis.

(4) An ice pack may be used on the abdomen prior to diagnosis to reduce pain because analgesics usually are not administered.

96. ❷ It would be most important to question the patient with Crohn's disease about diarrhea, determining the number of stools per day, their color, consistency, and odor. Ask specifically whether any blood has been seen in the stool.

(1) Nutritional intake is an important factor for a patient with Crohn's disease, but the percentage of meals eaten is only one factor in determining nutritional status.

(3, 4) These options are not related to Crohn's disease.

97. ❶ As a result of changes in the mucosa, the absorption of sodium bicarbonate and water is impaired, leading to watery diarrhea and potential acidosis.

(2) Ulcerative colitis would not affect the platelet count.

(3) The white blood cell count may be elevated due to inflammation and possible infection, but it is not as important as monitoring bicarbonate level.

(4) Ulcerative colitis may affect the hemoglobin level as a result of chronic GI bleeding, which may lead to iron deficiency anemia. Blood is lost and iron is poorly absorbed. The nurse needs to monitor the hemoglobin level, but it is not as important as monitoring the bicarbonate level.

98. ❹ Maintain the patient on bed rest during severe exacerbations to decrease peristalsis. Place a deodorizer in the room, and empty the bedpan immediately to control disagreeable and embarrassing odor.

(1, 2, 3) In the acute phase of Crohn's disease, the patient is NPO and is on bed rest to allow the intestine to heal. If the patient has diarrhea, stool softeners are not needed.

99. ❷ Symptoms of ulcerative colitis may develop gradually or have a sudden, acute onset, which sometimes follows a stressful event, minor infection, or even antibiotic therapy. The most frequent symptoms are rectal bleeding, diarrhea, abdominal pain, weight loss, and fever.

(1) Chronic blood loss from ulcerative colitis does not decrease cardiac output.

(3) The patient has chronic diarrhea and so is not constipated.

(4) Although patients have abdominal pain, they can move in bed and can cough, deep breathe, and get out of bed. Patients who have undergone abdominal or chest surgery cannot get out of bed for the first day after surgery; they usually will not turn, cough, and deep breathe as often because of incisional pain and may develop pneumonia. Note, however, that is not what the question asked.

100. ❸ Postural drainage and percussion are necessary to remove tenacious secretions from the lungs. This procedure should be done approximately 3 h after eating; this allows time for the food to be digested and eliminated from the stomach so that vomiting does not occur.

(1) If performed immediately after breakfast, it may cause the patient to vomit the breakfast meal.

(2) One hour after eating is too soon to perform postural drainage; the food will still be in the stomach, and vomiting may occur.

(4) Eight hours after eating would be before breakfast, and postural drainage would leave a bad taste in the patient's mouth. It is also a tiring procedure, so the patient may not feel like eating breakfast.

15 Cardiovascular and Peripheral Vascular Disorders

A. Cardiac Cycle

1. Systolic Pressure (Afterload)

   a. Systolic pressure is determined by the forces of ventricular contractions.

   b. Systolic pressure results when the heart contracts and forces unoxygenated blood out of the right ventricle, through the pulmonary artery (PA), and to the lungs, and forces oxygenated blood out of the left ventricle, through the aorta, and to the rest of the body.

2. Diastolic Pressure (Preload)

   a. Diastolic pressure results when the blood vessels and capillaries force oxygenated blood back from the lungs, through the pulmonary veins, and into the left atrium.

   b. The unoxygenated blood returns from other parts of the body, through the superior and inferior venae cavae, and into the right atrium.

   c. The blood from the atria then immediately flows into the ventricles for the systolic phase.

3. Cardiac Output

   a. Cardiac output is the amount of blood that the left ventricle pumps into the aorta (500 mL, or 5 qt/min).

   b. Output can be increased by increasing stroke volume and fluid volume and by decreasing afterload.

4. Drugs Used to Increase Cardiac Output

   a. Cardiac glycosides (e.g., digoxin) increase the force of contractions and push more blood out of the heart (stroke volume).

   b. Epinephrine and atropine increase heart rate stroke volume and, thus, increase cardiac output.

   c. Alpha-adrenergic blockers decrease peripheral vascular resistance (afterload) by causing vasodilation and blocking the effect of norepinephrine.

   d. Catapres, Aldomet, Minipress, Hytrin, Vasotec, Regitine, and Nipride will decrease afterload (systolic pressure) and preload (diastolic pressure).

5. Sympathetic Nervous System: Chemical Regulation

   a. The sympathetic nervous system activates the chemical activities of catecholamines (epinephrine, norepinephrine, and dopamine), which act as neurotransmitters in the body.

   b. Each of these hormones has a different purpose in the body.

   c. Most of the hormones are stored in the adrenal medulla, which is located on the kidney.

   d. Epinephrine.

   (1) This increases the heart rate and dilates the bronchioles because epinephrine attaches to beta receptors in the heart and in the bronchioles (Fig. 15–2).

   (2) Beta-blocking drugs, such as Inderal, block epinephrine, which slows the heart rate and causes bronchial constrictions (Fig. 15–3).

   e. Norepinephrine.

   (1) Norepinephrine causes peripheral vasoconstriction because norepinephrine attaches to alpha receptors in the peripheral vascular system (Fig. 15–4).

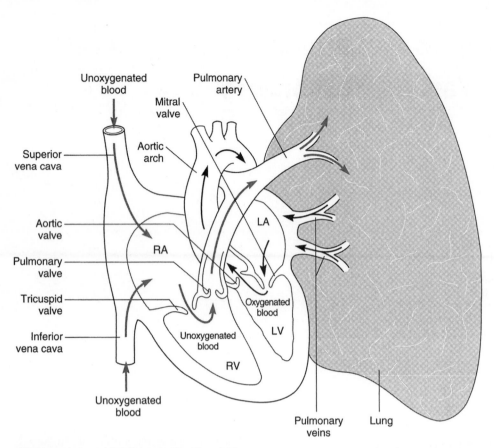

FIGURE 15–1 ◆ Cardiovascular Circulation

When the right side of the heart fails, blood backs into the peripheral vascular system because there are no valves on the superior or inferior vena cava. When the left side of the heart fails, blood backs into the lungs because there are no valves on pulmonary veins.

(2) Alpha-adrenergic blocking agents, such as Catapres, cause peripheral vasodilation because they block norepinephrine (Fig. 15–4).

f. Dopamine.

(1) Dopamine is used for neural transmission in the brain.

(2) It also causes vasoconstriction in the peripheral vascular system because dopamine receptors are in these locations (Fig. 15–5).

(3) A deficiency of dopamine causes Parkinson's disease.

II. PHYSIOLOGIC SHOCK

A. Types of Shock

1. Anaphylactic Shock

a. Gross vasodilation is caused by a severe allergic reaction (e.g., an allergic reaction to penicillin), which may be fatal, or by a spinal cord injury.

b. This results in a relative state of hypovolemia. Total fluid volume remains the same, but it is not moving within the vascular system due to a lack of vascular tone, decreased venous return to the heart, and decreased cardiac output.

c. Signs and symptoms of anaphylactic shock usually appear within minutes to 2 h of exposure to the drug or bee sting. Generally, the earlier the reaction, the worse it will be. The skin is almost always involved. A patient is likely to first complain of itching. Your exam often will reveal redness, swelling, and hives. As the reaction progresses, the hives may converge, so do not be deceived if the skin appears red without defined wheals. Angioedema and bronchospasm—swelling of the face and mucous membranes of the mouth and upper airway—are serious signs that may indicate impending airway blockage. Patients may complain of tightness or a "lump" in the throat, or they may try to clear their throats repeatedly. Their voice may become hoarse from laryngeal edema, and they may cough frequently. In severe cases, you may hear stridor—a late and ominous sign of upper airway obstruction.

d. Treatment consists of epinephrine, antihistamines, corticosteroids, and bed rest.

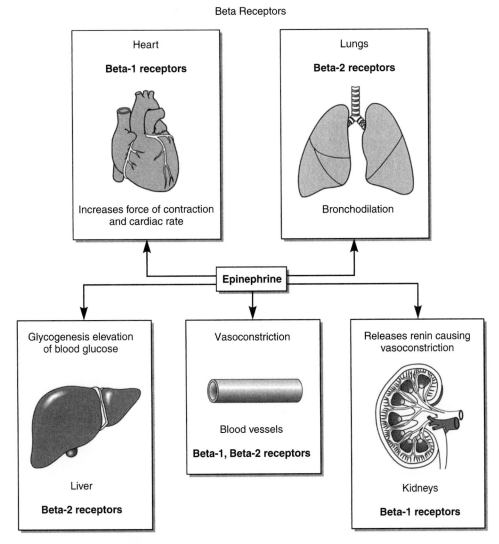

Beta Receptors

FIGURE 15–2 ◆ Beta Receptors

Epinephrine increases the heart rate and dilates the bronchioles because it attaches to beta receptors in the heart and lungs. Epinephrine also vasoconstricts blood vessels because it attaches to beta receptors in the blood vessels. It stimulates the release of renin angiotensin and causes vasoconstriction because it attaches to beta receptors in the kidney.

2. Hypovolemic Shock

a. Hypovolemic shock is caused by a severe decrease in oral fluid intake or significant fluid losses. Hypovolemic shock usually results from acute blood loss.

b. Treat promptly with adequate blood and fluid replacement to restore intravascular volume and raise blood pressure.

c. Ringer's lactate solution, along with plasma proteins (albumin) or other plasma expanders, may produce adequate volume expansion until whole blood can be matched.

d. Application of medical antishock trousers (MAST) may be helpful. These are body intermittent compression trousers used to counteract bleeding and hypovolemia by slowing or stopping arterial bleeding, forcing any available blood from the lower body to the heart, brain, and other vital organs.

3. Cardiogenic Shock

a. Any condition that causes severe dysfunction of the left ventricle, such as myocardial infarction (MI) or severe congestive heart failure (CHF), will cause cardiogenic shock.

b. Cardiogenic shock is discussed in this chapter (p. 166, 167).

4. Septic Shock

a. Bacteria or toxins in the blood will cause gross vasodilation.

b. Septicemia (sepsis) is an infection of the blood that can lead to a life-threatening condition called *septic shock.*

B. Nursing Implications

1. Signs and Symptoms

a. Cool moist skin, pallor, rapid breathing, and cyanosis of the lips, gum, and tongue.

Beta Blockers

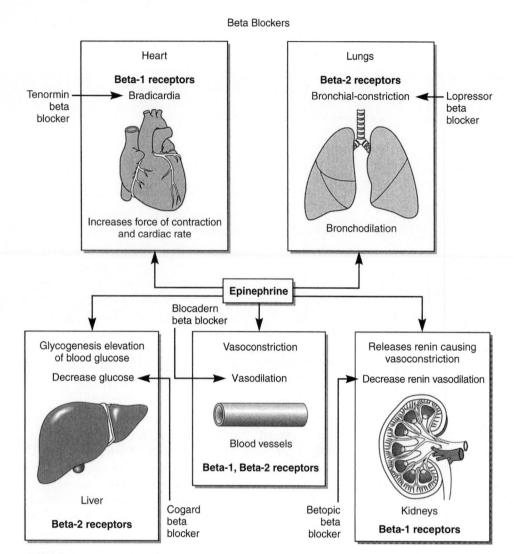

FIGURE 15–3 ◆ Beta Blockers

For example, Inderal blocks epinephrine, slowing the heart rate; causes bronchial constriction; decreases blood glucose, resulting in hypoglycemia; and causes vasodilation and a decrease in renin angiotensin, resulting in further vasodilation.

b. Rapid, weak, thready pulse, decreasing pulse pressure, and low blood pressure.

c. The heart cannot adequately perfuse itself in severe shock; thus, angina pain will occur.

d. The kidney is not adequately perfused; therefore, urine will be concentrated.

2. Treatment

a. Limit activities and monitor condition.

b. Monitor vital signs and hemodynamic changes.

c. Evaluate the effects of therapy.

d. Provide emergency equipment and intervention as indicated by the type of shock.

e. Inform the patient and family of the cause of the shock and the treatment to be administered.

f. Acquire laboratory data, especially the complete blood count (CBC) and electrolytes.

3. Assessment for Shock
Check the following:

a. Blood pressure, pulse, temperature, and respiration.

b. Arterial blood gases.

(1) Perform the Allen test to assess the collateral circulation before performing an arterial puncture on radial artery.

(2) To perform the Allen test, make the patient's hand blanch by obliterating both the radial and the ulnar pulses, then release the pressure over the ulnar artery only.

(3) If flow through the ulnar artery is good, flushing will be seen immediately.

(4) The Allen test then is positive, and the radial artery can be used for puncture.

(5) If the Allen test is negative (no flushing), repeat the test on the other arm.

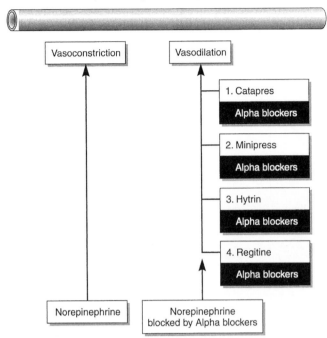

Blood vessel

Alpha-1 receptors and alpha blockers

Vasoconstriction

Vasodilation

1. Catapres
   Alpha blockers

2. Minipress
   Alpha blockers

3. Hytrin
   Alpha blockers

4. Regitine
   Alpha blockers

Norepinephrine

Norepinephrine blocked by Alpha blockers

FIGURE 15–4 ◆ Norepinephrine

Norepinephrine causes peripheral vasoconstriction by attaching to alpha-1 receptors in blood vessels. Alpha-adrenergic blocking agents (e.g., Catapres) cause peripheral vasodilation by blocking norepinephrine.

(**6**) If both arms give a negative result, choose another artery for puncture (e.g., femoral).

(**7**) Note that the Allen test ensures collateral circulation to the hand if thrombosis of the radial artery should follow the puncture.

(**8**) After drawing 3 to 5 mL of blood, remove needle and apply pressure to the arterial site for 3 to 5 min (10–15 min if the patient is on heparin).

c. Central venous pressure (CVP), pulmonary arterial pressure (PAP), pulmonary capillary wedge pressure (PCWP), and cardiac output, if appropriate vascular lines are in place.

d. Oral intake and urinary output.

III. CAUSES OF CONGESTIVE HEART FAILURE

A. Hypertension

1. Etiology

a. Early detection of hypertension is very important—it is a silent killer.

b. Hypertension is sustained elevated systolic blood pressure greater than 140 mm Hg and diastolic pressure greater than 90 mm Hg over at least a 3-day period.

c. Risk factors for essential primary hypertension are family history, race (most common in African-Americans), obesity, stress, high intake of saturated fat or sodium, use of oral contraceptives or tobacco, and aging.

2. Pathophysiology with Signs and Symptoms

a. When a patient has hypertension, the peripheral vascular system is constricted, which forces the left ventricle of the heart to work harder to get blood into the peripheral system.

b. Cardiac output and peripheral vascular resistance determine blood volume, stroke volume, and cardiac rate.

c. Peripheral vascular resistance may raise blood pressure, and the degree to which it is raised depends on many factors.

d. The heart muscle becomes stronger in the early stages of hypertension, but as the disease progresses, the ventricle hypertrophies, becomes ineffective, and fails as a pump.

e. When blood is not effectively pumped out of the left ventricle, it returns to the lungs, causing CHF.

f. Primary hypertension constitutes 90 to 95 percent of all cases of hypertension and is the leading cause of death and disability in adults. The cause is unknown.

g. Primary hypertension, a chronic elevation in blood pressure, occurs without evidence of any other disease process. Primary hypertension has no single known causative etiology, but the following risk factors have been identified: family history of hypertension, race (more common in blacks), stress, obesity, use of tobacco, oral contraceptives, sedentary lifestyle, high dietary intake of salt and saturated fats, and aging.

h. Secondary hypertension may result from renal vascular disease, primary hyperaldosteronism, Cushing's syndrome, hyperthyroidism, coarctation of the aorta, pregnancy, neurologic disorders, and pheochromocytoma (tumor on the adrenal gland).

i. Cardiac output and peripheral vascular resistance determine blood pressure.

3. Interventions

a. Monitor the patient's vital signs while the patient is lying, sitting, and standing.

b. Encourage the patient to rest frequently throughout the day to prevent fatigue and strain on the heart.

c. Instruct the patient to stop activity if it initiates episodes of chest pain or aggravated chest discomfort or causes dizziness indicating possible cardiac problems.

d. Use electrocardiogram (ECG) monitoring, especially if the patient experiences arrhythmias.

e. Review the results of laboratory studies and hemodynamic monitoring.

f. Check the patient's intake and output, observing for adequacy and balance.

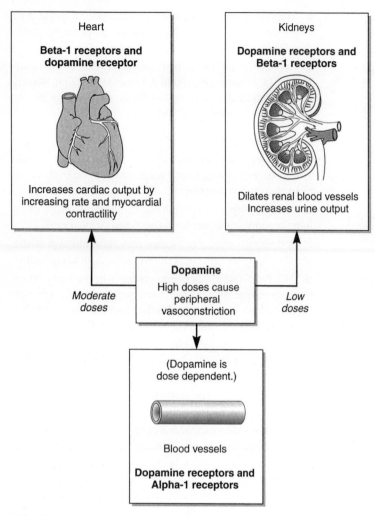

FIGURE 15–5 ◆

Relationship between dopamine and the heart, kidneys, and peripheral vascular system.

g. Educate the patient about foods high in sodium (e.g., milk, canned vegetables, soup, bacon, catsup, pickles).

h. Educate the patient about foods high in cholesterol (e.g., meat, eggs, cheese).

i. Instruct the patient on relaxation techniques and range of motion procedures to increase circulation while sitting or lying in bed.

4. Nursing Implications

a. Modification in diet and lifestyle may control hypertension.

b. Lifestyle and diet changes may include weight loss, restriction of sodium and saturated fat intake, relaxation techniques, regular exercise, avoiding smoking, and reducing or avoiding alcohol consumption.

c. Drug therapy usually begins with a diuretic if needed

   (1) Beta-adrenergic blockers (e.g., Inderal, Corgard), alpha-adrenergic blockers (e.g., Catapres, Aldomet),

angiotensin-converting enzyme (ACE) inhibitors, or other vasodilators are used as needed.

   (2) Therapy may also include calcium blockers (e.g., Cardizem, Procardia).

d. Treatment of secondary hypertension includes correcting the underlying cause and controlling the hypertensive effects. Secondary hypertension may be caused by, for example, renal stenosis, pregnancy, or prolonged administration of steroids or estrogen.

e. Assess the blood pressure while patient is lying, sitting, and standing, taking the measurements in both arms to determine the baseline and note any difference bilaterally.

f. Assess and palpate for edema in the extremities.

g. Auscultate for arrhythmias, tachycardia, and abnormal breath sounds that may indicate cardiac involvement.

h. Assess the patient's level of knowledge, stressors, and risk factors, such as smoking, obesity, and lack of exercise.

i. Determine if the patient is taking birth control pills, diet pills, amphetamines, cold medications, or alcohol that may be associated with hypertension.

j. Check the patient's family history for hypertension, other cardiovascular diseases, and diabetes.

k. Review the patient's dietary pattern: check caloric levels and the amount of fat, cholesterol, and sodium regularly consumed.

B. Myocardial Infarction

1. Contributing Factors

a. Family history of MI

b. Hypertension

c. Smoking or chewing tobacco

d. High-fat, high-cholesterol diet

e. Diabetes mellitus

f. Stress

g. Aging

h. Sedimentary lifestyle

i. Estrogen therapy

j. High salt intake

k. Overweight

2. Etiology and Incidence

a. Atherosclerosis builds up in the coronary arteries, and a blood clot develops in the same area and occludes the artery.

b. Severe angina that will not respond to treatment.

c. In the United States, approximately 1.5 million MIs occur each year and can cause CHF.

3. Diagnostic Procedures

a. Cardiac Enzymes

(1) Creatine kinase (CK) is an enzyme specific to cells of the brain, myocardium, and skeletal muscles. In an acute MI, inadequate oxygen is delivered to the myocardium, causing cell injury and the release of cardiac enzymes.

(2) The primary myocardium enzyme is CK, which is released from the myocardial muscles (CK-MB).

(3) Other cardiac specific enzymes are lactic acid dehydrogenases (LDH). If the serum concentration of LDH1 is higher than concentration of LDH2, the pattern is said to have flipped, signifying myocardial necrosis.

(4) Elevation of CK-MB may occur within 4 to 6 h and peaks 18 to 24 h after an acute MI.

(5) Eighty percent of individuals demonstrate elevated LDH1 within 48 h after MI.

(6) Of particular importance is the fact that up to a threefold elevation of CK-MB may follow an intramuscular injection; intramuscular injections should be avoided when treating a suspected MI.

(7) Blood for cardiac enzymes typically is drawn every 8 h for the first 24 h and followed daily for 3 days.

b. Cardiac Troponin

(1) A test made available in 1997 allows doctors to accurately diagnose mild heart attacks that might otherwise go undetected.

(2) The test measures two forms of cardiac troponin, which is a protein that is released into the bloodstream by dying heart cells.

(3) In mild heart attacks, CK-MB levels sometimes do not rise above the amount typically seen in the bloodstream of healthy people.

c. Cardiac Catheterization

(1) A procedure that allows study of the heart, great blood vessels, and coronary arteries.

(2) A catheter is passed into the heart through a peripheral vein or artery, depending on whether catheterization of the right or left side of the heart is being performed.

(3) Several weeks past infarct, the ECG will show a depressed T wave.

(4) Angina can cause ST-segment flattening and T-wave inversion.

4. Signs and Symptoms of MI

a. Intense, crushing, substernal pain of longer duration than angina pain. MI pain is not relieved with nitroglycerin nor with rest.

b. The pain may radiate to the left arm or jaw, with a feeling of a heavy weight on the chest, faintness (syncope), palpitations, and sweating (diaphoresis).

c. Hypotension and shock may occur.

5. Treatment

a. Give morphine for pain to reduce anxiety because pain causes the release of catecholamines, and catecholamines cause vasoconstriction that will increase the workload of the heart.

b. Lasix is not given after an MI unless there is fluid retention, which will occur if the heart fails as a pump.

c. Do not give digoxin in the first few weeks after an MI because the heart muscle is damaged, and forcing it to contract will cause more damage and arrhythmias.

d. Lidocaine is given to prevent or correct ventricle arrhythmias. Beta-blocking agents and calcium blockers also may be used to reduce the effects of epinephrine on the heart, allowing the heart to rest and heal.

e. Patient is NPO (nothing by mouth), IV KVO (keep vein open).

f. Give streptokinase, urokinase, or tissue plasminogen activator (t-PA) to dissolve clots, and give heparin to prevent clots. The greatest benefits occur when treatment is initiated within 6 h of symptoms.

g. Bed rest

(1) Have urinal or bedpan at bedside to decrease anxiety. Remember, anxiety will increase the release of catecholamines.

(2) For bowel movements, patient may use bedside commode, which is less stressful than using a bedpan.

h. Give stool softeners to avoid Valsalva movement (holding breath against a closed epiglottis and then releasing breath).

(1) This causes a large amount of blood to return to the heart at one time.

(2) Valsalva movement may occur when patients strain to have bowel movement or when lifting themselves with the hands and arms in bed, which drastically and suddenly perfuses the heart with blood and may cause cardiac arrhythmias.

i. No rectal temperatures are taken because the vagus nerve is in this area, and vagal stimulation may cause bradycardia or asystole (cardiac standstill). Remember, the vagus nerve slows the heart.

6. Nursing Implications

a. Immediately assess the patient for pain, determining duration, severity, and radiation.

b. Monitor the patient's ECG pattern.

c. Check the patient's respiratory status and cardiac rhythm.

d. Assess the patient's anxiety.

e. Monitor electrolytes, especially potassium.

f. Explain the medications and procedures used.

g. Provide a calm, quiet environment and comfort measures to ensure effectiveness of pain medications.

h. Teach the patient to use relaxation techniques for pain reduction and anxiety relief.

i. Check vital signs prior to administering medications.

j. Administer supplemental oxygen as needed.

k. Accept, but do not reinforce, the use of denial.

l. Treat life-threatening arrhythmias immediately.

m. Provide a bedside commode to decrease expenditure of energy that is required when ambulating to the bathroom or using a bedpan.

n. Allow the patient time to rest between treatments, and limit visitors and extra activity in the room.

o. Explain the diagnostic studies completed and the need for any follow-up studies after discharge.

p. Include the family in any of the teaching sessions when applicable.

q. Instruct the patient about medications, such as aspirin, beta blockers, and dietary modifications needed to reduce the risk of another MI in preparation for discharge from the hospital.

C. Coronary Artery Disease

1. Etiology and Incidence of Angina

a. Angina is the constriction of the coronary arteries causing ischemia, which produces pain.

b. Myocardial oxygen demands are increased by emotional stress, physical activity, smoking tobacco, eating, and exposure to cold weather.

c. Spontaneous angina occurs suddenly with no known cause. It can cause MI, which may lead to CHF.

d. As long as the coronary arteries can vasodilate, the increased blood supply needed for additional demands can be met; however, coronary arteriosclerosis (hardening and loss of elasticity of the wall of arteries) prevents adequate coronary vasodilation.

e. Atherosclerosis (accumulation of lipids in the media of the artery) also occludes the coronary arteries and prevents adequate perfusion of the heart.

f. This disease is near epidemic in the western world and is more common in men than in women and in the middle-aged and elderly.

2. Signs and Symptoms of Angina

a. Chest pain lasts from 2 to 5 min and occasionally from 5 to 15 min. It is relieved with rest in stable angina.

b. For unstable angina, the pain is not relieved, and hospitalization may be necessary.

c. The patient may complain of indigestion, tightness and heaviness in chest, sensation of strangling, and burning-type of pain.

d. Pain may radiate to left shoulder, down the inner side of the left arm, and to the jaw, tongue, or hard palate. The patient describes the pain as burning, pressing, choking, and aching.

e. The patient may complain of "gas" pain or "heartburn" or indigestion; the pain is not described as sharp, knifelike, or crushing pain, as described with an MI.

f. Unstable angina can lead to MI and then CHF.

g. Laser is used to stop stubborn angina pain.

(1) In the operation, a laser is used to bore 20 to 40 or more pencil lead-sized holes into the ventricle of the heart, creating routs for oxygenated blood to get to oxygen-deprived areas of the heart.

(2) This procedure relieves ischemia and, therefore, pain.

(3) The surgery is done on a beating heart by reaching through small incisions made under the left breast.

(4) It is an endoscopic procedure.

3. Treatment of Angina

a. With severe unstable angina, the patient must be hospitalized with prescribed bed rest.

b. Percutaneous transluminal coronary angioplasty (PTCA) may be performed during cardiac catheterization to compress fatty deposits and relieve occlusion in the coronary arteries.

c. Therapy consists primarily of nitroglycerin (given sublingually, PO, transdermally) or amyl nitrite (a nasal mist for acute angina), beta-adrenergic blockers (PO or IV), or calcium channel blockers (PO or IV).

d. Because coronary artery disease is so widespread, prevention is very important.

    (1) Dietary restrictions are aimed at reducing intake of calories (in obesity), cholesterol, salt, and fats.

    (2) Lifestyle changes include regular exercise, abstention from smoking tobacco, and reduction of stress.

4. Nursing Implications for Angina

    a. Ask patient to describe the chest pain in terms of location, intensity, duration, severity, and radiation.

    b. Check vital signs.

    c. Determine precipitating factors and relief method.

    d. Determine if patient is taking antiarrhythmic agents.

    e. Place patient at rest immediately upon the onset of chest pain.

    f. Administer oxygen and nitroglycerin or other prescribed medication, if available.

    g. Notify physician if pain is unrelieved.

    h. Document patient's description of pain.

    i. Monitor the patient's vital signs.

    j. Instruct the patient about pain relief measures and the use of the prescribed medications.

D. Mitral Valve Disorders May Cause CHF

1. Etiology and Incidence

    a. Prolapse or stenosis of the mitral valve can lead to arrhythmias and CHF.

    b. Mitral valve disorders are most common in women; most women older than 40 years have some degree of mitral valve prolapse.

    c. Prolapse of the mitral valve will cause blood to flow constantly from the atrium to the ventricle.

        (1) Prolapse occurs as the heart contracts, making the heart work harder and causing hypertrophy of the left ventricle.

        (2) It may cause arrhythmias or CHF.

    d. Stenosis of mitral valve causes hypertrophy of the left atrium and can lead to CHF.

        (1) When the mitral valve is stenosed, it is difficult for the left atrium to force the blood down through the mitral valve into the left ventricle.

        (2) The large amount of blood that remains in the left atrium backs into the lungs and cause CHF.

e. Rheumatic fever is a systemic inflammatory disease of childhood, which follows a group beta-hemolytic streptococcal infection of the nasopharynx.

    (1) Rheumatic heart disease refers to the cardiac manifestations of rheumatic fever and includes myocarditis, pericarditis, and endocarditis.

    (2) It can result in acute phase and chronic valvular disease.

    (3) Rheumatic fever has declined dramatically in the United States.

    (4) In many parts of the world, rheumatic heart disease is still the leading cause of death from heart disease in the 5- to 24-year age group.

f. Mitral valve prolapse is more common in women, with a peak incidence in the fourth decade.

g. Familial occurrence has been well established.

2. Signs and Symptoms of Mitral Valve Insufficiency

    a. Dyspnea, fatigue, angina, and palpitations.

    b. Tachycardia, moist rales, and pulmonary edema.

    c. Auscultation reveals a systolic murmur at apex.

    d. Mitral valve insufficiency may cause CHF.

3. Treatment of Mitral Valve Disorders

    a. Depends on the nature and severity of associated symptoms.

    b. Treatment includes anticoagulant therapy (heparin or Coumadin) to prevent thrombus formation around the diseased area or replaced mitral valve.

    c. Prophylactic antibiotics are used before and after surgery or dental care.

    d. Surgical treatment may include mitral valve replacement or open mitral valve commissurotomy during which the heart is surgically opened and the valve cleaned to remove vegetation. Cardiac arrhythmias may occur from this procedure.

    e. Closed mitral valve commissurotomy.

        (1) A small incision is made in the heart, and the physician uses a finger to clean out vegetation in the mitral valve.

        (2) Cardiac arrhythmias may occur from this procedure.

    f. Percutaneous mitral balloon valvuloplasty.

        (1) Involves passing a catheter into the left side of the heart through the femoral artery to the ascending aorta, through the aortic valve into the left atrium, and into the mitral valve.

        (2) The balloon is then inflated several times to enlarge the mitral valve.

        (3) Potential complications include ventricular arrhythmias and thrombus formation.

4. Nursing Implications for Mitral Valve Disorders

   a. Assess for dyspnea, weakness, fatigue, episodes of syncope, cough, and tachycardia.

   b. Check vital signs frequently.

   c. Review for history of rheumatic fever, streptococcal infections, or congenital heart problems that involve the valves.

   d. Auscultate the heart sounds, listening for a murmur.

   e. Assess the skin for paleness or cyanosis.

   f. Check the ECG for abnormal patterns in rate or rhythm.

   g. Instruct patient about dietary modifications needed to reduce risk of complications.

   h. Explain the effects and clinical cause of cardiac valve disease and the potential complications.

   i. Allow time for questions from the patient and family.

   j. Teach the patient to participate in a moderate exercise program to increase cardiac perfusion.

   k. If patient is to undergo surgery, explain preoperative and postoperative course.

   l. Teach the client the importance of taking anticoagulant medication as ordered by the physician, if the client has mitral valve disorder or a mitral valve replacement, and that the client will take this medication every day for the rest of his or her life.

   m. Evaluate any special discharge needs of the patient and family.

E. Cardiac Arrhythmias May Cause CHF

1. Etiology and Incidence

   a. Cardiac arrhythmias are disturbances in rate, rhythm, or conduction of the heart's electrical impulses and are the most common complication of MI. Acute ventricular arrhythmias can lead to CHF.

   b. Approximately 90 percent of all patients with acute MI exhibit arrhythmias of one type or another.

   c. Arrhythmias can lead to severe hemodynamic impairment, such as hypotension, MI, CHF, and shock.

   d. Causes of cardiac arrhythmias include myocardial ischemia and injury to the heart muscle, abnormal electrical conduction, hypertrophy of muscle fiber from hypertension, valvular heart disease, toxic doses of cardiac drugs (e.g., digoxin), degeneration of conductive tissue necessary to maintain normal heart rhythm (sick sinus node), and electrolyte imbalance (e.g., hypokalemia or hyperkalemia).

   e. Arrhythmias are among the most frequently encountered complications in patients with heart disease.

F. ECG Use for Diagnosing Arrhythmias

1. The ECG is a recording of the electrical activity in the heart through the electrodes on the skin.

   a. An ECG can be recorded on paper as a permanent record or visualized on a monitor.

   b. Each heartbeat produces a wave on the screen or paper.

   c. Cardiac waves are named P, Q, R, S, and T and represent specific action within the heart.

2. Normal ECG Waves

   a. P wave: shows depolarization of the atria.

   b. QRS complex: represents depolarization and contraction of the ventricles.

   c. T wave: indicates repolarization of the ventricles, the most vulnerable period of the heart cycle.

   d. PR interval: time the impulse takes to travel through the atria to the atrioventricular (AV) node, bundle of His, bundle branches, and ventricles.

   e. Intervals between these waveforms reflect the time an impulse takes to travel through the heart.

   f. Identification of rhythms, normal or abnormal, requires a careful systematic approach to interpretation.

   g. Determine the origin of cardiac impulse: sinus node, AV node, or foci (small pacemakers) in the atrial or in the ventricles.

   h. Determine whether or not the P waves are present, which will tell you if the impulse is coming from the sinus node (pacemaker).

   i. Calculate atrial (P waves) and ventricular (QRS complexes) rates.

   j. Always check the QRS complex. The QRS complex represents ventricular contraction and ventricular depolarization.

3. Abnormal ECG Waves

   a. ST segments and the T wave are elevated with an acute inferior MI.

   b. The T wave is depressed or inverted in old MI.

   c. Digitalis depresses ST segments and makes them sag (looks like an old MI).

     (1) Large doses can decrease the T-wave amplitude, causing sinus bradycardia (rate <50).

     (2) Large doses prolong the PR interval and can cause atrial, junctional, ventricular (bigeminy), and conduction abnormalities.

   d. Hypokalemia depresses T waves, and the ST segment is prolonged.

   e. Hyperkalemia depresses the ST segment, and T waves are narrow and peaked.

4. Types of Cardiac Arrhythmias

   a. Etiology

     (1) In *ventricular tachycardia,* the rate is greater than 100 bpm and usually is 140 to 250 bpm.

     (2) The rhythm is regular or slightly irregular.

     (3) P waves may be present but not associated with QRS complexes.

     (4) Ventricular tachycardia may result from a premature ventricular contraction (PVC) striking during the heart's vulnerable period.

(5) Conditions that lead to the occurrence of arrhythmias include hypoxemia, electrolyte imbalance, fever, emotional and physical stress, hyperthyroidism, caffeine, epinephrine, and atropine.

b. *Ventricular fibrillation* presents no recognizable QRS complexes.

(1) There is no cardiac output, and there is an absence of a pulse.

(2) Ventricular standstill can be distinguished from ventricular fibrillation only by ECG.

c. Ventricular fibrillation is caused by myocardial damage (e.g., MI), hypoxia, and contact with high-voltage electricity, electrolyte imbalance, and drug toxicity (e.g., digitalis or quinidine).

d. *PVCs* have wide QRS complexes not associated with the P wave.

(1) Other than those of the sinus node, PVCs are the most common of all arrhythmias.

(2) They are caused by irritable foci in the ventricle.

e. A ventricular impulse forms before the next expected impulse from the sinoatrial (SA) node and takes the place of the normal beat. PVCs result from hypoxia, hypokalemia, hyperkalemia, acidosis, toxic agents (e.g., digitalis, antidepressants), exercise, and intracardiac catheterization.

f. *Premature atrial contractions* (PACs) have an early P wave present (may merge into previous T waves). The QRS usually is normal and has a rapid heart rate that usually is greater than 150 bpm.

g. PACs are associated with stress, fatigue, alcohol, coronary artery disease, cardiac ischemia, heart failure, medications (e.g., digitalis, quinidine), pulmonary congestion, and pulmonary hypertension.

h. *Atrial fibrillations* are rapid irregular waves greater than 350 bpm.

(1) *Ventricular* rates vary but may increase to 150 bpm.

(2) The causes of atrial fibrillation include CHF, cor pulmonale, and organic heart disease.

i. *Atrial flutter* differs from atrial fibrillation in that it is an accelerated rhythm resulting from rapid firing of an ectopic atrial foci.

j. The hallmark of atrial flutter is the presence of a *sawtooth pattern* of rapid atrial activity producing a rate of 250 to 350 bpm.

(1) It is associated with coronary atherosclerotic heart disease, pulmonary embolism, and mitral valve disease.

(2) Cardioversion is highly successful in converting atrial flutter to sinus rhythm.

k. In *second-degree AV block* (Wenckebach), the PR interval progressively lengthens until the P wave is not followed by the QRS complex.

(1) Any drugs that slow AV conduction may cause a type I block, but these often are transient and reversible.

(2) Second-degree AV blocks are associated with acute anterior MI.

l. In *complete third-degree AV block,* there will be atrial flutter (rate 300 per minute) and a regular ventral rate of 33 per minute.

m. The AV node has become the pacemaker for the heart.

n. If the pacemaker was ventricular foci, the rate probably would not be regular.

o. *No* impulse from the sinus node can pass through the AV node.

p. Atria and ventricles beat independently.

q. The P waves have no relation to the QRS complexes.

r. Ventricular rate may be as low as 20 to 40 bpm.

s. QRS complex may be widened.

t. AV block is seen most often in acute anterior MI.

u. In bundle branch block, conduction is impaired in one of the bundle branches; thus, the ventricles do not polarize simultaneously.

v. In bundle branch block, the abnormal conduction pathway through the ventricles causes a wide and notched QRS complex.

w. The defect may result from inflammation, myocardial fibrosis, MI, or congenital anomalies.

5. Signs and Symptoms of Arrhythmias

a. Palpitations, dizziness, lightheadedness, chest pain, and syncope.

b. Skin, pallor, and diaphoresis.

c. Ectopic beats, tachycardia, bradycardia, and irregular rhythm.

d. Hypotension.

6. Treatment of Cardiac Arrhythmias

a. Give beta blockers, such as Inderal and Lopressor, which are used to slow the influence of epinephrine, thereby reducing cardiac oxygen consumption.

b. Lidocaine is the drug of choice for ventricular arrhythmias.

c. Digoxin is the drug of choice for atrial arrhythmias.

d. Give calcium blockers (e.g., verapamil, diltiazem).

e. Cardioversion using a defibrillator is the treatment of choice for any tachycardia causing severe hemodynamic impairment.

(1) Cardioversion is an elective procedure in which the physician delivers an electrical current to the heart to terminate a life-threatening arrhythmia.

(2) The electrical current causes the heart to stop momentarily and completely depolarize at the very moment of shock, which allows the sinus node to regain pacing control of the heart.

(3) The electrical discharge is synchronized by the physician or triggered by the patient's QRS complex (if ECG is computer driven) for the avoidance of accidental discharge during the ventricular repolarization phase (T wave).

(4) The T-wave phase of the cardiac cycle is highly vulnerable to the development of ventricular fibrillation.

(5) Cardioversion can terminate potentially dangerous or exhausting arrhythmias that have been refractory to pharmacologic intervention.

(6) A QRS complex must be present for successful conversion of the arrhythmia.

(7) The patient must sign an informed consent and then the intervention is scheduled. As with all informed consents, the patient must receive a full explanation of the benefits and dangers of the procedure from the physician.

(8) If the patient has been taking digitalis or a beta-blocking agent, the physician will withhold the drugs for 2 days before the procedure because drugs may predispose the patient to the development of ventricular arrhythmias during cardioversion.

(9) Hypokalemia or hyperkalemia increase the risk of lethal arrhythmias.

f. Defibrillation

(1) An emergency procedure in which the nurse or physician delivers an electrical current to the heart to terminate a life-threatening arrhythmia.

(2) Defibrillation delivers an electrical current (shock) of a preset voltage to the heart through paddles placed on the chest wall.

(3) Defibrillation is always indicated in ventricular fibrillation.

(4) It is also used in ventricular tachycardia when the patient is unconscious and pulseless.

(5) No QRS complex is present during ventricular fibrillation, so there is no need for electrical discharge to be synchronized.

(6) Defibrillation is also used after a patient has suffered an MI (if unconscious) to restore heartbeat.

7. Nursing Implications for Arrhythmias

a. Review patient's medical history and diagnostic data for the type of arrhythmia being exhibited.

b. Assess for unexplained fatigue and weakness.

c. Check vital signs and ECG monitoring.

d. Check circulation and urinary output.

e. Observe for signs of respiratory distress.

f. Assess for symptoms of palpitations, dizziness, lightheadedness, chest pain, and syncope.

g. Assess arterial pulse for ectopic beats, tachycardia, bradycardia, and rhythm.

h. Check skin for pallor and diaphoresis.

i. Assess for hypotension and mental status.

j. Explain the arrhythmia and treatment plan.

k. Allow patient to verbalize and ask questions.

l. Teach patient relaxation techniques.

m. Administer beta blockers, calcium blockers, and other antiarrhythmic agents as ordered by the physician.

n. Assist with cardioversion or defibrillation procedure if needed.

G. Pacemakers Used to Control Potentially Dangerous Arrhythmias

1. Etiology

a. The artificial pacemaker has become a leading modality in the control of potentially dangerous arrhythmias.

b. Pacemakers may be temporary or permanent.

c. Permanent pacing is used when the condition is recurrent or persistent.

d. The artificial pacing system consists of a battery-powered generator and a pacing wire that delivers the stimulus to the heart to control heart rate.

e. The pacing unit initiates and maintains the heart rate when the natural pacemakers of the heart are unable to maintain adequate circulation.

f. The lithium batteries used in most pacemakers last 6 years or more.

g. When the batteries fail, they must be replaced surgically.

2. Types of Pacemakers

a. There are two basic modes of artificial pacing: fixed rate and demand mode.

(1) In the *fixed-rate mode,* the pacemaker fires electrical stimuli at a preset rate regardless of the person's inherent rhythm.

(2) Because of the hazards of a pacing stimulus falling within the vulnerable period, the fixed rate is rarely used today.

(3) The *demand* or *standby mode* has an electrode at the tip of the pacing wire, which is able to sense the person's own heartbeats.

(4) The pacemaker produces a stimulus only when the person's own heart rate drops below the rate per minute preset on the generator by the physician.

(5) The *synchronous mode* is also a demand form of pacing but of a particular type. It uses two electrodes: a sensing device in the atrium and a stimulating electrode in the ventricle. The atrial sensing electrode perceives the patient's own atrial depolarization, waits for a present interval (stimulates the PR interval), and then triggers the ventricular pacemaker to fire. Normal cardiac sequence is best simulated when atrial activity and ventricular activity are synchronized. As a safety feature, should a rapid atrial rhythm occur that exceeds a certain rate limit, the ventricular pacemaker fires independently at a fixed rate.

b. *Universal, physiologic,* or *dual-chamber pacemakers* are the most sophisticated pacemakers available.

c. They consist of both atrial and ventricular circuits that sense and pace their respective chambers.

d. If spontaneous atrial activity does not occur, the atrium is paced.

e. Any sensed atrial activity inhibits the pacing function.

f. If ventricular depolarization does not occur in the preset time limit, the ventricle is paced.

g. The advantage of this mode of pacemaker is that it most closely mimics the normal heart.

h. Atrial kick occurs, which increases cardiac output by 30 percent.

   (1) The heart rate can be changed to meet metabolic demands.

   (2) The major risk of this mode of pacing is the development of pacemaker-induced tachycardia.

i. If a skeletal muscle activity is sensed, a ventricular beat may be triggered.

j. Temporary pacing may be used in emergency or elective situations that require limited, short-term pacing (under 2 weeks), but in this form of pacing, the pulse generator is external.

k. For temporary pacing, the pacer wire usually is passed transversely to the right atrium or ventricle.

   (1) The procedure usually is performed in a special procedure room using fluoroscopy or at the bedside.

   (2) The wires connect externally to a generator.

l. An implantable cardioverter-defibrillator (ICD) may be placed in patients who are chronically experiencing recurring symptoms of ventricular tachycardia or ventricular fibrillation.

   (1) More recent ICDs are capable of distinguishing ventricular tachycardia from ventricular fibrillation, thus delivering shocks only when absolutely necessary.

   (2) More recent ICDs are capable of pacing to treat ventricular tachycardia without resorting to cardioversion shocks unless necessary.

   (3) They are capable of providing backup for bradycardia and eliminating the need for a standard pacemaker.

   (4) They are capable of storing cardiac events so the data can be retrieved and the patient's response to treatment analyzed.

   (5) Batteries last 3 to 5 years.

   (6) When an ICD is placed (either through an epicardial or endocardial route), the device must be programmed and tested using electrophysiologic studies.

   (7) In essence, ventricular fibrillation is intentionally induced in a controlled environment.

   (8) The ICD is set to deliver shocks at the rate necessary to convert the ventricular fibrillation to a sinus rhythm.

   (9) If an epicardial route is selected, open heart surgery is necessary for placement.

      (a) Doctors are able to perform diagnostic checks by holding a wand over the chest where the device is implanted and reading images sent to a computer.

      (b) The device itself keeps a record of pacing and defibrillation activity, so with a few computer keystrokes, the physician can change settings if needed.

   (10) If the ICD is malfunctioning, it may be necessary to deactivate the device by applying a doughnut-shaped magnet over the ICD. Reapplying the magnet for 30 seconds will turn the device on again.

   (11) Deactivation should not be performed without a physician's order.

   (12) If the ICD is malfunctioning or if the heart is not responding to the delivered shocks, life support measures should be initiated.

   (13) During CPR, the rescuer may feel a mild shock if the device fires.

   (14) Education regarding the ICD for a patient who receives the device is extensive.

      (a) Patients must understand the difference between a heart attack and cardiac arrest.

      (b) The ICD will not prevent an MI (heart attack), but it will help prevent cardiac arrest.

      (c) Patients should be taught that the ICD is capable of pacing, cardioverting, and defibrillating (unless the device is an older model).

      (d) Patients should be taught to keep a diary of shocks received, activities before and after treatment, symptoms, and response after shock.

      (e) Patients should contact their physician when they receive a shock.

3. Complications of Pacemaker Insertion

   a. Pacemaker complications can occur from insertion.

   b. Complications include phlebitis at the site, pneumothorax, atelectasis, pericardial fluid accumulation, and arrhythmias.

   c. Complications can occur from malfunctioning of the pacemaker, for example, battery failure, oversensing or undersensing by the pacemaker, and lead displacement due to migration.

4. Complications of Pacemaker Therapy

a. Local infection or hematoma formation may occur at the venous cutdown site.

(1) With a permanent pacemaker, local infection at the suture line or sepsis may occur.

(2) The patient is monitored daily for any signs of inflammation or infection.

b. The pacemaker wire and electrode can irritate the ventricular wall and cause arrhythmias.

c. The most common causes of pacemaker failure are *displacement of the pacing wire electrode* and *battery failure;* both of these situations require minor surgery to repair them.

d. Special telephone monitoring of the patient's ECG may be performed occasionally on an outpatient basis, which provides information regarding the pacemaker and can determine battery weakness and failure.

5. Nursing Implications for a Patient with a Pacemaker

a. Assess pacemaker battery.

b. Assess ECG.

c. Check insertion site suture line for phlebitis, infection, and hematoma.

d. Teach patient to avoid electrical machinery that is not properly grounded.

e. Educate patient on how to check pacemaker battery function by using of a special phone.

f. Instruct patient on how to take vital signs.

g. Instruct patient to notify physician of palpitations, dizziness, or lightheadedness.

h. Instruct patient to carry a pacemaker identity card along with programming information.

H. Dilated Cardiomyopathy: A Common Cause of CHF

1. Etiology

a. The cause is unknown.

b. It occurs most frequently in multiparous women over age 30 years, particularly those with malnutrition or preeclampsia.

c. Predisposing factors include alcohol abuse, high blood pressure, infections, and pregnancy.

d. If associated with pregnancy, it may disappear.

e. Dilated cardiomyopathy probably is the most common cardiomyopathy, and it leads to CHF.

f. It is characterized by gross dilation of the heart with interference in systolic function.

g. Unlike hypertropic cardiomyopathy, in which ventricular filling is impaired, dilated cardiomyopathy is characterized by impaired systolic ejection function.

2. Signs and Symptoms

a. The most common symptom of the disease is dyspnea caused by elevated left ventricular end-diastolic pressure.

b. Angina, fatigue, and syncope are common symptoms.

c. CHF may occur but is less common.

I. Restrictive Cardiomyopathy: A Common Cause of CHF

1. Etiology and Incidence

a. The cause is unknown.

b. Filling of the ventricles is restricted because the ventricular walls are excessively rigid and impede ventricular filling.

c. Myocardial contractility usually is unaffected.

d. Fibrotic infiltration into the myocardium causes the ventricles to lose their ability to stretch.

e. Eventually the heart fails as a pump, and CHF occurs.

f. It occurs most often in young adults.

2. Signs and Symptoms

a. The earliest clinical finding in restrictive cardiomyopathy is exertional dyspnea that progresses to nocturnal dyspnea.

b. Ventricular dysfunction leads to pulmonary and systemic congestion and diminished perfusion.

c. A history of angina is common.

3. Treatment

a. For dilated and restrictive cardiomyopathies, the therapeutic goals and management are the same as for CHF.

b. Control of arrhythmias with antiarrhythmic drugs or pacemaker therapy to control life-threatening arrhythmias.

c. Heart transplant may be necessary.

d. Cardiomyopathy is not a systemic disease, so patients would be candidates for heart transplant.

4. Nursing Implications

a. Assessment and interventions are the same as for CHF.

b. These are discussed in this chapter on pp. 157–159.

J. Cardiogenic Shock (Pump Failure): A Common Cause of CHF

1. Etiology

a. Cardiogenic shock (pump failure) occurs when the heart can no longer pump blood efficiently to all parts of the body.

b. When CHF occurs, most patients die within 24 h of onset.

c. It reflects severe left ventricular failure and occurs as a serious complication in nearly 15 percent of all patients hospitalized with acute MI.

2. Sign and Symptoms

a. One of the most reliable signs of early compensatory shock is the patient's level of consciousness. Insidious changes in sensorium, usually in the form of restlessness, irritability, or apprehension, are frequently observed and are primarily due to hypoxia of brain cells.

b. The heart rate in early shock is slightly increased.

c. The pulse may be thready.

d. Respiration increases in rate and depth in an attempt to compensate for tissue hypoxia.

e. When the blood pressure begins to fall, the patient is no longer in early shock. Regardless of previous normal blood pressure, a *systolic pressure below 80 mm Hg* should be regarded as a danger signal.

f. Tachycardia is evident during this stage of shock, and the pulse is weak and thready.

g. Late or irreversible shock is the stage during which compensatory mechanisms is totally ineffective.

(1) Cellular necrosis and multiple organ failure occur.

(2) Attempts to restore the blood pressure fail, and death is imminent.

(3) The patient's skin is cold and clammy.

3. Treatment

a. Fluid replacement usually is the first therapeutic measure to be instituted, and it may include whole blood or volume expanders (e.g., dextran, Plasmanate, albumin).

b. The following medications may be given:

(1) Dobutamine (Dobutrex) increases myocardial contractibility without inducing marked tachycardia.

(2) Dopamine (Intropin) in large doses causes peripheral vasoconstriction and in low doses increases renal perfusion.

(3) Nitroprusside (Nipride) causes vasodilation (venous and arterial). This is used to increase venous return to the heart.

c. Increase oxygen intake and an intraaortic balloon pump (IABP) are used to reduce workload on the heart.

IV. OTHER CAUSES OF CHF

A. Atherosclerosis

1. Plaque buildup in arteries.

2. This is discussed with Peripheral Vascular in this chapter on p. 177.

B. Arteriosclerosis

1. Hardening of the arteries

2. This is discussed with Peripheral Vascular in this chapter on p. 177.

C. Rheumatic Fever

1. Caused by beta-hemolytic streptococci, which may damage the mitral valve, if early diagnoses is not made.

2. May lead to CHF.

3. This is discussed on p. 161.

D. Endocarditis or Pericarditis

1. Inflammation of the endocardium or pericardium may cause heart failure.

E. Myocarditis

1. Inflammation of the cardiac muscle.

2. Hyperthyroidism may cause myocarditis and cardiac failure.

F. Cardiac Tamponade

1. Acute compression of the heart.

2. Results from blood or fluid collection in the pericardial sac (i.e., from penetrating chest wound)

G. Digitalis Toxicity

1. Administration of excessive digitalis when the patient is hypokalemic can cause digitalis toxicity.

2. Do not give digoxin if apical pulse rate is below 60, because this may be a sign of digitalis toxicity.

3. Severe bradycardia can lead to CHF.

4. Dilantin and lidocaine are useful for treating digoxin-induced dysrhythmias.

H. Pericardial Effusion

1. Fluid in the pericardial sac and pulse paradoxus are signs of pericardial effusion.

2. Blood pressure is low on inspiration, and the heart sounds are difficult to hear.

3. Pericardial effusion can lead to CHF.

I. Syphilis

1. Syphilis can play an important role in the development of aortic disorders.

2. The patient may have aortic insufficiency or an aortic aneurysm, which can lead to CHF.

V. CONGESTIVE HEART FAILURE

A. Pathophysiology

1. Compensatory Mechanisms

a. When the heart fails as a pump, it cannot perfuse the kidney.

b. When the kidney is not perfused, it releases renin and aldosterone.

c. Aldosterone retains sodium (Na), which retains water, and this increases the amount of fluid saved.

d. Osmotic pressure is increased by the rising sodium concentration, leading to release of antidiuretic hormone (ADH).

e. ADH increases renal tubular reabsorption of water.

f. Renin is a powerful vasoconstrictor that causes hypertension and increases the workload of the heart.

g. The three mechanisms of compensation that enable the weakened heart to continue to meet the metabolic demands of the body are tachycardia, ventricular dilation, and hypertrophy of the myocardium.

2. Direct Causes of Left and Right Ventricular Failure

a. Although CHF may be acute as a result of MI, it is generally a chronic disorder that may develop into acute CHF.

b. Acute pulmonary edema is a medical emergency arising from severe left ventricular failure, and it usually results from prolonged strain on a diseased heart.

c. Hypertension is the major cause of left-sided heart failure.

d. Right-sided failure (cor pulmonale) usually is caused by left-sided heart failure (CHF).

    (1) This causes venous congestion in the systemic circulation, which results in peripheral edema, hepatomegaly, and splenomegaly.

e. The primary cause of right-sided failure is left-sided failure.

    (1) In this situation, left-sided failure results in pulmonary congestion and increases pressure in the blood vessels of the lung (pulmonary hypertension).

    (2) Eventually pulmonary hypertension results in right-sided failure.

f. Other causes of cor pulmonale include chronic obstructive pulmonary disease (COPD) and pulmonary emboli.

g. Emphysema (COPD) will cause the right ventricle to work harder to force blood into the lungs, which have bronchoconstriction and congestion.

B. Incidence

1. The American Heart Association estimates that between 2.3 and 3 million Americans have CHF and are alive.

2. Annually, 37,371 patients die of CHF.

C. Acute Heart Failure

1. Signs and Symptoms

  a. Patients with left-sided heart failure

    (1) Extreme breathing difficulty (dyspnea).

    (2) Lungs are fluid filled (coarse crackles).

    (3) The patient needs to sit in high Fowler's position and may need to lean over bedside table in order to breathe.

    (4) Patient may have extreme hypertension in acute CHF (e.g., blood pressure 200/100).

    (5) Respirations are rapid and noisy (audible wheeze, crackles).

    (6) Cough is productive of frothy, blood-tinged sputum.

    (7) Cyanosis, with cold clammy skin.

    (8) Tachycardia and arrhythmias.

  b. Patients with right-sided heart failure

    (1) A patient with advanced right-sided heart failure (cor pulmonale) will have coarse crackles after the left side of heart begins to fail.

    (2) Peripheral edema will develop, and jugular vein distention and hypertrophy of the right ventricle will occur.

    (3) Distended neck veins can be seen when a patient with right-sided failure is in a semirecumbent position and is due to increased pressure in the right atrium.

2. Diagnosis of CHF

  a. Arterial blood gas (ABG) studies are taken before oxygen is administered to obtain baseline.

  b. The ECG small electrodes are placed on the surface of the chest and extremities. A resting ECG helps to identify primary conduction abnormalities, cardiac arrhythmias, site and extent of MI, pacemaker performance, and effectiveness of cardiac drug therapy.

  c. The most commonly used PA flow-directed catheter is the Swan-Ganz, which has at least four lumens.

    (1) The proximal lumen terminates in the right atrium, allowing CVP measurement, fluid infusion, and venous access for blood samples.

    (2) The distal lumen terminates in the PA and measures PA pressure, PA diastolic pressure, mean pulmonary arterial pressure (PAP), and PCWP.

    (3) There is a small lumen used for the inflation and deflation of the balloon, but the balloon should be inflated only after it is in place and used to obtain PCWP readings.

  d. A Swan-Ganz catheter may be used to assess hemodynamic status (Fig. 15–6).

    (1) CVP reflects the pressure within the superior vena cava, which reflects the pressure under which the blood is returned to the superior and inferior venae cavae and the right atrium.

    (2) CVP is determined by vascular tone, blood volume, and the ability of the right side of the heart to receive and pump blood.

    (3) CVP also can be seen as a measure of preload on the right side of the heart (diastolic).

    (4) Preload refers to the filling of the ventricles just before ventricular contraction and reflects the load or stretch placed on the ventricles (systolic).

    (5) Normal CVP is 2 to 6 mm Hg.

    (6) A drop in CVP pressure indicates a decrease in circulating volume, which may result from hemorrhage or severe vasodilation and pooling of blood in the extremities with limited venous return.

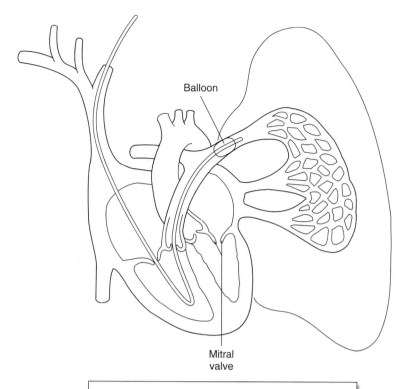

Pulmonary Artery and Pulmonary Wedge Pressures

1. PCWP 18 to 30 mm Hg—Left side of the heart
2. PS-Systolic 4 to 12 mm Hg
3. PA-Diastolic 1 to 10 mm Hg
4. CVP 2 to 6 mm Hg
5. CVP 2 to 12 H_2O—Right side of the heart

FIGURE 15–6 ◆

Swan–Ganz catheter is used to determine left and right heart failure and other hemodynamic problems.

(7) A rise in CVP indicates an increase in blood volume due to a sudden shift in fluid balance, excessive intervenous fluid infusion, renal failure, or sodium and water retention as seen in CHF.

(8) PAP indicates the peak pressure generated by the right ventricle.

(9) PCWP is a direct indicator of left ventricular pressure.

(10) Elevations in PCWP greater than 18 to 30 mm Hg indicate increased left ventricular pressure as seen in left ventricular failure and may indicate the onset of pulmonary edema and CHF (Fig. 15–6).

(11) PAP that climbs to more than 30 mm Hg generally heralds the onset of pulmonary edema and CHF.

(12) A low PCWP suggests insufficient blood volume and pressure in the left ventricle as seen in hypovolemic shock.

(13) Hemodynamic monitoring using the Swan-Ganz catheter allows for continuous monitoring of systolic, diastolic, and mean blood pressure pulse.

(a) It also allows assessment of the arterial pulse.

(b) It allows access for arterial blood sampling (ABGs), CVP, PCWP, cardiac output, and stroke volume.

3. Treatment

a. Administering oxygen in high concentrations by Venturi mask will give the most accurate amount of oxygen, and the rebreathing mask delivers the most oxygen.

b. Insert IV and Foley catheters.

c. Provide nasotracheal suction as needed.

d. Rotating tourniquets are put on all four extremities, which rotate and shut on and off on the extremities each time they rotate automatically, reducing the workload of the heart by pooling blood in the periphery.

e. A phlebotomy may be performed in case of acute CHF to draw blood from the patient because fluid overload overworks the heart and causes even further cardiac damage and decompensation.

f. Nothing by mouth (NPO) and bed rest for patients with acute CHF.

g. A temporary pacemaker may be needed during the acute phase of CHF.

   (1) Pacemakers are discussed in this chapter on pp. 164–166.

h. Bed rest, fluid restriction, NPO, IV KVO for medications in acute cases.

i. To correct the complications of CHF, the surgeon may use the IABP.

   (1) The IABP is a counterpulsation device that supports the failing heart by increasing coronary artery perfusion and reducing afterload.

   (2) The IABP consists of a sausage-shaped balloon catheter that is passed through the femoral artery and positioned in the descending thoracic aorta.

      (a) This catheter is attached to a power console, and the balloon is inflated during diastole.

      (b) Blood is pushed back into the aorta, and coronary artery perfusion is improved.

      (c) The balloon is deflated during systole.

      (d) Resistance is decreased, thereby reducing the workload of the heart (Fig. 15–6).

   (3) Timing of balloon inflation and deflation are critical so a registered nurse (RN) with specific education on use of the balloon pump is assigned to care for this patient.

j. Another intervention that provides mechanical support to the heart is the ventricular assist device (VAD), which is designed to assume a portion of the ventricular work by moving some blood from the heart to a pump and through the body.

   (1) The devices are used to support a failing left ventricle (left ventricular assist device [LVAD]), right ventricle (right ventricular assist device [RVAD]), or both ventricles (biventricular assist device [BVAD]).

   (2) Complications are common in patients with a VAD. The most common complication is formation of thrombi.

   (3) This leads to pulmonary emboli, stroke, MI, and thrombophlebitis. Clots tend to develop even with heparin therapy.

   (4) A VAD is considered to be only temporary therapy to sustain life for patients with severe cardiac failure or until a heart transplant is available.

4. Medications Most Commonly Used for Acute and Chronic CHF

a. Digitalis (Lanoxin) is very effective in increasing the force of the contraction; thus, it increases cardiac output and increases urinary output by increasing kidney perfusion.

b. Furosemide (Lasix) is a diuretic that mobilizes edematous fluid and reduces pulmonary venous pressure.

   (1) When excess vascular volume is excreted, blood volume returning to the heart is reduced and cardiac workload is decreased.

   (2) Diuretics act on the kidney by promoting excretion of sodium and water.

   (3) Thiazide diuretics usually are the first choices because of their safety and effectiveness.

   (4) Two potent diuretics are furosemide (Lasix) and ethacrynic acid (Edecrin).

   (5) A side effect is hypokalemia, so patients need a diet high in potassium or a potassium supplement.

   (6) Spironolactone (Aldactone) and triamterene (Dyrenium) are potassium-sparing diuretics that promote sodium and water excretion but block potassium excretion. Lasix and Aldactone may be given together to reduce potassium loss.

   (7) These are milder diuretics because of their potassium-sparing property.

c. Use of vasodilatory drugs has been particularly important in treating CHF patients. These drugs:

   (1) Reduce peripheral resistance (a factor affecting afterload) and pulmonary and peripheral venous pressure.

   (2) Reduce peripheral resistance, increasing left ventricular stroke volume and cardiac output.

   (3) Reduce pulmonary and peripheral venous pressure, causing a reduction in left ventricular preload.

   (4) Enhance myocardial function, lessening myocardial oxygen demand.

◆ An example of drugs that are used primarily is nitrates.

◆ The prototype of organic nitrates is nitroglycerin (Nitrostat).

d. Nitrates have three major effects:

   (1) First, dilation of veins, which reduces venous pressure and venous return to the heart, thus decreasing blood volume and pressure within the heart (preload), which in turn decreases cardiac workload and oxygen demand.

   (2) Second, nitrates dilate coronary arteries, which increase blood flow to ischemic areas of the myocardium.

   (3) Third, nitrates dilate arterioles, which lowers peripheral resistance (afterload), resulting in a lower systolic blood pressure and, consequently, reduced cardiac workload.

e. Arterial vasodilating drugs include hydralazine (Apresoline) and calcium channel blockers.

f. Drugs that have combined venous and arterial effects include nitroprusside (Nipride) and prazosin (Minipress).

g. Morphine is given to decrease anxiety so that the patient will breathe easier and reduce the workload on the heart.

h. Anxiety increases the release of epinephrine (Adrenalin), norepinephrine (Levophed), and dopamine (Intropin).

i. These are naturally occurring substances called *catecholamines* that function as neurotransmitters and hormones.

    (1) Norepinephrine acts only on alpha receptors, causing peripheral vasoconstriction and increasing blood pressure.

    (2) Epinephrine acts on both alpha and beta receptors.

◆ Beta-adrenergic activity includes increased heart rate and force of contraction and bronchial dilation.

◆ The alpha-adrenergic effect is vasoconstriction.

j. Dopamine, epinephrine, and norepinephrine cause vasoconstriction and increase cardiac output and urinary output by increasing kidney perfusion.

k. Dobutamine increases ventricular contractions, thus increasing cardiac output with a relatively minor effect on heart rate and peripheral blood vessels.

l. Atropine is used during acute CHF if bradycardia develops.

m. Lidocaine is used in acute CHF if ventricular arrhythmias develop.

n. Nitroprusside IV is the drug of choice.

    (1) It rapidly dilates both arterioles and venules, and it reduces both preload (diastolic) and afterload (systolic) pressure.

    (2) It may be used to reduce cardiac workload in cases of acute CHF.

o. Calcium blockers, such as nifedipine (Procardia), which is a potent peripheral vasodilator that reduces preload, are given in acute CHF.

5. Nursing Implications for CHF

  a. Assessment

    (1) Assess the patient's physical abilities, as the patient with CHF reports feeling fatigued to the point of exhaustion.

    (2) Ask about sleep and rest patterns, strength, endurance, and ability to complete activities of daily living.

    (3) Assess vital signs and note if the patient is dyspneic during activity, rest, or both.

    (4) Listen for crackles or wheezing because left-sided failure results in adventitious (acquired) lung sounds throughout the lung fields accompanied by a productive or nonproductive cough.

    (5) Assess peripheral pulses because they may be diminished because of the heart's decreased ability to perfuse the extremities.

    (6) Observe for edema of the ankles and sacrum and observe for liver or abdominal enlargement because right-sided failure results in peripheral edema.

    (7) Assess jugular vein for distention.

    (8) Check the blood pressure, which may be low, normal, or high depending on the degree of heart failure.

    (9) Assess capillary refill in the nailbed, which usually is slow in CHF.

    (10) Check for tachycardia and arrhythmias, such as atrial fibrillation, PVCs, and heart block.

    (11) Assess for fluid retention, which may cause the patient to complain of recent weight gain.

    (12) Note skin color, looking for paleness, cyanosis, or ashen appearance.

6. Interventions

  a. Monitor patient's vital signs both at rest and with activity, auscultate the apical pulse noting the rate and rhythm, and ask about any dyspneic episodes.

  b. Use telemetry monitoring whenever possible, especially if the patient experiences arrhythmias or if the patient is taking antiarrhythmic drugs.

  c. Review the results of laboratory studies and hemodynamic monitoring.

  d. Check the patient's intake and output, observing for adequacy and balance.

  e. Ask if the patient is getting enough rest and sleep and prevent disturbances in the room, especially at night.

  f. Encourage the patient to rest frequently throughout the day to prevent fatigue and strain on the myocardium.

  g. Administer digoxin, Lasix, and other prescribed medications.

  h. Monitor IV fluids closely to prevent fluid overload.

VI. MANAGEMENT OF PATIENTS WITH CARDIOVASCULAR DISORDERS

A. American Heart Association Guidelines

1. Cholesterol

  a. The American Heart Association's 2004 guidelines for lowering cholesterol targets low-density lipoproteins (LDLs), so-called "bad" cholesterol. The recommended LDL level for the *highest-risk* patients is less than 100 mg/dL. The highest-risk patients are those who have established heart disease and other conditions such as smoking or high blood pressure.

  b. The recommended LDL level for *high-risk* patients is less than 130 mg/dL. The high-risk patients are those with two or more risk factors.

  c. The recommended LDL level for the *moderate-risk* patient is less than 160 mg/dL. The moderate high-risk patient has one or no risk factors.

  d. No changes are recommended for patients at *low risk* for heart disease.

2. Statins

Statins are a category of drugs that decrease the liver's ability to synthesize cholesterol. Cholesterol serves as a precursor of various steroid hormones. Statin drugs have the potential to cause liver damage and are known to destroy liver cells, which explains why physicians recommend blood tests for liver function every few months. High-density lipoprotein (HDL), so-called "good" cholesterol, has a protective function. It transports cholesterol to the liver for catabolism and excretion by the gastrointestinal (GI) tract. The more HDL present in the liver, the greater the breakdown of LDL.

3. Nutrition and Lifestyle Changes

a. The first line of defense should include a diet low in saturated fat and carbohydrate and aerobic exercise. Including a large quantity of fiber in the diet is important because fiber helps to bind cholesterol in the intestines and flush it out of the system. In addition, several nutrients have been found to help lower cholesterol and other bad fats such as triglycerides. For example, extracts of red yeast rice have been found to decrease lipids: total cholesterol, LDL cholesterol, and triglycerides. These extracts have been used in China for food and medicine since 800 AD.

b. Foods recommended by the American Heart Association to help lower LDL include vegetables such as broccoli, carrots, red peppers, tomato, onions, cauliflower, okra, and eggplant; oats, barley, and psyllium; vegetable-based margarine; soy protein products such as soy milk and soy sausages, cold cuts, and burgers; and almonds.

c. To reduce triglycerides, limit alcohol and carbohydrate intake. Foods high in carbohydrates, which include bread, pasta, white rice, whole-wheat pasta, brown rice, barley, and oats, should be used in moderation.

d. Maintain a desirable body weight because obesity is shown to be a major cause of high triglyceride levels. If a patient is overweight, recommend weight loss by regular exercise and reducing total calorie intake. Daily exercise (e.g., walking, bike riding, or swimming) is a very important part of increasing HDL and decreasing LDL.

e. The major risk factors for stroke are hereditary, smoking, increasing age, high blood pressure, diabetes, heart disease, and sickle cell anemia. Secondary risk factors include high blood cholesterol levels, tobacco use, physical inactivity, and overweight.

B. Percutaneous Transluminal Coronary Angioplasty (Fig. 15–7)

1. Procedure

a. PTCA is a therapeutic procedure that can be performed during a coronary angiography in medical centers where open heart surgery is available.

b. During the procedure, a specially designed balloon catheter is introduced into the coronary arteries and placed across the stenosed area of the coronary artery.

c. The balloon is dilated to push the plaque against the wall of the artery.

d. The coronary arteriogram is repeated to document the effects of the forceful dilation of the stenosed area.

e. Procedures used to establish coronary patency are illustrated in Figure 15–7.

2. Complications

a. Potential complications include cardiac arrhythmias, perforation of the myocardium, rupture of the coronary artery, catheter-induced embolic stroke, MI, allergic reaction to the dye, and potential for bleeding from the femoral catheter insertion site.

b. The pulse distal from the insertion site must be monitored closely following the procedure.

C. Mitral Commissurotomy and Valve Replacement

1. Surgical Management

a. Surgical therapy for mitral valve stenosis can include valve commissurotomy or valve replacement.

b. Mitral commissurotomy is a surgical incision of the stenosed valve to increase the size of the orifice.

c. Repair or replacement of cardiac valves with acquired stenosis or incompetences is not considered curative but is generally seen as providing good and long-lasting palliation results.

d. Potential complications include risk of thrombus formation, especially in mechanical valves.

e. Patients with mechanical valve replacement require continuous anticoagulation therapy for the remainder of their lives.

f. The patients who are taking heparin while in the hospital are started on Coumadin before the heparin is discontinued because the anticoagulant effects of Coumadin are not immediate.

g. Prophylactic antibiotics are used for 6 months to 1 year when the patient has dental surgery or dental procedures.

D. Heart Transplant

1. Surgical Procedure

a. Cardiac transplantation is now a standard and effective treatment for patients with end-stage cardiac disease.

b. The surgical technique for heart transplant retains a large portion of the right and left atria in the recipient and implants the donor's ventricles to the atria. Cardiopulmonary bypass is used during the operation.

c. Basic criteria considered when determining whether or not a patient is a candidate for heart transplant are as follows.

(1) Presence of end-stage organ disease

(2) Inability of conventional therapy to treat the condition successfully

(3) Whether or not the problems caused by the condition are progressive despite careful management

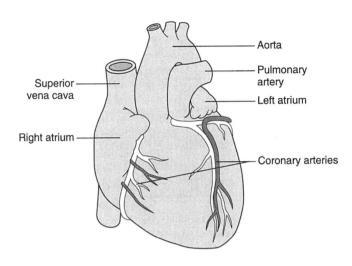

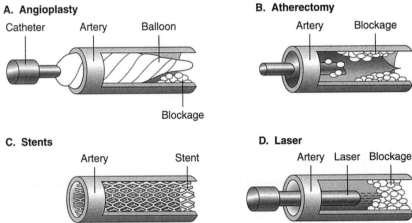

FIGURE 15–7 ◆ Technique for Clearing Clogged Arteries

Physicians have discovered a variety of alternatives to coronary bypass surgery.
A. Angioplasty. A catheter attached to a small sausage-shaped deflated balloon is
guided through the narrowed artery. The balloon is passed across the blockage and then
inflated to dilate the artery, crushing the fatty deposits and widening the blood vessel.
B. Atherectomy. Physicians use x-ray equipment and a specially designed catheter to
remove the blockage by shaving the cholesterol from the inner walls of the artery to
remove the blockage. **C.** Stents. A cylindrical wire mesh that works like scaffolding is
inserted into the blood vessel and expanded to hold the artery open. **D.** Laser. A variety
of lasers can be used to vaporize blockage in arteries. Using a catheter as a guide, laser
light is directed at the blockage in the arteries to vaporize the blockage.

d. Patients who meet these criteria are further evaluated to
determine their eligibility for transplant.

    (1) This includes assessment of the patient's ability to
recover from surgery and the patient's health.

    (2) Patients with terminal or chronic disease would not
be candidates for any transplant.

e. Other factors are based on age, psychological makeup,
family support, and the likelihood of adhering to the long-
term therapeutic regimen.

    (1) Age is not a major factor.

    (2) Health factors are most important.

f. The major obstacle to the complete success of a heart
transplant procedure is the management of the patient's immune response to the foreign organ.

    (1) Although immunosuppressant therapy that prevents
rejection traditionally is begun after transplantation,
some effort has been made to commence immunotherapy
prior to transplantation.

    (2) These efforts involve low-dose irradiation of the
lymphatic system, lymphatic drainage by the thoracic
duct, and administration of immunosuppressants.

g. All transplant recipients are at increased risk for opportunistic infections as a result of immunosuppressant therapy,

which they must take for as long as the transplanted organ functions.

(1) Opportunistic diseases are infections, which compromise the patient's weakened immune system.

(2) Following surgery, concern for nosocomial infections requires the use of aseptic technique in all of the patient's care.

h. Nursing care of a patient following transplant includes a major emphasis on assessment for rejection and subsequent care of the patient undergoing treatment for rejection.

i. Heart transplant patients may experience a phenomenon referred to as *pump psychosis,* which includes changes in mental status, such as confusion, disorientation, and depression.

(1) Pump psychosis may last for a few days or for as long as 1 month.

(2) Information on pump psychosis should be included in patient and family teaching.

E. Cardiomyoplasty

1. Cardiomyoplasty is being used in clinical trials as an alternative surgical technique for patients who are not candidates for cardiac transplantation.

2. Through low-frequency electrical stimulation, the pectoralis muscle is trained over many weeks to be more fatigue resistant and to contract in synchrony with ventricular systole.

3. When the skeletal muscle has been conditioned, the electrical stimulation is increased to cause the muscle to contract with sufficient force to augment the patient's cardiac output.

4. An advantage to this procedure is that the patient's own tissue is used, eliminating the problems of rejection.

5. The future potential of cardiomyoplasty offers new hope, but for now, a heart transplant remains the only choice for patients with end-stage heart failure.

F. Coronary Artery Bypass Graft

1. Etiology

a. This procedure is performed when coronary arteries are blocked.

b. A vein from the leg (saphenous) or from the breast (mammary) is used to bypass the blockage.

c. Development of calcium channel blockers and nonsurgical techniques, such as PTCA, have reduced the number of CABG surgeries performed.

d. Survival rates of patients with CABG have not been found to be significantly better than survival rates of medically treated patients.

e. Nevertheless, CABG remains a common surgery because it can reduce angina in 80 to 90 percent of patients by increasing cardiac perfusion, thus reducing the potential for an MI.

f. More than half of all CABG surgeries are performed on patients older than 65 years, and 75 percent of these patients are men.

g. Each patient remains hospitalized for an average of 3 to 4 days.

2. Preoperative Care

a. The patient is NPO and IV.

b. Heparin is given to prevent blood from clotting.

c. Streptokinase or other thrombolytic agents are used to dissolve blood clots.

d. Vitamin K reduces the potential for bleeding.

e. Steroids reduce inflammatory reaction.

f. Antibiotics are used prophylactically to prevent infections.

g. Preoperative teaching concerns about the surgery and postoperative expectations.

3. Postoperative Care in the Critical Care Unit

a. Mediastinal chest tube drains the surgical area and pleural chest tube maintains negative pressure in the lungs.

b. Heparin, thrombolytic agent, and antihypertensive agent.

c. Steroids and vitamin K.

d. Bed rest and NPO usually are required only for the first 8 to 24 h.

4. Planning

a. Continuous monitoring of heart rate, rhythm, and arterial blood pressure.

b. Intermittent monitoring of preload (systolic) when heart is contracting.

c. Continuous monitoring of electrolyte and hematologic values.

d. Continuous monitoring of mediastinal chest tube and pleural chest tube.

5. Assessment

a. Assess vital signs and electrolyte and hematologic laboratory values.

b. Assess for emboli, MI, and arrhythmias.

c. The nurse needs to assess mediastinal chest tube drainage (this tube is *not* in the pleural cavity); tube is milked periodically to maintain patency.

d. Assess pleural chest drainage for color, amount, and patency.

6. Analysis

a. A nurse never discontinues a chest tube that is used to reexpand the lungs because of the danger of pneumothorax or other complications of the lung.

b. The nurse can discontinue a mediastinal chest tube with an order from the physician.

c. The largest amount of drainage comes from the mediastinal chest tube.

   (1) There may be up to 100 mL of drainage during the first hour postoperative.

   (2) There may be up to 500 mL of drainage over the first 24 h.

7. Interventions

   a. Maintain blood pressure at 90/70 to prevent excessive pressure on the coronary artery graft.

   b. Maintain pulse rate at approximately 80 bpm.

8. Late Postoperative Care Following CABG

   a. Rehabilitation is started while the patient is in the cardiac care unit (CCU) to prevent anxiety, depression, and deconditioning.

   b. Patients usually are ambulatory 2 to 3 days after surgery.

   c. An important aspect of rehabilitation is to teach the patient to recognize the onset of adverse symptoms, such as shortness of breath, chest pain, palpitations, and dizziness.

   d. Patients should be taught to take their own pulse and blood pressure in the hospital while under a nurse's supervision.

   e. The objective of rehabilitation is to obtain and maintain optimal cardiac functional capacity.

VII. CARDIOPULMONARY RESUSCITATION

1. Purpose of cardiopulmonary resuscitation (CPR) is to restore, by artificial intervention, cardiovascular circulation and ventilation after cardiopulmonary arrest.

   The American Heart Association in 2005 simplified its (CPR) instructions, incorporating the latest available research, in an effort to make it even easier for medical professionals and people who have no medical training to perform CPR.

   a. People who are trained to use the technique are required to be regularly re-certified. Medical personnel can be expected to see changes in Basic Life Support training beginning sometime in 2006; they should expect it to be more in depth and to be held to a higher medical standard than a lay person.

   b. The new nationwide changes, American Heart Association expects will eventually result in significant upsurge in lives saved. In the United States, 225,000 people a year die because of an out-of-hospital cardiac arrest. Streamlining the CPR process could save one out of every five people in cardiac arrest every year, according to American Hospital Association officials.

   c. New guidelines eliminate the pulse check and urge people to look for alternative signs that someone's heart is beating, such as normal breathing, coughing, and movement. If no such signs are present, the guidelines instruct people to proceed to use chest compressions and rescue breathing in a ratio of 15 compressions to two breaths. This should be repeated in succession at a rate of 100 compressions a minute.

   d. Other changes in instructions include treating an unconscious choking victim. Instead of sweeping the mouth or using the Heimlich maneuver to dislodge a blockage, chest compressions only are recommended by the association. This purportedly lessens the chance that any blockage will be depressed further into the airway.

2. Assessment

   a. Check for signs of circulation, such as normal breathing, coughing, or response to stimulation. If unresponsiveness is established, call a code if in the hospital or 911 if not in a hospital. Use defibrillator if available; if not, start chest compressions.

Note: Do not conduct abdominal thrust or blind fingers sweep of the mouth.

3. Interventions: Start CPR

   a. Compressions: elbows straight in a locked position with shoulders directly over the patient's sternum so that the thrust for compressions is straight down on the sternum. Administer 15 chest compressions for every two rescue breaths, whether or not one or two rescuers are present.

   b. Assess for patient's response.

Note: A machine called an *automatic external defibrillator* (AED) can determine whether a victim's heart needs to be shocked and provide that shock if necessary. Seventy-five percent of people who suffer sudden cardiac arrest survive when an AED is available and used within minutes after cardiac arrest. AEDs are available in many public buildings, including sport stadiums, shopping malls, and airports.

VIII. CARDIAC DIAGNOSTIC TESTS

A. Cardiac Catheterization (Coronary Angiography)

1. Purpose

   a. Angiocardiography or coronary angiography is an x-ray procedure performed with contrast dye.

   b. Prior to the procedure, determine whether or not the patient has an iodine dye allergy.

   c. Purpose is to study the heart, great blood vessels, coronary arteries, and intracardiac pressure and volume.

2. Procedure

   a. A catheter is passed through a peripheral vein or artery into the right or left side of the heart.

   b. If the right side of the heart is being catheterized, the subclavian vein or femoral vein is used for vascular access.

   c. If left side of heart is being catheterized, the right femoral artery is used.

   d. A catheter is advanced into the desired position with appropriate guidance using a video camera.

   e. After pressures are obtained, angiographic visualization of the heart chambers, valves, and coronary arteries is performed with injection of radiographic dye.

   f. The patient is NPO for 4 to 8 h before the test.

B. Echocardiography (Ultrasound)

1. This is a noninvasive, painless study used to evaluate the structure and function of the heart.

2. Abnormal findings may be valvular stenosis, valvular regurgitation, mitral valve prolapse, pericardial effusion, poor ventricular muscle motion, or septal defects.

C. Exercise Stress Test

1. Purpose

a. This is a noninvasive study used to provide information about the patient's cardiac function.

b. A stress test is performed to determine if the heart can meet an increased demand for oxygen while under stress (work).

c. If it cannot, the arteries are not able to meet the heart's increased demand for oxygen. This is one indication that the heart is not being perfused adequately. Other tests will be performed.

2. Procedure

a. During stress testing, an ECG is used to monitor heart rate and blood pressure while the patient engages in some type of physical activity (stress).

b. Three common methods of stress testing are (1) climbing stair steps, (2) pedaling a stationary bike, and (3) walking on a treadmill.

c. *Note:* The coronary arteries branch off the aorta; therefore, when blood cannot be adequately pumped out of the heart through the aorta or when the coronary arteries are occluded or constricted, the heart will not be adequately perfused.

d. This may become obvious during the test if symptoms such as chest pain, dyspnea, tachycardia, cardiac arrhythmias, or hypotension develop or if the ECG changes.

D. Intravascular Ultrasound

1. Purpose

a. Intravascular ultrasound (IVUS) uses a flexible catheter with a miniature transducer at the distal tip to provide visual information about the interior of a coronary artery.

b. The results must be interpreted by a cardiologist.

2. Procedure

a. The catheter is inserted into a peripheral vessel and advanced over a guidewire into the coronary artery, much like a PTCA catheter is inserted.

b. The transducer is activated within the artery, where it emits high-frequency sound waves, which reflect off the arterial wall (or plaque) creating a two- or three-dimensional image of the vessel lumen.

c. An external console attached to the catheter records the image in shades of gray and displays the images on a video monitor.

3. Advantages of IVUS

a. For the last 3 decades, angiography has been the standard procedure used for assessing atherosclerotic lesions in coronary arteries.

(1) Compared with IVUS, the angiographic silhouette is not as reliable an indicator of plaque distribution and composition, arterial dissection, degree of stenosis in an occluded artery, or the full degree of stent expansion.

(2) All of these factors are used in either the cardiologist's diagnosis or the medical plan.

b. IVUS is also used when an atherectomy device is used to remove plaque by scraping it away from the coronary artery (Fig. 15–6).

(1) To avoid damaging the artery, the cardiologist needs to know how the plaque is distributed inside the arterial wall.

(2) Some studies have demonstrated that less arterial damage occurs when IVUS is used because visualization inside the artery is better.

c. If IVUS reveals a dissection of the vessel at the point of balloon expansion, an intracoronary stent will be inserted to tack up the dissected tissue and prevent platelets and fibrin from aggregating at the site where the intima has been exposed.

(1) Stents are also inserted into arteries to maintain patency.

d. Use of IVUS to assess stent deployment (Fig. 15–6) has decreased the risk of rethrombosis and the need for aggressive anticoagulation therapy (both are associated with inadequate stent expansion).

4. Postprocedure

a. Normally, during the first week after stent implantation, endothelial cells grow over the stent, and it becomes a permanent part of the vessel wall.

(1) If the stent does not fully expand and attach itself securely to the artery wall, endothelialization will not occur.

(2) Instead of a patent artery, a thrombus may form on the exposed stent, reoccluding the vessel.

(3) The stent could migrate, leading to a new occlusion in a different location in the coronary artery and possibly cause an MI.

(4) This is why an anticoagulant regimen combining aspirin, warfarin, and dipyridamole (Persantine) is generally prescribed for at least 1 month after stent implantation.

b. The stainless steel woven mesh stent is highly reflective on IVUS, so location and expansion are easily seen.

c. For many years, coronary angiography has been used to assess stent expansion after insertion.

(1) To achieve optimal coronary dilation, balloon expansion of the stent is commonly performed.

d. Studies suggest that angiography may detect only 20 to 30 percent of inadequately expanded stents that are visible by IVUS.

e. Given the risk for rethrombosis associated with inadequate stent expansion, many hospitals using IVUS during stent deployment are finding less need for aggressive post-procedural anticoagulation therapy.

PERIPHERAL VASCULAR

I. ARTERIAL DISORDERS

Patients with peripheral vascular disease must avoid using tobacco in any form (chewing or smoking).

A. Atherosclerosis of the Extremities

1. Etiology and Incidence

a. Atherosclerosis is the leading cause of occlusive arterial disease of the extremities in patients older than 40 years.

b. There is an increased prevalence of peripheral atherosclerotic occlusive disease in individuals with CHF, MI, hypertension, hypercholesterolemia, and diabetes mellitus and in cigarette smokers.

c. The pathology of the lesions includes atherosclerotic plaques with calcium deposits, destruction of muscle and elastic fibers, and thrombi composed of platelets and fibrin.

d. The primary sites are the femoral and popliteal arteries.

e. The highest incidence occurs in the sixth and seventh decades of life.

f. Atherosclerosis of the extremities is seen most frequently in elderly men.

g. Lipoproteins are proteins in the blood that can be grouped into the different lipoproteins.

(1) The purpose of HDLs is to remove the cholesterol from the peripheral tissue and transport it to the liver for excretion.

(2) HDLs may have a protective effect by preventing cellular uptake of cholesterol and lipids.

h. The purpose of LDLs is to deposit cholesterol into the peripheral tissues. It is associated with increased risk for arteriosclerotic occlusive disease.

i. The lipoprotein test is used to assess the risk of coronary artery disease.

(1) High levels of the "protective" HDL are associated with a decreased risk for coronary disease.

(2) High levels of LDL are associated with an increased risk for coronary occlusive disease.

j. Very low-density lipoproteins (VLDLs), to a lesser degree, are also associated with coronary occlusive disease.

k. Levels of HDL are increased in patients who engage in frequent physical activity or who drink a moderate amount of alcohol.

l. Genetic makeup, however, is the most important determinant of lipoprotein level.

m. For normal cholesterol levels in adults see pp. 171, 172.

2. Signs and Symptoms

a. The most common symptom of peripheral arterial occlusion is intermittent claudication, which is defined as pain, aches, cramps, and numbness in the leg muscles, that occurs during exercise but is relieved with rest.

(1) Intermittent claudication is severe pain in the calf muscle that occurs during walking but subsides with rest.

(2) It results from an inadequate blood supply, which may be due to arterial spasm, atherosclerosis, arteriosclerosis, or an occlusion.

b. Other symptoms are cold feet, thick toenails, and ulcers on the big toe (will turn black if gangrene develops). The feet will be cold to the touch with no edema.

3. Treatment

a. The legs should be kept level with the body, and bed covers should be kept off the feet by use of a bed (foot) cradle.

(1) Feet should receive meticulous care.

(2) Well-fitting shoes should be used to reduce trauma.

b. If the patient smokes cigarettes, education should include the importance of discontinuing cigarette smoking.

c. It is important to control blood pressure in hypertensive patients.

d. Patients with claudication should be encouraged to exercise regularly and to increase their regimen progressively.

e. Patients should be advised to walk 30 to 45 min daily, stopping at the onset of claudication and resting until the symptoms resolve before resuming ambulation.

f. Other forms of exercise, such as bicycle riding and swimming, provide overall cardiovascular and psychological benefits and often are tolerated better than walking.

g. Pharmacologic treatment of patients with peripheral arterial occlusive disease has not been as successful as medical treatment of coronary artery disease.

(1) In particular, vasodilators, as a class, have not proved to be beneficial.

(2) During exercise, peripheral vasodilation normally occurs distal to the site of arterial stenosis.

h. Platelet inhibitors, particularly aspirin, have been reported to decrease progression of atherosclerosis in patients with peripheral arterial occlusive disease.

i. Revascularization procedures, including nonoperative as well as operative interventions, usually are reserved for patients with progressive, severe, or disabling symptoms and ischemia at rest.

j. Nonoperative interventions include percutaneous transluminal angioplasty (PTA), laser angioplasty, atherectomy, and stent placement (Fig. 15–7).

k. PTA of the iliac artery is associated with a higher success rate than PTA of the femoral or popliteal arteries.

B. Occlusive Vascular Disorders: Thromboangiitis Obliterans

1. Etiology and Incidence

a. Thromboangiitis obliterans (Buerger's disease) is an inflammatory occlusive vascular disorder involving small- and medium-sized arteries and veins in the distal upper and lower extremities.

b. The disorder develops most frequently in men younger than 40 years.

c. The incidence is higher in Asians and individuals with Eastern Europe lineage.

d. The cause of thromboangiitis obliterans is not known, but there is a definite relationship to cigarette smoking.

2. Signs and Symptoms

a. Clinical features often include claudication of the affected extremity, Raynaud's phenomenon (see entry D), and superficial vein thrombophlebitis.

b. Claudication usually is confined to the lower calves and feet or forearms and hands.

c. In the presence of severe digital ischemia, atrophic nail changes, ulcerations, and gangrene may develop at the tips of the fingers or toes.

3. Treatment
There is no specific treatment except abstention from tobacco.

C. Raynaud's Disease

1. Etiology and Incidence

a. Raynaud's disease is diagnosed when secondary causes of Raynaud's phenomenon have been excluded.

b. More than 50 percent of patients with Raynaud's phenomenon have Raynaud's disease.

c. Distinction between the two disorders is difficult because some patients who experience mild symptoms of Raynaud's disease for several years later develop the overt connective tissue disease.

d. Women are affected approximately five times more often than men, and the age of presentation is usually between 20 and 40 years.

e. The fingers are involved more frequently than the toes.

f. The cause is unknown.

2. Signs, symptoms, and treatment are the same as for Raynaud's phenomenon (see entry D).

D. Raynaud's Phenomenon

1. Etiology and Incidence

a. Raynaud's phenomenon may be precipitated by emotional stress and is associated with several connective tissue disorders.

b. Raynaud proposed that cold-induced episodic digital ischemia was secondary to exaggerated reflex sympathetic vasoconstriction.

c. This theory is supported by the fact that adrenergic blocking agents decrease the frequency and severity of Raynaud's phenomenon in some patients.

d. Secondary causes of Raynaud's phenomenon include rheumatoid arthritis, systemic sclerosis (scleroderma), and systemic lupus erythematosus.

2. Signs and Symptoms

a. Characterized by episodic digital ischemia and manifested clinically by the sequential development of digital blanching, cyanosis, and rubor of the fingers or toes following cold exposure.

b. Typically, one or more digits appear white when the patient is exposed to a cold environment or touches a cold object.

c. The blanching, or pallor, represents the ischemic phase of the phenomenon and is secondary to vasospasm of the digital arteries.

d. With rewarming of cold hands, the digital vasospasm resolves, and blood rapidly flows into the dilated arterioles and capillaries.

E. Nursing Implications for Arterial Disorders

1. Assessment

a. Palpate distal pulses bilaterally, noting the rate and intensity.

b. Check extremities for temperature and cyanosis.

c. Assess for pain, noting the frequency, duration, intensity, location, and relief method.

d. Check for edema, lesions, and gangrene of the extremities.

e. Note if the patient is taking medication or smoking tobacco.

2. Nursing Interventions

a. Instruct the patient to stop smoking tobacco because smoking increases ischemia and exacerbates the disorder.

b. Instruct the patient to avoid wearing constricting clothing that interferes with circulation in the extremities.

c. Teach relaxation strategies and encourage frequent use of these techniques.

II. VENOUS DISORDERS

A. Superficial Venous Thrombosis

1. Etiology and Incidence

a. The presence of thrombosis within a superficial vein and the accompanying inflammatory response in the vessel wall is termed *venous thrombosis* or *thrombophlebitis*.

b. Factors that predispose to venous thrombosis include stasis, vascular damage, and hypercoagulability.

c. Venous thrombosis may occur in more than 50 percent of patients undergoing orthopedic surgical procedures, particularly those involving the hip or knee, and 10 to 40 percent of patients undergoing abdominal or thoracic operations.

d. The prevalence of venous thrombosis is particularly high in patients with cancer of the stomach, genitourinary tract, breast, pancreas, or lungs.

e. Risk for thrombosis is increased following trauma, such as fracture of the pelvis, femur, and tibia.

f. Immobilization, regardless of the underlying disease, is a major predisposing cause of venous thrombosis.

g. The incidence of venous thrombosis is increased during pregnancy, particularly in the third trimester and in the first month postpartum, and in individuals who use estrogen.

h. A variety of clinical disorders produce systemic hypercoagulability, including systemic lupus erythematosus and disseminated intravascular coagulation. These disorders may cause venous thrombosis.

2. Treatment

a. Prevention of pulmonary embolism is the most important reason for treating deep vein thrombosis because, in the early stage, the thrombosis may be loose and poorly adherent to the blood vessel wall.

b. The patient should be put on total bed rest, and the affected extremity should be elevated above the level of the heart until the edema and tenderness subside.

c. Anticoagulants prevent thrombosis formation.

d. Heparin may be administered intravenously.

e. Intermittent subcutaneous injections of heparin may be used as an alternative form of therapy.

f. It is important to overlap heparin treatment with oral anticoagulant therapy (Coumadin) for at least 4 to 5 days because the full anticoagulant effect of warfarin (Coumadin) is delayed.

g. Thrombolytic drugs, such as streptokinase, urokinase, or t-PA, also may be used, but there is no evidence that thrombolytic therapy is more effective than anticoagulants in preventing pulmonary embolism.

h. Do not rub the leg or ambulate the patient because this action may cause the clot to move (emboli).

i. If the patient demonstrates signs and symptoms of deep venous thrombosis, put the patient on bed rest, assess the patient carefully, and then notify the physician.

B. Deep Venous Thrombosis

1. Etiology and Incidence

a. The most important consequence of deep venous thrombosis of the iliac, femoral, or popliteal veins is pulmonary embolism.

b. Deep venous thrombosis occurs less frequently in the upper extremity than in the lower extremity.

2. Signs and Symptoms

a. Tenderness may be present along the course of the involved veins.

b. Various noninvasive tests are used to diagnose deep venous thrombosis, including venous ultrasonography.

c. Ultrasonography provides accurate visualization of the presence of deep venous thrombosis through the use of reflected sound waves.

d. Doppler ultrasound measures the velocity of blood flow in the veins.

e. Deep venous thrombosis can be diagnosed by venography.

(1) Contrast medium is injected.

(2) The presence of a filling defect or absence of filling of the deep vein is required to make the diagnosis.

3. Treatment is the same as for superficial venous thrombosis.

C. Phlebitis

1. Etiology and Incidence

a. Phlebitis is inflammation of the veins without thrombosis.

b. Inflammation of the veins is most often caused by infusion of an IV solution, especially IV medications such as potassium chloride.

c. Occurs most often in women and increases with age, affecting lower extremities most often.

d. Immobility for any reason can cause phlebitis.

e. Surgery can be another cause of phlebitis; therefore, support stockings are applied to the patient preoperatively and are maintained postoperatively. It is most important that the patient wear support stockings while in bed.

2. Signs and Symptoms

a. Reddened line along the inflamed vein can be seen.

b. Extreme tenderness along the course of the vein.

c. Inflamed area warm to touch.

3. Treatment

a. If an IV line is the cause, discontinue it. Apply warm compresses to affected site and elevate the arm.

b. Antiinflammatory agents may be used.

D. Varicose Veins

1. Etiology and Incidence

a. These are dilated tortuous superficial veins.

b. Varicose veins may be either primary or secondary.

c. Primary varicose veins result from a familial predisposition that leads to loss of elasticity of the vein walls and valvular incompetence.

d. Secondary varicosities occur with trauma, deep venous thrombosis, and inflammation-damaged valves.

e. Chronic venous insufficiency results from dysfunctional valves that reduce venous return, which increases venous pressure and causes venous stasis.

f. Chronic venous insufficiency follows severe cases of deep venous thrombosis, but it may take as long as 5 to 10 years to manifest.

g. Approximately 40 percent of patients with chronic venous insufficiency have no history of deep venous thrombosis.

2. Signs and Symptoms

a. Patients with venous insufficiency often complain of a dull ache in the legs that worsens with prolonged standing and resolves with leg elevation.

b. Examination demonstrates increased leg circumference, edema, and superficial varicose veins.

c. Erythema, dermatitis, hyperpigmentation, and stasis ulcers may develop around the ankle area.

3. Treatment

a. Varicose veins usually can be treated with conservative measures by elevating legs periodically, avoiding prolonged standing, and wearing elastic support hose.

b. An external sequential compression device may be used to increase venous return.

(1) This device is wrapped around the patient's legs and contracted intermittently.

(2) It can be used only while the patient is in bed.

(3) The sequential device is powered by electricity.

c. Small symptomatic varicose veins may be treated with sclerotherapy.

(1) A sclerosing solution is injected into the varicose vein and a compression bandage is applied.

(2) This procedure destroys the superficial varicose veins, and blood will flow through to deeper veins.

d. Surgical therapy usually involves extensive ligation and stripping of the greater and lesser saphenous veins. It should be reserved for patients who are very symptomatic, suffer recurrent superficial vein thrombosis, develop skin ulceration, or have a combination of these symptoms.

(1) Sclerosing therapy may be indicated for cosmetic reasons.

e. When a stasis ulcer is detected, no matter how small, treatment needs to begin immediately.

f. Some examples of treatments that can be used are Unna's boot, wet-to-dry dressing, DuoDERM, and compression wraps.

g. An open and draining ulcer should be cleansed with saline or hydrogen peroxide, dried well, and an appropriate dressing applied.

h. Treatment of a stasis ulcer is a long, slow healing process.

E. Nursing Implications for Venous Disorders

1. Assessment

a. Check lower extremities for edema, discoloration around ankles, and tenderness.

b. Ask patient about pain, and note its location, duration, and intensity.

c. Check for the presence of Homans' sign (calf pain with dorsiflexion of the foot).

d. Observe for signs of pulmonary embolism, such as sudden chest pain, dyspnea, restlessness, diaphoresis, and cyanosis.

2. Interventions

a. Instruct patient to stop smoking tobacco.

b. Instruct patient to avoid standing for long periods of time, and encourage the patient to walk for 30 to 60 min per day, resting if intermittent claudication occurs.

c. Have patient wear warm clothing to protect against vasoconstriction in the extremities.

d. Instruct patient to avoid crossing the legs because this position decreases circulation to the legs and feet and to elevate legs when sitting or while in bed.

EXAMINATION

1. Which of the following side effects are related to nitroglycerin?
   1. Bradycardia, syncope, hypertension, and nausea.
   2. Tachycardia, syncope, hypotension, and headache.
   3. Ocular irritation, headache, and constipation.
   4. Nervousness, dyspnea, headache, and rashes.

2. The nurse should instruct a male patient experiencing acute angina attacks to place one nitroglycerin tablet under his tongue and if pain persists to
   1. Repeat every 5 to 8 min for 15 min and, if pain persists, call physician.
   2. Wait 15 min and then put one more nitroglycerin tablet under his tongue; if pain persists call physician.
   3. Repeat every 15 min for one-half hour; if pain persists, call physician.
   4. Wait 10 min, put two nitroglycerin tablets under his tongue, and repeat every 15 min until pain disappears.

3. The nurse advises Mr. Vaughn on how to reduce future anginal attacks by advising him to
   1. Set up a regular exercise program, consisting of walking 15 min every day.
   2. Maintain a low-sodium diet and swim 2 h twice per day.
   3. Run a half mile and ride a bicycle 1 mile each day.
   4. Reduce the number of days he works in the factory.

4. The patient is diagnosed with MI and placed in the coronary care unit (CCU). Which of the following is the most common complication that the nurse should observe in this patient?

   1. Cardiac arrhythmia.
   2. Anaphylactic shock.
   3. Cardiac enlargement.
   4. Essential hypertension.

5. The patient is in the CCU on a cardiac monitor. The nurse observes ventricular irritability on the screen. Which of the following medications might the nurse expect to administer?

   1. Digoxin (Lanoxin).
   2. Lidocaine (Xylocaine).
   3. Furosemide (Lasix).
   4. Sodium bicarbonate.

6. The patient is released from the hospital and is taking Coumadin. It would be most important for the nurse to give him which of the following instructions?

   1. "Other medications do not interfere with the action of Coumadin."
   2. "Do not take Coumadin the day before you have a blood test."
   3. "Use a hard toothbrush to minimize bleeding of the gums that will occur because you are taking Coumadin."
   4. "Take one extra Coumadin dosage the day before a blood test."

7. When comparing the pain of angina pectoris with the pain of an MI, which statement is true?

   1. Angina pain is more intense than MI pain.
   2. MI pain is not relieved with rest, and angina pain is relieved with rest.
   3. Angina pain feels like a vise squeezing the chest.
   4. Angina pain radiates down the arm and affects the fingers more than the arm.

8. A 74-year-old woman is admitted to the hospital with a diagnosis of hypertension and CHF. The patient is receiving methyldopa (Aldomet) intravenously for control of hypertension. Her blood pressure before starting the infusion was 150/90. Fifteen minutes after the infusion begins her blood pressure rises to 180/100. The response to the drug would be described as

   1. A synergistic response.
   2. An individual hypersensitivity.
   3. An allergic response.
   4. A paradoxic response.

9. In which of the following cases will venous pressure be elevated?

   1. With hypovolemia.
   2. When pulmonary circulation is not maintained.
   3. With extensive bleeding from a stab wound.
   4. In CHF.

10. The rationale for giving 100 mg of Demerol to a patient with acute CHF is

    1. For coronary vasodilation.
    2. To relieve anxiety.
    3. To increase urinary output.
    4. To relieve painful breathing.

11. Chlorothiazide is the most useful group of diuretics because

    1. They will not cause sodium (Na) reabsorption.
    2. They are most useful in treating CHF.
    3. They have the most side effects but are the most effective.
    4. They are the most effective with the least amount of side effects.

12. The rationale for restricting fluid and sodium in a patient with CHF is that

    1. Sodium vasoconstricts and increases the workload of the heart.
    2. Sodium will increase potassium reabsorption and cause arrhythmias.
    3. Excessive fluid will cause hypokalemia and arrhythmias.
    4. Sodium causes water retention, which increases the workload of the heart.

13. In the clinical setting, especially in the very young and the elderly, the most common cause of cardiac overload is

    1. Forcing fluids by mouth (PO).
    2. Excessive intravenous infusion.
    3. Cardiac arrhythmias.
    4. Mitral valve disease.

14. Which of the following measures would best increase cardiac output in acute CHF?

    1. Epinephrine, Valium, and being in a semi-Fowler's position.
    2. Lidocaine, epinephrine, and being in a semi-Fowler's position.
    3. Digitalis, furosemide, and bed rest.
    4. Valium, oxygen, and moderate exercise.

15. Signs and symptoms that would best indicate acute CHF are

    1. Peripheral edema, localized cyanosis, and cardiac arrhythmia.
    2. Shortness of breath, chest pain, and cyanosis.
    3. A cardiac arrhythmia, ascites, and peripheral edema.
    4. Coarse crackles, shortness of breath, and generalized cyanosis.

16. The finding in the patient's laboratory report that would most likely increase her development of digitalis toxicity is a

1. Low sodium level.
2. Low potassium level.
3. High glucose level.
4. High calcium level.

17. The nurse is preparing to administer digitalis to this patient. Giving this drug would be contraindicated if the adult's
    1. Heart rate is less than 60 bpm and irregular.
    2. Heart rate is greater than 60 bpm and irregular.
    3. Heart rate is less than 70 bpm and very weak.
    4. Heart rate is greater than 60 bpm and is very strong but irregular.

18. Which of the following liquids, foods, or condiments are highest in potassium chloride (KCl)?
    1. Grapes, beef, lemons, and eggs.
    2. Apples, oranges, tomatoes, and instant tea.
    3. Bananas, prunes, oranges, instant coffee, and salt substitutes.
    4. Bananas, tea, catsup, fish, tuna, and liver.

19. Emma, a 60-year-old woman, diagnosed with coronary insufficiency, is receiving 20 mg of the coronary vasodilator Peritrate after meals. At the time of her afternoon dosage, she tells her nurse, "I feel so dizzy that I am afraid to get out of bed." The nursing action most appropriate for the nurse to take would be to
    1. Assist the patient to a chair and administer only half the prescribed dose of Peritrate.
    2. Instruct the patient not to get out of bed without assistance, administer this dose of Peritrate, and notify her physician.
    3. Instruct the patient not to get out of bed without assistance, do not give this dose of Peritrate, take the patient's blood pressure, and notify her physician.
    4. Assist the patient out of bed and ambulate her until she feels stronger but do not give this dose of Peritrate.

20. Fast-acting nitrates, such as amyl nitrate, usually are prescribed for the relief of acute pectoris pain. Amyl nitrate is administered
    1. By inhalation.
    2. Sublingually.
    3. Topically.
    4. Parenterally.

21. A 74-year-old woman with CHF and cardiac arrhythmias is hospitalized for digitalization. Prior to administering digoxin to this patient on the third day after her admission, the nurse takes the patient's apical pulse for 1 min. The patient's pulse rate is 55 bpm, but no new arrhythmias are noted. The nurse should do which of the following?
    1. Withhold the drug, chart the pulse rate, and inform the patient's physician as soon as he or she comes to see the patient.

2. Administer the drug, take apical pulse rate, and chart both radial and apical pulse rates.
3. Take apical pulse; if no arrhythmia is noted, administer the drug and chart both radial and apical pulse rates.
4. Withhold the drug, take apical pulse, chart pulse rates, and notify patient's physician immediately.

22. Which of the following effects is characteristic of digitalis?
    1. Stimulates the myocardium to contract more forcefully.
    2. Decreases angina pain.
    3. Increases cardiac rate and speeds conduction at the AV node.
    4. Increases blood pressure.

23. Some early signs and symptoms of digitalis toxicity are listed below. If a patient is 70 years old or older, the nurse should observe for
    1. Anorexia.
    2. Epigastric distress.
    3. Psychotomimetic effects.
    4. Change in rate, rhythm, and irritability of the heart.

24. A patient with sickle cell anemia needs to understand the physiology of cell sickling. The nurse should explain that
    1. Dyspnea will occur due to sickling.
    2. Nausea and vomiting will occur during sickling.
    3. Urinary failure will occur during sickling.
    4. Sickling is more likely to occur when oxygen levels are low.

25. A newborn with sickle cell anemia will be symptom-free because the
    1. High level of hemoglobin in fetal blood helps prevent sickling of the red blood cells.
    2. High level of oxygen in the blood helps prevent sickling of the red blood cells.
    3. Low number of red blood cells in fetal blood helps prevent sickling of red blood cells.
    4. Low number of platelets prevents the sickling of red blood cells.

26. An 82-year-old man is admitted to the emergency room complaining of pain in his right leg. The physician determines that the patient has thrombophlebitis in his right leg. Orders for this patient include heparin by continuous intravenous infusion, moist compresses to the affected leg, and elevation of the extremity. Before the nurse administers heparin to the patient on the second day of his hospitalization, the information most essential to obtain is
    1. The color of the patient's sclera.
    2. If petechiae appears on the patient's skin.
    3. The patient's partial thromboplastin time (PTT).
    4. The patient's prothrombin time (PT).

27. When applying warm compresses to the patient's leg, which of the following is the most essential procedure?

   1. Lubricating the skin before applying the compresses.

   2. Checking the temperature of the compresses on the radial aspect of the wrist.

   3. Covering the leg from ankle to mid-thigh with the compresses.

   4. Securing the compresses in place with a plastic sheet.

28. One morning, while a male patient is being ambulated, he complains of chest pain. The signs and symptoms that are most probably related to a pulmonary embolus would be

   1. Sharp, stabbing chest pain that intensifies on inspiration, dyspnea, low-grade fever, and tachycardia.

   2. Crushing, viselike chest pain that radiates to the jaw, fever, and hypotension.

   3. Dull, substernal pain that projects throughout the chest, fever, and bradycardia.

   4. Colicky, pericardial pain in the apex of the heart, fever, and hypertension.

29. A 64-year-old woman is admitted to the CCU with angina pain and CHF. She is receiving intravenous fluids KVO. Her vital signs are checked. Bed rest and medications, including digitalis and nitroglycerin, are prescribed. The nurse who has been caring for this patient for several days notes a significant decrease in the patient's respirations and the beginning signs of cyanosis. The nurse starts oxygen administration immediately. Which of the following statements concerning this situation is the correct one?

   1. The physician did not have the patient on oxygen so the nurse needs to get an order for oxygen.

   2. The physician should have been called for an order before oxygen was begun.

   3. The symptoms were too vague for the nurse to diagnose a need for oxygen.

   4. The nurse's observations were sufficient to begin administration of oxygen in the CCU.

30. After ambulating for 5 min, the patient states that she has anginal pain. The nurse realizes that angina pectoris is a sign of

   1. Myocardial ischemia.

   2. Myocardial infarction.

   3. Coronary thrombosis.

   4. Mitral valve insufficiency.

31. The nurse would tell the patient that she should suspect the nitroglycerin tablets to have lost their potency when

   1. Slight tingling is absent when the tablet is placed under her tongue.

   2. Onset of relief is delayed, but duration of relief is unchanged.

3. Pain occurs even after taking the tablet prophylactically to prevent the onset of pain.

4. Pain is unrelieved, and facial flushing is increased.

32. The patient has a Swan-Ganz catheter inserted into the subclavian artery to measure PAP. This provides useful information about

   1. Left and right ventricular malfunction and cardiac output.

   2. Left and right ventricular function and cardiac output.

   3. Left ventricular rate and rhythm and cardiac output.

   4. Right ventricular rate and rhythm and oxygen consumption.

33. Using a Swan-Ganz catheter, which reading of PCWP would indicate severe pulmonary edema?

   1. A reading of 6 to 15 mm Hg.

   2. A reading of 10 to 17 mm Hg.

   3. A reading of 18 to 20 mm Hg.

   4. A reading of 35 to 40 mm Hg.

34. Which of the following descriptions correctly defines cor pulmonale?

   1. Hypertrophy of the right ventricle; approximately 85 percent of these patients have COPD.

   2. Hypertrophy of the left ventricle; approximately 85 percent of these patients have CHF.

   3. Tetralogy of Fallot causing hypertrophy of the left and right ventricles.

   4. Ventricle septal defect permitting unoxygenated blood to mix with oxygenated blood.

35. The signs and symptoms of cardiogenic shock are

   1. A drop in systolic pressure 10 mm Hg below systolic baseline, with headaches and rapid shallow respirations.

   2. Rapid shallow respirations, polyuria, and a drop in blood pressure below patient's baseline.

   3. Cold pale skin, bounding pulse, hyperventilation, and tachycardia.

   4. Poor tissue perfusion, cold, pale, clammy skin, and a drop in systolic blood pressure of 30 mm Hg below baseline.

36. In caring for an elderly diabetic patient with varicose veins, the nurse would instruct the patient to

   1. Cut toenails with a sharp razor straight across and around the edges.

   2. Stand as much as possible on the unaffected leg, resting the affected leg.

   3. Keep lower extremities level with the body.

   4. Keep lower extremities elevated and warm.

QUESTIONS 37 TO 40

Match each mechanism of action with the appropriate drug.

37. ___ Dilates vein and arteries

38. ___ Hypertensive crisis

39. ___ Antihypertensive agent that dilates arterioles

40. ___ Is a calcium channel blocker

1. Diltiazem (Cardizem)

2. Nitroprusside (Nipride)

3. Hydralazine (Alazine)

4. Prazosin (Minipress) alpha blocker

End of Case

41. A 73-year-old female patient is admitted to the emergency room complaining of chest pain that radiates down her left arm and up into her left jaw. The results of diagnostic tests confirm that the patient has had an MI. She is admitted to the coronary care unit. Orders for this patient include complete bed rest and morphine sulfate for relief of pain every 3 h. Which of the following sequences of pathologic changes have occurred with this patient?
    1. Thrombosis of the carotid artery, followed by inflammation of the endocardium of the left ventricle.
    2. Occlusion of the coronary sinus, followed by reduced blood oxygen levels in the myocardium of the left atrium.
    3. Interruption of coronary circulation, followed by hypoxia of the myocardium and muscle damage.
    4. Formation of an atheromatous plaque in the pericardium, followed by an increased hypoxia of the major organs of the body.

42. Which coping mechanism will this patient be expected to use when dealing with the anxiety that accompanies a life-threatening illness?
    1. Suppression.
    2. Sublimation.
    3. Denial.
    4. Depression.

43. A female patient had an MI and has been in the cardiac care unit for 3 days. Her condition improves, and she is to be transferred to a medical unit. When informed of the transfer, she becomes upset and says, "Who will be there to take care of me?" To lessen the patient's anxiety, it is most important that the nurse's response would be
    1. "The unit nurses have experience in caring for patients from this unit."
    2. "I understand your concerns. Someone from this unit will visit you every day."
    3. "Can you tell me about your concerns? We will convey them to the nurses on the unit."

    4. "To recover, you should begin taking care of yourself so that you will be independent when you go home."

44. A male patient who had an MI has been in the cardiac care unit for 4 days. He complains of epigastric pain after eating a light supper. The nurse's evaluation of the patient's complaint should be based on an understanding of his condition at this time, which is
    1. An extension of an infarction can occur during the convalescent period.
    2. Elevated cholesterol levels can lead to gallbladder distress.
    3. Excitement increases gastric motility.
    4. Indigestion occurs in patients with heart disease.

45. The patient shows signs and symptoms of cardiogenic shock. The signs that are indicators of cardiogenic shock are
    1. Increased PCWP; cold, pale, clammy skin; drop in systolic pressure; and a weak, thready pulse.
    2. Decreased PCWP, nausea, hypertension, and increased respirations.
    3. Bradycardia, hypotension, and increased PCWP.
    4. Decreased PCWP, decrease in urinary output, and hypotension.

46. Which of the following functions is provided by a demand pacemaker?
    1. A continuous stimuli to the heart muscle, resulting in a fixed heart rate.
    2. Stimuli to the heart muscle only when the heart begins to beat irregularly.
    3. Stimuli to the heart muscle only when the heart rate falls below a specified level.
    4. Continuous stimuli to the heart muscle whenever ventricular fibrillation is present.

47. Systolic hypertension (systolic pressure >150 mm Hg) may develop as a result of
    1. An increase in the heart's electrical activity, causing hypertrophy of the heart muscle.
    2. Loss of elastic tissue or an aneurysm occurring in the aorta or other large blood vessels.
    3. Volume expanders administered too rapidly, renal stenosis, or increased salt intake.
    4. Anaphylactic shock or increase in electrical activity of the heart, causing the heart to hypertrophy.

48. Which of the following is the priority immediately following a coronary artery bypass graft?
    1. Patient teaching and assessing peripheral circulation.
    2. Assessing and stabilizing the patient.
    3. Assessing the patient's dressing for blood and pus.
    4. Maintaining blood pressure of 150 systole and 60 diastole.

49. Inserting a balloon-tipped catheter into the lumen of a coronary artery and inflating the balloon to push plaque back to the side of the artery is called a
1. Coronary artery bypass graft.
2. Aortocoronary bypass.
3. Cardiopulmonary bypass.
4. Percutaneous transluminal coronary angioplasty.

50. Postoperatively, the primary focus for the patient who has undergone a heart transplant is the prevention of
1. Rejection and MI.
2. Infection and rejection.
3. Hemorrhage and infection.
4. Stroke and rejection.

51. The patient requires surgery because of mitral valve incompetence. He is admitted to the hospital and states, "I need a new valve, an oil change, and a lube job!" What is the nurse's most appropriate response to the patient?
1. "I'm glad to see you're handling the situation so well."
2. "I'm sure you have a great deal to ask about this procedure."
3. "You really don't need to hide your anxieties."
4. "You've sure come to the right place for a valve job."

52. Which one of the following signs is the nurse most likely to observe *first* when a patient is developing digitalis toxicity?
1. Heart murmur, nausea, and vomiting.
2. Slow pulse rate.
3. Slow respiratory rate, nausea, and vomiting.
4. Drop in blood pressure.

53. Pulmonary embolism is a common cause of mortality among hospitalized patients. The nurse should recognize the grouping of symptoms of pulmonary embolism as
1. Fine rales throughout both lung fields and pink frothy sputum.
2. Dry persistent cough, restlessness, and drowsiness.
3. Viselike substernal pain and radiation to the left arm and jaw.
4. Chest pain that radiates like a knife through to the shoulders, dyspnea, tachycardia, and hemoptysis.

54. Which term describes intermittent third-degree heart block?
1. Stokes-Adams attack.
2. Leriche's syndrome.
3. Mobitz type I.
4. Mobitz type II.

55. The nurse should carefully evaluate the pulse and blood pressure reading prior to administering which of the following antihypertensive and antiarrhythmia drugs?
1. Sulfinpyrazone (Anturane) and calcitonin (Calcimar).
2. Propranolol (Inderal) and clonidine (Catapres).

3. Glucagon and pyridostigmine bromide (Mestinon).
4. Hydroxyzine (Vistaril) and prazosin hydrochloride (Minipress).

56. The patient has cardiac and renal damage related to his hypertensive condition. When teaching the patient about his diet, the nurse should advise him to
1. Drink plenty of whole milk and eat milk products.
2. Use salt substitutes, such as potassium chloride.
3. Increase the meat in his diet.
4. Decrease intake of processed foods and add fresh fruits and juices to diet.

57. The patient goes into hypertensive crisis. Diazoxide (Hyperstat IV) is ordered. The nursing action required during the time the drug is being administered is to
1. Monitor glucose levels.
2. Regulate infusion with a pump.
3. Place the patient in a semi-Fowler's position.
4. Cover the solution with aluminum foil.

QUESTIONS 58 TO 61

Match the clinical condition with its most likely cause.

58. ___ Aplastic anemia
59. ___ Sickle cell anemia
60. ___ Polycythemia Vera
61. ___ Thrombocytopenia (purpura)

1. Platelet destruction
2. Erythrocyte destruction
3. Bone marrow depression
4. Excessive production of erythrocytes

End of Case

QUESTIONS 62 TO 65

Match the condition with the phrase that most closely describes it.

62. ___ Raynaud's disease
63. ___ Disseminated intravascular coagulation
64. ___ Buerger's disease
65. ___ Pheochromocytoma

1. Excessive vascular blood clotting
2. Inflammation of arteries and veins
3. Intermittent spasms
4. Severe hypertension

66. A severely anemic patient is being treated with blood transfusions. The symptoms that are the first indications of hemolytic blood transfusion reaction are
1. Tachycardia, fever, chills, flushing, and lumbar pain.
2. Headache, hot flashes, arrhythmias, and dyspnea.
3. Tingling of fingers, cramping, headache, and vertigo.
4. Leg and abdominal pain, diarrhea, and uremia.

67. A patient complains of severe chest pain and left arm pain. The nurse should first
    1. Call the physician and place the patient on a cardiac monitor.
    2. Take the patient's blood pressure.
    3. Assess the patient and gather more information.
    4. Place the patient in a high Fowler's position and start oxygen.

68. The nurse on the day shift is a registered nurse, and she reports to the evening shift that a patient has experienced chest pain and cardiac arrhythmias throughout the afternoon. The nurse on the evening shift should first
    1. Tell the physician when he comes on the floor.
    2. Talk with the patient and help reduce her anxiety.
    3. Put the patient on a cardiac monitor immediately.
    4. Spend some time talking with and assessing the patient.

69. Which of the following groups of symptoms causes secondary hypertension?
    1. Obesity, high sodium intake, tobacco use, and renal artery stenosis.
    2. Renal artery stenosis, Cushing's syndrome, and pheochromocytoma.
    3. Fluid overload, high sodium intake, and stenosis of the aorta.
    4. Stress, high sodium intake, and an increase in blood pressures.

70. With nitroglycerin and modifications in lifestyle, a patient is able to control his angina attacks for several months. One night, however, he is awakened by excruciating chest pain that is not relieved by nitroglycerin. He is rushed to the hospital and admitted to the CCU with a diagnosis of an acute MI. Which priority of care is necessary for the patient with an acute MI?
    1. Reducing environmental stress.
    2. Relieving pain.
    3. Maintaining bed rest.
    4. Identifying emotional conflicts.

71. Several days after his MI, the patient expresses concern about the possibility of engaging in sexual intercourse in 1 month. The nurse should emphasize to the patient that
    1. Impotence is a major side effect of nitroglycerin.
    2. Sexual intercourse is contraindicated at this time but may be resumed after 5 months.
    3. Nitroglycerin should be taken before sexual intercourse.
    4. Before resuming sexual relations, the physician must be notified.

72. If the patient has an unmonitored cardiac arrest, the initial action by the rescuer, before starting cardiopulmonary resuscitation (CPR), is to
    1. Check for dilated pupils.
    2. Establish unresponsiveness.
    3. Palpate the carotid artery.
    4. Listen for breathing.

73. What is the rate of CPR when two rescuers are present?
    1. Provide 15 chest compressions for every 2 rescue breaths whether or not 1 or 2 rescuers are present.
    2. One lung inflation to 10 cardiac compressions.
    3. Two lung inflations to 15 cardiac compressions.
    4. Four lung inflations to 15 cardiac compressions.

74. During cardiac compression, manual pressure is applied to which area of the body?
    1. The area under the left nipple.
    2. The area halfway between the sternum and the left nipple.
    3. The lower half of the sternum.
    4. The midsternal area.

75. Many enzymes are released into the blood stream in increased quantities in response to an MI. The combinations of enzymes that are specific to the heart are
    1. Serum aminotransferase enzymes aspartate transaminase (AST), alanine transaminase (ALT), and creatinine phosphokinase (CK).
    2. Serum aminotransferase enzymes serum glutamic oxaloacetic transaminase (SGOT), serum glutamic pyruvic transaminase (SGPT), and CK.
    3. CK-MB isoenzymes and lactic dehydrogenase LDH1 is higher than LDH2.
    4. Lactic dehydrogenase LDH2 and serum aminotransferase enzymes AST and ALT.

76. Changes in the ECG or the cardiac monitor that indicate an MI are
    1. PVCs, absence of the P wave, and tachycardia.
    2. Prolonged PR interval and arrhythmias.
    3. Narrowing of the QRS complex and PVCs.
    4. Depressed ST segments, inverted T wave, and pathologic Q wave.

77. While in the CCU, the patient develops PVCs. The nurse should recognize that the greatest danger of this type of arrhythmia is that it can cause
    1. AV heart block.
    2. Sinus tachycardia.
    3. Paroxysmal atrial tachycardia (PAT) Preatrial contractions (PACs).
    4. Ventricular fibrillation.

78. The patient is given an IV bolus of lidocaine 75 mg, followed by IV administration of 250 mL of D_5W, which contains 1000 mg of lidocaine. The physician orders lidocaine to be administered at the rate of 1 mg/min. The drop (gtt) factor of the IV administration set is 60 drops/mL. The nurse should regulate the infusion (in gtt/min) at

1. Fifteen.
2. Thirty.
3. Forty-five.
4. Sixty.

79. When the patient returns to the clinic for his monthly checkup after having an MI, his wife states, "I don't know what is wrong with my husband. All he wants to do is sit around the house when he comes home from work. He said the physician told him to take it easy, but he does nothing!" The most appropriate action of the health team is to
    1. Caution the patient's wife that the patient should limit his daily living activity.
    2. Assist the patient and his wife in understanding that fear of heart disease may make him an invalid.
    3. Assist the patient in making plans to take more responsibility at home.
    4. Suggest ways and means for the patient and his wife to become more socially involved.

80. What is the expected outcome of lidocaine therapy?
    1. Elevated blood pressure.
    2. Controlled ventricular arrhythmias.
    3. Increased cardiac output.
    4. Relieved chest pain.

81. The nursing order states, "Observe for early signs of lidocaine toxicity." The group of toxic symptoms most often associated with lidocaine is
    1. Circumoral flush, dilated pupils, increased pulse rate, and dryness of the mouth.
    2. Constricted pupils, elevated blood pressure, coma, and respiratory arrest.
    3. Bradycardia, hypotension, confusion, and severe dizziness or fainting.
    4. Polyuria, tachycardia, headache, and increased salivation.

QUESTIONS 82 TO 85

Match the clinical condition with the phrase that is most related to it.

82. ___ Tetralogy of Fallot

83. ___ Myocarditis

84. ___ Rheumatic fever

85. ___ Secondary hypertension

1. Potential for mitral valve insufficiency
2. Children habitually squat when they feel short of breath
3. Inflammation of the cardiac muscle
4. Renal artery stenosis

End of Case

86. Which of the following phrases correctly describes cardiac tamponade?
    1. Restricted movement of the pericardial and vascular fluid.
    2. Compression of the chest wall against the heart and lungs.
    3. Compression of the heart and lungs as a result of thoracotomy.
    4. Compression of the heart as a result of increased fluid within the pericardial sac.

87. Syphilitic aortitis will result in regurgitation of blood into the
    1. Right ventricle with dilation and hypertrophy.
    2. Left atrium with dilation and hypertrophy.
    3. Left ventricle with dilation and hypertrophy.
    4. Left ventricle with dilation and regurgitation.

88. Which of the following conditions is caused by aortic stenosis?
    1. Decreased cardiac output, symptoms of angina, syncope on exertion, tachyarrhythmias, or bradyarrhythmias.
    2. Decreased cardiac contraction, right ventricular hypertrophy, angina pain, and fainting.
    3. Decreased cardiac contractions, hypertension, dyspnea, and hemoptysis.
    4. Right ventricular hypertrophy, angina, and dyspnea.

89. In which situation is contractility of the myocardium decreased?
    1. Increase in calcium intake.
    2. In the early stages of hypovolemic shock.
    3. Administration of epinephrine.
    4. In the later stages of MI (acidosis).

90. When PVCs are present, the stimulant for the heartbeat originates in the
    1. Atria.
    2. SA node.
    3. AV node.
    4. Ventricle.

91. When ventricular tachycardia is present, the atria and ventricles will characteristically beat
    1. Simultaneously.
    2. Very rapidly.
    3. Independently of each other.
    4. At the same rate that the patient breathes.

92. When a patient is receiving propranolol hydrochloride (Inderal), the nurse must observe for
    1. Ataxia.
    2. Bradycardia.
    3. Automaticity.
    4. Hypertension.

93. A dopamine (high dosage) drip is infusing. The expected action of this drug is

1. Decreased urine output and increased CVP.
2. Peripheral vasoconstriction, causing increased blood pressure.
3. Increased contractility of the heart and decreased blood pressure.
4. Decreased urine output and increased afterload.

94. Rapid supraventricular arrhythmias are dangerous because

1. They are often accompanied by chest pain.
2. They frequently progress to hypertension.
3. Ventricular filling is compromised.
4. They are chronic.

95. The patient states he had been told he has a mitral murmur, which can best be heard at the

1. Apex of the heart, at the fifth intercostal space.
2. Right posterior lung base below the heart.
3. Second intercostal space left of the sternum.
4. Third intercostal space to the right of the sternum.

96. A 65-year-old man has been diagnosed as having chronic CHF. The appropriate medications and procedures would be

1. Furosemide (Lasix), plasminogen, and liquid diet.
2. Nitroglycerin (Nitro-Bid), furosemide (Lasix), bed rest, and liquid diet.
3. Furosemide (Lasix), out of bed as desired, digoxin (Lanoxin), and low-sodium diet.
4. Ambulate every other day, no sodium in diet, IV set at KVO.

97. The most appropriate action taken before the nurse can perform postmortem care is

1. A physician has assessed the body, and the family has been notified.
2. A physician has ordered the IV and Foley catheter to be discontinued.
3. The death certificate has been signed, and the family has been notified.
4. The family and physician have left the room.

QUESTIONS 98 TO 100

98. Edward, a 58-year-old man, is admitted to the hospital with a diagnosis of hypertension and cardiac arrhythmias. The patient asks the nurse how hypertension is diagnosed. The nurse should explain that

1. Hypertensive blood pressure levels have been established by the American Heart Association.
2. Blood pressure must be elevated at three successive readings on separate days.

3. Coexisting symptoms of headache and nosebleeds confirm the diagnosis.
4. A diagnosis of hypertension can only be made when the cause is known.

99. At the time of Edward's physical examination, the finding that is indicative of hypertension is

1. Pupil changes on ocular examination.
2. Presence of second heart sound.
3. Sinus rhythm on auscultation.
4. Cardiac enlargement on percussion.

100. Laboratory studies to determine if surgical intervention will correct the patient's hypertensive condition would include levels of

1. Catecholamines.
2. Protein in the urine.
3. Blood urea nitrogen (BUN).
4. Triglycerides and cholesterol.

End of Case

ANSWERS AND RATIONALES

1. ❷ Side effects of nitroglycerin are tachycardia, syncope, headaches, and hypotension. Nitroglycerin is a coronary vasodilator, which is used as a long-term prophylactic in the management of angina pectoris. It can be administered sublingually or by extended-release tablets, buccal tablets, ointment, and by the transdermal system (skin patches).

(1, 3, 4) These options are incorrect as seen in rationale (2).

2. ❶ The nurse should instruct the patient that in an acute attack of angina pain, the patient should repeat medication (nitroglycerin) every 5 to 8 min for 15 min and, if pain persists, call the physician.

(2) If the pain persists, waiting 10 to 15 min could result in an MI. Blood would not be perfusing the heart at the area of vasoconstriction, and a cardiac arrhythmia could occur because the heart muscle becomes irritable when an area of the heart becomes hypoxic.

(3) If the pain is not relieved after 15 min of repeated use of nitroglycerin tablets, then the patient may be having an MI; therefore, he or she should call a physician immediately if pain is not relieved in 15 min. Nitroglycerin would not be repeated every 15 min for one-half hour (the patient may be having an MI).

(4) The patient may be having an MI; therefore, repeating the nitroglycerin until the pain is gone is not good advice.

3. ❶ A good way to reduce future angina attacks is to set up a regular program of exercise. In this way, the patient will gradually increase blood perfusion of the heart and strengthen the cardiac muscle, which will help reduce future attacks. Instruct the patient to establish a regular exercise program. Enhance activity tolerance by encouraging slower activity or shorter periods of activity with more rest periods. Most patients with angina pectoris can tolerate mild exercise, such as walking and playing golf, but exertion, such as running, climbing hills or stairs rapidly, and lifting heavy objects, causes pain. The regular exercise program may include walking 15 min or riding a bicycle every day and gradually increasing the time spent exercising.

(2) There is no reason for a patient to be on a low-sodium diet. This patient is not retaining fluids as he would be if he had CHF. Angina is the vasoconstriction of the coronary arteries, and when no blood reaches the heart, that part of the heart suffers from ischemia, which causes pain. Swimming 2 h twice per day will overwork the heart and cause angina pain, and it may cause an MI.

If a rubber band is put around a finger and is left on for a while, the tip of the finger will hurt because of obstruction (ischemia) to the tissue. When the rubber band is removed, the pain goes away. Removing the rubber band is like giving nitroglycerin: it causes coronary vasodilation and thus relieves the angina pain.

CHF is failure of the heart to work as a pump; therefore, the heart fails to perfuse the kidney. The kidney "thinks" the body is low on fluid so it releases renin-angiotensin, which stimulates the release of aldosterone, and aldosterone retains sodium. The sodium retains water, and the patient's CHF increases. The patient must be on a low-sodium diet.

(3) Running one-half mile and riding a bicycle 1 mile each day may cause an MI in a patient with angina. The patient may have severe angina pain after running one-fourth of a mile or less.

(4) Reducing the number of hours the patient works would not help to reduce angina attacks as much as increasing an activity level to improve the cardiovascular system. Some people enjoy working and may have less angina pain while working than when not working because they may experience less anxiety in the workplace than at home. Anxiety increases the release of catecholamines, which cause vasoconstriction and increase angina pain.

4. **①** One of the most common and most serious complications of an MI is a cardiac arrhythmia. The most dangerous is ventricular fibrillation, which may cause death.

(2) Anaphylactic shock is a generalized allergic reaction. For example, a patient may go into anaphylactic shock after receiving penicillin if they are allergic to it. The vascular system dilates and the patient's blood pressure falls, causing hypovolemia. (Total blood volume remains the same, but it is redistributed into smaller vessels. Without vasoconstriction, the blood pools in the extremities and the vital organs are *not* perfused.) The patient can die of anaphylactic shock.

(3) Cardiac enlargement may occur for many reasons. For example, in cardiomyopathy, there is gross dilation of the ventricles. The cause of most cardiomyopathies is unknown.

(4) Primary (essential) hypertension affects at least 15 percent of the adult population in the United States. Hypertensive disease constitutes the major risk factor for coronary, cerebral,

renal, and peripheral vascular diseases. Essential hypertension most commonly develops in middle-aged and older persons. The prevalence of hypertension among African-Americans is twice that of the white population. The cause of essential hypertension remains debatable. It is not a complication of an MI; it is a major cause of MI.

5. **②** Lidocaine is the drug of choice in treating ventricular arrhythmias.

(1) Digoxin (Lanoxin) is the drug of choice in treating CHF. It increases cardiac output by increasing the force of contractions. It is not used for ventricle irritability.

(3) Lasix is a diuretic and will increase urinary output. Lasix is used most often for CHF to help reduce excess fluid volume.

(4) Sodium bicarbonate is used in cases of metabolic acidosis.

6. **②** Coumadin should not be taken the day before a patient has a blood test because it would increase the risk of bleeding from the site where the blood was drawn. A patient in the hospital is closely monitored for bleeding, so blood may be drawn; however, a patient at home is not closely monitored. If a patient cannot be closely monitored for bleeding, he or she should not take Coumadin the day before a blood test.

(1) Other medications may interfere with the action of Coumadin. Barbiturates, oral contraceptives containing estrogen, and many other drugs may decrease or increase the anticoagulant response to Coumadin. Alcohol may also interfere with the action of Coumadin.

(3) A soft tooth brush minimizes gum bleeding; a hard tooth brush will increase bleeding.

(4) The patient usually is advised not to take Coumadin the day before having a blood test. Taking an extra Coumadin would increase the patient's risk for bleeding.

7. **②** MI pain is not relieved with rest; angina pain is relieved with rest.

(1) The pain of an MI is more intense than angina pain.

(3) The pain of an MI is acute, and the person complains of feeling a heavy weight on the chest. Angina pain is not as acute as MI pain.

(4) The pain of an MI may radiate from the left arm to the jaw. Angina pain may radiate to the arm but does not affect the fingers more than the arm.

8. **④** In a paradoxic response, the patient experiences an adverse effect that is opposite of the effect that the drug normally produces. In this situation, methyldopa (Aldomet) was given to decrease blood pressure, but instead it increased blood pressure, which is a paradoxic response. Aldomet is an alpha blocker; therefore, it causes peripheral vasodilation.

(1) In a synergistic response, two drugs work together to accomplish an effect.

(2, 3) In individual hypersensitivity, an individual is allergic to a substance (allergen) that does not normally cause a reaction. It is essentially an antigen–antibody reaction. The reaction is due to the release of a histamine substance from injured cells.

9. ❹ CVP will be elevated in CHF. The heart fails to perfuse the kidneys, so the kidneys "think" the body is low on fluid, and they release aldosterone to save sodium, which then causes water retention. Sodium and water retention by the kidneys causes increased venous pressure. The more fluid that is retained, the higher the CVP. A low CVP reading is seen in patients with severe vasodilation (shock) or hemorrhage.

The CVP measures the pressure within the superior vena cava. It reflects the pressure under which the blood is returned to the superior vena cava (right atrium). Normal CVP usually is between 4 and 10 cm H_2O, or 2 to 12 mm Hg. In the case of CHF, the CVP will be greater than 15 cm H_2O. CVP is a reflection of right heart function and is not a satisfactory means of determining the status of left heart function. (The most commonly used catheter for measuring left and right heart function is the Swan-Ganz catheter.)

There are at least three lumens. One lumen terminates in the right atrium to allow for CVP monitoring; one lumen is wedged in the PA to measure PCWP, which reflects left heart function; and the third lumen is the computer port in the PA. Normal PCWP is 8 to 13 mm Hg. Elevation greater than 18 to 20 mm Hg indicates a degree of left ventricular failure, if 30 mm Hg CHF is indicated.

Normal CVP measured by a Swan-Ganz catheter is 2 to 12 mm Hg, and normal CVP measured by water is 4 to 10 cm.

(1) Venous pressure would be decreased in the case of hypovolemia (low blood volume).

(2) When pulmonary circulation is not maintained, there would be a drop in CVP, as seen in neurogenic shock.

(3) A patient with extensive bleeding would have decreased CVP because blood is lost from the body; therefore, fluid volume is decreased.

10. ❷ Demerol is given to a patient with acute CHF to relieve anxiety. When patients feel as if they are suffocating, they become anxious and afraid that they are dying. Fear and anxiety release large amounts of epinephrine and norepinephrine, and this causes vasoconstriction and tachycardia, resulting in the heart having to work harder. Vasoconstriction reduces the blood supply to the lungs, causing increased dyspnea.

(1, 3, 4) Demerol does not cause coronary vasodilation or increase urinary output. The patient has difficulty breathing, not painful breathing.

11. ❹ Chlorothiazide is the most useful group of diuretics because it is the most effective with the least amount of side effects.

(1) Diuretics do not cause sodium (Na) reabsorption.

(2) Chlorothiazide is used to treat CHF; other types of diuretics are also used.

(3) Chlorothiazide has the smallest amount of side effects, not the most.

12. ❹ The rationale for fluid and sodium restriction in a patient with CHF is that sodium retains fluids, and fluid increases the workload of the heart. As fluid is retained, the heart has even more difficulty perfusing the kidney, more aldosterone is released, and sodium and fluid are retained.

(1) Sodium does not cause vasoconstriction; it will increase the workload of the heart by increasing fluid retention.

(2) If sodium is retained by the kidneys, then potassium is excreted by the kidneys.

(3) Too much fluid will not cause hypokalemia or arrhythmias. Hypokalemia occurs when potassium is lost from the GI tract or excreted in large amounts by the kidney. When the kidney retains sodium, it excretes potassium.

13. ❷ In the clinical setting, the most common cause of cardiac overload (CHF), especially in the very young and the elderly, is excessive intravenous infusion.

(1) Fluids by mouth should not be forced. It would be extremely difficult to cause fluid overload by oral intake unless the patient was in kidney failure.

(3) Cardiac arrhythmia cannot increase fluid in the body, so it cannot cause cardiac fluid overload. If the patient was in ventricular fibrillation, there may be pulmonary congestion because the heart is failing to move blood out of the pulmonary system.

(4) Mitral valve disease cannot increase fluid in the body, so it will not cause cardiac fluid overload. Mitral valve disease can cause arrhythmia and CHF.

14. ❸ Digitalis will increase the heart's force of contraction and increase cardiac output, reducing fluid congestion. Bed rest will cause diuresis; the reason is unknown, but it is believed that the kidney is better perfused when the patient is lying down, which increases urinary output.

(1) Epinephrine would increase the heart rate, which would somewhat increase cardiac output. However, the heart is failing as a pump, so speeding up the rate is of little use and may cause the heart to fail more. Valium would decrease the patient's anxiety, but its sedative effect on the body may reduce cardiac output. A patient in acute CHF cannot be placed in a semi-Fowler's position; the patient must be in a high Fowler's position, which allows the fluid in the lungs to drain to the base of the lungs, allowing the upper part of the lungs to move oxygen in and carbon dioxide out of the lungs. If a patient were to lie flat in bed, as in the case of acute CHF, he or she may drown in his or her own lung fluids.

(2) Lidocaine is used to treat ventricular arrhythmia and can be given intramuscularly (IM) or intravenously (IV). It should be given IM during transport to the hospital if IV lidocaine is not available. The use of epinephrine and being placed in a semi-Fowler's position in the case of a patient with CHF are discussed in rationale (1).

(4) Use of Valium in CHF is discussed in rationale (1). Administration of oxygen in CHF is very helpful because it reduces the possibility of the patient going into respiratory acidosis from excess carbon dioxide. Carbon dioxide is exchanged for oxygen in the lung, so increasing oxygen decreases carbon dioxide. Patients in acute CHF are unable to exercise because all of their energy is needed to breathe and stay alive.

15. **④** Rales (coarse crackles), shortness of breath, and generalized cyanosis are signs and symptoms of acute CHF. The rales are the sound of air moving through fluid in the lungs. Shortness of breath is caused by low oxygen and high carbon dioxide content in the lungs. The fluid in the lungs interferes with the adequate exchange of carbon dioxide for oxygen. Generalized cyanosis is caused by lack of oxygen in the peripheral circulation, because the heart is failing as a pump and is unable to perfuse the body with oxygen.

CHF is left-sided heart failure. When the left side of the heart fails, the blood backs into the lung through the pulmonary veins. The pulmonary veins carry blood from the lungs to the left atrium; however, there are no valves in these veins to stop the blood, so when the left side of the heart cannot pump the blood to the body, the blood backs up into the lungs.

The aorta (which pumps blood to the body) comes out of the left ventricle, which has a valve (aortic valve), so blood cannot back up in that direction. This valve is closed after the ventricle contracts and pushes oxygenated blood to the extremities. Peripheral edema is a sign of right-sided heart failure, not CHF, which is left-sided heart failure.

(1) In right-sided heart failure, there will be peripheral edema. When the right side of the heart fails as a pump, the blood backs up through the superior and inferior venae cavae because there are no valves in either vena cava. This blood then can back up into the periphery and cause peripheral edema.

The blood cannot back up into the lungs because the PA has a valve (pulmonary valve) that closes after the ventricle contracts and pushes unoxygenated blood into the lungs.

The venae cavae bring unoxygenated blood to the right atrium. When the right side of the heart fails, blood backs up through the venae cavae and into the body. Localized cyanosis means that there was cyanosis of the extremities, such as fingers and toes, which does not occur with CHF. Generalized cyanosis may occur in acute CHF and in ventricular arrhythmias.

(2) Shortness of breath is caused by a lack of oxygen. The fluid in the lung interferes with the exchange of carbon dioxide for oxygen. Chest pain is not a sign of CHF. Cyanosis is discussed in rationale (1).

(3) Cardiac arrhythmias are not a sign of CHF. CHF can cause arrhythmias because the heart has to work hard to move excess fluid that has accumulated as a result of the heart's failure as a pump. Ascites is not a sign of CHF. Ascites occurs when there is not enough protein (osmotic pressure) to hold fluid in the vascular system. The fluid will leak out of the vascular system and cause ascites (fluid in the peritoneal cavity). Peripheral edema is discussed in rationale (1).

16. **②** Low potassium levels will increase the development of digitalis toxicity. Potassium tends to maintain the effectiveness of digitalis. A low potassium level in the body allows digitalis to be much more effective and can cause digitalis toxicity.

(1, 3, 4) A low sodium level, high glucose level, or high calcium level will not cause digitalis toxicity.

17. **①** Digitalis should not be administered if the adult's heart rate is less than 60 bpm. Digitalis slows conduction at the AV node and, thus, reduces the heart rate. If the patient's heart rate falls below 60 bpm, this may be an indication of digitalis toxicity. (Digitalis should not be given to children with a heart rate below 70 bpm and should not be given to infants with a heart rate below 90 bpm.)

(2, 3, 4) These options are incorrect as seen in rationale (1). Digitalis normally is not withheld because of an irregular heart beat, unless the cardiac rate is less than 60 bpm. Digitalis is the drug of choice for atrial arrhythmias unless the arrhythmia is caused by digitalis toxicities; then propranolol (Inderal) or quinidine is used. Digitalis (Lanoxin) would be withheld if the ventricular arrhythmia was severe.

18. **③** The foods, condiments, and fluids highest in potassium chloride (KCl) are bananas, prunes, oranges, instant coffee, and salt substitutes.

(1, 2, 4) These foods are not high in potassium as are the foods in rationale (3).

19. **③** Peritrate is a nitrate that produces vasodilation. It dilates coronary arteries and improves collateral flow to ischemic regions, and it relieves anginal attacks and increases cardiac output. Peritrate may cause hypotension and dizziness (a sign of hypotension). Keep the patient in bed, do not give this dose of Peritrate, take the patient's pressure, and notify the physician if the blood pressure is unusually low. If the patient is allowed to get out of bed, he or she might faint because of orthostatic hypotension.

(1, 2, 4) These options are incorrect as seen in rationale (3).

20. **①** Amyl nitrate by inhalation usually is prescribed to relieve acute angina pain.

(2, 3, 4) Amyl nitrate cannot be administered sublingually, topically, or parentally.

21. **④** Digitalis is withheld if the adult apical pulse rate is 60 bpm or below. The physician should be notified immediately (stat). This pulse rate is especially dangerous when the patient is receiving digitalis. A slow pulse rate of 55 bpm may indicate digitalis toxicity and heart block because digitalis slows conduction of the AV node.

(1, 2, 3) These options are incorrect as seen in rationale (4).

22. **①** The therapeutic effects of digitalis are stimulation of the myocardium to contract more forcefully, increasing cardiac output, decreasing cardiac rate, and slowing conduction at the AV node.

(2, 3, 4) These options are incorrect as seen in rationale (1).

23. **③** The geriatric patient should be observed for psychotomimetic effects. The elderly use more medications than any other age group, averaging more than 13 prescriptions and renewals per year. Brain dysfunction in the elderly is secondary to any number of causes, including physical illness, drug or alcohol toxicity, dehydration, fecal impaction, malnutrition, infection, lack of environmental cues, and sensory deprivation or overload.

Older adults are particularly vulnerable to symptoms of delirium because of their marginal metabolic reserve, the high number of medications they usually take, and the reduced capacity of the liver to metabolize and the kidney to excrete the drugs. This lowers the ability and the efficiency of the circulatory system and the nervous system to cope with the effects of certain drugs.

The possibility of interaction between drugs is further magnified if the older person is also taking one or more over-the-counter (OTC) drugs. Because geriatric patients may have some senility along with other problems, it is important that the geriatric patient taking digitalis be monitored closely so that early signs of digitalis toxicity will be noticed. The first sign of digitalis toxicity may be psychotomimetic effects (hallucinogenic and strange illusions).

(1, 2, 4) These options are incorrect as seen in rationale (3).

24. ❹ When instructing a patient with sickle cell anemia, the nurse should explain that sickling (cell destruction) is more likely to occur when oxygen levels are low.

(1, 2, 3) Dyspnea, nausea, vomiting, and urinary failure are not caused by cell sickling.

25. ❶ A newborn with sickle cell anemia will be symptom-free because the high level of hemoglobin in fetal blood helps prevent sickling of the red blood cells.

(2, 3, 4) These options are incorrect as seen in rationale (1).

26. ❸ Before the nurse administers heparin on the second day of hospitalization, the information most essential to obtain is the patient's partial thromboplastin time (PTT).

The effect of heparin is immediate and short lived. This drug is often given during cardiac and vascular surgery to prevent intravascular clotting during clamping of the vessels.

The antidote used to reverse the effect of heparin is protamine sulfate. Because clotting factors II, IX, and X are vitamin K-dependent factors (produced in the liver), biliary obstruction, which interferes with the absorption of fat-soluble vitamins, such as vitamin K, will prolong the PTT.

Because coagulation factors are produced in the liver, liver diseases will also prolong the PTT, and bleeding may result. Drugs that prolong PTT test values include heparin, salicylates, ascorbic acid (vitamin C), and antihistamines.

Coumadin is slow acting, but its action may persist for 7 to 14 days after discontinuation of the drug. The action of Coumadin can be enhanced by drugs such as aspirin, quinidine, and sulfonamides.

The antidote used to reverse the effects of Coumadin is vitamin K. Vitamin K is administered parenterally, slowly over 12 to 24 h.

(1, 2, 4) These options are incorrect as seen in rationale (3).

27. ❷ Before applying a warm compress to a patient's leg, the most essential procedure is to check the temperature of the compresses on the radial aspect of the wrist to be sure the compress will not burn the patient's skin. Elderly patients have less sensation in their legs, and their skin is thin and fragile and can be easily burned.

(1, 3, 4) These options are incorrect as seen in rationale.

28. ❶ The signs and symptoms of a pulmonary embolus are sharp, stabbing chest pain that intensifies on inspiration, tachycardia, dyspnea, productive cough (sputum may be blood tinged), low-grade fever, and pleural effusion.

(2, 3, 4) These options are incorrect as seen in rationale (1).

29. ❹ Nurses working in the cardiac care unit (CCU) are educated and trained in the care of patients with serious cardiovascular problems. Each CCU has standing doctor's orders that allow the RN to treat a patient stat without waiting for a physician's order. When the nurse notes changes in a patient's condition that indicate the need for oxygen, the nurse must begin administering oxygen immediately.

(1, 2, 3) These options are incorrect as seen in rationale (4).

30. ❶ Angina pain is a sign of myocardial ischemia. When nitroglycerin is administered, it will cause vasodilation of the coronary arteries. This allows blood to flow to the heart, and pain will be relieved.

(2) A normal amount of activity will not produce the pain of a MI, but it can produce anginal pain because activity can constrict the coronary artery. When the patient rests, the coronary arteries will dilate and pain will stop.

(3) Coronary thrombosis is the same as an MI.

(4) If a patient has mitral valve insufficiency, exercise will not cause pain, but it may cause dyspnea.

31. ❶ If nitroglycerin tablets do not tingle when placed under the tongue, this indicates that the tablets have lost their potency and should be discarded.

(2, 3, 4) These options are incorrect as seen in rationale (1).

32. ❷ A Swan-Ganz catheter may be used to measure left and right ventricular function and cardiac output.

(1) A Swan-Ganz catheter is not used to evaluate right and left ventricular malfunction. An ECG is used to determine cardiac arrhythmias, which are malfunctions of the heart. A Swan-Ganz catheter may be used to measure cardiac output, making this part of the rationale correct.

(3, 4) A Swan-Ganz catheter is not used to measure right or left ventricular rate and rhythm; however, it may be used to measure cardiac rate. A stethoscope or an ECG is used to determine rate and rhythm of the heart. The second part of these two rationales is correct. The Swan-Ganz catheter can be used to measure cardiac output.

33. ❹ A measure of 30 to 45 mm Hg indicates severe pulmonary edema.

(1, 2, 3) A PCWP reading of 6 to 15 mm Hg [as in rationale (1)] or 10 to 17 mm Hg [as in rationale] on a Swan-Ganz catheter may indicate hypotension, and a PCWP reading of 18 to 20 mm Hg [as in rationale (3)] would indicate a normal PCWP reading.

34. ❶ Cor pulmonale (right-sided heart failure) is hypertrophy of the right ventricle, and 85 percent of these patients will have COPD. When there is emphysema in the lungs, this forces the right ventricle to pump constantly and more forcefully in order to move the venous blood from the right ventricle to the lungs. This constant workload on the right ventricle causes it to hypertrophy and fail as a pump. When the right ventricle fails, the blood backs up through the superior and inferior venae cavae and into the extremities, causing peripheral edema.

(2, 3, 4) These options are incorrect as seen in rationale (1).

35. ❹ Signs and symptoms of cardiogenic shock are a systolic pressure 30 mm Hg below the patient's systolic baseline reading, weak and thready pulse, cardiac arrhythmias, poor tissue perfusion, and pale clammy skin.

(1) A drop in systolic pressure 10 mm Hg below systolic baseline is not enough of a drop to indicate cardiogenic shock. Headache is not a sign of cardiogenic shock. Rapid shallow respirations would not indicate cardiogenic shock. Respirations may be rapid and deep, attempting to compensate for a decrease in oxygen and an increase in carbon dioxide. There will be a decrease in oxygen because the heart is unable to perfuse the body.

(2) In cardiogenic shock, the respirations are rapid but not shallow. Polyuria will not exist, but there may be anuria (no urine) or oliguria (little urine) if the kidney is not perfused. If the heart is not able to perfuse the kidney, then urine cannot be produced. How well the kidney produces urine in cardiogenic shock is an indication of the pumping ability of the left side of the heart. A drop in blood pressure below 5 mm Hg would be considered normal for either systolic or diastolic pressure (the rationale does not say how much the drop is). If the option gives you specific criteria, it is the wrong answer.

(3) In cardiogenic shock, the patient's skin would be pale due to poor tissue perfusion, and the pulse would be weak and thready. A pulse is bounding in fluid overload. There is no hyperventilation in cardiogenic shock. Hyperventilation is seen most often in hysteria and high levels of anxiety. Tachycardia may be present in cardiogenic shock, but it will produce a weak, thready pulse.

36. ❹ In caring for a patient with varicose veins, the nurse should instruct the patient to keep the lower extremities elevated and warm in order to increase the amount of blood returning to the heart. This procedure also reduces edema in the legs and allows any venous ulcers that may have developed around the ankle to heal.

(1) A diabetic patient with peripheral vascular problems needs to be very careful about cutting toenails with a sharp razor; if a toe is cut, it may not heal, and gangrene could develop. Diabetics usually have poor peripheral vascular circulation; therefore, an injured area will have difficulty healing because adequate nutrients and oxygen cannot reach the injured area. Also, white blood cells are slow to reach the injured area, increasing the chance of infection.

(2, 3) Standing increases edema, thus increasing the amount of unoxygenated blood in the legs. Standing on the unaffected leg would not help because gravity would keep blood in both legs, causing edema. Keeping legs level with the body does not allow excess fluid in the legs to return to the heart.

37. ❹ Prazosin (Minipress) alpha blocker is used in mild to moderate hypertension. Its action dilates both veins and arteries.

(1, 2, 3) These options are incorrect as seen in rationale (4).

38. ❷ Nitroprusside (Nipride) is used in the management of a hypertensive crisis or cardiogenic shock. It produces peripheral vasodilation by direct action on venous and arteriolar smooth muscle cells.

(1, 3, 4) These options are incorrect as seen in rationale.

39. ❸ Hydralazine (Alazine) is used in the management of moderate to severe hypertension. It is a direct-acting peripheral arteriolar vasodilator.

(1, 2, 4) These options are incorrect as seen in rationale (3).

40. ❶ Diltiazem (Cardizem) calcium channel blocker is used in the management of angina pectoris due to coronary insufficiency or vasospasm. It inhibits the transport of calcium into the myocardium and vascular smooth muscle cells, resulting in inhibition of excitation and subsequent contraction. Coronary vasodilation and a subsequent decrease in the frequency and severity of attacks of angina pectoris may decrease SA node and AV node conduction.

(2, 3, 4) These options are incorrect as seen in rationale (1).

41. ❸ The pathologic changes that occur with an MI are interruption of the coronary circulation, followed by hypoxia of the myocardium, which causes muscle damage.

(1) With an MI, there will be no thrombosis (blood clot) in the carotid artery, and there will be no inflammation of the endocardium of the left ventricle.

(2, 4) The coronary sinus is not occluded and there is no atheromatous plaque in the pericardium after an MI.

42. ❸ Denial is a coping mechanism commonly used after a life-threatening illness. To deny that an MI has occurred relieves the anxiety about possible complications, including death. Denial is unconsciously refusing to acknowledge to oneself a known fact that is uncomfortable to accept.

(1) Suppression is the conscious inhibition of an idea or desire, as distinguished from repression, which is an involuntarily (unconscious) forgetting of unacceptable ideas, impulses, or events.

(2) Sublimation is conversion of unwanted aggressive or sexual drives into socially acceptable channels, sometimes called "socialization of energy."

(4) In depression, there is a loss of interest in all usually pleasurable outlets, such as food, sex, work, friends, hobbies, or entertainment. Diagnostic criteria include poor appetite, insomnia, psychomotor agitation, loss of energy, fatigue, feelings of worthlessness, diminished ability to think, and recurring thoughts of death. At least four of the diagnostic criteria must be present and last for at least 2 weeks to make a diagnosis of depression.

43. ❸ When a patient is recovering from an illness and is being transferred out of the CCU, the patient may ask the nurse, "Who will be there to take care of me?" To lessen the patient's anxiety, the nurse would respond, "Can you tell me about your concerns? We will convey them to the nurses on the unit." This will allow the patient to express such concerns and reduce feelings of anxiety about being transferred to a medical unit.

(1) Telling a patient that a nurse has experience in caring for patients does not relieve the patient's anxiety. The patient needs to be encouraged to talk about these concerns in order to solve the problems.

(2) A nurse should never tell a patient that the nurse understands the patient's concerns when the nurse does not know what the patient's concerns are. If the nurse did know what the concerns were, it does not mean the nurse can understand them. Telling the patient someone from the unit will visit the patient every day leads the patient to believe the CCU is more caring than where the patient is being transferred.

(4) A nurse should never tell a patient what he or she should do. The patient is an adult and does not need someone telling him or her that he or she needs to be independent when he or she goes home. If the patient is a child, the parents will tell the child what needs to be accomplished each day. When answering this type of question, always look for the option that encourages patients to express and solve their own problems.

44. **1** After a patient has one MI, the chances of having another increases; therefore, if the patient complains of epigastric pain after eating, the nurse needs to assess the patient closely because pain that may seem like indigestion may be an MI.

(2) Elevated cholesterol levels will lead to cholelithiasis (gallstones). Cholesterol stones account for most gallbladder disease in the United States. Cholesterol, a normal constituent of bile, is insoluble in water. The cholesterol precipitates out of the bile to form stones. Women are four times more likely than men to develop cholesterol stones and gallbladder disease, and they are usually older than 40 years.

(3) Excitement decreases gastric motility because the blood is shunted away from the gut and to the brain and muscle in order to deal with the excitement.

(4) Indigestion does not occur more often in patients after an MI than before they had the MI.

45. **1** Signs and symptoms of cardiogenic shock are increased PCWP because the heart is failing as a pump. Therefore, the heart has difficulty moving the blood out of the pulmonary circulation and into the rest of the body; the blood becomes congested in the pulmonary system, increasing PCWP. The patient will have cold clammy skin because of poor peripheral blood circulation. Systolic blood pressure may fall 30 mm Hg or more below baseline level. The patient will have a weak, thready pulse.

(2, 3, 4) These options are incorrect as seen in rationale (1).

46. **3** A demand pacemaker functions by providing a stimulus to the heart muscle but only when the heart rate falls below a specified level.

(1, 2, 4) These options are incorrect as seen in rationale (3).

47. **3** Systolic hypertension (systolic pressure >150 mm Hg) may develop as a result of volume expanders. If volume expanders are administered too rapidly, they will increase the vascular volume to a point of fluid overload and systolic hypertension. Examples of volume expanders include albumin, dextran, and Plasmanate.

(1) An increase in the heart's electrical activity will cause arrhythmias, not systolic hypertension.

(2) Loss of elastic tissue is most noticeable in the skin of the elderly. An aneurysm is a balloonlike bulging out of an artery. This would not cause systolic hypertension.

(4) Anaphylactic shock would cause systolic hypotension, not systolic hypertension. See rationale (1) for an increase in electrical activity of the heart.

48. **2** The priority immediately following CABG is to assess and stabilize the patient.

(1) Patient teaching is not a priority immediately after surgery. The patient will not die if patient teaching is not received at this time, but the patient may die if not assessed and stabilized.

When answering this type of question, always look for the option that presents safe nursing practice. The NCLEX-RN examination wants to know if you will know what must be done to ensure the safety of the patient and keep the patient alive. Assessing the peripheral circulation is only a part of the assessment that must be done after CABG.

(3) Assessing the patient's dressing for blood and pus is only part of the assessment that must be done after CABG surgery.

(4) Maintaining a blood pressure of 150 systolic is too high. Blood pressure this high would rupture the new CABG. The blood pressure is kept low (110/80) after surgery and until the physician believes that the CABG is strong enough to allow the blood pressure to increase.

When answering questions like this, be sure to look for the "global answer." A total body assessment is obviously a better answer than assessing one bodily function.

49. **4** PTCA is the insertion of a balloon-tipped catheter to enlarge the lumen of an artery. The balloon is inflated and pushes plaque back to the side of the artery, allowing blood to flow more freely.

A percutaneous valvoplasty is the same procedure, except that the balloon is put into a valve (e.g., mitral valve) and inflated to open a stenosed valve.

(1) In CABG surgery, the saphenous vein is the most frequently used to bypass the obstructed coronary artery. The saphenous vein is attached to the obstructed coronary artery at a point past the obstruction and then attached to the aorta. The mammary artery is also used for CABG.

(2) Aortocoronary bypass, see rationale (3).

(3) Many cardiac surgical procedures are possible because of cardiopulmonary bypass (extracorporeal circulation). The procedure provides a mechanical means of circulating and oxygenating blood for the body while "bypassing" the heart and lungs. The heart–lung machine allows for a bloodless surgical field while maintaining perfusion to the other body organs and tissue.

Cardiopulmonary bypass is accomplished by inserting a cannula in the right atrium, vena cava, or femoral vein to withdraw blood from the body. The cannula is connected to tubing filled with Ringer's lactate solution. Venous blood removed from the body by this cannula is filtered, oxygenated, cooled or warmed (temperature controlled), and then returned to the body. The cannula returning the oxygenated blood to the body usually is in the ascending aorta, but it may be in the femoral artery.

Although cardiopulmonary bypass is a common technique in heart surgery, it is complex. The patient requires anticoagulation with heparin to prevent thrombus formation and possible embolization that could occur when blood contacts the foreign surfaces of the cardiopulmonary bypass circuit and is pumped into the body by a mechanical pump. After the patient is removed from the bypass machine, protamine sulfate is used to reverse the effects of heparin.

During the procedure, hypothermia is maintained. As the blood is cooled, it is returned to the body. The cooled blood slows the body's metabolic rate, thereby decreasing the body's demand for oxygen. Cooled blood has a higher viscosity; the blood is diluted with Ringer's lactate solution and used to prime the bypass tubing. When the surgical procedure is complete, the blood is rewarmed in the machine and returned to the body.

50. ❷ Postoperatively, the primary focus after heart transplant surgery is preventing infection and rejection. Patients who have heart transplants are constantly balancing the risk of rejection with the risk of infection. They must comply with a complex regimen of diet, medication, activity, follow-up laboratory studies, biopsies (to diagnose rejection), and clinic visits.

Most commonly, patients receive cyclosporine and corticosteroids to minimize rejection. These two drugs reduce the patient's ability to fight infections. Cyclosporine is an immunosuppressant drug. It reduces the patient's antibodies so that he or she will be unable to fight off the foreign body, in this case the heart. Corticosteroids reduce inflammation so that the heart muscle will not become inflamed and then rejected by the antibodies.

(1) As explained in rationale (2), infection is a major concern after a heart transplant; therefore, this part of the option is correct. Prevention of an MI is not a major focus after a heart transplant because an MI seldom is a complication after heart transplant surgery.

(3, 4) After a heart transplant, it is important to prevent hemorrhage [option (3)] and stroke [option (4)], but they are not the primary focus. Infection in option (3) and rejection in option (4) are correct. Therefore, parts of these options were correct, but all of the options were correct in rationale (1).

51. ❷ A patient waiting for heart surgery for mitral valve incompetence says to a nurse, "I need a new valve, an oil change, and a lube job." The nurse's most appropriate reply is, "I'm sure you have a great deal to ask about this procedure." This statement acknowledges the patient's concerns without belittling the patient and encourages the patient to talk about what is troubling them.

(1) The statement by the nurse, "I'm glad to see you're handling the situation so well," leaves the patient thinking, "If she only knew I am scared to death. I have no idea what they are going to do to me, and I don't know if I will live or die." The statement was not therapeutic because it did not help the patient deal with this concern.

(3) The nurse's statement, "You really don't need to hide your anxieties," is belittling to the patient and does not allow the patient to discuss his or her concerns in order to reduce anxiety.

(4) The nurse's statement, "You've sure come to the right place for a valve job," is not a professional statement and demonstrates a lack of understanding. It does not encourage the patient to discuss his or her concerns so they can be dealt with.

52. ❷ The first sign of digitalis toxicity is a slow pulse rate, which is a side effect of digitalis. Digitalis slows conduction at the AV node, and excessive intake of digitalis may slow conduction and cause AV block. Patients must have a certain amount of digitalis in their bodies before the digitalis is effective, and this level is reached near digitalis toxicity.

(1, 3, 4) These options are incorrect because they are not signs of digitalis toxicity.

53. ❹ Signs and symptoms of pulmonary embolism are chest pain that radiates like a knife through to the shoulders, dyspnea, tachycardia, and hemoptysis.

(1) Fine rales throughout both lung fields and pink frothy sputum may indicate pneumonia or CHF, not pulmonary embolism.

(2) Dry, persistent cough, restlessness, and drowsiness may be early signs of emphysema, not symptoms of a pulmonary embolism.

(3) Viselike substernal pain and radiation to the left arm and jaw may be symptoms of an MI but are not symptoms of a pulmonary embolism.

54. ❶ A term that describes an intermittent third-degree heart block is Stokes-Adams attack. A third-degree AV block (complete heart block) is associated with organic heart disease, digitalis toxicity, and MI. The heart rate may be markedly decreased, resulting in decreased perfusion to vital organs, such as the brain, heart, kidney, and skin. Atrial rate may be 110 bpm and ventricular rate 40 to 60 bpm.

The P wave will have no association with the QRS complexes because they are beating independently. The insertion of a pacemaker with conduction into the ventricles may be necessary to ensure perfusion of vital organs of the body.

A pacemaker is an electronic device that provides repetitive electrical stimuli to the heart muscle for control of the heart rate. It initiates and maintains the heart rate when the natural pacemakers of the heart are unable to do so. Pacemakers are generally used when a patient has a conduction disturbance that causes failure in cardiac output.

Permanent pacemakers are used most commonly for irreversible complete heart block. The AV pacemakers or so-called physiologic pacemakers are considered highly desirable because they can be programmed to mimic the patient's own intrinsic cardiac function, and they can stimulate a response in the ventricle, atrium, or both.

(2) Leriche's syndrome is the occlusion of the abdominal aorta at its bifurcation by a thrombus. This causes intermittent ischemia and pain, claudication in the lower extremities, impotence, and absent or diminished femoral pulses.

(3) Mobitz type I is a first-degree AV block. This block is often associated with coronary artery disease, congenital anomalies, and digitalis administration. If this is the only abnormal feature of an individual's ECG, it produces no symptoms and requires no intervention.

(4) Mobitz type II is a second-degree AV block and is more serious than Mobitz type I AV block. Mobitz type II more often progresses to a higher degree of AV block, especially in people with an anterior wall MI. This is a dangerous situation because complete heart block (third-degree AV block), a potentially life-threatening arrhythmia, may suddenly occur. A person with second-degree AV block requires close ECG monitoring for possible progression of the conduction defect.

Intervention includes administration of atropine (which speeds the cardiac rate), insertion of a pacemaker, and withholding cardiac depressant drugs such as digitalis.

55. ❷ The nurse should carefully evaluate pulse and blood pressure readings prior to administering Inderal. Inderal is a beta blocker used to treat hypertension and tachycardia, and it should not be given if the pulse is lower than 60 bpm or if the blood pressure is significantly lower than usual. Side effects of Inderal are bradycardia, CHF, pulmonary edema, hypotension, edema, depression, memory loss, insomnia, drowsiness, and dizziness.

Catapres, an alpha blocker, is used to manage mild to moderate hypertension. Side effects are drowsiness, nightmares, nervousness, depression, hypotension, and bradycardia.

(1) Anturane is used in the management of long-term gout. It decreases serum uric acid levels by decreasing renal reabsorption. Side effects are GI bleeding, nausea, vomiting, abdominal pain, kidney stones, and rashes.

Calcitonin is used to treat Paget's disease of the bone. It decreases the rate of bone turnover, lowering serum calcium. Side effects are headaches, nausea, vomiting, diarrhea, strange taste in the mouth, urinary frequency, rashes, and reaction at the injection site. Assess the patient for signs of hypocalcemic tetany.

(3) Glucagon is used to manage severe hypoglycemia when administration of glucose is not feasible. It is also used to terminate insulin shock therapy in psychiatric clients. Glucagon stimulates hepatic production of glucose from glycogen stores (glycogenolysis). Side effects include nausea, vomiting, and a hypersensitivity reaction.

Mestinon is used to increase muscle strength and improve muscle function in the patient with myasthenia gravis. Mestinon inhibits the breakdown of acetylcholine and prolongs its effects. Side effects include hypotension, seizures, dizziness, weakness, bronchospasm, and bradycardia. It is correct that the pulse and blood pressure should be taken before administering this medication because of the side effects of bradycardia and hypotension.

(4) Vistaril is used to treat anxiety, for preoperative sedation, as an antiemetic, and in the management of alcohol and drug withdrawal. It is often combined with a narcotic analgesic to potentiate the narcotic (synergistic) action, where the total effect is greater than the sum of the independent effect of the two

substances. Side effects include excessive sedation, drowsiness, dizziness, weakness, dry mouth, and urinary retention.

Minipress is used to treat mild to moderate hypertension. It dilates both arteries and veins by blocking alpha-adrenergic receptors. Therapeutic effects are lowering blood pressure and decreasing preload and afterload. Side effects are dizziness, drowsiness, syncope, depression, headache, weakness, nausea, and impotence. The blood pressure should be taken before administering Minipress but not before administering Vistaril, which makes this option wrong.

56. ❹ When a patient has cardiac and renal damage as the result of hypertension, the nurse needs to educate the patient about diet. The patient needs to know that processed foods are high in salt and that fresh fruit and juice are high in vitamins and low in salt.

(1) Milk and milk products are high in sodium. Patients with renal and cardiac damage should be on a low-sodium diet.

(2) Salt substitutes are high in potassium. Patients in renal failure have difficulty excreting potassium.

(3) Meat is high in protein. A patient in renal failure should not have a high protein intake but needs some protein for healing.

57. ❶ When a patient is in hypertensive crisis and is receiving Hyperstat to lower the blood pressure, the nurse needs to monitor the patient's glucose level because a side effect of Hyperstat is elevation of blood glucose level.

(2) An infusion pump is not used to administer Hyperstat. It may be given as an IV push in a hypertensive crisis. An infusion pump usually is used for long-term administration of medications, such as heparin.

(3) A patient in hypertensive crisis is very anxious and will move from one position to another. Breathing is not a problem for this patient; therefore, this patient would not need the bed in a high Fowler's position.

(4) Hyperstat does not have to be covered with aluminum foil; however, a sodium nitroprusside (Nipride) does need to be covered to protect it from light. Remember that plasma cyanide and thiocyanate levels should be monitored every 48 to 72 h when Nitride is being administered.

58. ❸ Aplastic anemia is the result of bone marrow depression, which results in a deficient red blood cell production due to bone marrow disorder. Approximately half of the cases are idiopathic (cause unknown), and they occur most often in adolescents and young adults. Exposure to chemical and antineoplastic agents and ionizing radiation can result in aplastic anemia.

(1, 2, 4) These options are incorrect as seen in rationale (3).

59. ❷ Sickle cell anemia is a hereditary, chronic form of anemia in which abnormal sickle-shaped or crescent-shaped erythrocytes are present. The sickled cells interfere with oxygen transport, obstruct capillary blood flow, and cause fever and severe pain in the joints and abdomen. The crisis is precipitated by decreased oxygen, as can occur during climbing a mountain at high altitudes without use of supplemental oxygen or any other activity where a large volume of oxygen is used. Sickle cell anemia is more common in the African-American population. The pathologic situation is compounded if dehydration is present.

(1, 3, 4) These options are incorrect as seen in rationale (2).

60. ❹ Polycythemia vera is the excessive production of erythrocytes (red blood cells). It usually develops between the ages of 40 to 60 years, particularly in men of Jewish ancestry. It rarely affects African-Americans and appears to be familial. Although the precise etiology remains unknown, it possibly is a form of malignancy analogous to leukemia.

The three major hallmarks of the condition are unrestrained production of erythrocytes, production of excessive melanocytes (leukocytes within the bone marrow), and overproduction of platelets.

The result of overproduction of these cells is an increase in blood viscosity; an increase in total blood volume, which may be two or even three times greater than normal; and severe blood congestion of all tissue and organs. Because of these three problems, the individual has numerous symptoms.

Thrombotic complications claim the lives of approximately 30 percent of those affected with polycythemia vera. Approximately 10 to 15 percent die of hemorrhage, and approximately 15 percent die from either myelogenous leukemia or myelofibrosis accompanied by pancytopenia (reduction of all cellular elements of the blood).

(1, 2, 3) These options are incorrect as seen in rationale (4).

61. ❶ Thrombocytopenia purpura is the most common cause of hemorrhage. (Purpura means a reduction in platelets below 200,000 mm³.) Because platelets are an important component of the clotting mechanism, hallmarks of thrombocytopenia are bruising easily, petechiae (fine red hemorrhagic rash), and a tendency to bleed readily, especially from the gums, perineal area, and GI tract.

(2, 3, 4) These options are incorrect as seen in rationale (1).

62. ❸ Raynaud's disease is characterized by vasospasm causing intermittent attacks of pallor and cyanosis of the fingers caused by exposure to cold or from emotional stimuli with bilateral involvement. Eighty percent of people with Raynaud's disease are women between the ages of 20 and 48 years. Raynaud's disease is of unknown etiology, although immunologic abnormalities seem to be present in many people with this disorder.

(1, 2, 4) These options are incorrect as seen in rationale (3).

63. ❶ Disseminated intravascular coagulation (DIC) means diffuse or widespread coagulation within arterioles and capillaries all over the body followed by hemorrhage.

DIC is a complex and important coagulation disorder characterized by two apparently conflicting manifestations: (1) widespread clotting and (2) hemorrhage from the organs, such as kidneys, brain, adrenals, and heart. Although the cause of the disease is unknown, it may be linked to metastatic cancer, obstetric complications, shock, sepsis, and tissue damage from burns, trauma, and snake bites. Platelets, prothrombin, and other clotting factors are consumed in the process, which leads to bleeding.

The onset of DIC usually is acute. Laboratory findings in severe cases of DIC indicate that the hemostatic mechanism has failed totally.

A prolonged prothrombin time (PT), very low platelet count, and incoagulable blood are typical findings. To reverse clotting in acute cases of DIC, the physician usually orders continuous IV heparin therapy.

During DIC, the platelets and coagulation factors consumed must be replaced by transfusion of platelets and fresh frozen plasma. Packed red blood cells are used to replace blood volume lost through hemorrhage.

The prognosis for a person with DIC varies. The condition may be chronic, acute, or self-limiting. On the other hand, in acute cases of DIC hemorrhage, organ damage or even death may occur in a few days.

(2, 3, 4) These options are incorrect as seen in rationale (1).

64. ❷ Thromboangiitis obliterans (Buerger's disease) is characterized by acute inflammatory lesions and occlusive thrombosis of the arteries and veins. This disease usually occurs in men younger than 40 years. Pain is the outstanding symptom.

Intermittent claudication is a common problem that occurs in almost all people at some stage of Buerger's disease. It is most common in the calf of the legs. Ulceration and gangrene are frequent complications, and they may occur early in the course of the disease. These lesions can appear spontaneously, but they often follow trauma.

Edema of the legs is fairly common in advanced cases. Intervention is generally the same as for other peripheral arterial disease.

Treatment is aimed at arresting the progress of the disease, producing vasodilation, relieving pain, and providing emotional support. Advise patients with Buerger's disease or any vascular disease to abstain completely and permanently from the use of tobacco in any form because tobacco is a vasoconstrictor.

(1, 3, 4) These options are incorrect as seen in rationale (2).

65. ❹ Pheochromocytoma is a tumor of the adrenal medulla resulting in release of excessive amounts of the catecholamines epinephrine and norepinephrine, which cause severe hypertension. The adrenal glands are small but vital endocrine structures that cap the top of each kidney. Each adrenal gland is composed of the medulla, which is the inner core, and the cortex, which makes up the outer shell of the gland.

Although both structures contribute to the individual's survival and well-being, only the adrenal medulla is essential for life. The brain, specifically the hypothalamus, controls the secretion of epinephrine and norepinephrine. Epinephrine attaches to beta receptors in the heart and increases the number of cardiac beats per minute; in the bronchi, it causes bronchodilation. Epinephrine attaches to a limited number of beta receptors in the peripheral vascular system. During stress reaction, epinephrine primarily acts to produce vascular constriction, thereby causing a rise in blood pressure.

Norepinephrine attaches to many alpha receptors in the vascular system. During stress reactions, norepinephrine primarily acts to produce extensive vascular constriction, thereby causing a marked rise in blood pressure. Both epinephrine and nore-pinephrine dilate pupils and inhibit GI functions.

(1, 2, 3) These options are incorrect as seen in rationale (4).

66. ❶ The first symptoms of a blood transfusion reaction are tachycardia, fever, chills, flushing, and lumbar pain. If these symptoms occur, stop the blood transfusion, keep the line open with normal saline, and notify the physician.

For a blood transfusion, use an 18-gauge or larger needle to prevent red blood cell damage and allow for an adequate flow rate. Blood must be administered with a filter set, which removes clots and aggregates of leukocytes and platelets. Never add any medications to a unit of blood or through the IV system because they may injure the red blood cells. Normal saline solution is used as the companion solution for administering blood.

(2, 3, 4) These signs and symptoms are not those of hemolytic blood transfusion reaction.

67. ❸ When a patient complains of severe chest pain and left arm pain, the patient may be describing the symptoms of an MI. The nurse needs to assess the patient and gather more information before notifying the physician.

(1) There is not enough information to call the physician. The physician will want to know the patient's vital signs and any other signs and symptoms the patient is having.

(2) Blood pressure is a minimal part of what the nurse needs to assess when a patient has chest pain.

(4) Placing the patient in a high Fowler's position and starting oxygen will not relieve the patient's symptoms. Also, this will not help the nurse to assess the patient's problem so that the physician can be notified before the patient becomes critically ill.

68. ❹ When a nurse reports to the RN on the next shift about a patient with chest pain and cardiac arrhythmias, the first thing the RN must do is spend time talking with and assessing the patient and then notify the physician if necessary.

(1) The patient may be dead if the nurse waits to tell the physician when he or she comes on the floor.

(2) Talking with a patient to reduce anxiety when the patient may be having an MI and needs immediate medical attention indicates very poor nursing assessment and endangers the patient's life.

(3) Putting a patient on a cardiac monitor immediately before the patient is assessed is poor nursing judgment. If the patient was in the CCU, the nurse would first assess the patient and possibly then place the patient on an ECG monitor, if the assessment indicated the need. The physician would be notified if the patient was having an MI.

69. ❷ Causes of secondary hypertension are renal artery stenosis, Cushing's syndrome, and pheochromocytoma.

Stenosis of the renal artery reduces blood flow to the kidney. The kidney will release aldosterone to retain sodium, so water will be retained. When the kidney is not being perfused, it will automatically help the body to retain fluid, causing secondary hypertension.

Cushing's syndrome results from overactivity of the adrenal cortex with oversecretion of steroids, aldosterone, and androgens. As stated previously, aldosterone will retain sodium, sodium will retain fluid, and glucocorticoid (steroids) will retain fluid. Body fluid is grossly increased, causing secondary hypertension.

Pheochromocytoma is a tumor of the adrenal medulla, and it causes excessive excretion of epinephrine and norepinephrine, which will cause severe secondary hypertension.

Renal artery stenosis and pheochromocytoma can be corrected by surgery, thus removing hypertension; therefore, they are referred to as secondary hypertension. Secondary hypertension occurs as a consequence of another condition. In primary hypertension, the etiology is unknown; therefore, hypertension cannot be removed.

(1) Obesity and high sodium intake are risk factors for primary hypertension, not a cause of secondary hypertension. The cause of primary hypertension cannot be removed. High sodium intake can reduce, but will not permanently remove, hypertension. It is a risk factor for hypertension, not a secondary cause of primary hypertension.

Tobacco is a risk factor for primary hypertension, but it is not a cause of secondary hypertension. Renal artery stenosis will cause secondary hypertension, making this part of the option correct.

(3) Fluid overload and high salt intake are risk factors for primary hypertension, not secondary hypertension.

(4) Stress and high sodium intake are risk factors for primary hypertension, not secondary hypertension. Hypertension is increased blood pressure; it is not a cause.

70. ❷ A priority of care for the patient with an acute MI is to relieve pain. Pain can be extreme and very frightening for a patient who believes that he or she may die.

Pain increases the production of epinephrine and norepinephrine, causing tachycardia and extreme vasoconstriction. This forces the already damaged heart to work harder than it is able to work, which will cause greater cardiac damage if the pain is not relieved.

(1) Reducing environmental stress will reduce the production of aldosterone and steroids. Steroids will increase glucose (sugar) in the body, and both of these hormones will increase fluid retention, which will cause the heart to work harder. This effect is significantly less damaging to the heart than the effects of pain. The effects of aldosterone and steroids take longer to develop than the effects of pain.

(3) A patient with excruciating chest pain will be on bed rest, but the priority of care for the patient is to relieve pain, as explained in rationale (2).

(4) When a patient is in a physical crisis, the patient cannot identify emotional conflicts. It is not a priority of care.

71. ❸ A person who has experienced an MI or severe angina pain should be educated to take nitroglycerin before having sexual intercourse. This will cause vasodilation of the coronary arteries and allow good cardiac perfusion. The person is less likely to experience angina pain during or after sexual intercourse.

(1, 2, 4) These options are incorrect as seen in rationale (3).

72. ② In an unmonitored cardiac arrest, the initial action by the rescuer, before starting cardiopulmonary resuscitation (CPR), is to establish unresponsiveness. Clinical manifestations of cardiopulmonary arrest are an abrupt and complete unconsciousness (no response to gentle shaking while asking, "Are you OK?"), apnea or gasping respirations, absence of heartbeat and blood pressure, patient's skin pallor or cyanosis, and an ECG that reveals asystole or ventricle fibrillation.

(1, 3, 4) These options are incorrect as seen in rationale (2).

73. ① Provide 15 chest compressions for every 2 rescue breaths, whether or not 1 or 2 rescuers are present.

(2, 4) These options are incorrect as seen in rationale (1).

(3) Two lung inflations to 15 cardiac compressions is the correct rate for one rescuer.

74. ③ During cardiac compression, manual pressure is applied to the lower half of the sternum. Perform cardiac compression by maintaining the elbows in a straight, locked position, with the shoulders directly over the person's sternum, so that the thrust for compressions is straight down on the sternum.

This method uses body weight rather than arm muscles and facilitates smooth, easy compressions. It avoids sharp, jerking motions, which are less effective. Allow the chest to return to its normal position after each compression. To prevent position migration (two rescuers), do not remove hands between compressions. By lightly maintaining hand position on the lower half of the sternum, compress the sternum 1.5 inches.

(1, 2, 4) These options are incorrect as seen in rationale (3).

75. ③ Cardiac enzymes are organ-specific enzymes that are present in high concentrations in myocardial tissue. Tissue damage causes a release of enzymes from their intracellular storage areas. Elevated levels of isoenzyme CK-MB and LDH are the enzymes most commonly used to detect MI. Increase in LDH1 greater than LDH2 indicates an MI.

Isoenzymes occur in various forms of CK and LDH and are identified by a process known as *electrophoresis*.

Eighty percent of individuals demonstrate elevations in LDH within 24 to 48 h after onset of chest pain (MI). These levels peak in 7 to 14 days and usually remain increased for 10 days. The CK-MB level increases 8 to 24 h after the onset of chest pain (MI), reaches a peak in 12 to 18 h, and returns to normal levels in 3 to 4 days.

(1, 2) The serum aminotransferase enzymes AST and ALT were previously designated SGOT and SGPT. They were used in the diagnosis of MI for many years, but they have fallen out of favor because it has been recognized that their course of elevation is intermediate between CK-MB and LDH, thus offering little advantage because of their lack of tissue specificity. Creatinine phosphokinase is the enzyme that is increased in MI, specifically isoenzyme CK-MB. Aminotransferase enzymes

AST and ALT are elevated to some degree in nearly all liver disorders.

(4) LDH is a specific enzyme in the heart; AST and ALT are liver enzymes.

76. ④ Depressed ST segments, inverted T wave, and pathologic Q waves are diagnostic indicators of cardiac ischemia (MI), but they need additional support from laboratory values of cardiac enzymes.

(1) An absence of a P wave would indicate failure of the atria to beat. The PVCs indicate the ventricles were contracting prematurely.

(2) A prolonged PR interval would indicate slowed conduction at the AV node.

(3) The QRS complex will not show narrowing in an MI, and PVCs are not an indication of an MI. See rationale (1) for a discussion of PVCs.

77. ④ The greatest danger of PVCs is that they may develop into ventricular fibrillation, which is life threatening.

(1) AV heart block is the failure of impulses to pass through the AV junction. Conduction of impulses from the atria to the ventricles slows or stops entirely, depending on the degree of the AV block. The person's ventricular rate will slow down, not speed up.

(2) In sinus tachycardia, the SA node is firing rapidly, so both atria and ventricles are beating rapidly. This could lead to ventricular fibrillation, but it usually does not. The sinus node (pacemaker of the heart) lies superior to the vena cava in the right atrium. The node is referred to as the *SA node*.

(3) In premature contractions (PACs), the atria are contracting before the ventricles. This will not cause ventricular fibrillation.

78. ① The nurse has available 250 mL of D_5W (dextrose 5% in water), which contains 1000 mg of lidocaine. The physician orders lidocaine to be administered at the rate of 1 mg/min. The drop (gtt) factor of the IV administration set is 60 gtt/mL. The nurse regulates the infusion (in gtt/min) at 15 gtt/min.

Divide 1000 mg of lidocaine into 250 mL of D_5W:

1000 mg/250 mL = 0.25 mg/mL.

Then multiply 0.25 mg/mL times 60 gtt factor:

$60 \times 0.25 = 15.00$ gtt/min.

(2, 3, 4) These options are incorrect as seen in rationale (1).

79. ② After having had an MI, a patient may become fearful of having another MI and dying. A nursing priority is to assist the patient and family in understanding that the fear of heart disease may make the patient an invalid. Cardiovascular exercise and diet should be the focus for the patient recovering from an MI.

(1, 3, 4) These options are incorrect as seen in rationale (2).

80. ② Lidocaine is the drug of choice for controlling ventricular arrhythmias. It is used for ventricular tachycardia and other ventricular arrhythmias. It also is used for patients with an

MI or digitalis toxicity, or for a cardiac catheterization procedure.

(1, 3, 4) These options are incorrect as seen in rationale (2).

81. ❸ Early signs of lidocaine toxicity are bradycardia, hypotension, confusion, and severe dizziness or fainting.

(1, 2, 4) These options are not signs and symptoms of lidocaine toxicity.

82. ❷ Children with tetralogy of Fallot develop blue spells that are characterized by dyspnea, deep, sighing respirations, bradycardia, fainting, seizures, and loss of consciousness. These children habitually squat when they feel short of breath.

Tetralogy of Fallot is a complex of four cardiac defects: ventricular septal defect (VSD), obstruction (pulmonary stenosis), right ventricular hypertrophy, and transposition of the aorta with overriding of the VSD. Blood shunts right to left through the VSD, permitting unoxygenated blood to mix with oxygenated blood, which results in cyanosis.

(1, 3, 4) These options are incorrect as seen in rationale (2).

83. ❸ Myocarditis is an inflammation of the cardiac muscle. Its occurrence may result from streptococcal invasion of the myocardium, endocardium, and pericardium. A patient's history reveals recent febrile upper respiratory infection, viral pharyngitis, or other systemic infection.

Although laboratory tests cannot confirm myocarditis, elevated cardiac enzymes, white blood cell count, and antibody titers support the diagnosis. Blood, stool, and throat cultures may identify bacteria or isolated virus. The most reliable diagnostic aid is ECG, with changes typically showing diffuse ST segments and T-wave abnormalities.

84. ❶ Rheumatic fever is a systemic inflammatory disease of childhood, often recurrent, that follows group A beta-hemolytic streptococcal infection.

Rheumatic heart disease refers to the cardiac manifestations of rheumatic fever and includes myocarditis, pericarditis, endocarditis, and chronic valvular disease. Later, mitral valve stenosis or prolapse will be especially noticeable. Long-term antibiotic therapy can minimize the recurrence of rheumatic fever, thereby reducing the risk of permanent valvular deformity.

(2, 3, 4) These options are incorrect as seen in rationale (1).

85. ❹ A cause of secondary hypertension is renal artery stenosis. When the kidney is not perfused, it "thinks" the body is low on fluid and produces aldosterone to retain sodium and sodium, causing water retention. The increase in body fluid increases blood pressure. The kidney also produces renin which causes vasoconstriction, which increases blood pressure. The excess fluid volume and vasoconstriction cause secondary hypertension.

Surgery can be performed on the renal artery to remove the stenosis. Any hypertension that can be corrected by surgery is called secondary hypertension. Other common causes of secondary hypertension are pheochromocytoma, Cushing's syndrome, dysfunction of the thyroid gland, and pregnancy. Essential hypertension, also called idiopathic or primary, accounts for more than 90 percent of cases of hypertension. This chronic elevation in blood pressure occurs without evidence of any other disease process. Essential hypertension has no single known causative etiology, but the following risk factors have been identified: family history, race (more common in African-Americans), stress, obesity, high dietary intake of salt and saturated fats, use of tobacco, oral contraceptives, sedentary lifestyle, and aging.

(1, 2, 3) These options are incorrect as seen in rationale (4).

86. ❹ Cardiac tamponade is the compression of the heart as a result of fluid increase within the pericardial sac. Two major complications that may result from acute pericarditis (the hallmark finding in acute cardiac tamponade is a pericardial rub) are pericardial effusion and cardiac tamponade. Pericardial effusion is generally a rapid accumulation of fluid from pericardial trauma (e.g., chest trauma).

Cardiac tamponade develops as the pericardial effusion increases in size. The patient with pericardial tamponade often is confused, agitated, and restless and has tachycardia and tachypnea with low cardiac output.

The neck veins usually are markedly distended because jugular venous pressure elevates, and a significant pulsus paradoxus is present. Pulsus paradoxus is an inspiratory drop in systolic blood pressure greater than 10 mm Hg.

There is a normal systolic drop of 10 mm Hg during respiratory inspiration; a drop greater than 10 mm Hg may indicate cardiac tamponade. The ECG changes in cases of acute pericarditis are key diagnostic clues and evolve over a period of hours to days and weeks. Pericardiocentesis is performed in the presence of acute cardiac tamponade.

(1, 2, 3) These options are incorrect as seen in rationale (4).

87. ❸ Syphilitic aortitis will result in regurgitation of blood into the left ventricle with dilation and hypertrophy.

(1, 2, 4) These options are incorrect as seen in rationale (3).

88. ❶ Aortic stenosis will result in decreased cardiac output, symptoms of angina, pain, tachyarrhythmias, or bradyarrhythmias. Cardiac output will be decreased because the narrowing of the aorta will allow only a small amount of output with each cardiac contraction.

There will be angina pain because the heart receives its blood from the aorta, and there may not be adequate output to perfuse the heart.

When the heart is not adequately perfused, there will be tachyarrhythmia or bradyarrhythmia and angina pain. Syncope is the result of low cardiac output, which reduces blood flow to the brain.

(2) The right ventricle will not hypertrophy because the aorta comes out of the left ventricle. It is the left ventricle that will hypertrophy because it has to work harder to get blood out through the stenosed aorta. There will not be a decrease in cardiac contraction. Angina pain results from inadequate perfusion of the heart because not enough oxygenated blood is coming out of the aorta. (Remember the coronary arteries come off the aorta.)

(3) Hypertension will not occur because of low cardiac output (because blood cannot be pushed out through the aorta), but hypotension may occur. Hemoptysis will not occur, and stenosis of the aorta will not cause bleeding in the lungs.

(4) The left ventricle will hypertrophy because the aorta comes out of the left ventricle, but the right ventricle will not hypertrophy.

89. ❹ Cardiac contractility is decreased in the later stages of acidosis, which explains why it is so difficult to save a person's life in a code situation. Acidosis causes bradycardia, which further complicates cardiac failure.

(1) When calcium intake is increased, it normally has no effect on the heart. A significant increase in the serum calcium level would increase cardiac contractility, and it may cause heart block. In severe calcium toxicity, cardiac arrest may occur.

(2) In the early stage of hypovolemic shock, cardiac contractility would be increased and the cardiac rate would increase to compensate for low blood volume.

(3) Epinephrine administered in a large dose would increase cardiac contractility.

90. ❹ When PVCs are present, the stimulant for the heartbeat originates in the ventricle. The foci (pacemaker in the ventricles) fires before the SA node fires (explaining the name premature ventricular contractions).

(1) Premature atrial contractions are called PACs.

(2) The SA node is where the sinus rhythm originates, and it is the normal pacemaker of the heart.

(3) The AV node is located between the atria and the ventricles and can take over as a pacemaker. It fires at approximately 40 bpm.

91. ❸ In ventricular tachycardia, the atria and ventricles characteristically beat independently.

(1) In normal sinus rhythm, the atria and ventricles beat simultaneously.

(2) In tachycardia, the atria and the ventricles beat simultaneously and rapidly.

(4) If the heart beats at the same rate as the patient breathes, bradycardia is occurring and the patient is in great danger of death; the heart would be beating at only 20 bpm or less.

92. ❷ A patient receiving Inderal must be observed for bradycardia. Inderal is a beta blocker, which blocks epinephrine from reaching the heart. Epinephrine speeds the heart; if it cannot reach the heart, the cardiac rate will slow.

(1) Ataxia is defective muscular coordination, especially manifested when voluntary muscular movements are attempted.

(3) Automaticity is the ability of cells to initiate an impulse spontaneously and repetitively without external neurohormonal control. Given proper laboratory conditions, the heart can beat outside the body via its own intrinsic control system.

In contrast, skeletal muscle must be stimulated by a nerve encoder to depolarize and contract. Heart muscle can depolarize spontaneously and stimulate its own contraction. Pacemaker cells have the highest rate of automaticity of all cardiac cells.

(4) Hypertension is a condition in which the person has a higher blood pressure than that judged to be normal.

93. ❷ Dopamine will peripherally vasoconstrict, increase cardiac contractility, and increase blood pressure. It is dosage dependent.

(1) Dopamine will increase urine output because it will increase kidney perfusion when administered in low dosage. It may increase CVP because it will vasoconstrict when administered in high dosage. However, dopamine is not given for either of these reasons. Dopamine is normally given to increase blood pressure.

(3) Dopamine will increase cardiac contractility of the heart, when given in moderate dosage, but it will not decrease blood pressure. It will increase blood pressure because it is a vasoconstrictor.

(4) Dopamine will not decrease urine out. It will increase afterload (systolic pressure) because it is a vasoconstrictor.

94. ❸ Rapid supraventricular arrhythmias are dangerous because ventricular filling is compromised. When the atria are contracting rapidly, there is insufficient time for the atria to fill with blood, which can result in reduced cardiac output.

(1, 2, 4) These are incorrect options as seen in rationale (3).

95. ❶ A mitral murmur can best be heard at the apex of the heart. The apex (at the bottom of the heart) is located at the fifth left intercostal space, approximately 3.5 inches from the middle of the sternum.

(2, 3, 4) These options are incorrect as seen in rationale (1).

96. ❸ The most common medication and procedure for a patient with chronic CHF is Lasix, OOB ad lib (get out of bed as desired), digoxin, and a low-sodium diet. Lasix will help in removing excessive fluid.

The patient's potassium level must be monitored closely because Lasix causes potassium loss in the urine. A low serum potassium level may cause serious cardiac arrhythmias.

Being OOB ad lib is important for the patient with chronic CHF. This helps the patient to cough and deep breathe and increases pulmonary circulation, so the patient will not develop pneumonia.

Digoxin increases cardiac output and, therefore, helps to reduce pulmonary congestion. A low serum potassium level will contribute to digitalis toxicity, so the patient must be monitored closely. A low-sodium diet will help to increase urinary output and reduce pulmonary congestion.

(1) Lasix would be used as discussed in rationale (3). Plasminogen is a protein found in many tissues and body fluids. It is important for preventing fibrin clot formation.

A patient with chronic CHF would not be NPO or on a liquid diet because chronic means the patient has CHF to some degree all of the time. Therefore, the patient would not be NPO or on a liquid diet all of the time.

(2) Nitroglycerin is used for angina pain, not CHF. The patient with chronic CHF would not be on bed rest because the patient needs to move around freely to help the patient to cough,

deep breathe, and get rid of some of the excessive pulmonary congestion. Otherwise, the patient may develop pneumonia.

(4) The patient would be ambulated if assistance is needed, but the patient could be OOB ad lib. The patient would not be on salt-free diet because everyone needs some sodium in the diet. The patient may have an IV KVO but usually will not need one.

97. ❸   The most appropriate actions taken before the nurse can perform postmortem care are to have the death certificate signed and ensure that the family has been notified.

(1, 2, 4) These options are incorrect as seen in rationale (3).

98. ❷   A patient is diagnosed as having hypertension if the blood pressure is significantly elevated at three successive readings on separate days.

(1, 3, 4) These options are incorrect as seen in rationale (2).

99. ❹   Physical findings on an examination of a patient that would be indicative of hypertension would be cardiac enlargement on percussion.

(1, 2, 3) These options are incorrect as seen in rationale (4).

100. ❶   Laboratory studies to determine if correction of a hypertensive condition is possible by surgical intervention would include the collection of a 24-h urine specimen to determine if the catecholamine level is high. A high level may indicate that the patient has a pheochromocytoma on the adrenal medulla. The adrenal medulla stores catecholamines, epinephrine, norepinephrine, and dopamine. All of these cause vasoconstriction and can produce hypertension, which is classified as secondary hypertension (because the cause is known and the condition can be corrected).

(2, 3, 4) These options are incorrect as seen in rationale (1).

Chapter 16

Respiratory Disorders

A. Fiberoptic Bronchoscopy

1. Allows the direct inspection of the larynx, trachea, and bronchi.

2. Also allows for biopsy and for collection of secretions through endotracheal or tracheostomy.

3. Foreign objects can be removed.

4. Prediagnostic

   a. Nothing by mouth (NPO), sedative, IV.

   b. Xylocaine sprayed in throat.

5. Postdiagnostic

   a. Observe for wheezing, dyspnea, hemoptysis, and pneumothorax.

   b. Observe for return of gag reflex before administering medications or food.

   c. Patient is placed on side or in semi-Fowler's position after procedure.

6. Nursing Implications

   a. Explain procedure and ensure that the physician has obtained the informed consent for this procedure.

   b. Check return of the swallow and cough reflexes following the procedure.

   c. Keep patient NPO after midnight on the day of the test.

   d. Observe for signs of complications, such as cyanosis, dyspnea, stridor, hemoptysis, hypotension, tachycardia, and arrhythmias.

   e. Assessing airway obstruction for signs and symptoms.

      (1) Noisy, wet respirations.

      (2) Restlessness.

      (3) Increased pulse and respirations.

      (4) Respiration may be labored.

      (5) Cyanosis is a late sign.

   f. Position the conscious patient in a flat or semi-Fowler's, side-lying position and instruct patient to let saliva drain out of the corner of the mouth into basin or tissue.

   g. Keep the patient NPO until swallow and cough reflexes return.

   h. Expect blood-streaked sputum for several hours if a biopsy is done, but report large amounts of blood (10–15 mL) to physician immediately.

B. Mediastinoscopy

Incision is made above the sternum for biopsy of the lymph node.

1. Prediagnostic

   a. NPO.

   b. Sedatives are administered.

2. Postdiagnostic

   a. Observe for complications, such as bleeding, vocal cord paralysis, pneumonia, cardiac arrhythmias, and myocardial infarction (MI).

3. Nursing Implications

a. Explain procedure to patient and be sure that the physician has obtained the informed consent for this procedure.

b. Keep the patient NPO after midnight on the day of test.

c. Administer preprocedural medications approximately one-half to 1 hour before the test as ordered.

d. Provide postoperative care as for any other surgical procedure.

C. Thoracentesis

Removal of fluid from pleural space. The procedure is painful.

1. Prediagnostic

a. Patient should be sitting up and leaning over a table during procedure.

2. Postdiagnostic

a. Apply pressure dressing.

b. Observe for hemoptysis and pneumothorax.

c. Bed rest for several hours.

3. Nursing Implications

a. Explain the procedure to the patient.

b. Ensure physician has obtained the informed consent for this procedure.

c. Patient is placed in a sitting position with arms and shoulders raised and supported on overhead table; this position spreads the ribs and enlarges the intercostal space for insertion of the needle.

d. Thoracentesis is performed under strict sterile techniques.

e. The needle is positioned in the pleural space, and the fluid is withdrawn.

f. Procedure is performed by a physician at the patient's bedside, in a procedure room, or in the physician's office in less than one-half hour.

g. Monitor patient's pulse for reflex bradycardia and evaluate the patient for diaphoresis and the feeling of faintness during procedure.

h. Label the specimen with the patient's name, date, source of fluid, and diagnosis.

i. Send promptly to laboratory.

j. Evaluate the patient for signs and symptoms of pneumothorax, tension pneumothorax, subcutaneous emphysema, diminished breath sounds, anxiety, restlessness, and fever.

(1) Diminished breath sounds could be a sign of pneumothorax.

k. If patient has no complaints of dyspnea, normal activity usually can be resumed 1 h after procedure.

D. Types of Airflow Assessment Test

1. Vital Capacity

a. Vital capacity is the maximum amount of air a person can exhale after one deep intake of air.

2. Tidal Volume

a. The tidal volume is how much air comes into and out of the lung with each normal respiration.

b. In adults, the average tidal volume is 500 mL.

3. Purpose of a Pulmonary Function Test

a. A preoperative evaluation of the lungs and the pulmonary reserve is a priority before thoracic surgery because surgery will result in loss of functional pulmonary tissue, as in lobectomy (removal of part of a lung) or pneumonectomy (removal of entire lung).

b. Evaluation of a response to bronchodilator therapy performed preoperatively; pulmonary function studies performed before and after bronchodilator are used to determine the amount of functional pulmonary tissue.

c. Differentiation between restrictive and obstructive forms of chronic pulmonary disease.

(1) Restrictive defects (e.g., pulmonary fibrosis, tumors, chest wall trauma) occur when ventilation is disrupted by limiting chest expansion.

(2) Obstructive defects (e.g., emphysema, bronchitis, asthma) occur when ventilation is disturbed by an increase in airway resistance. Expiration is primarily affected.

d. Pulmonary function tests routinely include determination of forced vital capacity and forced expiratory volume.

e. Arterial blood gases (ABGs) and many other tests can be performed.

4. Nursing Implications

a. Before a pulmonary function test, the physician must obtain an informed consent for this procedure.

b. Instruct the patient not to use any bronchodilators and not to smoke for 6 h before this test.

c. Withhold the use of inhalers and aerosol therapy before the study.

d. After the procedure, allow the patient to rest because patients with severe respiratory problems are exhausted after testing.

e. Before ABGs are drawn, explain the procedure to the patient. ABGs must be obtained before oxygen is started.

f. Perform the Allen test.

(1) Make the patient's hand blanche by obliterating both the radial and the ulnar pulses, and release the pressure over the ulnar artery only.

(2) If flow through the ulnar artery is good, flushing will be seen immediately.

g. The Allen test ensures collateral circulation to the hand if thrombosis of the radial artery occurs.

h. Note that arterial blood can be obtained from any area of the body where strong pulses are palpable but usually is obtained from the radial, brachial, or femoral arteries.

i. The femoral artery is used most often.

j. During the procedure, attach a 20-gauge needle to a syringe containing approximately 0.2 mL of heparin.

k. After drawing 3 to 5 mL of blood into the syringe, expel any air from the syringe and gently rotate it to mix the blood and heparin.

l. Indicate on the laboratory slip if the patient is receiving oxygen therapy or is attached to a ventilator.

m. Note that an arterial puncture is performed by laboratory technicians, physicians, respiratory therapists, or nurses.

n. After the procedure, place the arterial blood on ice and immediately take it to the chemistry laboratory for analysis.

o. Apply pressure to the puncture site for 3 to 5 min, and then apply a pressure dressing.

p. Frequently assess the puncture site for bleeding for the first 2 h (every 15–20 min).

q. If the patient is taking anticoagulants, apply pressure for a longer period (approximately 15 min) and assess more frequently.

r. Assess pulse distal to the arterial puncture site frequently (every 15–20 min for the first 3–4 h).

II. RESPIRATORY DISEASES

A. Chronic Obstructive Pulmonary Disease

1. Etiology and Incidence

a. Dead space increases in the lungs, trapping carbon dioxide.

b. In the United States, chronic obstructive pulmonary disease (COPD) remains one of the most critical health problems.

c. Both morbidity and mortality are increasing at an alarming rate.

d. An estimated 10 million Americans suffer from COPD.

e. Predominant COPD entities include asthma, chronic bronchitis, and emphysema.

f. Cigarettes, pollution, and allergens are causes.

g. The incidence is higher in men but is increasing in women, as more women choose to use tobacco.

2. Signs and Symptoms

a. Pursed lips.

b. Whistle sound.

c. Barrel chest.

3. Treatment

a. Do not give more than 2 L of oxygen; this will decrease respirations because the respiratory center has adjusted to a high CO_2.

B. Asthma

1. Etiology

a. Extrinsic causes are allergens (food, dust, pollen particles, etc.).

b. Intrinsic causes are infection and emotions.

2. Signs and Symptoms

a. Usually decreases with age.

b. Wheezing.

3. Treatment

a. Bronchodilators (e.g., epinephrine).

b. Steroids.

C. Bronchiectasis

1. Etiology

a. Chronic abnormal dilation of bronchi and destruction of bronchial walls.

2. Signs and Symptoms

a. Hemoptysis and pneumonia.

b. Chronic cough with foul-smelling, copious secretions.

3. Treatment

a. Antibiotics.

b. Steroids.

c. Trachea care PRN.

D. Legionnaire's Disease

◆ First case was diagnosed at a legionnaire's convention.

1. Etiology and Incidence

a. Legionnaire's disease is an acute bronchopneumonia produced by a gram-negative bacillus.

b. This disease may occur epidemically or sporadically, usually in late summer or early fall.

c. The disease ranges from mild to severe illness, with a mortality rate as high as 15 percent.

d. The milder illness subsides within a few days but leaves the patient fatigued for several weeks.

e. This milder form produces few or no respiratory symptoms and no pneumonia.

2. Treatment

a. Erythromycin is the drug of choice.

b. If erythromycin is not effective alone, rifampin can be added to the regimen.

E. Lung Abscess

1. Etiology and Incidence

The availability of effective antibiotics has make lung abscess considerable less common than it was in the past. The cause of lung abscess is generally the result of aspiration or oropharyngeal contents causing necrotizing pneumonia. Poor oral hygiene and dental or gingival (gum) disease is strongly associated with putrid lung abscess.

2. Signs and Symptoms

a. Cough produces bloody, purulent, foul-smelling sputum.

b. Pleuritic chest pain, dyspnea, fever, and chills.

3. Treatment

a. Put on affected side to encourage draining.

b. Prolonged use of antibiotics is necessary to eliminate a lung abscess.

F. Tuberculosis

1. Etiology and Incidence

a. Some drug-resistant strains exist now because patients failed to take tuberculosis (TB) medications over sufficiently long periods.

b. TB medications must be taken from 9 months to 1 year or longer.

c. Transmitted by *airborne* droplets.

d. Persons living in crowded conditions and those with a compromised immune system are at risk.

2. Diagnosis

a. Mantoux skin test. Purified protein derivative (PPD).

(1) Draw a circle around test and date it.

(2) Check within 48 to 72 h. An area of induration measuring 10 mm or more in diameter is interpreted as a significant indicator of TB, and further tests will be conducted.

b. Sterile sputum specimen (smear and culture).

(1) Obtain before breakfast (sputum smear or culture).

(2) If the tubercle bacillus is present, the diagnosis of TB is confirmed.

c. To obtain a sputum culture, instruct patient to take a deep breath and then cough.

3. Treatment

a. Includes isoniazid (INH) with streptomycin for 9 months to 1 year or more, vitamin B$_6$ (for peripheral neuropathy caused by INH).

b. Rifampin and pyrazinamide (PZA) may also be used to treat TB.

c. A private room with appropriate air handling and ventilation is particularly important for reducing the risk of transmission of microorganisms from a source patient to susceptible patients and other persons in hospitals when the microorganism is spread by airborne transmission.

G. Fungus Infection of Lungs or Coccidioidomycosis (Valley Fever)

1. Etiology and Incidence

a. Occurs especially between the San Joaquin Valley in California and southwestern Texas.

b. Caused by fungus *Coccidioides immitis* and occurs primarily as a respiratory infection.

c. Common in migrant farm laborers, dark-skinned men (e.g., African-Americans and Mexicans) and pregnant women.

2. Signs and Symptoms

a. Night sweats.

b. Chronic cough with or without sputum production.

c. Hemoptysis.

d. Fatigue.

3. Treatment

a. Chemotherapy (INH), amphotericin B, fluconazole (Diflucan), itraconazole (Sporanox), or ketoconazole (Nizoral)

4. Nursing Implications

a. Encourage bed rest and adequate fluid intake.

b. Record the amount and color of sputum.

c. Observe for shortness of breath, which may indicate pleural effusion.

d. Follow strict secretion precautions, wash hands frequently, and wear gloves when handling secretions.

e. Assess for side effects of INH, such as those caused by bone marrow depression, including bleeding, anemia, and infections.

f. Assess for side effects of amphotericin B and decreased urinary output; monitor laboratory results for elevated blood urea nitrogen (BUN), elevated creatinine, and hypokalemia.

H. Asbestosis

1. Etiology

a. Asbestosis results from the inhalation of respirable asbestos fibres, which assume a longitudinal orientation in the airway and move in the direction of airflow. The fibers penetrate respiratory bronchioles and alveolar walls. Sources include the mining and milling of asbestos, the construction industry, and the fireproofing and textile industries. Asbestos was also used in the production of paints, plastics, and brake and clutch lining. This disease develops in the general public as a result of expsure to fibrous dust or waste piles from nearby asbestos plants.

b. Asbestosis is a potent co-carcinogen, asbestos increases the risk of lung cancer in cigarette smokers.

2. Treatment

a. Hypoxemia requires oxygen administration by cannula or mask or by mechanical ventilation if arterial oxygen cannot be maintained above 40 mm Hg.

b. Cortisone.

c. Respiratory infection requires prompt administration of antibiotics.

d. Aerosol therapy, inhaled mucolytics, and increased fluid intake of at least 3 L daily to relieve symptoms.

I. Laryngeal Cancer

1. Etiology and Incidence

   a. Excessive alcohol intake, smoking, and chewing tobacco.

   b. Most frequent in men older than 40 years.

2. Signs and Symptoms

   a. Early signs include hoarseness.

   b. Late signs are dysphagia, dyspnea, muffled voice, weight loss, cough, and expectoration of blood.

3. Treatment

   a. Chemotherapy, radiation, and surgery.

   b. Total laryngectomy is most often performed.

   c. Preoperative

   (1) Plan for postoperative communication using pencil or pen.

   (2) Educate patient regarding stoma.

   d. Postoperative

   (1) Use alternative communication planned in preoperative teaching.

   (2) Assist with esophageal speech or voice prosthesis.

   (3) Stoma care is performed as required.

   (4) Patient airway is the number one priority.

4. Nursing Implications

   a. Tracheostomy tubes are used for long-term airway management.

   (1) They are inserted through a surgical opening (stoma) into the trachea.

   (2) The tracheostomy tube has three parts: an outer cannula, an inner cannula, and an obturator.

   (3) This surgery is known as a tracheostomy.

   b. Potential causes of patient anxiety include fear of suffocation, choking, death, inability to speak, need to learn new ways to communicate, possible rejection by friends, and inability to work.

5. Nursing Interventions for Posttracheostomy

   a. Provide opportunity for patient to express concerns and fears.

   b. Elevate head of bed to facilitate respirations and minimize stoma edema.

   c. Suction trachea as needed.

   d. Provide humidification and oxygen as needed.

   e. Keep suction catheters sterile.

   f. Change dressing around tracheostomy tube using sterile procedure as needed.

   g. Clean inner cannula (fits inside outer cannula) using sterile technique as needed.

   h. The obturator fits inside the inner cannula. It is removed immediately after the tracheostomy tube is inserted, and it is placed in a sterile container at bedside.

   i. Once a tracheostomy tube's obturator is removed, the inner cannula fits into the outer cannula of the tracheostomy tube. Lock it into place to prevent accidental removal (e.g., during sucking or coughing).

   j. The inner cannula maintains airway potency. It is removed easily for cleaning.

   k. Tracheostomy tubes may be cuffed or uncuffed.

   (1) Inflated cuffs permit mechanical ventilation.

   (2) They protect the lower airway by creating a seal between the upper and lower airway.

   l. A tracheostomy cuff will not hold the tube in place; rather, when inflated, it seals the area between the outer cannula and the tracheal wall.

   m. To inflate a tracheostomy or endotracheal tube cuff, inject air with a syringe through the one-way valve into the cuff.

   n. Once the syringe is removed, the one-way valve prevents air from escaping from the inflated cuff.

J. Lung Cancer

1. Etiology and Incidence

   a. Lung cancer is caused by cigarette smoking (tobacco in any form) and inhalation of carcinogenic pollutants by susceptible host.

   b. Lung cancer is the most common cause of cancer death in men and is quickly becoming the most common cause in women, even though the disease is largely preventable.

2. Signs and Symptoms

   a. Early-stage lung cancer usually produces no symptoms, and lung cancer is often in advanced stages before diagnosis.

   b. Early symptoms include smoker's cough and hoarseness.

   c. Later symptoms include chest pain, weight loss, anoxia, hemoptysis, and dyspnea.

3. Treatment

   a. Surgery (pneumonectomy), radiation, and chemotherapy.

   b. Chemotherapy consists of combination of 5-fluorouracil, vincristine, mitomycin, cisplatin, or vinblastine.

   c. Small-cell carcinoma is treated with a combination of cyclophosphamide with doxorubicin, vincristine, or etoposide.

4. Nursing Implications

   a. Offer psychological support by listening to patient's concerns.

   b. Preoperatively, teach patient about medications, therapy, and surgery.

   (1) Assess the patient's understanding of planned surgery and expected outcomes.

   (2) Teach the patient how to perform breathing exercises, coughing, splinting of chest with small pillow, and arm and shoulder exercises.

c. Postoperatively, check vital signs, central venous pressure (CVP) readings, and urinary output.

(1) Observe for signs of respiratory dysfunction, such as slow, rapid, shallow, or irregular respirations, or cyanosis.

(2) Check ABG values and chest X-ray results.

(3) Assess fluid and electrolyte status.

(4) Observe for signs of pulmonary edema.

(5) Observe for signs of mediastinal shift, severe dyspnea, rapid irregular pulse, cyanosis, and displacement of the trachea from the midline.

K. Histoplasmosis

1. Etiology and Incidence

a. Fungal infection of the organism *Histoplasma capsulatum,* which is found in the feces of birds and bats or in soil contaminated by their feces.

b. Transmission is through inhalation of *H. capsulatum* and is most common in men and in patients with immunosuppressant disorders.

2. Signs and Symptoms

a. Early Signs

(1) Mild respiratory illness similar to a severe cold or influenza.

(2) Typical clinical effects may include fever, malaise, headache, and myalgia (tenderness or pain in the muscles).

b. Late Symptoms

(1) Hepatosplenomegaly, generalized lymphadenopathy, anorexia, weight loss, and fever.

c. Chronic Pulmonary Histoplasmosis

(1) Mimics TB. Causes productive cough, dyspnea, and occasionally hemoptysis.

(2) Eventually, it causes weight loss, extreme weakness, breathlessness, and cyanosis.

3. Treatment

a. Antifungal therapy using amphotericin B, which is the drug of choice.

b. If disease does not respond, cancer chemotherapy may be used.

c. Surgery may be necessary, which includes resection to remove pulmonary nodules.

d. Supportive care consists of oxygen for respiratory distress and bed rest during the acute phase.

4. Nursing Implications

a. Administer drugs as ordered and inform patient regarding side effects of amphotericin B, which may include chills, fever, nausea, and vomiting. Give appropriate antiemetics.

b. Offer psychological support.

c. Supportive care includes oxygen for respiratory distress, parenteral fluids, and bed rest during the acute phase.

d. Teach patients in endemic areas to watch for early signs and to seek medical treatment promptly.

L. Influenza (Grippe, Flu)

1. Etiology and Incidence

a. Influenza, an acute, highly contagious infection of the respiratory tract, results from three different types of *Myxovirus influenzae.* It occurs sporadically or in epidemics (usually during the colder months). Epidemics tend to peak within 2 to 3 weeks after initial cases and subside within 1 month.

b. Although influenza affects all age groups, its incidence is highest in school-aged children. However, its severity is greatest in the very young, the elderly, and those with chronic diseases. In these groups, influenza may even lead to death.

2. Transmission

a. Transmission of influenza occurs through inhalation of respiratory droplets from an infected person or by indirect contact, such as use of contaminated drinking glasses.

3. Signs and Symptoms

a. Following an incubation period of 24 to 48 h, flu symptoms begin to appear: sudden onset of chills, temperature of 101°F to 104°F, headache, malaise, myalgia, nonproductive cough, and, occasionally, laryngitis, hoarseness, conjunctivitis, rhinitis, and rhinorrhea. These symptoms usually subside in 3 to 5 days, but cough and weakness may persist. Fever usually is higher in children than in adults.

4. Treatment

a. Treatment of uncomplicated influenza includes bed rest, adequate fluid intake, aspirin or acetaminophen (in children) to relieve fever and muscle pain, and an expectorant to relieve nonproductive coughing.

5. Nursing Implications

a. Watch for signs and symptoms of developing pneumonia, such as rales, temperature rise, or coughing accompanied by blood-stained mucus. Educate patients about influenza immunizations. For high-risk patients and health care personnel, suggest annual inoculations at the start of the flu season (late fall). Remember, however, that such vaccines are made from chicken embryos and must not be given to persons who are hypersensitive to eggs, feathers, or chickens. The vaccine administered is based on the previous year's virus and usually is approximately 75% effective.

M. Isolation Precautions in Hospital

1. Universal Precautions

◆ Universal precautions were designed by the Center for Disease Control and Prevention (CDC) for the prevention of nosocomial infections. The tenets of *standard precautions* are that *all* patients are considered infected with microorganism with or without signs or symptoms, and that a uniform level of caution should be used in the care of *all* patients. The standard precautions include hand washing, glove use, needle stick prevention, and avoidance of splash exposure (e.g., sneezing, coughing) using appropriate barriers.

◆ The standard precautions include blood, all body fluids, secretions and excretions except sweat (regardless of whether or not they contain visible blood), mucous membranes, and nonintact skin. Standard precautions are designed to reduce the risk of transmission of microorganisms from both recognized and unrecognized sources of infection in hospitals.

a. Hand Washing

◆ Wash hands after touching blood, body fluids, secretions, excretions, and contaminated items, whether or not gloves are worn. Wash hands immediately after gloves are removed, between patient contacts, and when otherwise indicated to avoid transfer or microorganisms to other patients or environments.

b. Mask, Eye Protection, Face Shield

◆ Wear a mask and eye protection or a face shield to protect mucous membranes of the eyes, nose, and mouth during procedures and patient care activities that are likely to generate splashes or sprays of blood, body fluids, secretions, or excretions.

c. Gown

◆ Wear a gown (a clean, nonsterile gown is adequate) to protect skin and prevent soiling of clothing during procedures and patient care activities that are likely to generate splashes or sprays of blood, body fluids, secretions, or excretions.

d. Transport of Infected Patients

◆ Limit the movement and transport of patients infected with virulent or epidemiologically important microorganisms and ensure that such patients leave their rooms only when absolutely necessary.

2. Transmission-Based Precautions

Microorganisms are transmitted in hospitals by several routes, and the same microorganism may be transmitted by more than one route. The routes that play the most significant role in the transmission of microorganisms are contact, droplet, and airborne.

a. Contact Transmission

◆ In addition to standard precautions, use contact precautions for patients known or suspected to have serious illnesses easily transmitted by direct patient contact or contact with items in the patient's environment. Contact transmission is the most important and frequent mode of transmission of nosocomial infections. Contact transmission is divided into two subgroups: direct-contact transmission and indirect-contact transmission.

(1) *Direct-contact transmission* occurs when a nurse turns a patient, gives a patient a bath, or performs other patient care activities that require direct personal contact.

Direct-contact transmission also can occur between two patients, with one serving as the source of the infectious microorganisms and the other serving as a susceptible host.

(2) *Indirect-contact transmission* involves contact of a susceptible host with a contaminated intermediate object, usually inanimate, such as contaminated instruments, needles, or dressing, or contaminated hands that are not washed and gloves that are not changed between patients. Hand washing is considered the single most important measure for reducing the risk of transmitting organisms from one person to another or from one site to another on the same patient. Wearing gloves does not replace the need for washing hands because gloves may have small inapparent defects or may be torn during use, and hands can become contaminated during removal of gloves.

b. Examples of Illnesses Spread by Transmission Direct and Indirect Contact

(1) Abscess

(2) Hemorrhagic fever (e.g., Ebola)

(3) Resistant bacteria (multidrug-resistant)

(4) Scabies

(5) Methicillin *Staphylococcal aureus* infection

(6) Mononucleosis

(7) Herpes simplex virus (neonatal or mucocutaneous)

(8) Impetigo

(9) *Staphylococcal furunculosis* (boils)

(10) Herpes simplex (type I) cold sores

(11) Pediculosis (lice)

(12) Rubella (German measles) transmitted through direct and indirect contact with the blood, urine, stool, or nasopharyngeal secretions of infected person

(13) *Staphylococcus aureus* (group A streptococcus) causes the formation of foils.

(14) Zoster (shingles). Shingles results from the reactivation of varicella-zoster virus that has lain dormant in the cerebral nerve roots since a pervious episode of chicken pox.

Note: Congenital varicella may affect infants whose mothers had acute chicken pox infection in their first trimester of pregnancy. It can cause serious birth defects.

Note: Contact with infected body secretions is a major means of disease transmission.

c. Droplet Transmission

◆ Droplet transmissions are generated from the person infected, primarily during coughing, sneezing, and talking, and during the performance of certain procedures such as suctioning and bronchoscopy. Transmission via large-particle droplets will occur only when there is *close contact* with the infected person. Close contact with the infected person is required for transmission to occur because the droplets are propelled a very short distance through the air and deposited on the host's conjunctivae, nasal mucosa, or mouth. The nurse should wear a mask when suctioning the patient who is on droplets precautions and during a bronchoscopy. Because droplets are large and do not remain suspended in the air, special air handling and ventilation are not required to prevent droplet transmission. Droplet transmission must not be confused with airborne transmission.

d. Examples of illness spread by *droplets* contact transmission include

(**1**) Influenza (flu)

(**2**) Mumps droplets and contact with saliva

(**3**) Meningococcal (meningitis)

(**4**) Pneumococcal droplets and contact with infected respiratory secretions

(**5**) *Haemophilus influenzae* (infants and children, any age)

(**6**) *Streptococcus pneumoniae* (pneumococcal pneumonia) droplets and contact

(**7**) Respiratory syncytial virus droplets and direct or indirect contact with infected respiratory secretions

(**8**) *Bordetella pertussis* (vaccination is available)

e. Airborne Transmission

◆ Airborne transmission occurs by the same route as droplet transmission, but the airborne droplets are *very small* and are propelled a *long distance* through the air.

(**1**) Chicken pox (varicella) can be transmitted by airborne droplets, but it is transmitted primarily by respiratory secretions and less commonly from skin lesions. Chicken pox is caused by the varicella-zoster virus. A patient with chicken pox should be kept in a private room.

(**2**) TB is transmitted by airborne droplets. A patient with TB must be in an isolated, well-ventilated room until no longer contagious.

Note: Legionnaire's disease is an acute bronchopneumonia that is transmitted into the air by air conditioners. It is not spread from person to person.

N. Patient Placement

1. Appropriate patient placement is a significant component of isolation precautions. A private room is important to prevent direct-contact or indirect-contact transmission when the source patient has poor hygienic habits, contaminates the environment, or cannot be expected to assist in maintaining infection control precautions to limit transmission of microorganisms (i.e., infants, children, and patients with altered mental status). When possible, a patient with highly transmissible or epidemiologically important microorganisms is placed in a private room with hand washing and toilet facilities, to reduce opportunities for transmission of microorganisms.

2. When a private room is not available, an infected patient is placed with an appropriate roommate. *Patients infected by the same microorganism usually can share a room, provided they are not infected with other potentially transmissible microorganisms and the likelihood of reinfection with the same organism is minimal.* Such sharing of rooms, also referred to as *cohorting patients,* is useful especially during outbreaks or when there is a shortage of private rooms. When a private room is not available or cohorting is not achievable or recommended, it is very important to consider the epidemiology and mode of transmission of the infecting pathogen and the patient population being served in determining patient placement. Under these circumstances, consultation with infection control professionals is advised before patient placement.

III. OTHER RESPIRATORY DISORDERS

A. Pulmonary Embolism

Occlusion of a pulmonary artery.

1. Etiology and Incidence

a. Pulmonary emboli are fairly common.

b. Most pulmonary emboli originate in the deep veins of the lower extremities or pelvis.

c. Predisposing factors include venous stasis, vascular damage, and increased blood coagulability after surgery or other injury.

2. Signs and Symptoms

a. Pleuritic chest pain and mild to severe cough, with or without hemoptysis, tachycardia, and tachypnea.

b. Sharp pain clear through chest to the shoulder.

3. Treatment

a. The best treatment is prevention through use of one adult low dose 81 mg aspirin per day.

b. If patient is at high risk for pulmonary emboli, Coumadin PO every day.

c. Heparin and Coumadin to prevent clots; tissue-type plasminogen activator (t-PA) and streptokinase to dissolve blood clots.

d. Prevention of pulmonary emboli includes good hydration and early ambulation by elevation, exercise, elastic stockings, or electrical leg compression device to prevent venous stasis.

e. Assess for dyspnea, chest pain, tachypnea, cough, hemoptysis, cyanosis, and apprehension.

f. Place the patient in semi-Fowler's position to facilitate breathing, and administer oxygen as ordered.

g. Give analgesics as ordered to foster good ventilation because pain usually is pleuritic.

h. Implement the prescribed medical regimen of anticoagulant or thrombolytic therapy; start range-of-motion exercises.

i. Monitor respiratory status, including lung sounds, ABGs, prothrombin time, and partial thromboplastin time.

j. Check the patient for signs of bleeding.

k. Instruct the patient on self-administration of prescribed anticoagulants and related precautions prior to discharge.

B. Drug-Induced Pulmonary Edema

1. Etiology and Incidence

a. Most common cause is overdose of heroin, methadone, cocaine, or acetylsalicylic acid (aspirin).

b. Incidence has increased with increased use of these drugs.

2. Signs and Symptoms

a. The first symptom of an overdose is respiratory depression.

b. Other signs include hypotension, lethargy, and drowsiness.

c. In acute intoxication, pulmonary edema, pinpoint pupils, and coma may be present.

3. Treatment

a. Narcotic overdose is treated with naloxone (Narcan) administered intravenously.

b. Treatment of aspirin overdose includes administration of ipecac syrup to produce vomiting. Enemas may be given, and nasogastric (NG) suctioning may be performed.

c. For any of these treatments to be effective, they must be given before the drug is absorbed into the bloodstream.

d. Hemodialysis may be used to remove toxin from the bloodstream.

4. Nursing Implications

a. If drug overdose was intentional, patient needs psychological support by the nurse and counseling from a psychologist.

C. Respiratory Acidosis

1. Etiology and Incidence

a. Predisposing factors include COPD and pneumonia (failure to rid lungs of carbon dioxide).

2. Signs and Symptoms

a. Increase in pH (compensation), increased carbon dioxide.

b. Early: confusion, headache, tachypnea.

c. Late: papilledema (inflammation of optic nerve), depressed reflexes, hypoxemia, hypoventilation, coma, and death.

3. Treatment

a. Sodium bicarbonate

b. Mechanical ventilation

c. Bronchodilators

d. Prophylactic antibiotics

D. Respiratory Alkalosis

1. Etiology

a. Hyperventilation

2. Signs and Symptoms

a. Decrease in pH (compensation) and increased bicarbonate (too much carbon dioxide exhaled).

b. Tachypnea, lightheadedness, paresthesias, and dizziness.

3. Treatment

a. Place paper bag over head to rebreathe carbon dioxide.

E. Spontaneous Pneumothorax

1. Young men are more prone to develop this disease.

2. Surgery may be necessary.

3. Surgeon will rough up pleura so that it sticks together.

4. Chest tubes will be used to reexpand the lungs.

F. Mediastinal Shift

1. Can be caused by tension pneumothorax, where one lung pushes over and pushes trachea over.

2. Patient will have difficulty breathing.

3. During total pneumonectomy (removal of a lung), no chest tubes are used so that the compartment will fill up with blood and prevent the remaining lung from pushing the trachea over (mediastinal shift).

G. Crepitus

1. Subcutaneous emphysema can be caused by displaced trachea tube as air blows up underneath the skin.

2. Patient can die from the condition.

3. If the trachea tube becomes dislodged and comes out of the trachea, a sterile hemostat is needed to hold the trachea open.

IV. MANAGEMENT OF CHEST TUBES

A. Description of Chest Tubes

1. The drainage chest tube is closest to the patient, next is the water-seal compartment, and then the suction unit.

2. All three components are in a unit called a *Pleur-evac.*

3. The suction unit is hooked to wall suction.

4. The amount of suction is determined by the physician.

B. Function of Chest Tubes

1. Tidaling

a. Tidaling is the rise and fall of fluid in the water-seal compartment with inspiration and expiration, respectively.

b. Tidaling occurs during the first 3 to 4 days after the chest tube is inserted. It occurs during this period because the pleural leak has not healed.

c. If tidaling does not occur during the first 3 days, follow these steps to locate the occlusion.

(1) Check to be sure the tube is not kinked or compressed.

(2) If tube is not kinked, ask the patient to take a deep breath and cough; this may clear the tubing.

(3) If tubing remains occluded, notify the physician.

(4) It has been a practice to "milk" the drainage tube to remove the source of occlusion when tidaling was not occurring during first 3 days.

(5) This practice is usually not recommended because of the potential for a pressure pneumothorax caused by occluding the chest tube while milking it.

(6) Tidaling will stop after the pleural leak has healed and the lung has reexpanded approximately 4 to 6 days after chest tube was inserted.

2. Bubbling

a. Intermittent bubbling should occur in the water-seal compartment during the first 3 to 4 days after chest tube is inserted.

b. Bubbling occurs during expiration.

c. Continuous bubbling that occurs in the water-seal chamber during both inspiration and expiration indicates that air is leaking into the drainage system or pleural cavity.

d. This situation must be corrected because air entering the system also enters the pleural space.

e. Locate the source of the air leak and repair it if possible. First, find the source of the air leak and then institute the following steps.

(1) If a catheter is loose, gently squeeze the skin up around the catheter, secure it with sterile petrolatum gauze, and tape firmly around the catheter and onto the skin.

(2) Determine whether or not this step stops the continuous bubbling in the bottle.

(3) If this step does not stop the bubbling, check all connections.

(4) Check the tubing inch by inch and seal with tape if a leak is found.

(5) Rapid bubbling in the water-seal compartment in the absence of an air leak indicates a considerable loss of air, such as from a tear in the pulmonary pleura.

(6) Notify the physician immediately so that appropriate intervention can be taken to prevent collapse of the lung.

3. Absence of Bubbling

a. Absence of continuous bubbling in the suction control compartment indicates the system is not functioning properly and the correct level of suction is not being maintained.

b. Possible reasons

(1) Mechanical problems with the suction source or leak in the drainage connection.

(2) Large amounts of air leaking into the pleural space or drainage compartment.

c. To find the cause, follow these steps:

(1) Briefly clamp the chest drainage tube.

(2) If bubbling begins in the suction control compartment, there is nothing wrong with the drainage connection or the suction source; the problem is an air leak into the pleural space around the chest tubes.

(3) If the air leak cannot be sealed off (e.g., with petrolatum gauze), notify the physician immediately.

(4) If bubbling does not begin in the suction control compartment when the chest drainage catheter is clamped, the problem is in the drainage connection or the suction source.

4. Understanding the Concept of Bubbling

a. To understand the concept of bubbling, put a straw in a glass of water and blow air through it; the water bubbles.

b. Now kink the straw and blow air; no bubbling occurs.

c. If your mouth heals shut (joke), no air can come out through the straw, so there is no bubbling.

d. This is the process when the hole in the pleural cavity heals and the lung reexpands.

e. If no air can come out of the pleural cavity, no bubbling will occur in the water-seal compartment, and there is no tidaling fluctuation in the tubing in the water-seal compartment.

5. Understanding the Concept of Tidaling

a. If there is a hole in the pleural cavity, then when the patient takes a breath it pulls water up in the water-seal compartment, which is the same as pulling water up a straw.

b. When the patient breathes out, the water goes back down into the water-seal compartment.

c. When you blow air into the straw, water goes back down the straw.

d. This continues until the hole in the pleural cavity is healed and the lung is reexpanded.

e. About the fourth or fifth day, the chest tube can be pulled out of the pleural space by the physician.

6. Drainage

a. Usually as much as 50 to 1000 mL of drainage occurs in the first 24 h after chest surgery.

b. Between 100 and 300 mL of drainage may accumulate during the first 2 h.

c. After this period, drainage should gradually decrease.

7. Removing the Chest Tube

a. Prior to removing the chest tube, give the patient an analgesic if there is an order for PRN pain medication because the procedure is very painful.

b. Have petrolatum gauze ready for pressure dressing as soon as the physician removes the chest tube (use sterile gloves).

c. Physician will change the dressing 3 days later or remove it.

8. Accidental Removal

a. If the chest tube is removed accidentally, make a flutter valve by cutting a finger off a latex glove and holding it over the incision site or tape it over the incision site.

b. Call the physician immediately.

c. Do not cover the chest tube incision with a pressure dressing because it may cause a pressure pneumothorax.

d. If the chest tube becomes disconnected from the Pleur-evac, immediately place tubing in a bottle of sterile saline solution and notify the physician immediately.

e. Have a Pleur-evac available for reattachment.

EXAMINATION

1. A patient is admitted to the hospital with a tentative diagnosis of bronchogenic tumor in the left lung area. The physician's admission orders include sending the sputum specimen to laboratory for cytology, scheduling a bronchoscopy, and scheduling pulmonary function tests. Cytologic examination of the patient's sputum is done to determine the presence of

1. Mucous casts.
2. Blood cells.
3. Malignant cells
4. Pathogenic bacteria.

2. The *primary* purpose for conducting a variety of pulmonary function tests prior to surgery is to

1. Evaluate the extent of the spread of the lung cancer.
2. Estimate the amount of anesthesia needed for surgery.
3. Determine the amount of lung tissue that will need to be removed.
4. Calculate whether or not the contemplated surgery will leave enough functioning lung tissue.

3. A patient asks the nurse the purpose of intermittent positive-pressure breathing (IPPB) therapy. The nurse correctly replies that the *primary* purpose for using preoperative IPPB therapy for the patient is to

1. Dilate the bronchioles.
2. Aerate dead air spaces in the lungs.
3. Reduce the carbon dioxide in the blood.
4. Clear the airway to the greatest extent possible.

4. After receiving a sedative, a patient says to the nurse, "I guess you are too busy to stay with me." The best response in this circumstance is

1. "I have to see other patients because we are short staffed, but I'll check on you in a few minutes."
2. "The medication will help you, and you will be just fine."
3. "I have to go now, but I will come back in 10 minutes."
4. "You will feel better. I will increase your oxygen, and if that doesn't help, put your light on and I will bring you an analgesic."

5. A patient has surgery to remove the tumor in his left lung. He returns from the recovery room with a left chest tube hooked to a Pleur-evac. Suction is being used. The statement that would correctly explain intermittent bubbling in the water-seal compartment and fluctuation (tidaling) in the compartment is

1. The lung has not reexpanded.
2. The water level has dropped too low in the drainage bottle.
3. The chest tube has slipped out of the patient's chest.
4. The tube connecting the drainage bottle with the patient's chest catheter has developed a leak.

6. The Pleur-evac is hooked to suction, and continuous bubbling in the suction bottle occurs. This would indicate that

1. There is a lack of suctioning by the wall suction.
2. The wall suction is not working.
3. The chest tube is kinked.
4. There is active suctioning.

7. The patient complains of pain at the chest tube insertion sites. The nurse should

1. Check the tube for kinks.
2. Check the tube for patency.
3. Call the doctor immediately.
4. Administer Demerol 100 mg IM as ordered.

8. On the patient's third postoperative day, the intermittent bubbling stops and the fluctuation in the water-seal container stops. The most probable cause of this finding is

1. The tubing is loose at the insertion site.
2. The lung has reexpanded.
3. There is leakage of air in the seal.
4. The tubing needs to be irrigated.

9. On the third postoperative day, the physician removes the patient's posterior chest tube. The nurse would immediately place which of the following directly over the wound when the chest tube is removed?

1. A Montgomery strap.
2. An OpSite dressing.
3. A petrolatum gauze dressing.
4. A fine-mesh gauze dressing.

10. The dressing applied after a chest tube is removed should be
    1. Changed during each shift.
    2. Looked under during each shift but not removed.
    3. Changed after 5 to 6 days.
    4. Taken off on the third or fourth day and left off.

11. A patient who has repeated upper respiratory infections is diagnosed as having bronchiectasis. The nurse explains to the patient that bronchiectasis is characterized by
    1. A growth of malignant cells that have spread through the lungs.
    2. Extensive inflammation of the lungs.
    3. An incurable inflammation of the bronchial tree.
    4. Permanent dilation of the bronchi with a collection of copious amounts of a foul-smelling mucopurulent secretion.

12. When assessing a patient with bronchiectasis, the nurse recognizes which of the following as the most outstanding sign(s) of bronchiectasis:
    1. Low-grade fever in the afternoon.
    2. Copious amounts of foul-smelling sputum.
    3. Watery eyes and nasal discharge.
    4. Nonproductive cough.

13. A primary nursing intervention for a patient with bronchiectasis would be
    1. Frequent assessment of vital signs.
    2. Frequent oral hygiene care.
    3. Respiratory isolation.
    4. Alternating periods of rest and activity.

14. A patient with a long history of cigarette smoking is admitted to the hospital with mild respiratory distress. The doctor performs diagnostic studies to determine the causative factors of his symptoms. The physician orders sputum cultures. The nurse understands that these cultures should be done
    1. Early in the morning, 3 to 4 days after the antibiotic is started.
    2. Before antibiotics are initiated.
    3. Immediately after antibiotics are initiated.
    4. Any time sputum is produced.

15. A patient has a bronchogram performed. In order to determine when to offer fluids to the patient, the nurse will note when
    1. The gag reflex returns.
    2. Two hours after the procedures have passed.
    3. The patient has expectorated all of the dye.
    4. The patient's vital signs are stable.

16. A patient is diagnosed with right lower lobe viral pneumonia. The nursing care plan for the patient includes the following: do not stimulate the patient to talk, feed in small quantities, and help the patient move in bed. The rationale for these actions would be to
    1. Increase the patient's need for oxygen.
    2. Decrease the patient's intake of oxygen.
    3. Conserve the patient's need for oxygen.
    4. Increase the patient's awareness of his or her oxygen needs.

17. A patient who is acutely ill and has a diagnosis of pneumonia is admitted to the hospital. Oxygen by nasal cannula is to be administered. The *least* important data the nurse collects when a patient is admitted with a diagnosis of pneumonia is
    1. Information about the patient's diet.
    2. Observing the skin color.
    3. Obtaining the respiratory rate.
    4. Auscultating for chest sounds.

18. A patient says to the nurse, "I started with a cold and used nose drops but after a while they made me even stuffier." The nurse judges that the effect the patient has experienced from the repeated use of nose drops is a (an) ____ effect.
    1. Rebound.
    2. Synergistic.
    3. Antagonistic.
    4. Accumulative.

19. The appropriate nursing intervention to be used by a nurse when wishing to obtain a sputum specimen from a patient is to
    1. Teach the patient how to cough deeply to produce sputum.
    2. Help the patient decrease fluid intake temporarily.
    3. Have the patient fast for several hours prior to obtaining the specimen.
    4. Teach the patient to expectorate whatever is in his or her mouth for the specimen.

20. It is necessary to supply humidity through a tracheostomy because
    1. Periods of dyspnea will occur as oxygen dries the lungs.
    2. The nose and pharynx are bypassed, and oxygen dries secretions.
    3. Periods of apnea occur and the mouth will become dry.
    4. All of the above.

21. When suctioning the respiratory tract, it is recommended that the nurse wait for several minutes if it is necessary to repeat the procedure because the rest period allows time for
    1. The irritated mucous membrane to recover.
    2. The body to replenish itself with oxygen.
    3. The patient to overcome fatigue because the procedure is tiring.

4. The patient to overcome pain because the procedure is painful.

22. A female patient is brought to the emergency room (ER) by her sister following a day spent outside doing spring yard work. She is experiencing dyspnea, coughing, and tachycardia. A diagnosis of asthma is made. In assessing the patient during her asthmatic attack, the nurse would expect that the patient's respirations would be characterized by a (an)

1. Absence of breath sounds in the lower lobes of lung.
2. Asymmetric movements of the chest.
3. Prolonged expiratory breathing with wheezing.
4. Increased rate and depth of respirations.

23. A patient with asthma is given aminophylline to

1. Induce sleep and rest.
2. Relax the pulmonary vessels.
3. Cause dilation of the bronchi.
4. Decrease the body's inflammatory reaction to an allergen.

24. The physician orders epinephrine 1:1000 solution 1 mL SC stat at 10:00 AM and then every 4 h PRN for respiratory distress. At 2:00 PM, the patient develops dyspnea and respiratory wheezing. The nurse's *best* action would be to

1. Administer the epinephrine promptly as ordered.
2. Administer all medications IM because they would be better absorbed.
3. Verify the medication order with the physician and then give the medication stat.
4. Notify the physician of the change in the patient's condition.

25. The disease that has decreased in frequency and severity with the increased use of antibiotics is

1. Bronchitis.
2. Emphysema.
3. Bronchiectasis.
4. COPD.

26. The most effective treatment of TB is

1. Chemotherapy isoniazid (INH).
2. Dobutamine.
3. Adriamycin.
4. Streptomycin.

27. The procedure that allows for the *direct* inspection of lungs and the biopsy of lymph nodes is

1. Mediastinoscopy.
2. Bronchography.
3. Bronchoscopy.
4. Thoracentesis.

28. When suctioning via a tracheostomy tube, the nurse must

1. Insert the catheter approximately 8 to 15 inches to ensure the bronchi are cleared.

2. Apply suction while inserting and withdrawing the catheter.
3. Suction 30 seconds per entry to prevent severe hypoxia.
4. Rotate the catheter while applying suction and withdrawing the catheter.

29. A patient is admitted to the unit with a diagnosis of chronic emphysema and acute bilateral pneumonia. He is confused, agitated, dyspneic, and cyanotic. Which of the following concerning his need for oxygen would be true?

1. A high flow rate of oxygen.
2. An oxygen tent.
3. A low flow rate of oxygen.
4. A high oxygen concentration.

30. In emergency situations, the method of choice for oxygen administration is

1. Oxygen tent until the immediate danger is over.
2. Nasal cannula at a high flow rate.
3. Nonrebreathing masks.
4. Nasal catheter lubricated with water-soluble lubricant.

31. The primary purpose of an incentive spirometer is to

1. Encourage the patient to exhale.
2. Arouse and stimulate the patient.
3. Increase respiratory volume.
4. Measure tidal volume and inspiratory reserve volume.

32. A patient is admitted with a diagnosis of pneumonia. As a general rule, the test most valuable in the selection of an antibiotic is the

1. Schilling test.
2. Leukocyte count.
3. Serologic test.
4. Culture and sensitivity test.

33. Physical assessment of a patient reveals rhonchi and wheezes in the left lung and some wheezes in the right lower lobe. Rhonchi and wheezes are due to

1. Total obstruction of small bronchioles.
2. Partial obstruction of bronchi and bronchioles.
3. Fluid in the alveoli.
4. Inflammation of the pleura.

34. The nurse explains to a patient that a bronchoscopy is

1. An X-ray procedure that allows for multiple views of the lungs.
2. A procedure using a flexible fiberoptic scope to observe the walls of the trachea, mainstem bronchus, and major bronchial tubes, larynx, and alveoli.
3. A diagnostic test during which a radiopaque substance is inserted into the tracheobronchial tree for clear visualization.

4. A needle puncture of the lung mass identified on X-ray film with aspiration of cells for microscopic examination.

35. A male patient is admitted with a history of asthma. The physician prescribes isoetharine hydrochloride (Bronkosol) per air-driven nebulizer for 20 min q4h. The nurse should observe the patient for the following side effects of Bronkosol:
    1. Pallor, dyspnea, and sweating.
    2. Bradycardia, diplopia, and gastrointestinal bleeding.
    3. Diarrhea, pulmonary edema, and weakness.
    4. Headache, anxiety, and arrhythmias.

36. The nurse should suspect the provoking factor for an asthmatic attack is that the patient
    1. Wore a new suit made of synthetic material 2 days ago.
    2. Ate strawberries.
    3. Used a new kind of cough medicine.
    4. Slept on a new feather pillow.

37. A male patient is scheduled for pulmonary function tests. The nurse should instruct him that the purpose of these studies is to
    1. Determine his tolerance for exercise.
    2. Determine which areas of his lung are affected.
    3. Evaluate the extent of his ventilatory deficiency.
    4. Evaluate the adequacy of his cardiopulmonary circulation.

38. A male patient has an acute asthmatic attack. Epinephrine hydrochloride (Adrenalin) is administered. Following administration of Adrenalin, the nurse should observe the patient for Adrenalin's vasoconstricting effects. These would include
    1. Drowsiness and hypotension.
    2. Throbbing headache, muscle tension, and hypertension.
    3. Flushed face, increase in body temperature, and headache.
    4. Polyuria, urticaria, and hypertension.

39. During the asthmatic attack, the patient spontaneously assumes an upright sitting position. The nurse provides an over-bed table for the patient to lean on. Implementation of this nursing measure will promote the positive effect of
    1. Reducing the intracellular pressure of the diaphragm.
    2. Stimulating initiation of the pleural reflex.
    3. Increasing the muscle tone of the bronchioles.
    4. Permitting a more efficient use of the muscles of respiration.

40. A nursing history reveals that a male patient had all of the diseases listed below during his childhood. The nurse should recognize that one of these diseases has a relationship to asthma. That disease is
    1. Rheumatic fever.
    2. Otitis media.
    3. Chicken pox.
    4. Eczema.

41. A male patient has a partial glossectomy with dissection of the left cervical lymph nodes. When he returns from the recovery room, he has a cuffed tracheostomy tube and a nasogastric feeding tube in place. His postoperative prescriptions include special mouth care. The nurse provides the patient's mouth care during the postoperative period. The most therapeutic approach would be to
    1. Cleanse his suture line with cotton balls moistened with saline.
    2. Wash his tongue with antiseptically saturated sterile gauze pads.
    3. Have him gargle and rinse his mouth with warm water.
    4. Irrigate his mouth with dilute hydrogen peroxide solution.

42. When a patient has a tracheostomy, the nursing measure that will be *essential* is
    1. Detecting the need for suctioning.
    2. Keeping the suction apparatus patent and turned on at all times.
    3. Removing the inner cannula each time suctioning is required.
    4. Changing the dressing around the tracheal opening each shift.

43. A male patient with a 30-year history of COPD is admitted to the intensive care unit with symptoms of pallor, cyanosis, tachypnea, orthopnea, restlessness, and confusion. He has a spontaneous left pneumothorax, and chest tubes are inserted. After the nurse makes an overall assessment of the patient, the nurse will
    1. Milk the tubing to prevent accumulation of fibrin and clots.
    2. Raise the Pleur-evac to bed height to assess accurately the meniscus level.
    3. Attach the chest tubes to the bed linen to ensure that air flow and drainage are unhindered by kinks.
    4. Mark time and amount of drainage in the collection bottle.

44. The nurse observes that a patient has an increase in rales (coarse rhonchi), anxiety, and tachypnea. The first nursing intervention will be to
    1. Call the doctor.
    2. Perform tracheobronchial suctioning.
    3. Increase the oxygen flow rate and call the doctor.
    4. Administer a bronchodilator.

45. A patient has a chest tube, and on the third postoperative day, fluctuation in the water-seal compartment stops. Auscultation of the patient's upper left chest indicates the lung has reexpanded. The physician orders a chest X-ray film to assess the degree of reexpansion. To transport the patient safely to the radiography department, the nurse would

1. Assist the physician to remove the chest tubes, immediately covering the incision site with a sterile petrolatum gauze to prevent air from entering the chest.
2. Disconnect the Pleur-evac from the chest tube, covering the catheter tip with a sterile dressing to prevent contamination.
3. Send the patient to the radiography department with the chest tube clamped but still attached to the drainage system to prevent air from entering the chest wall if the bottles are accidentally broken.
4. Send the patient to the radiography department with the chest tube attached to the Pleur-evac, taking precautions to prevent breakage of the Pleur-evac or tube separation.

46. A patient was involved in a serious automobile accident. He has been taken to the hospital where it has been determined that he has multiple traumas and a possible skull fracture. While monitoring this patient initially, the nurse is particularly alert for signs and symptoms of

1. Increased intracranial pressure (ICP) and shock.
2. Shock and infection.
3. Peritonitis and pulmonary edema.
4. Shortness of breath and hypertension.

47. A patient with hematuria after a serious car accident alerts the nurse to observe for

1. Tachycardia and hypotension.
2. Symptoms of peritonitis.
3. Hypertension and renal failure.
4. Symptoms of urinary infection.

48. Hematuria after an automobile accident most likely means that there is an injury to

1. The urethra.
2. The kidney.
3. The bladder.
4. The ureters.

49. The nurse would help a terminal breast cancer patient deal with her depression by

1. Asking the physician for a patient-controlled analgesia (PCA) pump for the patient.
2. Suggesting that she have her minister come and talk with her.
3. Cheering her up by talking about things that interest her.
4. Recognizing her grief and helping her express it.

50. When evaluating a patient with breast cancer and on chemotherapy, the nurse knows that the *least* important value to monitor is that the patient's

1. White blood cell (WBC) count is significantly lower than it was 2 days ago.
2. Red blood cell (RBC) count is significantly lower than yesterday.
3. Platelet count is significantly lower than yesterday.
4. Serum protein is significantly lower than yesterday.

ANSWERS AND RATIONALES

1. ❸ Assessment of a person suspected of a bronchiogenic tumor of the lung includes serial cytologic sputum assessment to determine if the cells are benign or malignant; bronchial brushing during bronchoscopy washing; and percutaneous needle biopsy of a mass previously located by chest Xray film, tomogram, or computed tomographic (CT) scan.

(1, 2, 4) A cytologic examination would not be done to determine the presence of mucous casts, blood cells, or pathogenic bacteria.

2. ❹ The primary purpose for conducting a variety of pulmonary function tests prior to surgery is to determine whether or not the contemplated surgery will leave enough functioning lung tissue. If insufficient functioning lung tissue will be left after surgery for the patient to have adequate gas exchange, there would be no reason to perform the surgery.

(1) A pulmonary function test will evaluate the ability of the lung to function; the test will not determine metastasis of the cancer. Lymph node biopsy and blood work are needed to determine metastasis.

(2) Pulmonary function tests are not used to estimate the amount of anesthesia needed for the surgery.

(3) The concern is not how much tissue will be removed during surgery but rather how much functional lung tissue will remain.

3. ❶ The primary purpose of IPPB is to dilate the bronchiole.

(2) Dead air space cannot be aerated.

(3) IPPB does not directly reduce the carbon dioxide in the patient's blood, but if there is an accumulation of carbon dioxide in the blood then dilating the bronchioles will increase gas exchange, which would help reduce the carbon dioxide in the blood. IPPB is given to increase gas exchange in the lungs and to decrease the potential for lung infections.

(4) IPPB does *not* clear the airway. Nasotracheal suctioning and postural drainage would help prevent airway obstruction and help clear the airway.

4. ❸ When the patient says to the nurse, "I guess you are too busy to stay with me," the nurse's best response is to give a time when she or he will return. This allows the patient to feel safe and cared for because the patient knows when the nurse will return.

(1) A nurse should never tell a patient that they are short staffed because this makes the patient feel unsafe and a burden to the nurse.

(2) Telling the patient that the medication will help and that the patient will be just fine is false reassurance. The nurse cannot be sure the medication will help or that the patient will be fine.

(4) Again, telling a patient that he or she will feel better is not appropriate, as stated in rationale (2). A nurse cannot increase the patient's oxygen without a physician's order. These orders would have to be written in the stem of the question. The patient is not in pain. The patient just wants someone to spend some time talking and listening to him or her.

5. ❶ The Pleur-evac is a three-chamber system used most often for closed-chest drainage. Intermittent bubbling in the water-seal compartment indicates the puncture into the pleural cavity has *not* healed and air is still leaking from the lung into the pleural cavity, down the tubing, and into the water-seal compartment (continuous bubbling would indicate an air leak). To check to see if the lung has reexpanded, shut the suction off. No tidaling or bubbling should occur in the water-seal compartment if the lung has reexpanded. If continuous bubbling occurs in the water-seal compartment in the absence of suction, there may be air leaking from the pleural space at the point where the tube enters the chest. If the leak is where the tube enters the chest, this leak can be sealed off by the nurse with a petrolatum jelly gauze and by taping the tubing. If it is not leaking there, check the rest of the tubing for leaks.

(2) There is no water in the drainage bottle (compartment). This compartment is for drainage from the lungs, and each shift the nurse must mark the level of drainage on the drainage compartment of the Pleur-evac.

(3) If a chest tube has slipped out of the patient's chest, there would be no bubbling and no fluctuation because the Pleur-evac is no longer connected to the pleural space. This is an emergency situation.

(4) If a leak developed, there would be continuous bubbling in the *water-seal bottle*. The *drainage chamber* is connected to suction, so it will have continuous bubbling because of the suction.

6. ❹ Continuous bubbling in the drainage compartment will occur when the Pleur-evac is hooked to suction and the suction is turned on.

(1, 2, 3) If there is lack of suction by the wall suction or the chest tube was kinked, there would be little or no bubbling.

7. ❹ It is normal for the chest tube to hurt at the site of insertion, and pain medication is given as ordered. This is a large tube stitched to the chest wall, which causes irritation and pain; therefore, there is no need to call the doctor or check the tubing for kinks or patency. Administer analgesics as ordered.

(1, 2, 3) These options are incorrect as seen in rationale (4).

8. ❷ When fluctuation (tidaling) and intermittent bubbling stops in the water-seal compartment after the third postoperative day, this is an indication that the lung has reexpanded.

(1, 3) If the tubing was loose at the insertion site or there was leakage somewhere else in the tubing, there would be continuous bubbling in the water-seal compartment.

(4) Chest tubes are never irrigated.

9. ❸ Immediately after the physician removes the chest tube, a petrolatum gauze dressing is taped over the site to serve as a pressure dressing to prevent air from reentering the pleural space.

(1, 2, 4) None of these items would be used over a wound after a chest tube was removed.

10. ❹ After the third or fourth day, the wound where the chest tube was removed will be healed and the dressing usually is removed by the physician.

(1, 2) The dressing is a pressure dressing, so it is not changed each shift or looked under.

(3) Five to six days is longer than a chest tube dressing should stay on.

11. ❹ Bronchiectasis is characterized by permanent dilation of the bronchi with a collection of copious, foul-smelling, mucopurulent secretions.

(1, 2, 3) These options are not characteristic of bronchiectasis.

12. ❷ The most outstanding sign of bronchiectasis is copious amounts of foul-smelling sputum.

(1, 3, 4) These options are not signs of bronchiectasis.

13. ❷ Frequent oral hygiene care is a very necessary nursing intervention because of the copious amounts of foul-smelling sputum that the patient continually coughs up.

(1) Assessment is not an intervention. When the question asks for a nursing intervention, then be test-wise and look for an appropriate nursing intervention and not an assessment.

(3) There is no need for respiratory isolation because bronchiectasis is not contagious. This disease results from conditions associated with repeated damage to bronchial walls and poor mucociliary clearance. Such conditions include cystic fibrosis and inadequately treated bacterial infections, such as TB or pneumonia.

(4) Alternating periods of rest and activities will be what the patient does for himself or herself because most of the patient's energy will be used in coughing up sputum and fighting the infection.

14. ❷ It is important that the sputum culture be obtained before antibiotics are started because the antibiotics will begin to destroy the microorganism and the culture may not reflect the seriousness of the disease or the main bacteria causing the disease. The physician needs to know what organism needs to be destroyed so that the antibiotic that will be most effective against that bacteria will be ordered.

(1, 3, 4) These options are incorrect as seen in rationale (2).

15. ❶ After a bronchogram, the nurse must determine if the patient's gag reflex has returned before offering fluids to the patient. If fluids are given before the gag reflex returns, the patient could aspirate them.

(2, 3, 4) These options are incorrect as seen in rationale (1). The return of the gag reflex will determine when the patient can have fluids by mouth.

16. ❸ When a patient is in respiratory distress, it is a priority to conserve the patient's oxygen and energy so that the patient can recover.

(1) The nurse would not want to increase the patient's need for oxygen.

(2) The nurse cannot decrease the patient's intake of oxygen without a physician's order.

(4) The patient is well aware of his or her need for oxygen and will not need anyone to tell her or him.

17. ❶ The least important information to collect on a patient admitted with acute pneumonia is about the patient's diet.

(2, 3, 4) When a patient is admitted with acute pneumonia, it is most important to collect data on the patient's skin color to determine if the patient is cyanotic, determine the respiratory rate, and auscultate the chest sounds to assess the patient's degree of respiratory distress.

18. ❶ The continual use of nose drops causes a rebound effect, meaning it causes more nose congestion rather than clearing up the congestion.

(2) "Synergistic" means acting together (enhancing the effect of the Pleur-evac on another agent). This effect does not occur with the repeated use of nose drops.

(3) "Antagonistic effect" refers to a substance that interferes with the normal action and use of another substance. This effect does not occur with repeated use of nose drops.

(4) "Accumulative effect" refers to the effect of drugs given together over a period of time working together. This is not what happens with repeated use of nose drops.

19. ❶ It is important that the nurse instruct the patient to cough deeply so that the material coughed up is sputum and not spit.

(2) Decreasing the patient's fluid intake temporarily would have no effect on sputum formation. Fluid taken in large amounts over several days will help liquefy the sputum and make it easier for the patient to cough it up, but physicians prefer a thick sputum for a specimen so that it is filled with whatever organism that is causing the infection.

(3) There is no need for the patient to fast for several hours prior to obtaining a sputum specimen, but it is important to get the sputum specimen before breakfast because there usually is a large accumulation of tenacious mucus in the lungs during the night. Never have the patient cough up a sputum specimen after eating because the patient may vomit.

(4) If a patient expectorates whatever is in his or her mouth, the patient may expectorate spit or food.

20. ❷ It is necessary to supply humidity through a tracheostomy because oxygen is very drying and the nose and pharynx are bypassed.

(1, 3, 4) These options are all incorrect. Apnea (transient cessation of breathing) and dyspnea (difficulty breathing) are not caused by the mouth or lungs becoming dry.

21. ❷ When suctioning the respiratory tract, the nurse must wait for several minutes before resuctioning. This waiting period allows the body to replenish itself with oxygen.

(1) An irritated mucous membrane will not recover in several minutes.

(3) Respiratory tract suctioning is very uncomfortable for the patient; however, the patient will not be overcome with fatigue because the suctioning is done for a very short time and repeated only as needed.

(4) Suctioning causes discomfort but not pain.

22. ❸ During an asthmatic attack, the patient will have prolonged expiratory breathing. The patient may have difficulty getting air out of the lungs and may develop a barrel chest.

(1) An absence of breath sounds would indicate atelectasis, which would indicate collapse of alveoli. It can occur in segments of lobes or an entire lung. Air would not be heard moving through this area.

(2) Asymmetric movement of the chest may be an indication of a collapsed lung (pneumothorax) but not of an asthma attack.

(4) Increased rate and depth of respirations are not seen in a patient with an asthma attack. This is seen any time a patient is in respiratory acidosis.

23. ❸ Aminophylline is given to patients with asthma or emphysema because it dilates the bronchi, allowing the patients to breathe easier.

(1) Aminophylline will not induce sleep and rest. It is a bronchodilator.

(2) Aminophylline does not cause relaxation of the pulmonary vessels. It is a bronchodilator.

(4) Aminophylline is a bronchodilator, not an antiinflammatory agent.

24. ❶ Epinephrine is a bronchodilator and would be used to reduce dyspnea and respiratory wheezing. It should be administered promptly as ordered. The order is written for administration every 4 h PRN; it was given at 10:00 AM and was needed at 2:00 PM, which is 4 h.

(2) Epinephrine is given subcutaneously (SC), not IM (that was how it was ordered in the stem of the question). Some medications are absorbed better by SC than IM. Epinephrine can be administered SC, IM, or IV. In this case, it was ordered SC.

(3) The physician's order for epinephrine is a normal dosage, so there is no need for verification of the medication.

(4) The physician ordered the epinephrine stat and every 4 h PRN for respiratory distress, so there is no need to notify the physician of the patient's condition at this time.

25. ❸ The number of cases and severity of bronchiectasis have decreased with the use of antibiotics.

(1) Bronchitis is an inflammation of the bronchi, not an infection. An inflammation is treated with steroids, and antibiotics would be used prophylactically to prevent infection.

(2, 4) COPD includes asthma and emphysema. The specific causes of COPD are not clearly identified; however, numerous irritants in cigarette smoke stimulate excess mucus production and destroy ciliary function. Tobacco is related to lung cancer.

The destructive changes occurring with emphysema permanently overdistend the air spaces beyond the terminal respiratory bronchioles and destroy alveolar walls. As lung tissue destruction progresses, the area available for gas exchange decreases. Initially, dyspnea develops only on exertion. As the condition worsens, dyspnea occurs even at rest and orthopnea develops (dyspnea occurs but is less in upright positions).

26. ❶ The most effective treatment of TB is chemotherapy, and isoniazid (INH) or rifampin taken for at least 9 months usually cures TB. There are some very resistant strains of TB because the treatment was discontinued too soon by patients.

(2, 3, 4) These medications are not used to treat TB.

27. ❶ Mediastinoscopy allows the direct inspection of lungs and the biopsy of lymph nodes.

(2) Bronchography is an X-ray examination of the tracheo-bronchial tree produced after installation of an iodinated dye into the bronchi via a catheter attached to a bronchoscope. Bronchography is used to diagnose bronchiectasis.

(3) Bronchoscopy permits endoscopic visualization of the larynx, trachea, and bronchi by a flexible fiberoptic bronchoscope.

(4) Thoracentesis is a procedure that entails the insertion of a needle into the pleural space for removal of fluid for both diagnostic and therapeutic purposes. All of the procedures in these options are invasive procedures.

28. ❹ When suctioning via a tracheostomy tube, the nurse should rotate the catheter while applying suction and withdrawing the catheter. This will pull the secretions out of the tracheo-bronchial tree while the catheter is being withdrawn.

(1) Inserting the catheter 8 to 15 inches into the tracheo-bronchial tree is too deep and could cause damage.

(2) Suction is never applied while inserting the catheter into the trachea because this action would tend to push secretions back into the tracheobronchial tree.

(3) Suctioning 30 seconds causes anoxia followed by severe cardiac arrhythmia.

29. ❸ A patient with emphysema would stop breathing if administered a high rate of oxygen because the medulla oblongata (respiration center) is only stimulated by a low oxygen content and higher carbon dioxide content.

(1, 2, 4) These options have procedures that would increase oxygen intake too fast and may cause the patient to stop breathing.

30. ❸ In emergency situations, the method of choice for administration of oxygen is the nonrebreathing mask because the one-way valve prevents expired air from mixing with supplemental oxygen.

(1, 2, 4) These methods of administrating oxygen are not as efficient as a Venturi mask.

31. ❸ The primary purpose of an incentive spirometer, if properly used, is that each deep breath is a very potent bronchodilator and is essential for effective coughing, which helps to clear the lungs of mucus. An incentive spirometer is most effective if taught to the patient preoperatively. The purpose of an incentive spirometer is to encourage the patient to maximize deep breathing. Another procedure to clear lungs of mucus is cough, turn, and deep breathe. Slow, deep breaths with an inspiratory hold of 3 to 5 seconds will significantly reduce the incidence of pulmonary complications. This procedure will increase inspiratory volume.

(1, 2, 4) The incentive spirometer is not used to encourage the patient to exhale; it is not used to arouse or stimulate the patient; and it does not measure tidal volume or inspiratory reserve volume. Pulmonary function studies are used for this purpose.

32. ❹ The test most valuable in the selection of an antibiotic is the culture and sensitivity test. This is a test to determine which antibiotic will be most effective in killing the organism that is causing the patient's illness.

(1) The Schilling test is used to determine vitamin B_{12} absorption.

(2) An elevated WBC count usually indicates inflammation, infection, tissue necrosis, or leukemic neoplasia.

(3) Serologic testing is performed to determine if the patient has syphilis.

33. ❷ The sounds of the rhonchi and wheezing in the lungs are due to partial obstruction of bronchi and bronchioles.

(1) If the small bronchioles are totally obstructed, no air can move through them, so no sound is heard.

(3) If there is fluid in the alveoli, then there will be the sound of air moving through water. This is called coarse rhonchi, formerly called rales.

(4) If the patient's pleura is inflamed, it is called pleurisy.

34. ❷ Bronchoscopy is a procedure using a flexible fiberoptic scope to observe the walls of the trachea, mainstem bronchus, and major bronchial tubes, larynx, and alveoli.

(1) An X-ray procedure is a noninvasive procedure that allows pictures to be taken of the lungs for diagnostic purposes.

(3) A diagnostic procedure that inserts radiopaque dye into the tracheobronchial tree is called a bronchogram. X-ray films are taken to demonstrate the outline and structure of the trachea, bronchi, and entire tracheobronchial tree. This procedure is used to diagnose bronchiectasis.

(4) A needle puncture of the lung mass with aspiration of cells is called a lung biopsy. This procedure is performed to diagnose cancer and other lung diseases.

35. ❹ Bronkosol is a bronchial dilator used for bronchospasm and asthma. Side effects of Bronkosol are headache, nervousness, arrhythmias, tremors, and anxiety. The headache results because Bronkosol, like nitroglycerin, causes some vasodilation in the brain.

(1, 2, 3) These options are incorrect because Bronkosol does not cause these side effects.

36. **④** Asthma may result from sensitivity to specific external allergens. Allergens, which cause extrinsic asthma, include pollen, animal hair, and feathers.

(1) Synthetic materials are not known to cause an allergic reaction.

(2, 3) Strawberries and cough medicine are not as likely to cause an allergic reaction in the general population, as do feathers.

37. **③** Pulmonary function studies are used to evaluate the extent of ventilatory deficiency.

(1) To determine a patient's tolerance for exercise, a cardiac stress test would be used.

(2) To determine which area of the lung is affected, an X-ray film or CT scan would be used.

(4) To evaluate the adequacy of cardiopulmonary circulation, a Swan-Ganz catheter would be used to measure CVP and pulmonary capillary wedge pressure. An echocardiogram along with pulmonary function studies and ABGs would also be used.

38. **②** Adrenalin, which is the same as epinephrine, will speed the heart, dilate the bronchioles, and vasoconstrict the peripheral vessels. The latter effect causes a throbbing headache, muscle tension, and hypertension.

(1, 3, 4) Epinephrine (Adrenalin) will not cause any of the side effects listed in these options.

39. **④** During an asthmatic attack, the patient will spontaneously assume an upright sitting position. It is helpful to have the patient lean over a bed table because this position permits more efficient use of the muscles of respiration.

(1, 2, 3) These options are incorrect as seen in rationale (4).

40. **④** Most extrinsic asthma begins in children and usually is accompanied by other manifestations such as eczema and allergic rhinitis (inflammation of the nasal mucosa). Why these diseases have a relationship with asthma is not understood.

(1, 2, 3) These diseases do not have a relationship with asthma.

41. **④** After a glossectomy (tongue resection), special mouth care includes irrigating the mouth with dilute hydrogen peroxide solution. It decomposes readily, liberating oxygen to the injured tissue. It is also a mild antiseptic germicide and cleansing agent.

(1, 2) Suture lines should not be cleaned with either cotton balls moistened with saline or an antiseptically sterile gauze pad because these materials will catch and stick on the suture lines and may be aspirated.

(3) To gargle and rinse the mouth with warm water after a glossectomy is not harmful, but it is not helpful either. It serves no purpose.

42. **①** When a patient has a tracheostomy, it is essential that the nurse detect the need for suctioning or the patient will die of respiratory obstruction.

(2) It is important to keep the suction apparatus patent, but it is *not* necessary for the suction machine to be on all of the time. It is of no use to have the suction equipment ready if the nurse cannot recognize when to use it.

(3) The inner cannula is not removed and cleaned after each suctioning. This is unnecessary and would cause tracheal irritation.

(4) The dressing around the tracheal opening is changed as needed, not once per shift.

43. **④** It is very important that at the beginning and the end of the shift, the nurse knows the amount of drainage in the collection compartment. That is why the nurse marks the amount of drainage on the collection bottle. The nurse needs to know if there is too much drainage, which may indicate bleeding. If there is no drainage, the nurse should be sure the tubes are patent. If the tubes are not patent, the patient could develop a tension pneumothorax, and the increased pressure may collapse the lung (atelectasis) either partially or totally.

(1) Milking the chest tubes is seldom permitted because forcing the chest tube closed during milking may cause a tension pneumothorax. Chest tubes are clamped only when the Pleur-evac is changed, and this is done quickly. A special clamp or padded forceps must be used when changing chest tubes to prevent puncturing them.

(2) The Pleur-evac should never be raised to the height of the bed because this would allow fluid from the Pleur-evac to flow back into the lungs.

(3) The chest tubes should never be attached to the bed linen because if the bed linen is pulled by the patient or the nurse, the chest tubes may be pulled out of the patient's chest.

44. **②** If the patient develops increased sounds of rales (coarse rhonchi), anxiety, and tachypnea (rapid respirations), these are signs of pulmonary congestion. The nurse should perform deep tracheobronchial suctioning to pull off some of the fluid, thus reducing pulmonary congestion.

(1) There is no reason to call the physician at this point. If the patient continues to have respiratory distress after suctioning, the physician should be notified. Always assess before calling the physician.

(3) Increasing the oxygen flow rate is not an independent nursing action. The reason for not calling the physician is discussed in rationale (1).

(4) Administering a bronchodilator is not an independent nursing action and would *not* be effective until excessive pulmonary fluid was removed.

45. **④** When sending a patient with a chest tube to the radiography department, the chest tubes should remain attached to the Pleur-evac. Precaution must be taken to prevent damage to the Pleur-evac and to ensure that the chest tubes remain intact and patent.

(1) The physician would not remove the chest tubes until lung reexpansion had been verified.

(2) The chest tube is not disconnected from the Pleur-evac except when a new Pleur-evac is needed for some reason.

(3) The chest tube is not clamped because air cannot escape from the lungs; this could cause a pressure pneumothorax. Air

pressure in the pleural space could cause the lung to collapse (atelectasis) either partially or totally.

46. ❶ A patient with a skull fracture needs to be monitored closely for increased ICP and shock. The skull is a "closed container" and contains a fixed volume of blood, cerebrospinal fluid, and brain tissue. An increase in volume of any one of these may cause increased ICP because the skull is a rigid sphere with little room (or slack) for expansion of its contents. The volume of its contents normally almost fills the sphere, and in healthy individuals the total volume remains nearly constant.

When the patient's skull is fractured, there is trauma to the brain tissue; swelling and edema may cause increased ICP. Symptoms of ICP are related to the brain location most affected.

If the blood pressure increases and the pulse decreases, this would indicate ICP. Normally, if blood pressure increases, the heart rate also increases; as a compensatory measure, when blood pressure drops, the pulse rate increases.

47. ❶ Hematuria may indicate internal bleeding, so it would be important for the nurse to observe for signs of shock from bleeding, tachycardia, and hypotension.

(2, 3, 4) Hematuria would not indicate peritonitis, hypertension, renal failure, or urinary infection.

48. ❷ Hematuria after multiple trauma most likely indicates that the kidney has been injured.

(1, 3, 4) Injury to the bladder, urethra, or ureters may cause some hematuria, but after a serious automobile accident, an injury to the kidneys is more likely because they are in a vulnerable position and easily injured compared with the bladder, urethra, or ureters, which are more protected.

49. ❹ Recognizing the patient's grief and helping her express it is the best way to help her deal with the loss of her breast and relieve her depression.

(1) The patient is depressed, not in pain.

(2) The patient may not have a minister with whom she would want to discuss her feelings. The patient needs someone now, not sometime in the future.

(3) When a person is depressed, he or she needs to talk about what is causing the depression. The nurse has no way of knowing the patient well enough to really know what interests her, and even if the nurse did, it would not change the fact that the patient is depressed and needs to discuss her feelings with someone.

50. ❹ A significantly lower than usual protein level is important to monitor, but it is not as life threatening as are significantly lower WBC, RBC, or platelet counts.

(1) A significantly lower than usual WBC count is very important because the patient will be more susceptible to infections.

(2) A significantly lower than usual RBC count is very important because the patient may develop anemia.

(3) A significantly lower than usual platelet count may indicate a side effect of chemotherapy, such that a drop in the platelet count causes bleeding to become a serious problem. *Note:* Chemotherapy will cause WBC, RBC, and platelet levels to drop significantly, and chemotherapy may have to be stopped for a while to allow the bone marrow to rebuild itself.

Chapter

17

Orthopedic Disorders

TOPICAL OUTLINE

I. DIAGNOSTIC STUDIES

A. Arthrography

1. Description

   a. X-ray film of joint after injecting the joint cavity with radioactive contrast medium, air, or both.

   b. Joint is moved through range of motion (ROM) as x-ray series is performed.

   c. Usually requires local anesthesia.

2. Purpose

   Visualization of articulating surfaces to diagnose trauma to the joint capsule or supporting ligaments.

3. Preparation

   a. Assess patient for allergy to local anesthetics, iodine, seafood, or dyes.

   b. Advise of necessity for remaining still during procedure.

B. Arthroscopy

1. Description

   Endoscopy is an examination of joints (hip, knee, shoulder, elbow, and wrist) under local anesthesia in an operating room setting as an outpatient.

2. Purpose

   a. Assess and repair articular cartilage abnormalities.

   b. Remove loose bodies and biopsy tissue.

3. Preparation

   a. Same as for any preoperative patient.

4. Postprocedure care

   a. Keep extremity elevated.

   b. Assess neurovascular status of affected extremity.

   c. Activity as directed by surgeon.

   d. At discharge, instruct patient to report elevated temperature, inflammation of incision site, increased swelling of joint, or calf pain (indicative of thrombophlebitis).

C. Synovial Biopsy (Arthrocentesis)

1. Description

   Needle aspiration of joint capsule fluid under local anesthesia.

2. Purpose

   a. To recover synovial fluid for differential diagnosis of joint disease, to remove fluid to relieve pain, to culture for identification of bacterial infection, or to instill medication.

   b. Normal fluid is straw-colored and clear with the viscosity of motor oil.

   c. Turbid, thin fluid indicates inflammation or infection.

3. Preparation

   a. Teach patient regarding procedure.

4. Postprocedure care

   a. Maintain compression bandage (Ace wrap) and joint rest for 8 to 24 h.

   b. Assess affected extremity for neurovascular status.

   c. Postdischarge activity as directed by surgeon.

D. Electromyography

1. Description

   a. Insertion of needle electrodes into skeletal muscle.

   b. No anesthesia.

2. Purpose

   a. To detect myopathic conditions or peripheral nerve disease.

3. Preparation

   a. Explain procedure.

   b. Advise patient that insertion of needles is uncomfortable.

   c. Instruct patient not to take any stimulants or sedatives 24 h prior to procedure.

4. Postprocedure care

   a. None.

E. Bone Scanning

1. Description

   a. X-ray film 2 h after intravenous injection of radioisotopes, which are absorbed by bone. Only tracer doses are used, so no precautions are needed.

2. Purpose

   a. To detect malignancies, osteomyelitis, osteoporosis, and some fractures.

   b. The isotope collects in areas of abnormal bone metabolism called *hot spots*.

3. Preparation

   a. Explain that the procedure is not painful, and there are no harmful effects from radioisotopes.

   b. Patient will be required to lie still for approximately 1 h.

4. Postprocedure care

   a. As with all procedures using a visualization medium, the patient must increase fluid intake to excrete medium.

F. Myelography

1. Description

   a. X-ray film of spinal cord and vertebral canal following injection of contrast medium via lumbar puncture into subarachnoid space.

2. Purpose

   a. To visualize intervertebral discs, spinal cord, and nerve roots for diagnosis of herniated disc, tumors, nerve root avulsion, or cord pathology.

3. Preparation

   a. Hydration for 12 h prior to procedure.

   b. Teach patient to expect mild discomfort from local anesthetic at puncture site.

   c. Patient will be secured to table, which will be tilted to various positions to allow dye to move up and down spinal column.

4. Postprocedure care

   a. Maintain head of bed elevated 15 to 30 degrees (if water-soluble dye was used) or flat (if oil-soluble dye was used) for 8 to 12 h.

   b. Encourage extra fluids.

   c. Assess neurologic status compared to preprocedure status.

   d. Administer analgesics and antiemetics as needed for spinal headache, back pain, and nausea and vomiting.

   e. May require intravenous hydration if unable to tolerate oral fluids.

II. OSTEOPOROSIS

A. Patients at Risk

1. All elderly patients are at risk for primary osteoporosis, as are all postmenopausal women. In fact, postmenopausal decreases in bone density due to estrogen loss average 1 to 3 percent per year, with the greatest losses occurring during the first eight postmenopausal years.

2. Hyperparathyroidism, long-term drug therapy, and bone marrow disorders such as myeloma or leukemia can put men and women of various ages at risk for secondary osteoporosis.

3. Glucocorticoid-induced osteoporosis is the most common type of secondary osteoporosis. Approximately 30 percent of all adults receiving glucocorticoid drugs, such as prednisone (Deltasone, Orasone, others), for 5 years or more may have a low-trauma fracture, that is, a fracture that occurs from a fall from standing height or lower.

4. In light of who is at risk, the National Osteoporosis Foundation recommends testing the bone mineral density in all postmenopausal women and men over age 65 years. Patients younger than 65 years who have one or more risk factors for osteoporosis other than menopause also should be tested.

B. Interventions

1. Education on preventing falls is especially important for elderly patients. Teach them to avoid sedatives, have their vision corrected, and have adequate lighting in all areas of their homes. Encourage the proper use of crutches, canes, walkers, and handrails. Falls are the number one cause of death in the elderly.

2. Smoking, a cause of osteoporosis that is independent of a bone mineral density, puts a patient at high risk for hip fracture.

3. A diet low in protein is linked to calcium deficiency and low bone density. In fact, protein malnutrition, common in the elderly, is more severe in patients with hip fracture.

4. When calcium (1200 mg/day in those 51 years or older) and vitamin D are not sufficient to treat patients with established osteoporosis; pharmacologic intervention is necessary. Estrogen has the potential to cause severe side effects but is very effective in the prevention of postmenopausal osteoporosis. At any age, estrogen can prevent bone loss for as long as it is being taken. Bone loss resumes when estrogen is discontinued. High-calcium diet and weight-bearing exercise (pressure on long bones necessary for bone absorption) are very important for calcium absorption.

Note: Very-low dosage estrogen patches are now available; in addition, low-dosage oral calcium may be prescribed. Because of the many serious side effects of estrogen, patient teaching will be very important.

5. Bisphosphonates inhibit bone resorption, possibly by inhibiting osteoclast activity and promoting osteoclast cell apoptosis. This action leads to decreased release of calcium from bone and decreased serum calcium level (e.g., alendronate [Fosamax]).

C. Fractures

1. *Articular (joint):* fracture involving a joint surface

2. *Closed (simple):* uncomplicated fracture with intact skin over the site

3. *Comminuted:* more than one fracture line exists, and fragments are crushed or broken into several pieces

4. *Complete:* fracture extends through the entire bone substance

5. *Compound (open):* bone is broken, and there is an external wound leading down to the fracture or a bone fragment that protrudes through the skin

6. *Compression (impacted):* one bone fragment is forcibly driven into another adjacent bone fragment; often involves vertebrae

7. *Displaced:* bone fragments are separated at the fracture line

8. *Epiphyseal:* fracture involving ossification center at the end of long bones; may result in alterations in bone growth

9. *Extracapsular:* fracture near a joint but not entering the joint capsule

10. *Greenstick:* fracture in which one side of the bone is broken and the other side is bent; usually seen in children, whose bones are more pliable

11. *Hairline:* minor, hairlike fracture in which all portions of bone are in perfect alignment (no separation of fragments)

12. *Intracapsular:* fracture within a joint capsule

13. *Linear:* fracture line runs parallel to the bone's long axis

14. *Oblique:* fracture line is at approximately 45 degrees to the shaft (axis) of the bone

15. *Pathologic:* fracture occurs at a site weakened by a preexisting disease, such as osteoporosis or bone tumor

16. *Spiral:* fracture line forms a spiral, encircling the bone

17. *Stress (fatigue):* caused by sudden, violent force or repeated, prolonged stress

D. Clinical Manifestations

1. Pain: immediate, severe pain at the time of injury

2. Loss of function: may result from instability of bone, pain, from muscle spasm or from a combination of these

3. Obvious deformity: alignment and contour change due to muscles pulling on bone fragments

4. Excessive motion (new "joint"): movement of part that is normally immobile

5. Crepitus: grating sensation and sound when fractured part is moved against another bone

6. Edema: may appear rapidly from serous fluid at fracture site or from bleeding into adjacent soft tissue

7. Ecchymosis: from subcutaneous bleeding

8. Loss of sensation (numbness): may result from nerve damage by bone fragments or nerve entrapment due to edema or bleeding

9. Fracture appears on x-ray film; bone scan for fractures that are difficult to find

10. Shock: may occur due to blood loss or intense pain

E. Immediate Management

1. Splint: to stabilize fracture

2. Elevate: to decrease amount of edema

3. Apply ice (first 24 h after fracture, for 20 min of each hour): to decrease edema. Remember continuous ice application will cause severe vasoconstriction.

4. Observe for neurocirculatory impairment; report to physician immediately

5. Observe for early signs of shock; notify physician immediately

6. Analgesics as needed for pain

    a. Assess quality and quantity of pain prior to each dose to determine if pain is due to an increase in bleeding or neurocirculatory impairment.

    b. Administer before pain becomes severe. A patient controlled analgesia pump (PCA) may be used.

F. Secondary Management

1. Simple Fracture

    a. Closed reduction or open reduction, traction, and external fixation.

    b. Examples include cast, splint, or external traction device.

2. Compound Fracture

    a. Culture, surgical debridement, and open reduction is performed (may leave wound open and packed, to be closed at a later date when there are no signs of infection), along with the administration of antibiotics and tetanus toxoid prophylactically.

    b. Monitor carefully for infection.

    c. May develop gangrene or osteomyelitis.

G. Factors Impeding Callus Formation (Results in Nonunion of Fracture)

1. Inadequate reduction of fracture

2. Decreased supply of nutrients due to excessive edema or interruption of arterial blood flow

3. Excessive bone loss

4. Inefficient immobilization

5. Infection

H. Complications

1. Osteomyelitis

   a. Infection within the bone, most likely following an open, compound fracture.

   b. Clinical manifestations include localized redness, warmth, edema, pain, leukocytosis, and signs of systemic infection.

   c. Treatment includes long-term, organism-specific, antibiotic therapy; surgical incision and drainage; immobilization of the affected bone; and analgesics.

   d. Isolation may be ordered.

   e. The condition can be seen in patients without fractures, in whom it results from soft-tissue infection (e.g., decubitus ulcers) that is transported in the blood to a bone.

2. Compartment Syndrome

   a. Neurocirculatory impairment resulting from edema.

   b. Clinical manifestations include edema, severe pain on passive stretching, numbness, lack of pulse, pallor, and cool to touch.

   c. Treatment includes early recognition, elevation of extremity, ice, removal or loosening of dressing or cast, and fasciotomy (surgical incision and division of fascia surrounding muscle).

3. Fat Emboli

   a. Associated with fractures of long bones.

   b. Clinical manifestations include petechiae, decreased level of consciousness (LOC), and respiratory distress.

   c. Treatment includes oxygen, anticoagulants, and steroids.

III. PAGET'S DISEASE

A. Etiology and Incidence

1. Affects approximately 2.5 million people over age 40 years (mostly men). Its exact cause is unknown.

B. Signs and Symptoms

1. Paget's disease is a slowly progressive metabolic bone disease characterized by an initial phase of excessive bone resorption (osteoclastic phase), followed by a reactive phase of excessive abnormal bone formation (osteoblastic phase). The new bone structure, which is chaotic, fragile, and weak, causes painful deformities of both external contour and internal structure.

2. Paget's disease usually localizes in one or several areas of the skeleton (most frequently the lower torso), but occasionally skeletal deformity is widely distributed. It can be fatal, particularly when it is associated with congestive heart failure (widespread disease creates a continuous need for high cardiac output), bone sarcoma, or giant-cell tumors.

3. Other deformities include kyphosis (spinal curvature due to compression or fracture of vertebrae), accompanied by a barrel-shaped chest and asymmetric bowing of the tibia and femur, which often reduces height.

4. Bony impingement on the cranial nerves may cause blindness and hearing loss with tinnitus and vertigo. Other complications include hypertension, renal calculi, hypercalcemia, gout congestive heart failure, and a waddling gait (from softening of pelvic bones).

C. Treatment

Primary treatment consists of drug therapy and includes one of the following:

1. Calcitonin (synthetic human calcitonin [Cibacalcin]) is a hormone secreted by the thyroid. Calcitonin inhibits bone resorption, lowers elevated serum calcium level in patients with Paget's disease, and increases excretion of filtered phosphate, calcium, and sodium by the kidney.

2. Etidronate (Didronel) slows normal and abnormal bone formation; decreases serum calcium level.

IV. TRACTION

A. Skin

1. Definition

   a. Application of pulling force on underlying skeletal structure using adhesive-backed materials. Examples are Buck's traction, Russell's traction, halters, and slings.

2. Types

   a. Buck's Traction

      (1) Exerts straight pull on one or both legs.

      (2) Used to immobilize a limb temporarily prior to surgical reduction.

   b. Russell's Traction

      (1) Modification of Buck's traction.

      (2) Vertical pull is added by placing a sling under the thigh.

(3) Allows for easier mobility in bed.

(4) Used to reduce or immobilize hip fractures.

V. EXTERNAL FIXATORS

A. Definition

1. Series of pins inserted in bone fragments and maintained in position through attachment to a rigid portable frame.

B. Purpose

1. Used to manage open fractures with soft-tissue damage and provide stable support for severe comminuted fractures, while permitting active treatment of damaged soft tissue.

C. Advantages Over Skeletal Traction

1. Facilitate patient comfort, early mobility, and active exercise of adjacent joints

2. Decrease length of hospitalization

3. Minimize complications of disuse and immobility

D. Nursing Care

1. Assess pin sites for infection.

   a. Cleanse as prescribed.

   b. Expect serous drainage around pins.

2. Never adjust frame.

3. Weight bearing usually can be encouraged; check physician orders.

4. Monitor neurovascular status of extremity distal to fracture.

5. Observe soft tissue for signs of infection.

VI. CASTS

A. Purpose

1. Immobilization of fracture

2. Prevention or correction of deformity

B. Types

1. Short arm extends from palm and thumb to mid-forearm

2. Long arm extends from palm to axillae

3. Short leg extends from foot to below knee

4. Long leg extends from foot to groin

C. Casting Materials

1. Plaster

   a. Can be used for severely displaced fractures.

   b. It is easily molded and inexpensive.

   c. Plaster, however, is slow drying, heavy, and easily weakened by moisture.

2. Synthetic used most often

   a. Lightweight, quick drying, and moisture resistant.

   b. Increased chance of skin maceration if not dried properly.

   c. These casts are expensive.

D. Nursing Care

1. Support wet casts with palms to avoid indentation.

2. Turn patient frequently.

3. Expose cast to air and rest on absorbent material to aid drying.

4. Elevate casted body part on pillows until danger of swelling is over (24–48 h).

5. Inspect cast edges and underlying skin for irritation.

6. Instruct patient not to insert objects beneath cast because objects may abrade skin and cause infection.

7. If patient's complaints of discomfort are not relieved by positioning or if neurocirculatory impairment is noted distal to the cast, notify the physician immediately because the cast may require bivalving.

8. Upon discharge, instruct patient to report fever, increased pain, altered sensation, drainage, or odor.

VII. JOINT REPLACEMENTS

A. Total Hip

1. Most likely candidates are patients with rheumatoid arthritis, osteoarthritis, or intracapsular hip fracture.

2. Postoperative complications may include hemorrhage, infection, thrombus formation, or prosthesis dislocation.

3. Postoperative positioning

   a. Avoid flexion greater than 60 degrees for 6 to 10 days, then 90 degrees for 2 to 3 months.

   b. Maintain hip abduction for 6 to 10 days, then no adduction beyond midline for 2 to 3 months.

   c. No extreme internal or external rotation.

4. Instruct the patient not to sit on low chairs or low toilet seats

5. Instruct the patient to avoid crossing legs or bending over to put on socks and footwear.

6. Alendronate sodium (Fosamax) may be prescribed for osteoporosis, especially in postmenopausal women.

   a. Instruct patient to drink two glasses of water after taking Fosamax to prevent esophageal damage. Client cannot bend over for 15 minutes after taking medication. This medication can cause damage to the esophagus if not taken with water.

   b. Fosamax increases bone mineral density.

B. Total Knee

1. Most likely candidates are patients with rheumatoid arthritis or osteoarthritis.

2. Postoperative complications may include hemorrhage, infection, thrombus formation, or prosthesis dislocation.

3. Postoperative positioning

   a. Elevate leg on pillows first 24 h.

   b. Passive ROM exercises as prescribed.

   c. Patient may return from surgery with a continuous passive motion (CPM) machine, which flexes and extends leg within prescribed limits. This is a painful activity.

4. Discharge instructions

   a. Activity restrictions as prescribed.

   b. After surgery the knee usually is protected with a knee immobilizer and elevated when the patient sits in a chair. Weight-bearing limits are prescribed by the physician.

   c. After discharge from the hospital the patient may have to continue to use a CPM device. The CPM promotes healing by increasing circulation and movement of the knee joint. The rate and amount of extension and flexion are prescribed by the physician.

   d. This can be a very painful procedure for the first few days it is used.

   e. Patient must observe partial weight-bearing restriction and use ambulatory aid for approximately 2 months.

VIII. AMPUTATION

Surgical removal of all or part of an extremity

A. Etiology

Most likely candidates are patients with peripheral vascular disease (often secondary to diabetes mellitus) and patients with traumatic injury.

B. Types

1. Open (guillotine) method: used when wound is infected

   a. Stump is left open, allowing the wound to drain freely and to be irrigated with antibiotic solutions. Used when wound is infected.

   b. Once infection is eradicated, a second surgery is required to close the wound.

2. Closed (flap) method: stump is closed

C. Dressings

1. *Soft:* greater potential for hemorrhage, and rehabilitation period is longer; however, better able to assess for hemorrhage and infection

2. *Rigid:* facilitates earlier ambulation but more difficult to assess

D. Postoperative Complications

1. May include hemorrhage, infection, and contracture of proximal joint

E. Nursing Care

1. Elevate stump first 24 h postoperatively to decrease edema and bleeding, then keep flat to prevent contracture

2. Keep tourniquet at bedside

3. Position in prone position as tolerated to prevent hip contracture

4. Assist with grief reaction and phantom-limb pain

IX. RHEUMATOID ARTHRITIS

A. Etiology

1. Chronic, systemic, progressive, inflammatory connective tissue disorder, resulting in symmetric distribution of joint inflammation

2. Unknown etiology

3. Theories suggest viral origin or immunologic aberration

B. Signs and Symptoms

1. General: fatigue, anorexia, weight loss, rheumatoid nodules, vasculitis, peripheral neuropathy, myopathy, cardiopulmonary involvement, and ischemic skin ulcerations

2. Joints: generalized stiffness, pain, limitation of motion, heat, swelling, and deformity

C. Diagnosis

1. Elevated erythrocyte sedimentation rate (ESR).

2. Serum rheumatoid factor present in titers greater than 1:160 in almost 80 percent of cases.

3. Positive antinuclear antibody test (ANA) and lupus cell test are found in some patients.

4. Synovial fluid analysis shows increased volume and turbidity and increased number of white blood cells.

5. X-ray film may show degenerative changes later in disease process.

D. Treatment

1. Comprehensive Pharmacotherapy

   a. Methotrexate, salicylates, nonsteroidal antiinflammatory drugs (NSAIDs), corticosteroids, immunosuppressives, and remission-inducing agents (e.g., gold salts, chloroquine, penicillamine).

   b. Side effects include dermatitis, gastrointestinal distress, blood dyscrasias, and nephrotoxicity.

2. Heat and Cold Application for Pain

3. Physical therapy to strengthen weakened muscles and improve function

E. Nursing Implications

1. Encourage balance between rest and exercise

2. ROM exercises to maintain maximum joint mobility; however, if joints are warm and swollen, limit ROM to once daily

3. Advise patient to take salicylates, NSAIDs, and corticosteroids with food

X. OSTEOARTHRITIS

A. Etiology

1. Degenerative joint disease, affecting primarily the large, weight-bearing joints (hips and knees)

B. Signs and Symptoms

1. Pain on motion and weight bearing that is relieved by rest

2. Progressive loss of function, crepitation, and malalignment

3. Heberden's nodes (bony overgrowth in distal interphalangeal joints)

C. Treatment

1. Rest and joint protection

2. Heat, cold, and exercise

3. Mild analgesics (salicylates, NSAIDs)

4. Arthrodesis (surgical fusion of the joint), osteotomy, or total joint replacement

XI. GOUT

A. Etiology

1. Overproduction or retention of uric acid

B. Signs and Symptoms

1. Dusky or cyanotic inflamed joints, which are extremely tender and painful

2. Can affect any joint but usually occurs in joints of the feet and the great toe

3. Renal calculi

C. Treatment

1. Joint immobilization

2. Local application of heat or cold

3. Drug therapy

  a. Colchicine

    (1) Used during acute attacks to relieve pain and between attacks prophylactically.

    (2) Inhibits uric acid production.

  b. Probenecid (Benemid) increases renal excretion of uric acid.

  c. Corticosteroids decrease joint inflammation.

  d. Intraarticular corticosteroid injections.

4. Dietary restriction of foods high in purines (e.g., sardines, sweetbreads, liver, kidney, venison, and meat soups).

EXAMINATION

1. Passive range-of-motion (ROM) exercises will prevent

  1. Loss of muscle mass.

  2. Decubiti.

  3. Loss of body nitrogen.

  4. Contractures.

2. Which part of the joint is initially affected by rheumatoid arthritis?

  1. Bursa.

  2. Synovial membrane.

  3. Cartilage.

  4. Ligaments.

3. When caring for a bedridden patient with arthritis, the head of the bed should be kept flat in order to

  1. Make position changes easier.

  2. Decrease edema around the joints.

  3. Prevent flexion deformities of the hip.

  4. Increase the circulation of blood to the brain.

4. Mrs. Crane, a 32-year-old woman, is admitted to the hospital with rheumatoid arthritis. She states that her knees and wrist joints have been intermittently painful for the past 3 months. The nurse would expect to receive a medication order for

  1. Codeine 30 mg q4h.

  2. Aspirin (acetylsalicylic acid [ASA]) 0.6 g q4h.

  3. Amitriptyline (Elavil) 25 mg tid.

  4. Pentobarbital (Nembutal) 90 mg q4h PRN.

5. The bed of a patient in traction is often kept in a flat position, which will produce

  1. Less pull.

  2. Unequal balance.

  3. Countertraction.

  4. Balanced suspension.

6. To be effective, weights for traction must

  1. Hang 12 inches from the floor.

  2. Hang freely at all times.

  3. Weigh a minimum of 4 lb.

  4. Consist of sandbags.

7. To proceed up the stairs with crutches, the patient should first advance

  1. The weaker extremity.

2. The stronger leg.

3. The crutches.

4. Both extremities.

8. When caring for a patient 5 days after a total hip replacement, the nurse should

   1. Avoid adduction of the patient's affected leg past the body's midline, and instruct the patient to avoid crossing legs.

   2. Discourage quadriceps sets, gluteal sets, and exercise of the upper extremities.

   3. Keep the head of the bed flat at all times, and instruct the patient to avoid using the overhead trapeze.

   4. Keep the affected leg adducted, and maintain a trochanter roll in place.

9. Mr. Blackman, age 60 years, sustained a compound fracture of the right femur in a car accident. Two days after the accident, he becomes agitated and confused. The nurse notes petechiae across his chest and in the axillary area. These symptoms are most likely the result of

   1. Sensory overload.

   2. Fat emboli.

   3. Narcotic analgesics.

   4. Sepsis.

10. Avascular necrosis may occur in the head of the femur following a hip fracture. This condition results from

    1. Wound contamination and infection.

    2. Immobilization.

    3. Circulatory impairment.

    4. Weight bearing before the fracture is healed.

11. Mrs. Smith has sustained a fractured right femur. Prior to surgery, she is placed in Buck's traction. The primary purpose of this traction is to

    1. Correct the deformity.

    2. Immobilize the patient.

    3. Relieve muscle pain and spasm.

    4. Stretch tight muscles.

12. Mrs. Sculley has an open reduction internal fixation (ORIF) of the right hip. When assisting her into a side-lying position, the nurse ensures that a firm wide pillow is placed between the patient's thighs and that the entire length of the patient's upper leg is supported. The most important reason for this is to

    1. Make the patient more comfortable.

    2. Prevent strain on the fracture site.

    3. Prevent flexion contracture of the hip joint.

    4. Prevent bone surfaces from rubbing together.

13. A regimen of rest and physical therapy for a patient with arthritis will

    1. Halt the inflammatory process.

2. Provide for return of joint motion after fibrous ankylosis becomes a problem.

3. Decrease joint pain during ROM exercises and other physical activity.

4. Help prevent the crippling effects of the disease.

14. The joints that would most likely be affected in a patient with osteoarthritis are the

    1. Ankles and metatarsals.

    2. Fingers and shoulders.

    3. Hips and knees.

    4. Cervical spine and shoulders.

15. The main reason for using Crutchfield tongs or a halo jacket in treating a cervical injury is to

    1. Prevent cervical hyperextension and occipital decubitus.

    2. Prevent further damage to the spinal cord.

    3. Allow freedom of movement.

    4. Give the patient a sense of security.

16. The nurse should encourage all patients in a cast to perform

    1. Isometric exercises.

    2. Quadriceps exercises.

    3. Passive ROM exercises.

    4. Active ROM exercises.

17. Mr. Howard has a long leg cast on his right leg. During the nurse's assessment, she notes that his right toes are cold and pale. The nurse's best initial action is to

    1. Notify the physician.

    2. Assess vital signs.

    3. Check pedal pulses.

    4. Elevate the right leg.

18. Which of the following would cause a nurse to suspect that an infection has developed under a cast?

    1. Complaint of paresthesia.

    2. Cold extremity distal to the cast.

    3. Loss of sensation distal to the cast.

    4. A foul odor.

19. Mr. Jackson has a medical diagnosis of gout. He has been placed on a purine-restricted diet in an effort to decrease his uric acid level. The nurse should recommend that he avoid

    1. Potatoes, sardines, and shellfish.

    2. Oats, barley, and rye.

    3. Beans, milk, and red meats.

    4. Liver, anchovies, and clams.

20. Following a right-above-the-knee amputation, John experiences phantom-limb sensations and tells the nurse that his right foot is throbbing. The most appropriate response for the nurse would be to

    1. Agree with the patient's statements, recognizing that he is expressing a psychological need.

2. Consistently stress the absence of the lower leg.

3. Disagree with the patient, and reorient him to reality.

4. Keep the patient as active as possible, and encourage self-expression.

21. Following an amputation, a rigid plaster dressing may be preferred over a traditional soft compression dressing because the rigid dressing

1. Creates a socket for immediate postoperative prosthetic fitting.

2. Allows for better inspection of the stump.

3. Prevents the potential complication of hemorrhage.

4. Prevents residual limb edema.

22. Two of the most difficult complications in long-term rehabilitation of an above-the-knee stump are flexion and abduction contractures. To prevent these complications, the nurse would encourage

1. Lying in the prone position several times a day.

2. Elevation of the stump on pillows at all times.

3. Lying in a semi-Fowler's position with the foot of the bed elevated.

4. Doing Buerger-Allen exercises.

QUESTIONS 23 TO 25: CASE HISTORY

Betty Myers, a 16-month-old child, is admitted to the hospital with a fractured femur and placed in Bryant's traction. Her parents state that Betty was injured when she fell down a flight of stairs.

23. Mrs. Myers asks the nurse why both of Betty's legs are in traction when only one leg was broken. The nurse should respond that Bryant's traction is used for children under the age of 2 years because

1. The child's weight is insufficient to provide adequate countertraction; therefore, their entire body weight must be used.

2. The child's bones are not fully calcified, and the traction is needed to maintain pressure on the long bones for calcium absorption.

3. The child is not old enough to understand why she must lie quietly; therefore, the additional restraint helps maintain immobilization.

4. The child would crawl out of bed, pulling the traction with her if both legs were not immobilized.

24. The nurse checks Betty's traction. Proper body alignment is being maintained if her legs are perpendicular to her trunk and her buttocks are

1. Raised on a pillow.

2. Lower than her head.

3. Flat on the mattress.

4. Raised off the bed.

25. The nurse checks Betty's feet for adequate circulation. When the foot of the uninjured leg feels colder to the touch than the broken leg, the nurse should

1. Encourage Mrs. Myers to wiggle Betty's toes every 3 h.

2. Assess the injured leg; if it is warm to the touch, circulation in the body is adequate.

3. Cover the uninjured foot with a sock and recheck its temperature in 1 hour.

4. Report this finding to the physician because the strapping may be wrapped too tightly.

End of Case

26. Sally, age 13 years has just been placed in a plaster hip spica cast. When turning her, the nurse must observe all of the following principles except

1. A minimum of three staff members is necessary so that the cast can be adequately supported by the palms of their hands.

2. Points over body pressure areas must be supported to prevent the cast from weakening and perhaps crackling.

3. The abduction bar should be used to lift her weight up off of the bed and ensure moving the lower extremities as a unit.

4. The patient should be encouraged to use the trapeze or bed rail to assist with repositioning.

27. A patient in a body cast complains of severe nausea. Assessment of the abdomen reveals absent bowel sounds. Which of the following would be the nurse's best course of action?

1. Place the patient in a side-lying position and reassess.

2. Notify the physician so that he or she can give an order for a nasogastric tube.

3. Encourage slow, deep breathing.

4. Suggest watching television or listening to the radio as diversionary activities.

QUESTIONS 28 TO 32: CASE HISTORY

Mr. Morris Black, a 78-year-old man, is admitted to the hospital after a car accident. He is diagnosed as having a compound fracture of the right femur and the right fibula and tibia. He is placed in skeletal traction.

28. Which one of the following phrases correctly describes skeletal traction?

1. Direct application of traction to bones by transversing the affected bone with a pin (Steinmann's pin or Kirschner's wire).

2. Direct application of traction to the skeletal system through the skin and soft tissue, using the body as countertraction.

3. Manual or mechanical application of a steady pulling force to reduce a fracture and minimize muscle spasms.

4. Indirect application of traction to the bone by a steady pulling force to reduce a fracture.

29. When Mr. Black asks the nurse, "Can I move in bed while hooked up to this traction?" the nurse's correct response should be:

1. "You can move to your unaffected side to relieve the pressure on your back, but you cannot raise the head of your bed."

2. "You can move to either side to get off your back; I will lift the weights just enough to allow you to move, about every 2 to 3 hours."

3. "You can sit up on the left side of the bed and allow your left leg to touch the floor, but you must be careful not to fall."

4. "You can use your trapeze and pull yourself up off the bed, and the head of your bed can be elevated."

30. Mr. Black asks the nurse if he can exercise in bed. The correct response by the nurse is:

1. "You can do any exercise you like with your upper body; you can lift weights as long as you keep your back flat on the bed."

2. "You can lift weights when you sit on the side of the bed and perform active ROM exercises with all the joints on your right side."

3. "You can flex and extend your right foot, do isometric exercises with your right leg, and do active ROM exercises with all the joints on the left side of your body."

4. "Exercise is not a good idea while you are in traction; your body will get out of alignment and prevent good callus formation of the fracture sites."

31. The diet Mr. Black's physician will place him on will be a

1. Regular diet.

2. Low-sodium diet.

3. High-calcium diet.

4. High-potassium diet.

End of Case

32. A patient presents to the emergency department after a fall in which he injured his right hip. If the hip is fractured, assessment findings will reveal a right leg that is

1. Internally rotated and abducted.

2. Externally rotated and shortened.

3. Internally rotated and adducted.

4. Externally rotated and abducted.

33. A patient is scheduled for an arthrogram of her right knee. She is asking what to expect. The nurse can best describe this procedure as

1. An x-ray film of the joint, which is taken after air, dye, or both are injected into the joint.

2. An endoscopic examination of the joint, during which the physician may repair cartilage abnormalities and biopsy tissue.

3. A simple x-ray film of the joint requiring no invasive procedures.

4. A noninvasive technique used to measure joint ROM.

34. A patient has just returned from the radiology department following a myelogram. Metrizamide, a water-soluble dye, was used for the procedure. Which of the following nursing interventions is appropriate?

1. Limit fluid intake for the next 8 h.

2. Encourage ambulation and prepare for discharge.

3. Maintain the head of the bed in a flat position of 8 to 12 h.

4. Assess neurologic status and compare to preprocedure status.

35. Crepitus, which may be noted following a fracture, can best be defined as

1. Movement of a part that is normally immobile.

2. Muscle spasm associated with movement.

3. Grating sensation and sound when injured part is moved.

4. Alignment and contour changes due to muscles pulling on bone fragments.

36. All of the following factors may impede callus formation *except*

1. Excessive bone loss.

2. Infection.

3. Pain.

4. Inefficient immobilization.

37. Clinical manifestations of osteomyelitis include

1. Localized redness, pain, and fever.

2. Numbness, lack of pulse, and pallor.

3. Limited ROM and severe pain on passive stretching of the muscle.

4. Ecchymosis, loss of function, and numbness.

38. A male patient, age 24 years, had an arthroscopy of his right knee this morning to repair a torn meniscus. The nurse should expect which of the following physician's orders for this patient?

1. Apply warm, moist compresses to right knee for the next 8 h.

2. Encourage active ROM exercises with right knee every 2 h.

3. Keep right leg elevated on pillows.

4. May ambulate ad lib after recovery from anesthesia.

39. A patient is scheduled for an electromyogram. Select the true statement concerning this procedure.

1. It involves the insertion of needle electrodes into skeletal muscles.
2. It is a noninvasive procedure that measures peripheral nerve conduction times.
3. It is performed to stimulate bone growth when a fracture displays evidence of delayed union.
4. It is used to stimulate muscle contraction in paralyzed extremities.

40. A patient, age 62 years, is admitted with a fractured left femur and is placed in Russell's traction. Nursing care of this patient should include

1. Advising the patient not to try to move around in bed without assistance.
2. Assessing the traction device to ensure that knots in the ropes are against the pulleys.
3. Monitoring color, temperature, and sensation in left foot when assessing vital signs.
4. Adding additional weights to the traction device if the patient complains of muscle spasms.

41. A patient, age 17 years, is admitted to the hospital with a spiral fracture of the femur. The fracture is reduced, and the patient is placed in skeletal traction with balanced suspension. Nursing care of this patient should include

1. Removing the weights when pulling the patient up in the bed.
2. Routinely inspecting pin sites for redness and drainage.
3. Discouraging use of the trapeze bar.
4. Encouraging active ROM of the affected extremity every 4 h.

42. Select the true statement regarding compartment syndrome.

1. Treatment includes application of warm moist compresses.
2. Clinical manifestations include severe pain on passive stretching, pallor, and numbness.
3. This syndrome occurs only in patients who are placed in full body casts.
4. It occurs when venous return is obstructed by thrombus formation.

43. Hip prosthesis dislocation is a potential problem associated with total hip replacement surgery. Which of the following activity limitations is necessary to prevent this complication?

1. The bed must be maintained in a flat position.
2. Extension of the operative hip is not allowed.
3. Hip abduction is prohibited.
4. Stooping over to tie shoes is prohibited.

44. A patient has sustained a hip fracture and is placed in Buck's traction. When caring for this patient, the nurse must

1. Remove the traction apparatus every 4 h to inspect for skin breakdown.
2. Monitor the neurovascular status of the extremity proximal to the fracture.
3. Keep linen and clothing off of ropes and traction setup.
4. Encourage the patient to provide complete self-care.

45. External fixator is used more often than skeletal traction in the management of complicated fractures because

1. There are no pin sites that may lead to infection.
2. Complications related to disuse and immobility are minimized.
3. Neurovascular impairment is not a concern.
4. Soft-tissue injuries are completely covered and less likely to become infected.

46. Which of the following is true concerning the nursing care of a patient in an external fixator device for a compound fracture of the tibia?

1. Weight bearing is not allowed.
2. Pin site care is not necessary.
3. The fixator frame can be adjusted as needed for comfort.
4. Serous drainage around the pin sites should be cultured.

47. Jamie, age 7 years, has a new plaster cast to his right forearm. The nurse should include which of the following information when providing discharge teaching for his parents?

1. Notify the physician if his fingers are cool to touch.
2. You may use a backscratcher to rub inside the cast gently if itching occurs.
3. Keep his arm elevated for the next 24 h.
4. If the cast gets wet when showering, use a hair dryer on a cool setting to dry it.

48. Mrs. White, age 48 years, has rheumatoid arthritis. A synovial biopsy and fluid analysis are performed on her left knee. Findings consistent with her medical diagnosis would include

1. Increased fluid volume and viscosity.
2. Absence of white blood cells.
3. Increased fluid viscosity.
4. Clear, yellow appearance of fluid.

49. Clinical manifestations of osteoarthritis include which of the following?

1. Generalized, symmetric joint pain and stiffness.
2. Anorexia, fatigue, and weight loss.
3. Heberden's nodes and joint malalignment.
4. Positive antinuclear antibody test.

50. Colchicine is prescribed for treatment of gout. This medication acts by

1. Inhibiting uric acid production.

2. Increasing renal excretion of uric acid.

3. Binding with foods high in purines to prevent absorption.

4. Directly suppressing the inflammatory response.

ANSWERS AND RATIONALES

1. ❹ Passive ROM exercises (moving a patient's limb without the patient's assistance) will prevent contractures. When a patient does not use muscles over a period of weeks, contractures may develop. Contractures occur because the contractor muscles are stronger than the extender muscles.

(1) Passive ROM exercise will not prevent loss of muscle mass. The patient must be working the muscles (active ROM exercise) to maintain the muscle mass.

(2) ROM exercise will not prevent the development of decubiti. Decubiti occur as a result of prolonged pressure, usually over a bony prominence.

(3) Prolonged bed rest, illness, and increased protein (nitrogen) catabolism can cause a negative nitrogen balance. ROM exercise will not correct this condition.

2. ❷ The part of the joint initially affected by rheumatoid arthritis is the synovial membrane. The involved joint's synovial membrane becomes inflamed, and as the tissue thickness with edema and congestion, fibrous ankylosis (immobility and fixation of the joint) develop.

(1, 3, 4) These options are incorrect as seen in rationale (2).

3. ❸ Keeping the bed flat for a bedridden patient with arthritis helps to prevent flexion deformities of the hip. Extension is important to combat flexion contractures. Place a small pillow or folded towel under the patient's head. A small pillow may be placed under the ankles to straighten the knees. Use sandbags or trochanter rolls as necessary to maintain proper body alignment.

(1, 2, 4) These options are incorrect as seen in rationale (3).

4. ❷ Salicylates, such as aspirin (ASA), are the mainstay of pharmacologic therapy for arthritis. These drugs act as analgesics and antiinflammatory aids, and they are relatively safe. Frequent doses (three to four times daily) are required (even if pain is not present) to keep the salicylate levels high enough for the antiinflammatory effect. If aspirin becomes ineffective or is not tolerated, then NSAIDs (e.g., Motrin, Naprosyn, Feldene) are used. If NSAIDs are ineffective, adrenocorticosteroid (e.g., prednisone) is often used, then gold salts. This progression is often referred to as the pyramid of therapy for rheumatoid arthritis.

(1, 3, 4) These options are incorrect as seen in rationale (2).

5. ❸ The bed of a patient in traction is often placed in a flat position in order to provide countertraction, which prevents the patient's entire body from being pulled toward the traction weights. The bed usually is elevated or tilted under the part of the body in traction. For example, the foot of the bed may be elevated when traction is applied to the lower extremities. If the bed is not properly elevated, countertraction from the patient's body weight is inadequate and the patient slides down, making the traction ineffective. With some types of traction, countertraction is applied with ropes and pulleys in a direction opposite that of the traction.

(1, 2, 4) These options are incorrect as seen in rationale (3).

6. ❷ To be effective, weights must hang freely at all times. If the weight falls against the bed, then part of the traction pull is being transferred to the bed instead of the patient, and the patient experiences only partial pull from the weights.

(1) It is not necessary for the weights to be exactly 12 inches from the floor, but they must not be allowed to touch the floor.

(3) The weight of the traction is determined by the physician. *Skin traction* may be continuous or intermittent and usually requires 2 to 7 lb of weight. *Skeletal traction* is continuous and may use 15 to 25 lb. The amount of weight required will decrease after the initial application as the muscle spasms diminish. Always assume that traction is continuous unless the physician specifically states that it should be intermittent.

(4) Traction weights may be in the form of sandbags or metal disks.

7. ❷ To proceed up the stairs with crutches, the patient should first advance the stronger leg. If the patient advances the weak leg first, the patient would be forced to put all of his or her weight on the weak leg to advance up the stairs.

(1, 3, 4) These options are incorrect as seen in rationale (2).

8. ❶ After hip surgery, the nurse must avoid adduction of the patient's affected leg past the body's midline. Instruct the patient to avoid crossing the legs, because this action will pull the affected hip out of its socket.

(2) The nurse would assist the patient with quadriceps and gluteal setting (isometric) exercises to maintain muscle tone in the affected leg, and exercise of the upper extremities is important to strengthen the arms in preparation for ambulating with a walker. Most exercises of the affected extremity begins on the fifth postoperative day.

(3) The head of the bed can be elevated up to 30 degrees without placing too much stress on the operative site. Use of the overhead trapeze is encouraged because this strengthens the upper extremities.

(4) The affected leg must be maintained in abduction, not adduction.

9. ❷ Symptoms of fat emboli include petechiae, altered level of consciousness, and respiratory distress, including dyspnea, tachypnea, wheezes, crackles, and large amounts of tenacious white sputum. Fat emboli are associated with fractures of long bones, pelvic fractures, multiple fractures, and crushing injuries. At the time of the fracture, fat globules move into the blood, where they combine with platelets to form emboli. The onset of symptoms usually is within 48 h after injury, but it may occur up to a week after injury. Immediate immobilization of fractures and minimal fracture manipulation may reduce the likelihood of developing fat emboli.

(1, 3, 4) These options are incorrect as seen in rationale (2).

10. ❸ Avascular necrosis of the femoral head occurs most frequently with intracapsular fractures, where the fracture interrupts the flow of arterial blood through the femoral neck into the femoral head.

(1, 2, 4) These options are incorrect as seen in rationale (3).

11. ❸ The primary purpose of Buck's traction is to relieve muscle pain and spasm. Traction can be used to immobilize a limb for a short period of time (e.g., a fractured hip prior to internal surgical fixation).

(1, 2, 4) These options are incorrect as seen in rationale (3).

12. ❷ When moving a patient after an open reduction internal fixation (ORIF) of the right hip, the nurse must place a firm pillow or abduction splint between the patient's thighs and support the entire length of the upper leg. The most important reason is to prevent strain on the fracture.

(1) Turning the patient may make her more comfortable, but the use of the firm pillow or abductor splint is specifically to prevent strain on the fracture site.

(3) Assisting the patient into a side-lying position in this way will not prevent hip flexion or flexion contracture of the hip joint.

(4) The pillow or abductor splint will prevent the knees from rubbing together; however, this is not the main reason for using these objects, as seen in rationale (2).

13. ❹ A regimen of rest and physical therapy for a patient with arthritis will help prevent the crippling effects of the disease. ROM exercises must be instituted to maintain mobility of joints; however, overuse of the joints may tend to keep the joint inflamed. For this reason, rest along with exercise is important.

(1) Rest and physical therapy will not halt the inflammatory process.

(2) Physical therapy cannot return joint motion after ankylosis has developed. Ankylosis means the joint is locked and cannot move.

(3) Pain will be increased during physical activities and ROM exercises.

14. ❸ The joints that would most likely be affected by osteoarthritis are the hips and knees. They are the weight-bearing joints and undergo the most stress.

(1) Although the ankles and metatarsals are weight-bearing joints, normal motion is not as great as in the hips and knees; thus, there is less degeneration.

(2) Fingers and shoulders are not weight-bearing joints, so they are not as affected as hips and knees.

(4) The cervical spine and shoulders are not weight-bearing joints, so they are not as affected as hips and knees.

15. ❷ The chief reason for using Crutchfield tongs or a halo jacket when treating cervical injury is to prevent further damage to the spinal cord. These devices immobilize the cervical vertebra so that fractured pieces cannot move and place pressure on or injure the cord.

(1, 3, 4) These options are incorrect as seen in rationale (2).

16. ❶ The nurse should encourage all patients in casts to perform isometric exercises. Isometric contraction is the contraction of a muscle without shortening the muscle. Tension is developed, but no mechanical work is performed. This type of exercise helps maintain muscle mass, which otherwise tends to diminish when an extremity is casted.

(2, 3, 4) These exercises cannot be performed by all patients who have casts; for example, ROM exercises cannot be done on a leg or arm that is fractured.

17. ❸ If the nurse notes that the toes are cold and pale when assessing a patient in a long leg cast, the nurse should check for a pedal pulse. If the pedal pulse is not palpable, a Doppler should be used to listen for the pulse. If the pulse is not audible, then the nurse should notify the physician immediately. The nurse should never notify the physician until a thorough assessment has been completed.

(1, 2, 4) These options are incorrect as seen in rationale (3).

18. ❹ A foul odor may be detected when an infection develops beneath a cast. Other signs and symptoms may include an increase in pain, warmth, an elevated white blood cell count, and fever.

(1, 2, 3) Paresthesia, coldness, and loss of sensation distal to the fracture are symptoms of neurocirculatory impairment that may result from edema. These are not indications of infection.

19. ❹ Gout results from impaired metabolism of purines. The dietary intake of foods high in purines must be restricted. These foods include sardines, sweetbreads, liver, kidney, venison, and meat soups.

(1, 2, 3) These options are incorrect as seen in rationale (4).

20. ❹ When a patient experiences phantom-limb sensation following an above-the-knee amputation, the most appropriate nursing response would be to encourage self-expression of the feelings the patient is experiencing related to body image and to keep the patient as active as possible. The increase in activity actually diminishes the sensations.

(1, 2, 3) These options are incorrect as seen in rationale (4).

21. ❶ The rigid dressing technique is used as a means of creating a socket for immediate postoperative prosthetic fitting. It provides uniform compression, controls pain, and helps prevent hip flexion contractures by adding weight to the stump and keeping it extended when the patient is in a recumbent position.

(2) The rigid dressing makes wound inspection more difficult than the soft dressing.

(3) The rigid dressing decreases the risk of hemorrhage but does not prevent it.

(4) The rigid dressing decreases soft-tissue edema but does not prevent it.

22. ❶ To prevent long-term complications in stump rehabilitation, the nurse would encourage the patient to lie in the prone position several times per day in order to prevent hip flexion and abduction contractures from occurring.

(2, 3, 4) These options are incorrect as seen in rationale (1).

23. **①** When very young children fracture a femur, both legs are put in Bryant's traction because the child's weight is inadequate to provide sufficient countertraction; therefore, the whole body weight must be used.

(2, 3, 4) These options are incorrect as seen in rationale (1).

24. **④** Proper body alignment and traction pull are being maintained for a child in Bryant's traction if the legs are perpendicular to the trunk and the buttocks are barely lifted off the bed.

(1, 2, 3) These options are incorrect as seen in rationale (4).

25. **④** When checking the child's feet in Bryant's traction for adequate circulation, if the unaffected foot feels colder to the touch than the affected leg and foot, the nurse should report this finding to the physician. The strapping (elastic bandage) around the unaffected leg may be so tight that it is preventing adequate arterial circulation into that foot.

(1) Encouraging the child to wiggle her toes will not correct the problem.

(2) Assessing the injured leg will not improve the circulation in the uninjured leg.

(3) Covering the toes on the uninjured foot may provide additional warmth to the foot, but rechecking in 1 h is too long to wait if circulation is inadequate.

26. **③** The abductor bar on a hip spica cast should never be used to lift the patient when turning. This will weaken the structure of the cast and perhaps cause it to break.

(1, 2, 4) These principles should all be observed whenever turning a patient in a hip spica cast.

27. **②** When a patient in a body cast complains of severe nausea and has absent bowel sounds, the patient is most likely developing cast syndrome and a paralytic ileus. The nurse should notify the physician and expect an order for a nasogastric tube to wall suction.

(1) Placing the patient in the side-lying position will not correct the problem, as seen in rationale (2).

(3) Encouraging slow, deep breathing may diminish the nausea momentarily but will not correct the problem.

(4) Diversionary activities will not correct the problem, as seen in rationale (2).

28. **①** Skeletal traction is the direct application of traction to bones. It is accomplished by surgically inserting metal wires (Kirschner's wires) or pins (Steinmann's pins) into the bone distal to the fracture and attaching a bow to the wire or pin. The traction ropes and weights are connected to the bow and provide a direct pull on the bone.

(2, 3, 4) These options are incorrect as seen in rationale (1).

29. **④** The patient can move in bed when in skeletal traction and can use the trapeze to pull himself up off the bed. The head of the bed can be elevated into a semi-Fowler's position.

(1, 2, 3) These options are incorrect as seen in rationale (4).

30. **③** Exercises are valuable in maintaining muscle strength and tone and in promoting circulation. The patient who is in skeletal traction for a compound fracture of the right femur, fibula, and tibia can flex and extend the ankles, can do isometric exercises (e.g., quadriceps sets and gluteal sets) with the affected leg, and can do active ROM with all joints on the unaffected side.

(1, 2, 4) These options are incorrect as seen in rationale (3).

31. **①** The patient who is confined to bed and in traction because of bone fractures will be on a regular diet unless other health problems dictate a specific dietary restriction.

(2) patient with bone fractures has no reason to be on a low-sodium diet, unless the patient is retaining sodium for some other reason.

(3) The patient who is confined to bed develops hypercalcemia as a result of removal of calcium from the bones into the blood and therefore should not be on a high-calcium diet.

(4) There is no reason for this patient to be on a high-potassium diet.

32. **②** Clinical manifestations of a fracture hip include pain, swelling, loss of control of the leg, shortening, and external rotation of the leg.

(1, 3, 4) These options are incorrect as seen in rationale (2).

33. **①** An arthrogram is an x-ray film of a joint following injection of the joint cavity with air, dye, or both. This provides better visualization than a routine x-ray film. It usually requires local anesthesia.

(2, 3, 4) These options are incorrect as seen in rationale (1).

34. **④** A myelogram is a series of x-ray films of the spinal cord and vertebral canal, taken after a contrast medium is injected via a lumbar puncture into the subarachnoid space. Following the procedure, neurologic status should be monitored and compared to preprocedure status to ensure that the nerve roots have not been damaged. If a water-soluble dye is used, the patient is kept in a semi-Fowler's position for 8 to 12 h to prevent the dye from migrating upward toward the base of the brain, which could result in seizure activity. If an oil-soluble dye is used, the head of the bed is kept flat, for the same reason. The water-soluble dye is heavier than the cerebrospinal fluid, and the oil-soluble dye is lighter.

(1) Fluids should be encouraged following a myelogram to aid in eliminating the contrast medium, which is excreted in the urine.

(2) The patient usually is kept in the hospital overnight and ambulation is allowed only as tolerated to the toilet and back.

(3) This option is incorrect as seen in rationale (4).

35. **③** Crepitus is a grating sensation and sound that is noted when moving an extremity that has a fracture.

(1, 2, 4) These options are incorrect as seen in rationale (3).

36. **③** Although pain occurs with fractures, it has no effect on callus formation.

(1, 2, 4) Callus formation and bone healing may be impeded by inadequate reduction of the fracture, inefficient immobilization, excessive bone loss, decreased nutrient supply secondary to interruption of arterial blood flow, and infection.

37. **①** Osteomyelitis is an infection of the bone resulting from direct invasion of microbes in a compound fracture or from bacteria in the blood, which is transported from a decubitus ulcer. Clinical manifestations include localized redness, warmth, edema, pain, leukocytosis, and signs of systemic infection.

(2) Numbness, lack of pulse, and pallor are not associated with osteomyelitis, but they would be manifestations of circulatory impairment.

(3) Limited ROM and severe pain on passive stretching of the muscle are not symptoms of osteomyelitis but are seen in patients who develop compartment syndrome.

(4) These symptoms are not seen in osteomyelitis.

38. **③** Care of the patient following an arthroscopy includes keeping the extremity elevated, application of ice, maintenance of a compression dressing, and immobilization for 8 h up to several days, depending on what surgical repairs were performed.

(1) This option is incorrect as seen in rationale (3).

(2) Following an arthroscopy, the affected knee is immobilized. Active ROM is not allowed.

(4) Following an arthroscopy of the knee, the patient is not allowed to ambulate ad lib.

39. **①** An electromyogram involves the insertion of needle electrodes into skeletal muscle to measure peripheral nerve conduction and muscle response. It is a very uncomfortable procedure and is performed without sedatives or anesthesia.

(2, 3, 4) These options are incorrect as seen in rationale (1).

40. **③** When a patient is in a traction setup, the color, temperature, sensation, and movement of the affected extremity must be monitored to ensure that there is no neurocirculatory impairment resulting from the device or the fracture.

(1) The patient in Russell's skin traction is able to move about in bed by pulling up on the overhead trapeze. The suspension device under the leg is intended to make movement easier.

(2) If the knots are against the pulleys, this will prevent the weight from pulling on the extremity and will negate the effect of the traction.

(4) The amount of weight applied to the traction setup is prescribed by the physician and cannot be increased or decreased without a physician's order.

41. **②** A major disadvantage of skeletal traction is the potential for infection. Pin sites must be routinely inspected for redness, warmth, and drainage, which would indicate the presence of infection.

(1) The weights on a traction device are never to be removed without a physician's order.

(3) Use of the overhead trapeze is to be encouraged so that the patient can move around in bed.

(4) Active ROM exercises are not allowed or possible for the extremity that is in skeletal traction.

42. **②** Compartment syndrome is a neurocirculatory impairment resulting from edema within the fascia or beneath a dressing or cast. Clinical manifestations include edema, severe pain on passive stretching of the muscle, numbness, lack of pulse, pallor, and cool to touch. Treatment includes early recognition, elevation of the extremity, and ice. The physician will remove or loosen the dressing or cast, or do a fasciotomy (surgical incision and division of the fascia surrounding the muscle).

(1, 3, 4) These options are incorrect as seen in rationale (2).

43. **④** Activity limitations following a total hip replacement include avoiding flexion greater than 60 degrees (sitting only in chairs with raised seats and no stooping over), maintaining hip abduction (no crossing legs), and no extreme internal or external rotation.

(1, 2, 3) These options are incorrect as seen in rationale (4).

44. **③** When caring for a patient in traction, the nurse must be sure to keep all bed linens and clothing off of the ropes so that the traction device can function maximally.

(1) Buck's traction cannot be removed unless the physician specifically states that it is to be intermittent.

(2) The neurovascular status of the affected extremity must be monitored distal to the fracture, not proximal.

(4) It is not possible for the patient with a hip fracture in Buck's traction to provide total self-care.

45. **②** External fixator device is used more often than skeletal traction because the patient is not confined to bed, and the complications associated with disuse and immobility are minimized.

(1) The external fixator requires pin sites, just as does the skeletal traction device.

(3) Neurovascular impairment is always a concern with a fracture, regardless of whether the treatment involves skeletal traction or an external fixator device.

(4) Soft-tissue injuries are open and more accessible for treatment, but they are not necessarily covered or protected from infection.

46. **①** When a patient has an external fixator device for a fractured tibia, weight bearing is not allowed; crutches are used.

(2) Pin site care is necessary for the patient with an external fixator device, just as it is for skeletal traction. The procedure and solution used should be specified by the physician.

(3) The fixator frame cannot be adjusted for the patient's comfort. It is only adjusted as directed by the physician.

(4) Serous drainage around the pin sites is expected and does not need to be reported to the physician.

47. **③** The patient in a new plaster cast for a fracture should be instructed to keep the extremity elevated for the first 24 to 48 h to prevent swelling, which could result in compartment syndrome and require bivalving the cast.

(1) If the fingers are cool to touch, a more thorough assessment of the neurovascular status of the hand should be done, including noting the color, presence of pulses, sensation, and movement. If those findings suggest an impairment, then the physician should be notified.

(2) The parents and child should be instructed not to insert anything inside the cast to relieve itching. This could tear the padding and cause lumps in the padding that would place pressure on the skin and result in decubiti. Also, the skin might be scraped by the backscratcher or any other device, increasing the potential for infection.

(4) The child's parents should be instructed to keep the plaster cast dry. Allowing it to get wet will weaken the cast and may cause maceration and infection of the underlying skin.

48. ❶ The synovial fluid from a patient with rheumatoid arthritis would be cloudy and have white blood cells, and there would be an increase in the fluid volume and the viscosity.

(2, 3, 4) These options are incorrect as seen in rationale (1).

49. ❸ Clinical manifestations of osteoarthritis or degenerative arthritis include pain with motion and weight bearing (which is relieved by rest), progressive loss of function, crepitation, Heberden's nodes (bony overgrowth in distal interphalangeal joints), and malalignment.

(1, 2, 4) These are symptoms of rheumatoid arthritis, which is a systemic disease.

50. ❶ Colchicine is prescribed for the treatment of gout. It acts by inhibiting uric acid production.

(2, 3, 4) These options are incorrect as seen in rationale (1).

Chapter

18 Neurologic Disorders

TOPICAL OUTLINE

I. NEUROLOGIC ASSESSMENT

A. Level of Consciousness

1. This is the single most valuable neurologic indicator

2. The following are terms used to describe level of consciousness (LOC): alert, lethargic, stuporous, semicomatose, and comatose

B. History and Evaluation of Mental Status

1. The purpose of the history is to determine past and present health status and to obtain a description of onset of the current illness.

C. Physical Examination

1. Used to detect abnormalities in neurologic functioning.

2. LOC determines how detailed the examination can be.

3. Vital signs and the Glasgow Coma Scale assessments are first priority when performing a neurologic examination.

    a. They offer quick and accurate assessment of the patient's neurologic status.

    b. An example is disorientation to time, place, and person as seen in a severe head injury.

    c. These problems may be recognized early and treated.

4. An example of a neurologic change seen in vital signs is the rise in systolic blood pressure and drop in diastolic blood pressure (widen blood pressure) that accompany a rise in intracranial pressure (ICP).

5. A patient with a neurologic disorder may have difficulty coping with daily living (ability to meet basic needs).

    a. A patient may have problems breathing, eating, seeing, hearing, walking, or talking.

    b. These problems may be permanent or temporary.

    c. The patient will be frustrated trying to do the things most people take for granted.

D. Assessing Motor Function

1. Ask the patient to touch his or her nose with each index finger, alternating hands.

2. Test balance; check gait and muscle tone.

3. Evaluate muscle strength.

    a. Have the patient grip your hands and squeeze.

    b. Ask the patient to push against your hand with his or her foot.

4. Compare muscle strength on each side using a 5-point scale (where 5 is normal strength and 0 is complete paralysis)

E. Assessing Sensory Function

1. Test for superficial pain perception with cotton; if no response, pin prick.

2. Test for thermal sensation.

3. Assess for tactile sensation.

    a. Ask patient to close the eyes and tell you what is felt when you touch the patient lightly on the hand, wrist, arm, thigh, lower legs, and feet.

4. Have patient close the eyes and assess for sense of position.

  a. Move patient's toes or fingers up, down, and to the side.

  b. Have the patient tell the direction of movement.

F. Assessing Cranial Nerve Function

1. Olfactory Nerve (I)

  a. With patient's eyes closed, have the patient identify common smells, such as coffee, beer, and cinnamon.

2. Optic Nerve (II)

  a. Examine the patient's eyes with an ophthalmoscope.

  b. Have patient read the Snellen eye chart. To test peripheral vision, ask patient to cover one eye and fix his or her other eye on a point directly in front of him or her. Then ask if he or she can see you wiggle your finger in the four quadrants; you'd expect him or her to see your finger in all four quadrants.

3. Oculomotor Nerve (III)

  a. Compare the size and shape of pupils and the equality of pupillary response to a pin light (flashlight) in a darkened room.

4. Trochlear Nerve (IV) and Abducens Nerve (VI)

  a. Both of these are responsible for lateral eye movement.

  b. Ask patient to follow your finger with his or her eyes, as you slowly move it from the patient's far right to the far left.

5. Trigeminal Nerve (V): Trigeminal Neuralgia (Tic Douloureux)

  a. Test all three portions of this cranial nerve. Test facial portion by stroking the patient's jaws, cheeks, and forehead with a cotton ball, the point of a pin, or test tube filled with hot or cold water. Testing for a blink reflex is no longer commonly performed because the test is irritating to the patient.

6. Facial Nerve (VII): Bell's Palsy

  a. To assess facial motor function ask patient to raise the eyebrows, wrinkle the forehead, and open the mouth.

  b. Facial nerves are also involved in taste, so place sugar or salt on the tongue.

7. Acoustic Nerve (VIII)

  a. Ask the patient to identify common sounds, such as a person whispering or a tapping noise.

  b. A tuning fork can be used to test air and bone conduction.

8. Glossopharyngeal Nerve (IX)

  a. Use a tongue depressor to test gag reflex.

9. Vagus Nerve (X)

  a. The vagus nerve slows the heart rate.

  b. It can increase gastrointestinal (GI) peristalsis, and it controls swallowing.

  c. To assess the patient's ability to swallow, look for symmetric movement of palate when the patient says "Ah."

10. Spinal Accessory Nerve (XI)

  a. Assess shoulder muscle strength.

  b. Ask the patient to shrug shoulder against resistance.

11. Hypoglossal Nerve (XII)

  a. Ask the patient to stick out tongue and inspect for tremor, atrophy, or lateral deviation. To test for strength, ask the patient to move tongue from side to side while you hold a tongue blade against it.

II. DIAGNOSTIC TESTS TO ASSESS NEUROLOGIC STATUS

A. Computed Tomographic Scan

1. Description

  a. Computed tomography (CT) is performed by passing x-ray beams through the brain in many slices to provide a cross-sectional picture.

  b. CT is a noninvasive x-ray technique used to diagnose pathologic conditions of the head, neck, spine, chest, abdomen, kidneys, and adrenals.

  c. An oral or intravenous iodinated contrast dye may be administered prior to the test for better visualization.

B. Nursing Implications

1. Assessment

  a. Note vital signs for baseline data.

  b. Check for allergies to iodinated dye or shellfish if contrast medium is used.

  c. Note if an informed consent has been obtained, if required by the institution.

  d. Check that nothing by mouth (NPO) status has been maintained for 4 h prior to the procedure.

2. Diagnostic Procedure

  a. Some patients feel claustrophobic during the procedure.

  b. They should be assured that it is possible to communicate with the technologist during the scan.

  c. The examination takes approximately 1 h.

3. Postprocedure Care

  a. Encourage the patient to drink increased amounts of oral fluids to promote dye excretion and prevent renal complications.

  b. Observe the color, consistency, and amount of urinary output.

  c. Assess for dyspnea, tachycardia, flushing, rashes, or wheals, which may indicate a reaction to the contrast dye.

C. Magnetic Resonance Imaging

Diagnostic tool similar to CT scan.

1. Advantages

a. Provides a more anatomically detailed picture than provided by a CT scan.

b. Does not have the associated radiation exposure (x-ray) as occurs with the CT scan.

(1) It uses magnetic fields and radio waves analyzed by computer to produce two- and three-dimensional cross-sectional images of body.

(2) It reveals subtle variations in structure, such as tumor masses, degenerative changes, areas of necrotic tissue, and blood flow, which often cannot be identified with other types of diagnostic procedures.

c. A magnetic resonance imaging (MRI) scan looks like an anatomic slice of the brain, spinal cord, or other body system.

2. Prediagnostic Preparation

a. Before the examination, remove all objects from the hair, including wigs, rings, barrettes, earrings, and any hair pins.

(1) The patient's hair should be combed smoothly so that hair is not pulled up in one pile.

(2) Such a hair pile and objects in hair would show up on the scan and may interfere with the reading of the scan.

b. Patient will be positioned supine and the head placed into the donut-shaped ring of the scanner.

c. The patient should expect a loud noise from the scanner as it scans.

3. Nursing Implications

a. Prediagnostic Preparation

(1) Inform patient that he or she must tolerate close surroundings.

Note: Some of the newer MRI machines are open, eliminating the claustrophobic problem.

(2) Patient must lie very still during the entire procedure.

(3) Assess patient to be sure no metal is in the patient's body, such as eye or ear implant, pacemaker, cardiac valve replacement, joint replacement, or metal fragments.

(4) The powerful magnet in the MRI machine can interfere with the function and position of metal devices.

(5) The patient is not NPO prior to the examination.

(6) An MRI can be done with or without contrast medium because it is a paramagnetic enhancement agent that crosses the blood–brain barrier.

(7) No dietary restrictions are necessary before using contrast medium.

(8) If contrast agent is planned, the nurse should ask the patient if he or she is allergic to iodine or tends to become nauseated easily; a light breakfast may be given to reduce nausea.

4. During Diagnostic Procedure

(1) Some patients feel claustrophobic during the procedure.

(2) The patient should be assured that it is possible to communicate with the technologist during the scan.

(3) The examination takes approximately 1 h.

D. Lumbar Puncture

1. The procedure consists of the insertion of a needle into the subarachnoid space in the lumbar region of the spine below the level of the spinal cord.

a. Cerebrospinal fluid (CSF) can be withdrawn or substance injected into this space; for example, a myelogram can be performed by a lumbar puncture.

b. A myelogram is an x-ray study of the spinal cord using a contrast material.

c. CSF can be removed to reduce intracranial pressure.

(1) This must be performed with great care because the change in pressure might allow the brain to drop (herniate) into the spinal cord, causing sudden death.

2. Nursing Implications

a. Prediagnostic Preparation

(1) Prior to the procedure, the bowel and bladder should be emptied.

(2) The patient will need to lie on one side with the legs pulled up onto the abdomen and head tucked into chest in order to open the spaces between the vertebrae.

(3) The patient must lie still during the procedure.

(4) The patient may develop a throbbing headache following lumbar puncture.

(5) In an attempt to prevent a throbbing headache, the patient must remain flat in bed for 3 h.

(6) Fluids should be encouraged to replace spinal fluid lost in the procedure.

III. PATHOPHYSIOLOGY OF DECREASED LEVEL OF CONSCIOUSNESS

A. Etiology

1. Decreased LOC is most often due to disorders in the reticular activating system of the brainstem and thalamus.

2. A blow to the head is a common cause of decreased consciousness and coma.

3. Metabolic disorders, such as hyperglycemia and hypoglycemia, can produce a coma.

4. Infections of the brain, such as encephalitis, which is an inflammation of the brain, can affect LOC.

5. Overdose of sedative drugs suppresses the central nervous system (CNS).

6. Failure of the liver, kidney, and lungs allows metabolic waste to accumulate, which poisons the neurons.

B. Metabolic Needs with Coma

1. The metabolic needs of the patient in a coma are markedly increased.

2. Malnutrition can lead to increased risk for infection, pressure sores, stress ulcers, weight loss, skeletal muscle wasting, starvation, and death

3. The brainstem and cerebellum remain intact and functioning so that vital functions, such as heart, lungs, and GI, continue.

4. Patients can remain in an irreversible coma for years.

C. Assessing Level of Consciousness

1. LOC is a valuable indicator of neurologic function. It can vary from alertness (response to verbal stimulus) to coma (failure to respond even to painful stimulus). The Glasgow Coma Scale, which assesses eye opening as well as verbal and motor responses, provides a quick, standardized account of neurologic status. In this test, each response receives a numerical value. For example, if the patient readily responds verbally and is oriented to time, place, and person, he scores a 5; if he is completely unable to respond verbally, he scores a 1.

D. Levels of Consciousness

1. Levels of consciousness can vary from the normal alert state of consciousness to deteriorating stages, each with its own definition.

   a. *Confusion* is the loss of the ability to think rapidly and clearly, that is, an impairment in judgment and decision making.

   b. *Disorientation* is the beginning of loss of consciousness.

   ◆ Disorientation "to time" is followed by disorientation "to place" and an inability to recognize others.

   ◆ The last step in disorientation is the inability to know the self ("What is your name?").

   ◆ These are referred to as "disoriented times three" to time, place, and person.

   c. *Lethargy* is the lack of spontaneous movement or speech.

   ◆ The patient is easily aroused with speech or touch but is not oriented to person, place, or time.

   d. *Stupor* is a condition of deep sleep or unresponsiveness from which a patient may be aroused only with vigorous, painful stimulation to which the patient responds by withdrawing.

   e. *Coma* is the state where the patient has no motor or verbal response to the environment or any stimuli and does not respond even to deep pain.

E. Brain Death

1. *Brain death* is irreversible damage to the cerebrum, cerebellum, and brainstem.

2. *Irreversible coma,* also called *cerebral death,* is due to damage to the cerebral hemisphere.

3. These patients, and the maintenance of their feeding and fluids, have inspired great ethical and legal debates.

IV. NEUROLOGIC DISORDERS

A. Brain Abscess (Secondary to Other Infections)

1. Etiology

   a. Otitis media, tooth abscess, sinus infection, bacterial endocarditis, and head wounds

2. Signs and Symptoms

   a. Early: nausea, vomiting, and headache

   b. Late: decrease LOC and seizure (increased ICP).

3. Treatment

   a. Dilantin, Valium, phenobarbital (to prevent seizures), mannitol (to decrease ICP)

   b. Antibiotics

   c. Assess for increased ICP and prepare for surgery (Burr holes) if ICP develops.

4. Diagnosis

   a. CT

   b. MRI

B. Bell's Palsy: Cranial Nerve VII (Facial)

1. Signs and Symptoms

   a. Difficulty closing eyes, unilateral facial weakness, mouth droops causing saliva drool, looks like stroke (brain attack).

   b. Subsides spontaneously and recovers in 1 to 8 weeks or becomes a chronic and painful condition.

2. Treatment

   a. Treatment consists of prednisone, an oral corticosteroid that reduces facial nerve edema and improves nerve conduction and blood flow.

   b. If severe pain continues, alcohol injections are given into cranial nerve VII to stop pain.

   c. Injections must be repeated every 8 to 12 months until recovery occurs.

   d. If recovery does not occur, surgery is used to cut cranial nerve VII.

C. Cerebral Aneurysm

1. Etiology and Incidence

   a. Dilation of the cerebral artery.

   b. Results from a weakness in the arterial wall.

   c. The vessel ruptures and causes subarachnoid hemorrhage or cerebrovascular accident (CVA), stroke (brain attack).

   d. Congenital defect or degenerative process (hypertension and atherosclerosis are contributing factors).

   e. Occurs most often in patients older than 50 years.

2. Signs and Symptoms

  a. Headache, nuchal rigidity (back of neck), stiff back and legs

  b. Nausea and vomiting

  c. Altered consciousness or deep coma

3. Treatment

  a. Bed rest, quiet room, no stimulants.

  b. Hydralazine hydrochloride (Apresoline hydrochloride) or other hypotensive agents or calcium channel blockers if patient is hypertensive to prevent rupture of the aneurysm (CVA) or to reduce bleeding if a CVA has occurred.

  c. Corticosteroids to reduce edema.

  d. Phenobarbital or other sedative.

D. Brain Attack (Stroke)

1. Etiology and Incidence

  a. Strokes are now called *brain attacks.*

  b. A stroke (brain attack) results from one of four events:

  ◆ Blood clot within a blood vessel of the brain or neck (thrombosis)

  ◆ Blood clot or other material carried to the brain from another part of the body (cerebral embolism)

  ◆ Decrease of blood flow to an area of the brain, causing death to brain cells (prolonged ischemia)

  ◆ Rupture of cerebral blood vessel with bleeding into the brain tissue or space surrounding the brain (CVA)

  c. Third most common cause of death in the United States.

2. Risk Factors

  a. Diabetes (atherogenesis)

  b. Oral contraceptive (blood clots)

  c. Cholesterol

  d. Severe hypertension (CVA)

  e. Cardiovascular disease (cerebral embolism)

3. Signs and Symptoms

  a. Paralysis of one side of the body due to brain attack on the opposite side of brain

  b. Inability to perform a previously learned task (apraxia)

  c. Loss of speech (aphasia), defective speech (dysphasia)

4. Treatment

  a. Anticoagulants (e.g., heparin)

  b. Thrombolytic agents (e.g., streptokinase)

  c. Adequate oxygenation of blood to the brain

  d. Head of bed slightly elevated to lower cerebral venous pressure

  e. Monitor vital signs and treat hypertension

  f. Monitor for bleeding

  g. Osmatic diuretic (e.g., mannitol)

  h. Corticosteroids (e.g., dexamethasone)

E. Epilepsy and Convulsive Disorders

1. Etiology and Incidence

  a. The epilepsies are a group of disorders characterized by chronic, recurrent, paroxysmal changes in neurologic function caused by abnormalities in the electrical activity of the brain.

  b. Each episode of neurologic dysfunction is called a *seizure.*

  c. Seizures may be convulsive when they are accompanied by motor manifestations or may be manifested by other changes in neurologic function (e.g., sensory, cognitive, emotional events).

  d. They are estimated to affect between 0.5 and 2 percent of the population and can occur at any age.

  e. Epilepsy can be acquired as a result of neurologic injury or a structural lesion, or as a part of many systemic medical diseases.

  f. Epilepsy also occurs as an idiopathic form in an individual with no history of neurologic insult or other apparent neurologic dysfunction and may have a genetic cause.

  g. Isolated, nonrecurrent seizures may occur in otherwise healthy individuals for a variety of reasons; under these circumstances, the individual is not said to have epilepsy.

  h. In adolescents and young adults, head trauma is a major cause of focal epilepsy.

  i. Epilepsy can be caused by any kind of serious head injury; the likelihood of developing recurrent seizures is proportional to the extent of the damage.

2. Signs and Symptoms

  a. The neurologic manifestations of epileptic seizures range from a brief lapse of attention to a prolonged loss of consciousness with abnormal motor activity.

  b. The proper classification of the kinds of seizures that an individual is experiencing is important for an appropriate diagnostic workup, prognostic evaluation, and selection of therapy.

  c. The major underlying premise of the seizure classification is that some seizures (partial or focal seizures) start in one area of the brain (cortex) and either remain localized or secondarily generalize (e.g., spread throughout the brain), whereas other seizures appear to be generalized from their earliest manifestation.

  d. Glassy-eyed staring, picking at clothes, aimless wandering, chewing motion, unintelligible speech before seizure, and an aura precedes an attack (the patient's psyche is aware that something is amiss).

  e. Mental confusion may last several minutes after seizures.

  f. Patient will sleep several hours after a seizure.

3. Treatment

a. Treatment of the patient with a seizure disorder is directed at eliminating the cause of the seizures, suppressing the seizures, and dealing with the psychosocial consequences that may occur as a result of the neurologic dysfunction underlying the seizure disorder or from the presence of a chronic disability.

b. If the seizure discomfort is a result of a metabolic disturbance, such as hypoglycemia or hypocalcemia, restoration of normal metabolic function usually is accompanied by cessation of the seizures.

c. If the seizures are caused by a structural brain lesion, such as a brain tumor, arteriovenous malformation, or cerebral cyst, removal of the offending lesion may eliminate the seizures.

d. Dilantin (does not mix with dextrose solution and cannot be given IM), diazepam (Valium), carbamazepine (Tegretol), phenobarbital (Luminal), sodium valproate (Depakene), or divalproex sodium (Depakote ER).

  (1) Dilantin often can produce effective control with no sedation and very little, if any, intellectual impairment.

  (2) Phenytoin (Dilantin), however, produces gum hyperplasia in some individuals, coarsening of facial features, and mild hirsutism, which can lead to a long-term change in appearance, which is especially unpleasant for young women.

4. Nursing Implications

a. Avoid restraining patient; loosen tight clothing during seizure.

b. Do not force any object into the patient's mouth during seizure.

c. Turn head so if patient vomits, the patient will not aspirate.

d. Protect patient from injury by padding bed with pillows or blankets.

e. Stay with patient during seizure.

5. Alternative to Medication

a. Vagus nerve stimulation (VNS) therapy involves a generator implanted in the left side of the chest that sends precisely timed and measured mild electrical pulses to the left vagus nerve, which then activates various areas of the brain. The vagus nerve is the leading information highway to the brain from the thorax and the abdomen. Approximately 40 percent of patients on VNS therapy experienced a reduction in their seizures by 50 percent or more over 2 to 3 years, according to Cybernetics, Inc, September 4, 2003.

b. The device has been approved by the FDA for use in adults and children older than 12 years since 1997. A study also indicates that the therapy is effective and well tolerated in children. Approximately 20,000 people have undergone device implantation, according to Cybernetics.

c. Therapy is not intended for every person who has seizures. It is primarily useful for patients with uncontrollable seizures.

F. Guillain-Barré Syndrome

1. Etiology and Incidence

a. Acute, rapidly progressive, and potentially fatal form of polyneuritis.

b. Causes muscle weakness.

c. Demyelination of peripheral nerves.

d. The cause is unknown, possible autoimmune attack on peripheral nerves.

e. Occurs between ages 30 to 50 years and occurs equally in men and women.

2. Signs and Symptoms

a. Muscle weakness usually appears in legs first and then ascends to arms and facial nerves within 24 to 72 h.

b. If chest muscles are involved, a respirator is needed.

c. Febrile illness or flu vaccination usually precedes Guillain-Barré syndrome.

3. Treatment

a. Supportive, endotracheal, or trachea intubation as needed.

b. Recovery is spontaneous and complete in 95 percent of patients.

G. Herpes Zoster ("Shingles")

1. Etiology and Incidence

a. Acute, unilateral (one-sided), segmented inflammation of the dorsal root ganglia (follows along nerve endings).

b. Herpes caused by herpes zoster also causes chicken pox; the person who has *not* had chicken pox is susceptible to shingles.

c. Relatively common infection caused by herpes virus.

2. Signs and Symptoms

a. The first symptoms are small, red nodular skin lesions that erupt and spread unilaterally around the thorax.

b. Within 2 to 4 days, severe pruritus and paresthesia develop, usually on the trunk and occasionally on the legs and arms.

c. Shingles last 2 to 4 weeks.

d. Onset is fever, malaise, itching, and pain.

3. Treatment

a. Benadryl and baking soda bath or calamine lotion may be used to relieve itching and make lesions less painful.

b. Analgesics are prescribed to relieve pain.

c. Acyclovir is administered in the acute phase and Neurontin for postherpetic neuralgia.

4. Nursing Interventions

a. Occasionally, herpes zoster involves cranial nerves, especially the trigeminal (V) nerve, causing eye pain and possible corneal damage.

H. Huntington's Disease

1. Etiology and Incidence

   a. Hereditary disease of the CNS.

   b. Occurs between ages 25 and 55 years.

   c. Death in 10 to 15 years.

   d. More common in men than in women.

2. Treatment

   a. No cure.

   b. Treatment is supportive care.

3. Diagnosis by MRI or CT scan

I. Malignant Brain Tumors (Glioblastoma Multiforme)

1. Etiology and Incidence

   a. Cause is unknown.

   b. Occurs most often in adults aged 40 to 60 years and children aged 2 to 12 years.

   c. It is one of the most common causes of death in children.

   d. Glioblastoma multiforme occurs twice as often in men than in women.

   e. It is highly malignant.

2. Signs and Symptoms

   a. Clinical features generally result from ICP.

   b. Symptoms vary with type and location of tumor and degree of invasion.

   c. Onset usually is insidious.

3. Treatment

   a. Includes surgical removal, radiation, chemotherapy, decompression of ICP with osmotic diuretics, and corticosteroids.

   b. Possible intrathecal infusion of methotrexate or other antineoplastic agent.

   c. Nitrosourea agents (cancer drugs) include carmustine, lomustine, and semustine, which are used because they can cross the blood–brain barrier.

   d. Cytarabine (Cytosar-U), also an antineoplastic agent, crosses the blood–brain barrier.

J. Multiple Sclerosis

1. Etiology and Incidence

   a. Characterized by exacerbation and remission.

   b. Demyelination of the myelin sheath in brain and spinal cord may cause signs and symptoms resembling those of spinal cord injury (muscle dysfunction).

   c. Increased incidence in women aged 20 to 40 years and increased in high socioeconomic groups.

2. Signs and Symptoms

   a. Numbness and tingling, muscle weakness or paralysis, ataxia (defective muscle coordination), spastic or hyper-reflexia if demyelination occurs in spinal cord, urinary incontinence, blurred vision, mood swings, and intentional tremors.

3. Treatment

   a. Prognosis is poor and variable. Disease may progress rapidly or slowly.

   b. Seventy percent of patients can lead active and productive lives.

   c. Adrenocorticotropic hormone (ACTH) releases steroids from adrenal gland. Prednisone or dexamethasone is used to reduce edema.

   d. Physical therapy promotes emotional stability.

   e. Help patient maintain optimal function.

K. Myasthenia Gravis

1. Etiology and Incidence

   a. Progressive weakness of skeletal muscle system.

   b. Myasthenia gravis is an autoimmune disease that causes a failure in transmission of nerve impulses because of ineffective acetylcholine release.

   c. Occurs between ages 40 and 50 years in men and women.

2. Signs and Symptoms

   a. Usually affects the muscles of the tongue, lips, face, and throat, which are muscles that are innervated by cranial nerves, causing muscle weakness.

3. Treatment

   a. Worsens with exercise and improves with administration of anticholinesterase (e.g., physostigmine and Mestinon).

   b. This drug prevents the breakdown of acetylcholine.

   c. There is no cure.

   d. Acute exacerbations that cause severe respiratory distress require emergency treatment. Tracheotomy, ventilation with a positive-pressure ventilator, and vigorous suctioning to remove secretions usually result in improvement in a few days. Because anticholingeric drugs (e.g., mestinon) drugs are not always effective in myasthenic crisis, they are discontinued until respiratory function begins to improve. Remember that the concentration of acetylcholine at the sites of cholinergic transmission prolongs and exaggerates the effect of acetylcholine by reversibly inhibiting the enzyme acetylcholinesterase, thus facilitating transmission at the skeletal neuromuscular junction. Such crisis may require immediate hospitalization and vigorous respiratory support.

L. Lou Gehrig's Disease (Amyotrophic Lateral Sclerosis)

1. Etiology and Incidence

   a. Chronic progressive debilitating disease.

   b. Each year 5000 new cases are diagnosed.

c. Lou Gehrig's disease (amyotrophic lateral sclerosis [ALS]) is an autoimmune disease that occurs between ages 40 to 70 years.

d. It is the most common motor neuron disease causing muscle atrophy in the United States.

e. It is fatal within 4 to 12 years after onset, usually as a result of aspiration pneumonia or respiratory failure.

f. More common in whites than in blacks.

2. Signs and Symptoms

a. Ultimately loss of all muscle control; cannot even blink.

b. No facial expressions.

c. No mental deterioration.

d. Patient accumulates lung secretions, also dysphagia.

3. Treatment

a. Supportive.

b. Death within 2 to 5 years.

M. Parkinson's Disease

1. Etiology and Incidence

a. Parkinson's disease strikes 2 in every 1000 persons in the general population, most often developing in those older than 50 years; however it can occur in children and young adults.

b. Higher incidence in men.

2. Signs and Symptoms

a. Produces progressive muscular rigidity, akinesia, involuntary tremors, pill rolling, mask face, shuffle gait, and monotone voice.

b. Intellect is totally intact.

3. Treatment

a. Levodopa (dopamine replacement).

b. Use carbidopa plus levodopa (Sinemet).

c. Now can surgically remove part of adrenal gland and put in brain.

d. Adrenal medulla contains dopamine, epinephrine, and norepinephrine.

4. Diagnosis

a. Based on history, age, and clinical picture.

N. Reye's Syndrome

1. Etiology and Incidence

a. Acute childhood illness that causes fatty infiltration of the liver with hyperammonemia, increased ICP, and encephalopathy.

b. Reye's syndrome almost always follows an acute viral infection, such as chicken pox or respiratory infection.

c. Possibly linked to aspirin, so best to give acetaminophen (Tylenol) for arthritis and to treat pain in children.

d. Reye's syndrome occurs mostly in white children older than 1 year and adolescents.

e. Occurs equally in male and female children.

2. Signs and Symptoms

a. Vomiting, irritability, agitation, lethargy, delirium, confusion, and hepatic dysfunction (monitor LOC).

b. Hyperventilation, hepatic dysfunction, increased blood pressure and pulse rate.

c. Coma, deep coma, seizure, and death.

3. Diagnosis

a. Liver biopsy contains fatty droplets.

b. Prothrombin time (PT) and partial thromboplastin time (PTT) prolonged.

c. Serum glutamic oxaloacetic transaminase (SGOT) and serum glutamic pyruvic transaminase (SGPT) elevated to twice normal levels.

d. Serum ammonia level elevated.

4. Prognosis

a. Depends on CNS depression.

5. Treatment

a. Osmotic diuretic to decrease ICP.

b. Vitamin K or fresh frozen plasma.

O. Spinal Cord Injury

1. Etiology and Incidence

a. The most common causes are motor vehicle accidents, falls, diving into shallow water, and gunshot wounds.

b. Occurs most often in young men.

2. Signs and Symptoms

a. The most obvious initial symptoms are muscle spasm and back pain, which become more severe with movement.

b. Patient may have suffered mild paresthesia to quadriplegia and shock.

3. Treatment

a. Treatment after spinal cord injury is immediate immobilization of the patient to stabilize the spine and prevent cord damage.

b. Place cervical injury sand bags on both sides of patient's head, place a hard cervical collar around neck, place in skeletal traction with skull tongs (Crutchfield tongs), or use a halo device to stabilize cervical area.

c. An unstable dorsal or lumbar fracture requires a plastic cast, turning frame, and, in severe fractures, a laminectomy and spinal fusion.

d. A tilt table will be used to place pressure on the long bones for calcium absorption and to overcome hypotensive problems.

P. Spinal Hyperreflexia (Autonomic Dysreflexia)

1. Etiology and Incidence

a. Occurs most in quadriplegics and is an emergency.

b. Requires immediate attention.

c. Autonomic dysreflexia is an exaggerated autonomic response that may occur with spinal cord injury.

d. Severe hypertension, bradycardia, and a pounding headache usually are triggered by bladder distention.

e. Exaggerated autonomic responses in CNS autonomic dysreflexia.

f. Most common with cervical and high thoracic injuries.

g. Distended bladder or bowel initiates hyperreflexia.

h. Hyperreflexia is very common in quadriplegics.

2. Signs and Symptoms

a. Severe hypertension, possibly as high as 300/160.

b. Severe headache.

c. Profuse diapiresis above the level of the lesion or break.

d. Blurred vision, nausea, and bradycardia.

3. Treatment and Prevention

a. Empty bowel or bladder on a regular basis and immediately if hyperreflexia occurs.

b. Atropine given to raise heart rate for bradycardia.

c. Emotional support.

d. Antihypertensive drugs.

4. Nursing Interventions: Teaching Bowel and Bladder Care

a. Patients catheterize their bladder q4–7 h for the first 2 weeks and then as needed but must be performed before bladder becomes distended and hyperreflexia occurs.

b. Teach self-catheterization; when patient self-catheterizes it is not a sterile procedure, but when a nurse does it, the procedure is.

c. Drink 2000 to 3000 mL fluid per day to prevent constipation and urinary tract infection.

d. After catheterization, perform Crede maneuver (fist over bladder with a kneading, gentle motion) to empty bladder into Foley.

e. Bowel training or stimulating bowel.

(1) Start 3 days after injury or when peristalsis returns (may not return).

(2) Provide for privacy.

(3) Provide suppository and finger rectal stimulus until a bowel movement occurs.

(4) Use stool softeners and increase bulk in diet.

Q. Tetanus

1. Etiology and Incidence

a. Anaerobic spore-forming, gram-positive bacillus *Clostridium*.

b. Transmission is through a puncture wound that is contaminated with soil, dust, or animal excretions containing *Clostridium tetani*.

c. Occurs at any age in men and women.

2. Signs and Symptoms

a. Incubation period is 3 to 4 weeks in mild tetanus and less than 2 days in severe tetanus.

b. When symptoms occur within 2 days after injury, death is more likely to occur.

c. Signs are spasm and increased muscle tone near wound.

d. It tetanus is generalized, marked muscle hypertonicity, profuse sweating, boardlike abdominal rigidity, and locked jaw will occur.

3. Treatment

a. Within 72 h after puncture wound, a patient who has not had tetanus immunization within 10 years needs a booster injection of tetanus toxoid.

b. If tetanus develops, patient will require airway maintenance and a muscle relaxant, such as diazepam (Valium or Flexeril), to decrease muscle rigidity and spasm.

c. High doses of antibiotics, such as penicillin IV, should be given if the patient is not allergic to penicillin; if allergic, tetracycline can be used.

R. Trigeminal Neuralgia (Cranial Nerve V)

1. Etiology and Incidence

a. Cause is unknown.

b. Occurs most often in women older than 40 years.

2. Signs and Symptoms

a. Very painful burning for 1 to 15 minutes after touching face.

3. Treatment

a. Carbamazepine (Tegretol) or Dilantin may temporarily relieve pain episodes.

b. Microsurgery to relieve pressure on cranial nerve V.

S. Transient Ischemic Attack

1. Etiology and Incidence

a. In transient ischemic attack (TIA), microemboli are released from a thrombus and probably temporarily interrupt blood follow, especially in the small distal branches of the arterial tree in the brain. Small spasms in these arterioles may impair blood flow and precede TIA. Predisposing factors are the same as for thrombotic strokes.

The most distinctive characteristics of TIAs are the transient duration of neurologic deficits and complete return of normal function.

2. Signs and Symptoms

a. Double vision, speech deficits (slurring or thickness), unilateral blindness, staggering or uncoordinated gait, unilateral weakness or numbness, falling because of weakness in the legs, and dizziness.

3. Treatment

a. During an active TIA, treatment aims are to prevent a complete stroke and consists of aspirin or anticoagulants to minimize the risk of thrombosis. After or between TIA attacks, preventive treatment includes carotid endarterectomy or cerebral microvascular bypass.

EXAMINATION

1. A male patient lost control of his motorcycle and struck the car in front of him. His diagnosis is head injury. He has a history of partial occlusion of the left common carotid artery and epilepsy. He has been taking phenytoin (Dilantin) for 12 years. The fact that the patient cannot close his left eye can be explained by nonconduction of the
   1. Fourth cranial nerve (trochlear).
   2. Third cranial nerve (oculomotor).
   3. Seventh cranial nerve (facial).
   4. Second cranial nerve (optic).

2. A patient has a slightly dilated left pupil. This can be explained by nonconduction of the
   1. Seventh cranial nerve (facial).
   2. Fourth cranial nerve (trochlear).
   3. Third cranial nerve (oculomotor).
   4. Fifth cranial nerve (trigeminal).

3. A male patient is scheduled for an arteriogram at 9 AM and is NPO before the test. His Dilantin is scheduled for oral administration at 7 AM. The nurse should
   1. Ask the physician if the drug can be given IV.
   2. Omit the 9 AM dose of the drug.
   3. Administer the drug with little or no water.
   4. Administer the drug with 30 mL of water at 7 AM.

4. An 85-year-old man is scheduled to receive a 100-mg Dilantin capsule 100 orally at 3 PM. He is having difficulty swallowing capsules. The nurse should
   1. Give him a Dilantin suspension containing 100 mg/5 mL.
   2. Insert a rectal suppository containing 100 mg of Dilantin.
   3. Obtain a change in the prescribed administration route to allow IM administration.
   4. Open the capsule and sprinkle the powder into 30 mL of water.

5. The nurse plans health teaching and emphasizes meticulous oral hygiene because Dilantin
   1. Increases plaque, which increases cavities.
   2. Increases bacterial growth.
   3. Causes hypertrophy of the gums.
   4. Causes bleeding of the gums.

6. The physician changed the anticonvulsant drug (Dilantin) to Valium after Mr. Adams was diagnosed with folic acid anemia. The most likely reason for this change is that
   1. Dilantin may decrease absorption of folic acid.
   2. Dilantin is incompatible with folic acid.
   3. Folic acid given with Dilantin may cause neuropathy.
   4. Folic acid greatly increases the absorption of Dilantin.

7. Immediately following a car accident, a female patient is diagnosed as a quadriplegic. She is critically ill and is admitted to the hospital's intensive care unit (ICU). The quadriplegic patient is placed on a tilt table for one-half hour while the head of the table is elevated to 30 degrees. Each day the angle is increased and the time spent on the table increased. The nurse explains to the patient that the *main* purpose for this procedure is to
   1. Prevent hypotension.
   2. Prevent loss of calcium from the bones.
   3. Improve circulation to the extremities.
   4. Prevent pressure sores.

8. The nurse explains to a male patient that he is placed on a Stryker frame to
   1. Help prevent contracture and increase cardiac output.
   2. Increase respiratory function and decrease hypotension.
   3. Allow horizontal turning of the patient and prevent pressure sores.
   4. Allow vertical turning of the patient to increase calcium absorption.

9. Before releasing the pivot pins and turning the Stryker frame, the nurse should
   1. Secure all bolts and straps to ensure patient safety.
   2. Observe the patient for hypotension.
   3. Get another nurse because the procedure requires two people.
   4. Tell the patient to hold on to the frame.

10. A male patient has been in the hospital with a diagnosis of cerebral thrombosis. His symptoms include right-sided paralysis and complete motor aphasia. The patient is very withdrawn and refuses to assist in feeding himself or performing personal hygiene. The patient's wife insists on doing everything for him when she visits and rarely leaves his side. The nurse would assess the patient as
    1. Depressed as a result of the cerebral edema caused by the thrombus.
    2. Feeling guilty about being a burden to his wife.
    3. Being unable to participate in his care and will continue to require total care from his family.
    4. Feeling depressed by his loss of independence.

11. A patient has dysphasia. As part of long-term planning the nurse should
    1. Help the patient accept this disability as permanent.
    2. Consult with physician concerning a speech therapy program.
    3. Ask the patient questions and wait as long as it takes for him to respond verbally.
    4. Begin associating words with physical objects.

12. A female patient is diagnosed with a CVA in the left hemisphere. The nurse explains to the patient that her cerebral accident (stroke) occurred in the left hemisphere of her brain; therefore, she will have paresis (weakness) on
    1. The right side of the body and the left side of her face.
    2. The four extremities of the body.
    3. The right side of the body.
    4. The left side of the body.

13. A male patient is diagnosed with injury to the left hemisphere of his brain. The damage makes speaking difficult, although he is able to communicate through gestures. When writing nursing notes about this patient, the term that best describes the patient's symptom is called
    1. Alopecia.
    2. Allergen.
    3. Albinism.
    4. Dysphasia.

14. The action *least* helpful when communicating with a patient diagnosed with injury to the left hemisphere of the brain is
    1. Conversing in a slow manner.
    2. Using gestures to accompany the spoken word.
    3. Giving him directions on a one-at-a-time basis.
    4. Speaking in a louder-than-usual tone of voice.

15. A male patient recovering from a CVA is receiving oxygen therapy. The action the nurse should take before starting oxygen therapy is to
    1. Keep the patient's head slightly elevated and clear his mouth of secretions.
    2. Position the patient so that he feels comfortable and have him cough several times.
    3. Turn the patient on his side and percuss his back over the area of the lungs.
    4. Place the patient in a supine position and have him deep breathe and cough up any secretions in his trachea.

16. While the nurse is administering sterile eye drops for a corneal abrasion, the patient asks, "What do you think caused my eye injury?" The correct response by the nurse is, "The most common cause of corneal abrasion is _____."
    1. Continuous glare of overhead lighting in a room.
    2. Trauma from a fall.
    3. Facial nerve damage.
    4. A foreign body.

17. The nurse admitting a male patient with Parkinson's disease to the hospital records that the patient has a shuffling and propulsive gait. If the nurse is using the term propulsive gait correctly, she has observed that the patient's walk is characterized by
    1. Slumping forward while walking.
    2. Walking with increasingly quicker steps.
    3. Walking erect on the balls of his feet.
    4. Having a tendency to lean backward while walking.

18. When the nurse asks a male patient with Parkinson's disease to undress, the nurse observes that the patient's upper arm tremors disappear as he unbuttons his shirt. Which of the following statements would be best to guide the nurse when analyzing her observation?
    1. The tremors probably are psychological and can be controlled by will.
    2. This type of tremor usually disappears with purposeful and voluntary movements.
    3. The tremors usually decrease in severity when attention is diverted by some activity.
    4. There is no explanation for the observation, which probably is a chance happening.

19. The signs and symptoms seen in Parkinson's disease result from the fact that the patient's body suffers from a
    1. Depletion of dopamine.
    2. Sustained relaxation of nerve impulse activities.
    3. Blockage of depolarization at motor nerve plates.
    4. Absence of acetylcholine.

20. A female patient taking Sinemet tells the nurse she does not feel well when she moves about or tries to sit up in bed. The nurse correctly decides that the patient most probably is moving too fast when the specific complaint is that she
    1. Feels faint when she first stands up and start to walk.
    2. Has back pains while walking.
    3. Feels excessively warm while sleeping.
    4. Has heart palpitations when she tries to bathe herself.

21. The male patient with Parkinson's disease tells the nurse he enjoys the activities given below. The nurse should judge which one of the following activities is most beneficial for the patient and encourage him to continue this activity as much as possible?
    1. Building model cars.
    2. Playing Scrabble.
    3. Growing vegetables in her garden.
    4. Discussing current events with her family.

22. Which of the following nursing goals is most realistic and appropriate in caring for a patient with Parkinson's disease?
    1. Cure the disease in 3 to 5 years.
    2. Maintain optimal functioning of the body.
    3. Begin preparations for terminal care at this time.
    4. Stop the progression of the disease at this time.

23. A physician discontinued levodopa but then reordered it but in combination with carbidopa. One of the major advantages in using this combination called Sinemet is that

1. The levodopa can be prescribed in lower doses.
2. Symptoms are better controlled and side effects are reduced.
3. It will eliminate problems of intolerance to levodopa.
4. Levodopa can be discontinued safely.

24. A patient is admitted to the hospital with a disease characterized by rapid development of symmetric weakness and lower motor neuron flaccid paralysis that ascends to the upper extremities. The nurse recognizes these are characteristics of which of the following diseases?
    1. Huntington's disease.
    2. Guillain-Barré syndrome.
    3. Multiple sclerosis.
    4. Myasthenia gravis.

25. The physician orders neostigmine (prostigmin) and pyridostigmine (Mestinon). The nurse knows that these drugs are used to treat a disease that is the result of impaired synthesis or storage of acetylcholine, which is
    1. Myasthenia gravis.
    2. Guillain-Barré syndrome.
    3. Multiple sclerosis.
    4. Huntington's disease.

26. A 35-year-old male patient is hospitalized with a disease characterized by chronic progressive chorea and mental deterioration. The nurse recognizes these characteristics as a disease resulting in degeneration of the basal ganglia and cerebral cortex called
    1. Myasthenia gravis.
    2. Huntington's disease.
    3. Multiple sclerosis.
    4. Guillain-Barré syndrome.

27. An RN teaching a class on neurologic problems would be correct in stating that the most common cause of neurologic deficit in the United States and the major cause of chronic disability is
    1. Myocardial infarction (MI).
    2. Stroke (brain attack).
    3. Cancer.
    4. Congestive heart failure (CHF).

28. The *primary* goal of nursing care for the patient 3 days after a subarachnoid hemorrhage is the prevention of
    1. Urinary failure.
    2. Contractures.
    3. Increased ICP.
    4. Hypotension.

29. In assessing a patient after a severe concussion, the nurse is aware that a late development will be
    1. ICP
    2. Hypertension.

3. Cyanosis and decreased level of consciousness.
4. Coma.

30. A 21-year-old female patient is admitted to the hospital because she has had two seizure attacks in the past week. It has been 2 months since the patient sustained a head injury in an automobile accident. The nurse would consider which of the following admission protocols as most valuable in helping to establish the patient's diagnosis?
    1. An x-ray examination of the patient's skull.
    2. A complete blood study.
    3. A complete history of her seizures and monitoring her closely for seizures.
    4. A neurologic examination and obtaining an order for Dilantin.

31. The patient has some knowledge about her seizures but tells the nurse that she is unclear about what an aura is. The nurse correctly defines an aura when she explains that it is a
    1. Postseizure state of amnesia.
    2. Hallucination during a seizure.
    3. Premonition of an impending seizure.
    4. Feeling of relaxation as the seizure begins to subside.

32. A male patient tells the nurse he is afraid that he will not be able to drive a car again because his seizures seem to occur more often now. The nurse responds correctly by telling him that driving will depend on local laws but most laws require
    1. That the person drives only during daytime hours.
    2. Evidence that the seizures are under medical control.
    3. Evidence that the seizures occur only every 6 months.
    4. That the person carries a medical identification card at all times.

33. Mannitol is used to reduce ICP and to
    1. Reduce intraocular pressure.
    2. Decrease the excretion of uric acid.
    3. Reduce pulmonary edema.
    4. Treat and prevent seizures.

34. A patient suffered a spinal cord injury in a swimming accident that resulted in quadriplegia. The nurse recognizes that the one major early problem for a quadriplegic will be
    1. Patient education.
    2. Learning to use mechanical aids.
    3. Relearning how to control his bladder.
    4. Diarrhea.

35. The nurse anticipates that the primary signs and symptoms caused by hypopituitarism are
    1. Deepening and coarsening of the voice.
    2. Demineralization of the bone.
    3. Decreased libido and impotence.
    4. Difficulty sleeping and anxiety.

36. After a hypophysectomy, a patient complains of postnasal drip. The physician suspects that CSF is leaking through the nasal passages. The nurse would confirm this by testing the nasal drainage for
1. Blood.
2. Glucose.
3. Protein.
4. Acidity.

37. The nurse knows that persistent CSF leaks are initially treated by
1. Bed rest with the head of the bed elevated to decrease pressure on the operative site.
2. Keeping the patient in supine position preoperatively and performing immediate surgical repair of operative site.
3. Keeping the patient in supine position. The physician will order Mannitol and methylprednisolone (Solu-Medrol) stat.
4. Keeping patient in supine position. The physician will pack the nasal cavity and will write preoperative orders.

38. After a hypophysectomy, the patient began to demonstrate signs and symptoms of diabetes insipidus. Which of the following would the nurse anticipate observing?
1. Blood glucose level greater than 200 mg/100 mL and nausea.
2. Polyuria, polydipsia, and urine specific gravity between 1.001 and 1.006.
3. Decreased urine output, urine specific gravity of 1.040, and diarrhea.
4. Urine high in ketones and glucose.

39. Treatment for diabetes insipidus includes
1. Regular insulin given subcutaneously (SC) and restriction of carbohydrate intake.
2. Increased fluid intake and administration of corticosteroids (e.g., ACTH).
3. Administration of vasopressin (Pitressin) IM, prevention of dehydration, and monitoring of urine specific gravity.
4. Administration of oxytocin and mannitol IV, prevention of dehydration, and monitoring of urine specific gravity.

40. A male patient expresses concern about the effect the surgery will have on his sexual ability. The *most* accurate information concerning the physiologic effects of a hypophysectomy is
1. Potency will be restored but decreased libido will persist.
2. Exogenous hormones will be needed to restore potency and fertility.
3. Removal of the source of estrogen and progesterone production will restore the patient's natural potency and fertility.
4. Potency will depend on the patient's ability to regain his psychological belief in his ability to perform sexually.

41. The nurse should be aware that spinal shock is seen in patients who have suffered a complete transection of the spinal cord. The nurse should assess for signs and symptoms of
1. Hypotension and tachycardia.
2. Hypertension and bradycardia.
3. Ventricular arrhythmias and tachypnea.
4. Hypotension and bradycardia.

42. The nurse needs to assess for signs and symptoms of autonomic dysreflexia (hyperreflexia), which are
1. Hypertension, bradycardia, and severe headache.
2. Hypotension, tachycardia, and headache.
3. Respiratory distress and headache.
4. Ventricle arrhythmias and hypotension.

43. A female quadriplegic complains of severe headache and is extremely anxious. The nurse checks her blood pressure and finds it to be 240/110. The nurse should then
1. Check for incontinence of stool.
2. Check the patency of the urinary catheter.
3. Administer Aldomet per physician's order.
4. Administer aspirin per physician's order and retake blood pressure in 15 minutes.

44. A 16-year-old female patient suffered a head injury in a gymnastics accident. She was immediately taken to the emergency room of the local hospital. When the nurse assesses this patient and takes a nursing history, the finding(s) indicative of the most serious head injury is(are)
1. Unconsciousness for 20 minutes and temporary amnesia when conscious.
2. A large contusion of the scalp with profuse bleeding.
3. Severe headache and blurred vision.
4. Nausea, vomiting, and blurred vision.

45. After the physician assessed and treated a patient with a severe head injury, the physician orders meperidine (Demerol) 25 mg IV stat every 3 h as necessary for pain. The nurse should
1. Administer the medication only when the patient requests it.
2. Administer the medication every 3 h if the patient complains of a severe headache.
3. Administer the medication as ordered provided that the blood pressure is 150/80.
4. Question the physician about the advisability of administering the Demerol to a patient with a head injury.

46. When the nurse performs a neurologic check, the nurse should recognize findings that are late signs of increased ICP, which are
1. Increased lethargy, widened pulse pressure, elevated temperature, bradycardia, and irregular respirations.
2. Hypotension, bradycardia, increased lethargy, and tachycardia.

3. Apprehension, hypertension, tachycardia, and a 15 on the Glasgow Coma Scale.

4. Increased lethargy, tachycardia, tachypnea, and a 3 on the Glasgow Coma Scale.

47. After a patient is treated for a severe head injury and is being released from the emergency room, the teaching that should be stressed by the nurse is

1. The need to sleep in a supine position.

2. The importance of notifying the physician immediately of decreased level of consciousness.

3. The importance of blowing the nose to keep the passage clear.

4. The use of aspirin as needed to relieve headache and notify the physician immediately if the patient complains of being tired.

48. Formation of urinary calculi is a complication that may be encountered by a paraplegic patient. The major factor that contributes to this condition is _____. To decrease this problem, the patient should _____.

1. An increased intake of calcium; decrease protein intake.

2. Inadequate kidney functions; decrease fluid intake.

3. Increased loss of calcium from the skeletal system; increase fluid intake.

4. Hypoparathyroidism; increase fiber intake.

49. Three days after a male patient is diagnosed as a paraplegic, he asks the nurse if he will be able to have sexual intercourse. The *most* knowledgeable response is

1. "You are a paraplegic and have lost all motor control below your waist."

2. "It is too early to make that determination."

3. "That should not even be discussed this early in your recovery."

4. "No, I really don't think you will every have sexual intercourse again."

50. When planning care for a paraplegic, the nurse is aware that

1. Rehabilitation should be left up to the patient.

2. It is not necessary to begin rehabilitation while the patient is in the hospital, but it should be started in a rehabilitation facility.

3. Rehabilitation should begin as soon as the patient is stabilized.

4. Rehabilitation should begin as soon as the patient is admitted to the hospital.

ANSWERS AND RATIONALES

1. **②** The third cranial nerve (oculomotor) innervates the upper eyelid. If this nerve is damaged, the eyelid would not close. It also is responsible for pupil dilation.

(1) The fourth cranial nerve (trochlear) is responsible for extraocular movement.

(3) The seventh cranial nerve (facial) innervates the eyebrow and lower lid.

(4) The second cranial nerve (optic) is responsible for acuity and visual field.

2. **③** Damage to the third cranial nerve (oculomotor) may cause pupil dilation.

(1, 2) The seventh and fourth cranial nerves are discussed in rationale (1).

(4) The fifth cranial nerve, if injured, will cause pain or loss of sensation in the face, forehead, temple, and eyes. Motor root injury will cause difficulty chewing.

3. **①** When a patient is NPO and has been on Dilantin PO, the nurse needs to consult with the physician to find out if the Dilantin should be given IV. The nurse knows that it would be dangerous to skip a scheduled dose of Dilantin.

(2, 3, 4) These options are incorrect as seen in rationale (1).

4. **①** If patient has difficulty swallowing a Dilantin capsule after a procedure, the nurse can substitute a Dilantin oral suspension without a physician's order because they are both the same medication given by the same route PO.

(2) Dilantin is not made in suppository form.

(3) Dilantin is not given IM.

(4) A capsule should not be opened and content removed because the capsule allows the medication to be absorbed slowly. (Exception may be made when a medication must be administered through a nasogastric [NG] or percutaneous endoscopic gastrostomy [PEG] tube). Usually the physician will change the order to IV.

5. **③** Because Dilantin may cause hypertrophy of the gums, meticulous oral hygiene is needed to reduce inflammation and prevent infection of the gums.

(1, 2, 4) These options are incorrect as seen in rationale (3).

6. **①** Another side effect of Dilantin is that it tends to decrease absorption of folic acid, which may cause folic acid anemia.

(2) Dilantin interferes with the absorption of folic acid, but it is not incompatible.

(3) Folic acid and Dilantin given together will not cause neuropathy.

(4) Folic acid does not increase or decrease the absorption of Dilantin, but Dilantin does interfere with the absorption of folic acid.

7. **②** In order for the body to absorb calcium, there must be pressure on the long bones. The tilt table allows the patient to be in a standing position, which puts pressure on the long bones.

(1) The tilt table is raised slowly to prevent hypotension, but this is not the purpose of the tilt table. The blood pressure may drop significantly when a quadriplegic is in an upright position because there is no vasoconstriction and blood pools in the lower extremities. Inadequate blood supply to the brain causes cerebral hypoxia.

(3) Using a tilt table will increase circulation to the extremities, but this is not the main purpose of the tilt table. Turning the patient in bed will increase circulation.

(4) Using a tilt table may help prevent pressure sores, but this is not the main purpose of the tilt table. Turning the patient in bed will help to prevent pressure sores. Special beds that constantly rotate to prevent pressure sores are available.

8. ③ A Stryker frame has two metal frames (anterior and posterior) with a taut canvas cover and a thin protective padding over each frame.

The frames are supported on a movable cart with a pivot apparatus at each end. By securing one frame over the patient while he or she lies on the other, two people can turn the person from back to abdomen and vice versa. During turning, the patient is briefly "sandwiched" between the frames and is kept from falling or sliding by the straps secured around both frames.

Patients who can use their arms are told to fold them around the frame during turning. Strap the arms of a patient who cannot use them alongside the body to prevent injury.

Once the patient is safely turned, the uppermost frame is removed. A small canvas strip across the middle of the posterior frame (the one the patient is on when supine) is removable for bedpan use. The anterior frame has a space for patient's face so that, when lying prone, the person can rest, read, or eat without turning the head.

The Stryker frame allows horizontal turning of the patient. This helps prevent pressure sores and increases circulation to prevent blood clots and respiratory problems.

(1) To prevent contracture, require passive range of motion and have patient wear tennis shoes to prevent foot drop. To some degree, increase cardiac output.

(2) Turning the patient on a Stryker frame will not increase respiratory function but to some degree will increase blood flow to the lungs.

(4) Vertical positioning of the patient would be putting him or her in a standing position as is accomplished with a *tilt table*. This would increase calcium absorption, but the question was about a *Stryker frame*.

9. ① Before releasing the pivot pin and turning the Stryker frame, the nurse should secure all bolts and straps to ensure the patient's safety.

(2) The patient will not experience hypotension when turned horizontally.

(3) Most of the time, two nurses will work together in turning a patient on a Stryker frame, but it is more important to be sure the patient is secured before turning the Stryker frame (or else the patient may fall on the floor).

(4) The patient does not have to hold onto the frame. All the patient has to do is to keep the hands near the body so they will not be injured when the Stryker frame is turned.

10. ④ A cerebral thrombosis is the most common cause of brain attack. It is a blood clot that occludes blood vessels in the brain. Occlusion of cerebral vessels by an embolus causes necrosis and edema. The edema may cause greater dysfunction than the infarct itself.

The edema may subside in a few hours or sometimes after several days. As the edema subsides, the patient begins to improve and may regain some functions that were impaired by the edema.

The symptoms of paralysis and complete motor aphasia can be very devastating to a patient. The patient may become depressed because of the loss of independence and the patient's new dependence on others to do everything for them (including communicating for him or her) until the patient can establish an adequate means of communication. The patient knows that some effects of the stroke may be permanent.

(1) Edema does not cause depression.

(2) When a patient becomes totally dependent on others because of a stroke, the patient knows it is not his or her fault, so he or she will not feel guilty but may be depressed.

(3) It takes several weeks, even months, before the permanent damage from a stroke can be determined. If the stroke is not severe, most or all of the paralysis may disappear, and the patient may regain speech slowly.

11. ② Long-term planning for a patient with dysphasia includes consultation with the patient's physician regarding a speech therapy program. It is very upsetting for the patient, and the patient needs therapeutic assistance.

(1) It is too early to know the residual disabilities that the patient will have to live with, so there is no reason for the patient to accept his or her disabilities as permanent.

(3) A patient with dysphasia cannot respond, and to ask the patient a question and expect a response would be very emotionally upsetting for the patient.

(4) This patient had motor dysphasia, which is impairment of the ability to communicate through speech. The inability to associate words with objects is called anomic aphasia.

12. ③ When a patient had a CVA in the left hemisphere, there will be paresis (weakness on the right side). This is because the pyramidal motor tracts cross over at the medulla oblongata. Therefore, the left side of the brain controls the motor activity of the right side of the body and the right side of the brain controls the motor activity of the left side of the body.

(1) The right side of the body and the right side of the face will have paresis with a CVA in the left hemisphere.

(2) The four extremities of the body would *not* be affected by a left CVA.

(4) The left side of the body would *not* have paresis because the CVA was on the left side of the brain and paramedial motor tracts cross over at the medulla oblongata. Therefore, the right side of the body would have paresis. Remember when feeding patients with strokes to feed them on the *unaffected* side of the mouth.

13. ④ Dysphasia is the term used to describe impairment of speech, but the patient can communicate through gesture.

(1) Alopecia is the absence of hair, especially of the head.

(2) An allergen is any substance that causes manifestation of an allergy.

(3) Albinism is a congenital total absence of pigment in skin, hair, and eyes.

14. **④** This question is asking which one of these options is the *least* correct. Rationales (1), (2), and (3) are correct, which leaves rationale (4) as the incorrect option. Speaking in a louder-than-usual tone of voice is of no help to a stroke patient. These patients do not have a hearing problem. They have a speech problem, so speaking louder is not helpful.

(1) Conversing in a slow manner allows the patient time to comprehend what is being said.

(2, 3) Using gestures and giving directions on a one-at-a-time basis will help the patient better understand the message being communicated. After a stroke, the patient may be slower to comprehend, and gestures will help.

15. **①** Before starting oxygen on a patient recovering from a CVA, it is important to clear the patient's mouth of secretions and slightly elevate the head of the bed because the patient may have difficulty swallowing and could easily aspirate on oral secretions.

(2) It is more important to position the patient so that he or she will not aspirate than to put the patient in a comfortable position. The patient may be unable to cough because of the weakness of abdominal and throat muscles caused by the stroke.

(3) Turning the patient on the side and percussing the back over the area of the lung serves no purpose because the lungs are not congested. Allowing the patient to lie flat in bed is dangerous because the patient may aspirate on oral secretions.

(4) Allowing the patient to lie in a supine position and encouraging the patient to cough up secretions is very dangerous because the patient may aspirate on secretions. A patient will have secretions in the mouth and throat after a CVA but does not have lung congestion.

16. **④** The nurse knows that the most common cause of corneal abrasions is a foreign body.

(1) The continuous glare of overhead lighting will not cause corneal abrasion.

(2) Trauma from a fall is not a common cause of corneal abrasion.

(3) Damage to seventh cranial nerve (facial) would not cause corneal abrasion.

17. **①** A patient with Parkinson's disease will have a shuffling and propulsive gait. In other words, the patient will walk with the body bent forward. Other signs and symptoms include muscle rigidity, akinesia (complete or partial loss of muscle movement), and insidious tremors that begin in the fingers (unilateral pill-roll tremor; high-pitched, monotone voice; drooling; masklike facial expression).

(2, 3, 4) These options are incorrect as seen in rationale (1).

18. **②** The unilateral pill-roll tremors will disappear with purposeful and voluntary movement.

(1) These tremors are not psychological. They are caused by the depletion of dopamine, a neuromuscular transmitter.

(3) Diverting will not decrease tremors because they are not psychological.

(4) These tremors are not a chance happening. They are caused by depletion of dopamine.

19. **①** Signs and symptoms of Parkinson's disease are caused by depletion of dopamine.

(2, 3, 4) These options are incorrect as seen in rationale (1).

20. **①** Carbidopa/levodopa (Sinemet) is given to replace dopamine, and with this neuromuscular replacement, the patient can now move faster. This may cause orthostatic hypotension (blood pressure drops), and the patient will feel faint.

(2, 3, 4) These options are incorrect. Levodopa will not cause back pain, feelings of excessive warmth, or heart palpitations.

21. **①** A patient with Parkinson's disease needs to exercise the hands so that he or she will not lose use of them because they are constantly involved in unilateral pill-rolling tremors. These tremors stop with purposeful movement. Building model cars would engage the hands in purposeful movement and rest the hands from tremors.

(2) Playing Scrabble would be too demanding for a patient with hand tremors because the game is competitive.

(3) Growing vegetables in a garden would be almost impossible for a patient with a propulsive gait, who is bent forward and has muscle rigidity. The patient would not be working the soil because he or she would be lying on the ground.

(4) Discussing current events with the family would be very difficult for a patient with a high-pitched monotone voice and drooling from the mouth.

22. **②** The most realistic and appropriate goal for a patient with Parkinson's disease is to maintain optimal functioning of the body.

(1) Parkinson's disease is not curable, so that is not a goal.

(3) Terminal care should not be a goal this early in the disease process.

(4) The progression of the disease cannot be stopped; there can be only a reduction in symptoms using levodopa and carbidopa.

23. **②** Drug therapies usually include levodopa because it is converted to dopamine in the CNS, where it serves as a neurotransmitter and is most effective in the early stages. This drug is given in increasing doses until symptoms are relieved or side effects appear. Carbidopa prevents peripheral destruction of levodopa, so more is available to the CNS. The therapeutic effect is the relief of the tremors and rigidity associated with Parkinson's disease. Because the side effects can be serious, levodopa can be given in lower doses when given with carbidopa, thus reducing the side effects and better controlling the symptoms. Sinemet is the name of the drug containing both carbidopa and levodopa.

(1) Levodopa is given in a lower dosage, but this option does not explain why it is given in a lower dosage. Always choose the option that gives the most complete answer, and that option usually is the longest option.

(3) There is not intolerance to levodopa; rather, the side effects need to be reduced.

(4) Carbidopa is not given with levodopa, so levodopa can be discontinued.

24. ❷ Guillain-Barré syndrome is an acute, rapidly progressive, potentially fatal form of polyneuritis that causes muscle weakness and mild distal sensory loss.

This syndrome is most common between the ages of 30 and 50 years. It affects both sexes equally. Recovery is spontaneous and complete in approximately 95 percent of patients, although mild motor or reflex deficits in the feet and legs may persist.

The precise cause of Guillain-Barré syndrome is unknown, but it may be a cell-mediated immunologic attack on peripheral nerves in response to a virus.

Muscle weakness, the major neurologic sign, usually appears in the legs first (ascending type), then extends from the legs to the arms and facial nerves in 24 to 72 h.

(1) Huntington's disease is a hereditary disease in which degeneration in the cerebral cortex and basal ganglia causes chronic progressive chorea (involuntary muscle twitching) and mental deterioration, ending in dementia.

(3) Multiple sclerosis (MS) is characterized by progressive demyelination of the white matter of the brain and spinal cord. It is the major cause of chronic disability in young adults. Prognosis is variable. Multiple sclerosis may progress rapidly, disabling the patient by early adulthood or causing death within months of onset. However, 70 percent of patients lead active, productive lives with prolonged remissions.

Onset occurs between the ages of 20 and 40 years. The exact cause of MS is unknown, but theories suggest a slow-acting viral infection or an autoimmune response of the nervous system.

(4) Myasthenia gravis produces progressive weakness of skeletal muscles, which become weaker with exercise.

25. ❶ Myasthenia gravis produces progressive weakness of skeletal muscles, which become weaker with exercise. Muscle strength improves with administration of anticholinesterase drugs, such as neostigmine and pyridostigmine. These drugs decrease the ability of cholinesterase to break down acetylcholine. Acetylcholine is a neuromuscular transmitter necessary for normal muscle function.

Myasthenia gravis causes a failure in transmission of acetylcholine at the neuromuscular junction. The cause of myasthenia gravis may be an autoimmune response.

(2) The major neurologic sign of Guillain-Barré syndrome usually appears in the legs first (ascending type), as explained in answer 24, rationale (2).

(3) Multiple sclerosis is the major cause of chronic disability in young adults, as explained in answer 24, rationale (3).

(4) Huntington's disease is a hereditary disease in which degeneration in the cerebral cortex and basal ganglia causes chronic progressive chorea (involuntary muscular twitching of the limbs or facial muscles) and mental deterioration, ending in dementia.

26. ❷ Huntington's disease is a hereditary disease in which degeneration in the cerebral cortex and basal ganglia causes chronic progressive chorea (involuntary muscle twitching) and mental deterioration, ending in dementia (deteriorative mental state due to organic brain disease). Huntington's disease usu-

ally strikes persons between the ages of 25 and 55 years. The cause of Huntington's disease is unknown. Onset is insidious. The patient eventually becomes totally dependent emotionally and physically through loss of musculoskeletal control. Death usually results 10 to 15 years after onset.

(1, 3, 4) Myasthenia gravis is explained in answer 25, rationale (1), multiple sclerosis is explained in answer 24, rationale (3), and Guillain-Barré is explained in answer 24, rationale (2).

27. ❷ The most common cause of neurologic deficit in the United States and the major cause of chronic disability is stroke.

(1) MI reduces blood flow through one or more coronary arteries. The result is myocardial ischemia and necrosis. This is a cardiovascular problem, not neurologic, so it cannot be the most common cause of a neurologic deficit.

(3) Cancer, a malignant tumor, is the rapid reproducing of immature cells and tends to metastasize (spread) to new sites. Cancer may affect the brain, but it is not a neurologic disease.

(4) CHF means the heart has failed as a pump. It is not a neurologic disease.

28. ❸ The primary goal of nursing care for the patient with a subarachnoid hemorrhage is to prevent increased ICP. Intracranial hemorrhage may require a craniotomy or burr holes to locate and control bleeding and to aspirate blood to help prevent increased ICP. Mannitol is administered IV to help control ICP.

(1) Urinary failure is not associated with a subarachnoid hemorrhage.

(2) Prevention of contractures is not a primary goal 3 days after a subarachnoid hemorrhage.

(4) Hypotension is not associated with a subarachnoid hemorrhage, but hypertension is.

29. ❶ Increased ICP is a late development after a cranial fracture. It will occur as edema caused by the injury increases.

The first neurologic signs after a concussion are a brief loss of consciousness, immediately followed by confusion and memory loss. Usually, there are no other abnormal neurologic findings. The signs and symptoms of ICP become evident as the brain swelling and edema increase.

(3) Decreased level of consciousness is an early sign.

(2, 4) These options are incorrect as seen in rationale (1).

30. ❸ A patient with a head injury who has experienced two seizure attacks before admission to the hospital needs to be monitored closely for seizure activity. The nurse would assist the physician in establishing the patient's diagnosis by obtaining a complete history of the patient's seizures.

(1, 2) Obtaining x-ray films of the patient's skull or a complete blood study is not an independent nursing action.

(4) A nurse may perform a neurologic examination, but there may be no neurologic deficit other than seizures. This procedure would not help establish the patient's diagnosis. Normally, patients who have seizures will not show a neurologic deficit when a nurse performs a neurologic examination.

31. ❸ An aura is a premonition of an impending seizure.

(1, 2, 4) These options are incorrect as seen in rationale (3).

32. ❷   Most laws require that a person who experiences seizures show evidence that the seizures are under medical control before the person is allowed to drive a car.

(1, 3, 4) These options are incorrect as seen in rationale (2).

33. ❶   Mannitol is an osmotic diuretic used for decreasing increased ICP and intraocular pressure.

(2, 3, 4) Mannitol does not decrease excretion of uric acid, reduce pulmonary edema, or prevent seizures. It increases the excretion of uric acid.

34. ❷   The nurse recognizes that one major early problem for a quadriplegic is learning to use mechanical aids. Most quadriplegics are young adults who are accustomed to living very active lives and depending on no one to help them. Now they must tediously begin to relearn many motor skills using mechanical aids.

(1) Because the average quadriplegic is young and may be in high school or college, education usually is not a problem. If they are of school age, home teaching is available in most states.

(3) A quadriplegic has no bladder control and will have to learn to catheterize himself or her.

(4) A quadriplegic has a paralytic ileus so diarrhea is not a problem, but constipation is a major problem.

35. ❸   Hypopituitarism will cause decrease in progesterone and testosterone, the primary hormone responsible for male masculinization. A low testosterone level will result in decreased libido and impotence. Levels of follicle-stimulating hormone (FSH) and luteinizing hormone (LH) are decreased. These hormones stimulate gametogenesis (gamete is a mature male or female reproductive cell, the spermatozoon or ovum) and sex steroid production in males and females. Levels of antidiuretic hormone (ADH), thyroid-stimulating hormone (TSH), ACTH, oxytocin, and prolactin also are decreased.

(1, 2, 4) These options are incorrect as seen in rationale (3).

36. ❷   Hypophysectomy is the removal of the pituitary gland. Because the pituitary gland lies proximal to the nose, CSF could leak through the nasal passages. CSF contains glucose. Surgery for a hypophysectomy is performed through the roof of the mouth.

(1, 3, 4) These options are incorrect as seen in rationale (2).

37. ❶   CSF leaks usually heal spontaneously if there is decreased pressure on the operative site. If the head of the bed is elevated, this reduces the pressure of blood returning to the brain. If the head of the bed is flat, the force of blood returning to the brain is increased.

(2, 3, 4) These options are incorrect as seen in rationale (1).

38. ❷   Diabetes insipidus occurs when the posterior lobe of the pituitary fails to secrete ADH. There will be an increase in urinary output (polyuria), increased thirst (polydipsia), and the concentration of urine will be very low with a specific gravity between 1.001 and 1.006. Normal adult specific gravity is 1.005 to 1.030 or 1.025.

(1, 3, 4) These options are incorrect as seen in rationale (2).

39. ❸   Pitressin, a synthetic pituitary hormone, promotes reabsorption of water by acting on the renal collecting ducts. Pitressin can be administered by IM route, by nasal spray, or by dropper.

(1, 2, 4) These options are incorrect as seen in rationale (3).

40. ❷   People who have undergone a hypophysectomy must take a cortisone replacement for the rest of their lives. They also will have to take exogenous hormones, which are needed to restore the patient's natural potency and fertility. The pituitary secretes many different stimulating hormones, such as ACTH, which stimulates the release of cortisone from the adrenal cortex.

(1, 3, 4) These options are incorrect as seen in rationale (2).

41. ❶   Spinal shock is seen in patients with complete transection of the spinal cord. The main problem is impairment of the vasomotor mechanism (nerves having muscular control of the blood vessel walls), which causes hypotension and tachycardia. The increase in heart rate is a compensatory reaction.

(2, 3, 4) These options are incorrect as seen in rationale (1).

42. ❶   Signs and symptoms of autonomic dysreflexia are hypertension, bradycardia, and severe headache.

(2, 3, 4) These options are incorrect as seen in rationale (1).

43. ❷   When a patient with complete transection of the spinal cord at the fourth thoracic (T4) level complains of a severe headache and has a blood pressure of 240/110, these are signs of autonomic dysreflexia. A major cause of this is a distended bladder, so the nurse must check the patency of the urinary catheter.

(1, 3, 4) These options are incorrect as seen in rationale (2).

44. ❶   A patient with a serious head injury may be unconscious for 20 minutes or longer, and amnesia may occur temporarily when the patient is conscious.

(2) A large contusion of the scalp will cause profuse bleeding but is not indicative of a serious head injury.

(3) Severe headache and blurred vision may be temporary effects of head trauma but are not indicative of serious head injury.

(4) Nausea, vomiting, and blurred vision may be temporary effects of head injury but are not indicative of severe head injury.

45. ❷   After a head injury has been assessed and treatment started, the physician may order a low dose of analgesic, such as Demerol 25 mg IV. This should be administered *PRN* as ordered because pain will cause vasoconstriction and may increase ICP.

46. ❶   Late signs of increased ICP are increased lethargy, widened pulse pressure, increased temperature, and irregular respirations (a random sequence of deep and shallow breaths). The Glasgow Coma Scale is used to detect early signs of increased ICP.

This scale encompasses three types of behaviors that are used to assess the patient's level of responsiveness: verbal responses, motor responses, and eye opening. The criteria that best reflects the patient's response are selected, and a numerical value is assigned to those criteria.

The Glasgow Coma Scale has three areas of assessment: the best eye opening response (scale 1–4) if "spontaneous" eye opening response will receive a 4; the best motor response to painful stimuli (scale 1–6) if "obeying a verbal command" will receive a 6; and the best verbal response (scale 1–5) "oriented (×3)" will receive a 5. The higher the score, the better the client is responding.

(2, 3, 4) These options are incorrect as seen in rationale (1).

47. ❷ After a patient has been treated for a head injury and sent home, it is important for the nurse to stress to the patient that the physician should be notified immediately if there is a decrease in the level of consciousness.

(1, 3, 4) These options are incorrect as seen in rationale (2).

48. ❸ Paraplegic patients tend to develop urinary calculi because these patients cannot put pressure on their long bones. Pressure on the long bones is necessary for calcium absorption. When there is no pressure on the long bones, the calcium is lost from the skeletal system, which causes an increase in the serum calcium level and can cause renal calculi. Increased fluid intake helps eliminate some of the serum calcium and reduces urinary calculi.

(1, 2, 4) Renal calculi usually are not caused by an increased intake of calcium, inadequate kidney function, or hypoparathy-roid imbalance. The parathyroid glands regulate calcium and phosphate metabolism, increase absorption of bone, and thereby maintain normal serum calcium levels. Hypoparathyroid will produce a low serum calcium level, so renal stones will *not* develop. A decrease in protein intake or an increase in fiber intake will not decrease urinary calculi.

49. ❷ Three days after a spinal cord injury would be too early to make a determination about a male patient's ability to have sexual intercourse.

(1, 3, 4) These options are incorrect as seen in rationale (2).

50. ❸ Rehabilitation should begin as soon as the patient is stabilized after a spinal cord injury.

(1) Rehabilitation cannot be left up to the patient because the patient is depressed and not interested in rehabilitation at this early time in the recovery.

(2) Valuable time would be lost in rehabilitating the patient if it was not started until the patient was in a rehabilitation facility. Some body functions that might have been restored could be lost forever.

(4) Rehabilitation cannot begin until the patient recovering from a spinal injury is stable because these activities may kill the patient when he or she is in the crisis time of recovery.

Chapter
19

Obstetric, Neonatal, and Gynecologic Disorders

TOPICAL OUTLINE

Obstetric and Neonatal Disorders

I. MENSTRUAL CYCLE

A. Gonadotropin-Releasing Hormone

Gonadotropin-releasing hormone (GnRH) is produced by the hypothalamus and transmitted to the anterior pituitary, where the gonadotropins follicle-stimulating hormone (FSH) and luteinizing hormone (LH) are produced.

B. First Half of Cycle (Follicular Phase)

1. *FSH*: Follicles ready for maturation are stimulated to develop by release of FSH

2. *Estrogen* level (produced on the graafian follicle)

    a. Peaks on approximately day 8 or 9, halting production of FSH.

    b. On approximately day 14, a surge of LH triggers rupture of the follicle and ovulation (extrusion of the ovum) occurs.

C. Second Half of Cycle (Luteal Phase)

1. LH stimulates luteinization of the granulosa cells and formation of the corpus luteum.

2. These cells produce progesterone, which peaks on approximately day 23 or 24.

3. If impregnation does not occur, estrogen and progesterone levels decline, reaching critical lows on approximately day 28 when endometrial bleeding (menstruation) occurs.

4. The low estrogen and progesterone levels trigger FSH production in the anterior pituitary gland.

5. If impregnation does occur, estrogen and progesterone levels continue to rise.

6. LH maintains the corpus luteum during the first 2 to 3 months of gestation.

II. NORMAL PREGNANCY

A. General Considerations

1. The lifespan of sperm is 48 to 72 h in the female reproductive tract.

2. The life span of ovum is 24 to 36 h post ovulation.

3. Conception usually occurs 12 to 24 h post ovulation.

4. Implantation occurs within 6 to 9 days after conception.

B. Pregnancy Tests

1. Human Chorionic Gonadotropin

    a. Levels can be measured in blood or urine. Within 7 to 10 days after conception, tests for detecting human chorionic gonadotropin (hCG) in the urine and serum usually are positive. A pelvic examination at this stage can yield various finding, such as Hegar's sign (cervical and uterine softening), Chadwick's sign (bluish coloration of the vagina and cervix resulting from increased venous circulation), and enlargement of the uterus. A pelvic examination will help estimate gestation age, but vaginal sonography is more accurate.

b. *Note:* High levels of hCG can result from a pathologic condition (hydatidiform mole or chorionic epithelioma, cancer of the chorionic villi or uterus).

2. Ultrasound is accurate approximately 3 weeks after the first menstrual period.

C. Signs and Symptoms

1. Presumptive

a. Amenorrhea, breast sensitivity, breast enlargement, nausea and vomiting, frequent urination, quickening, fatigue, skin pigmentation, and striae

2. Probable

a. Hegar's sign (softening of the lower uterine segment), Goodell's sign (softening of the cervix), uterine enlargement, ballottement, and Braxton Hicks contractions

3. Positive

a. Fetal heartbeat (at 5 weeks via ultrasound and at 10 weeks via Doppler ultrasound).

b. Fetal movement on palpation (18 to 20 weeks).

D. Functional and Structural Maternal Changes

1. Uterus

a. Becomes round and upright, the cervix softens, and the lower uterine segment becomes soft.

b. The broad, round ligaments stretch and elongate.

2. Vascular

a. Blood volume increases 25 to 40 percent.

b. The increased ratio of plasma to red blood cell mass may cause the hematocrit to drop to 36 to 37 percent and the hemoglobin to drop to 11 to 13 percent late in pregnancy (physiologic dilutional anemia of pregnancy).

3. Cardiac

a. Rate increases 15 to 20 bpm in the second trimester.

b. Cardiac output increases 33 to 50 percent.

4. Renal

a. Increased glomerular filtration rate.

b. Pressure of the fetus and uterus on the bladder causes frequent micturition and dilated ureters.

c. Slight proteinuria and glucosuria are not uncommon.

5. Respiratory

a. The diaphragm rises approximately 4 cm during pregnancy. and the circumference increases 5 to 7 cm to compensate for this rise.

b. The respiratory rate may increase by two breaths per minute in the third trimester.

6. Breasts

a. Enlarge due to progesterone and estrogen production.

b. Montgomery's glands (surrounding the nipple) enlarge, and the areola darkens.

7. Skin

a. Pigmentation changes include linea nigra (brown or black line from the umbilicus to the mons pubis), chloasma gravidarum (dark blotches on face), and striae gravidarum (stretch marks).

8. Gastrointestinal

a. Nausea and vomiting during the first trimester

b. Heartburn, primarily during the third trimester, due to increased gastric acid production

9. Endocrine

a. Neurohypophysis (posterior lobe of the pituitary gland) produces oxytocin, which stimulates contraction of the uterus during labor and delivery.

b. Oxytocin is secreted during suckling, causing milk release from the mammary glands.

c. The placenta (at 8 weeks) secretes hCG, estrogen (responsible for breast enlargement and fat deposition, promotes sodium and water retention), and progesterone (produces relaxation of smooth muscles, raises body temperature, promotes fat deposition).

10. Psychosocial

a. High levels of estrogen cause emotional lability.

11. Weight Changes

a. Weight gain directly related to the pregnancy is approximately 14 lb, from the placenta, amniotic fluid, enlarged uterus, breast tissue, and blood volume.

b. Other weight gain can be attributed to fluid retention and fat accumulation.

c. Recommended weight gain for women who are ideal weight is 24 to 32 lb and generally is less for overweight women.

III. PRENATAL CARE

A. Laboratory Tests

1. Initial Visit

a. Complete blood cell (CBC) count with differential; screen for anemia, active infection, idiopathic thrombocytopenic purpura (ITP).

b. Rubella titer: if nonimmune, avoid exposure, especially during first trimester, and vaccinate postpartum.

c. Rapid plasma reagin (RPR): initial screen for syphilis.

d. Blood type and Rh with antibody screen: predicts Rh disease and ABO incompatibility and identifies irregular antibodies.

e. Urinalysis

(1) Assess for protein and glucose.

f. Other tests

(1) Culture for beta-hemolytic streptococci, gonorrhea, chlamydia, or genital herpes simplex virus type 2 (HSV-2).

(2) Screen for sickle cell anemias (thalassemia).

(3) Hepatitis B and human immunodeficiency virus (HIV).

(4) Pap smear.

(5) Drug screen.

2. At 16 to 18 weeks

a. Maternal serum alpha-fetoprotein (MSAFP) levels are measured at 16 weeks.

(1) If elevated, assess for possible neural tube defect (or for twins or inaccurate gestational age).

(2) If low, assess for trisomy 21 (Down syndrome).

(3) *Note*: May be normal neonate with elevated MSAFP.

b. Ultrasound.

(1) Generally performed in either the first or second trimester for verification of gestational age and to identify major congenital anomalies.

(2) Amniocentesis may be performed later in the pregnancy in conjunction with an ultrasound to assess amniotic fluid for phospholipids, lecithin to sphingomyelin (L/S) ratio, and phosphatidylglycerol, which may indicate fetal lung maturity.

3. At 27 weeks

a. Glucose tolerance test (obese women are screened at first prenatal visit).

B. Genetic Testing (Optional)

1. Chorionic Villus Sampling

a. Prenatal diagnosis of many genetic disorders is feasible at 8 to 12 weeks of gestation using this method.

b. Risks include spontaneous abortion, limb-reduction defect, and serious infection.

2. Amniocentesis

a. Prenatal diagnosis performed at 14 to 16 weeks.

b. Risk of spontaneous abortion.

C. Assessment

1. Obtain Medical History

a. Identify estimated date of confinement (EDC).

(1) Use Nägele's rule (subtracts 3 months from first day of last menstrual period [LMP] and adds 7 days).

b. Record baseline vital signs.

c. Identify religious and cultural implications to pregnancy (e.g., Jehovah's witness: no blood products).

2. Identify Pelvic Structure

a. Gynecoid (most common and favorable for childbirth): oval inlet, straight side walls, nonprominent ischial spines, wide subpubic arch, and concave sacrum.

b. Android (malelike): wedge-shaped inlet, convergent side walls, prominent ischial spines, narrow subpubic arch, lower one third of sacrum is inclined anteriorly.

c. Platypelloid (flat pelvis, rare): wide transverse diameter of inlet.

d. Anthropoid (ape-type pelvis); oval inlet, pelvic side walls diverge, and sacrum is inclined posteriorly.

3. Fundal Height (McDonald's)

a. Begin at or before 16 weeks.

b. At 20 to 22 weeks, the height of the fetus should equal gestational age.

c. Measure in centimeters from the symphysis pubis to the fundus.

4. Review of Past Pregnancies

a. Establish gravidity.

(1) Total number of pregnancies, including ectopic pregnancies and hydatidiform moles (molar pregnancies are 10 times more common in women older than 45 years).

(2) Multiple gestation counts as one pregnancy.

b. Establish parity.

(1) Birth of an infant, dead or alive, weighing more than 500 g or 24 weeks of gestation or greater if weight is unknown.

(2) Multiple gestation counts as a single experience.

c. Establish number of abortions, which is any pregnancy that terminates at less than 24 gestational weeks or a fetus weighing less than 500 g.

d. Establish the number of living children.

e. Identify any previous diagnosis of incompetent cervix (pregnancy loss without labor), treatment by cerclage.

5. Evaluation of Fetal Well-Being

a. Maternal weight, fetal growth, and fetal heart rate (FHR) each visit.

b. First trimester: auscultation of FHR and maternal weight gain.

c. Second trimester: measurement of fundal height, FHR, fetal movement (quickening), and maternal weight gain.

d. Third trimester: same as second trimester plus electronic fetal monitoring, if indicated.

6. Emotional Status and Support Systems

a. Maternal adjustment: developmental tasks.

(1) First trimester: ambivalence, acceptance of pregnancy.

(2) Second trimester: role and change in body image.

(3) Third trimester: acceptance of body image and its potential impact on sexual activities; preparing for labor, delivery, and parenting.

b. Paternal adjustment: developmental tasks.

(1) First trimester: ambivalence, role transition.

(2) Second trimester: developing father image, difficulty relating to fetus.

(3) Third trimester: changing self-concept, fears.

c. Sibling adjustment: normal rivalry dependent on developmental maturity.

d. Nursing interventions.

(1) Assess attitude toward pregnancy, emotional status, and available support system.

(2) Consult with social worker as indicated.

(3) Establish a plan of care, which includes ongoing assessment and evaluation of effectiveness of interventions.

(4) Avoid being judgmental and provide emotional support.

7. Nutritional Needs

a. Prenatal vitamins are prescribed for increased vitamin and mineral demands.

b. Nursing interventions.

(1) Assess weight and diet history.

(2) Identify harmful eating habits, such as pica (eating nonfood substances).

c. Educate regarding basic four food groups and need for an additional 300 calories, 30 g of protein, and 30 to 60 mg of iron daily.

D. Discomforts of Pregnancy

1. Nausea, Vomiting, or Both

a. Etiology: possibly due to increasing levels of hCG.

b. Treatment

(1) Intractable vomiting (hyperemesis gravidarum) may require correction of fluid and electrolyte imbalances.

(2) Antiemetics are prescribed only when absolutely indicated.

c. Nursing implications

(1) Educate patient to eat five or six small meals daily, with liquids 30 to 60 min after meals.

(2) Avoid having an empty stomach and eating fatty foods and foods that are difficult to digest.

(3) Observe for hyperemesis gravidarum.

2. Heartburn

a. Etiology: gastric acid reflex from displacement of the stomach and duodenum by the uterine fundus.

b. Treatment: antaci

c. Nursing implication: educate patient to avoid fatty and spicy foods.

3. Constipation

a. Etiology: relaxation of smooth muscle, iron ingestion, or pressure on the lower bowel from enlarging uterus.

b. Treatment: stool softener.

c. Nursing implications

(1) Educate regarding increased intake of fruits, vegetables, and fluids.

(2) Exercise.

4. Hemorrhoids

a. Etiology: straining at stool.

b. Treatment

(1) Consult physician.

(2) Surgical treatment is rarely indicated during pregnancy.

c. Nursing implications

(1) Educate patient to prevent constipation by increasing intake of fruits, vegetables, and fluids.

(2) Exercise.

5. Leg Cramps

a. Etiology: may be due to reduced level of diffusible serum calcium or an increased serum phosphorus level.

b. Nursing implications

(1) Educate patient to decrease phosphate intake (less milk) and increase calcium intake (calcium carbonate or calcium lactate).

(2) May massage affected leg muscle, gently flex the feet, or apply warm towel.

6. Fatigue

a. Etiology: extra weight carried and altered body posture, especially in the third trimester.

b. Nursing implications: educate patient to take frequent rest periods.

7. Urinary Frequency, Urgency, and Stress Incontinence

a. Etiology

(1) Usually due to reduced bladder capacity because of pressure from growing fetus.

(2) Suspect urinary tract infection if above symptoms is accompanied by dysuria or hematuria.

b. Nursing implications

(1) Assess for dysuria and hematuria.

(2) Educate patient to restrict evening fluids, empty bladder frequently, and perform daily Kegel exercises.

8. Varicose Veins

a. Etiology

(1) Increased pressure on the venous return from the legs by the enlarging uterus, smooth muscle relaxation, weakness of the vascular walls, and dysfunctional valves.

b. Nursing implications: educate patient to avoid restrictive clothing, wear support hose, and elevate extremities frequently.

9. Ankle Swelling

a. Etiology: lower extremity edema due to water retention and increased venous pressure in the legs.

b. Nursing implications

(1) Educate patient to elevate legs several times per day.

(2) Avoid excessive salt intake.

(3) Wear support hose for varicose veins.

10. Backache

a. Etiology: posture changes to accommodate altered center of gravity from enlarging uterus may cause fatigue, muscle spasm, or postural back strain.

b. Nursing implications

(1) Educate patient to improve posture by wearing low-heeled shoes and perform back exercises.

(2) Recommend sleeping on a firm mattress.

11. Dizziness and Faintness

a. Etiology: vasomotor instability largely due to proges-terone-related relaxation of vascular smooth muscle.

b. Treatment: sit and place head between knees.

c. Nursing implications

(1) Educate patient to avoid sudden position changes, standing for long periods, and hot crowded environ-ments, and to lie on side rather than on back.

(2) Eat six small meals per day instead of three large meals.

12. Increased Nonirritating Vaginal Discharge (Leukorrhea)

a. Etiology: estrogen stimulation of cervical mucus.

b. Nursing implications: educate patient to clean perineum daily and wear underwear with cotton crotch.

13. Breathlessness

a. Etiology: effect of progesterone and enlarging uterus dis-placing diaphragm.

b. Nursing implications: educate patient to avoid lying flat by elevating head in bed with pillows.

14. Headache

a. Etiology: usually due to tension.

b. Nursing implications

(1) Acetaminophen 10 g orally may be prescribed.

(2) Assess for signs and symptoms of preeclampsia-eclampsia, now referred to as pregnancy-induced hyper-tension (PIH: proteinuria, generalized edema, increased blood pressure).

15. Abdominal Discomfort

a. Etiology: may be due to pelvic pressure from the weight of the uterus on pelvic supports and the abdominal wall, tenderness of the round ligament due to traction by the uterus, or uterine contractions.

b. Nursing implications

(1) Educate patient to rest frequently (preferably in the lateral recumbent position) and apply heat.

(2) Assess for contractions and determine if they are Braxton Hicks (infrequent, irregular, and brief) or actual labor.

IV. FETAL GROWTH AND DEVELOPMENT

A. First Trimester (First 12 to 13 Weeks)

1. All organs formed

2. Major congenital anomalies occur during the first 8 weeks

B. Second Trimester (End of First Trimester Through 27 weeks)

1. Sex of fetus can be distinguished

2. Eyelids separate

3. Movement perceived by the mother by approximately 20 weeks

C. Third Trimester (End of Second Trimester Through Term or 40 Weeks)

1. Fetus gains muscle and fat

2. Alveoli develop and secrete surfactant by week 26 to 28

V. TERATOGENIC AGENTS

A. Etiology

Any agent or influence that causes physical defects in the devel-oping embryo

B. Ionizing Radiation

1. At greater than 15 rads fetal exposure, there may be an in-creased incidence of childhood leukemia in children.

2. Nursing Implications: educate patient to notify X-ray person-nel that she is pregnant and to use safety shielding to decrease exposure, especially during period beginning after week 28 of pregnancy through day 28 following birth.

C. Perinatal Infections

In the period beginning after week 28 of pregnancy through day 28 following birth.

1. Viruses include cytomegalovirus, hepatitis, herpes simplex virus, HIV, human parvovirus B19, mumps, poliomyelitis, rube-ola, rubella, vaccinia, varicella zoster, variola, and Venezuelan equine encephalitis virus

2. Spirochetes include syphilis

3. Bacteria include gonorrhea, streptococcus (beta-hemolytic), listeriosis, and tuberculosis

4. Protozoan includes malaria and toxoplasmosis

5. Nursing Implications

a. Educate patient to avoid exposure to people known to have the listed infections and encourage use of latex condoms and water-based lubricant if not in a monogamous relationship.

b. Instruct to seek medical attention for signs or symptoms of infection because the listed infections can cause fetal conditions ranging from growth retardation to death.

D. Maternal Diseases

1. Diabetes mellitus increases the incidence of fetal death and fetal defects, especially cardiac anomalies

2. Thyroid Disorders

a. May result in fetal goiter formation.

b. Possibly fatal neonatal thyrotoxicosis if untreated.

3. HELLP Syndrome

a. Hemolysis, elevated liver enzymes, and low platelet (count) (HELLP).

b. May cause pancytopenia (reduction in all cells in the blood) at birth requiring platelet and red blood cell transfusions.

4. Systemic Lupus Erythematosus (SLE)

a. Increases the rate of fetal loss.

b. May result in cardiac arrhythmias (with complete heart block being most common).

5. ITP (decrease in platelets) may cause thrombocytopenia that could last up to 4 months after birth.

6. Nursing Implications

a. Assess for above maternal diseases.

b. Educate regarding the signs and symptoms, especially bleeding.

E. Drugs

1. Fetotoxic (anything that is toxic)

a. May cause fetal anomalies.

b. Aminoglycosides, androgens, anticonvulsants, antineoplastic agents, antithyroid agents, amphetamines, benzothiadiazides, chloroquine, chlorpropamide, cocaine, Coumarin (warfarin), diethylstilbestrol, ethanol, isoniazid (INH), isotretinoin (Accutane), lithium, narcotics (heroin, morphine, methadone), oral hypoglycemics, phenothiazine, phenytoin (Dilantin), sulfonamides, tetracycline, thalidomide, trimethadione, vitamins A and D.

2. Nursing Implications

a. Educate regarding the risks as well as the benefits (where applicable) of the listed drugs.

b. Allow patient to verbalize concerns and participate in development of plan of care.

F. Other Agents

1. Alcohol

a. Safe consumption levels have not been established.

b. Use of alcohol should be discouraged to prevent fetal alcohol syndrome.

2. Tobacco

a. Increases carbon monoxide levels.

b. Causes vasoconstriction.

c. May cause growth retardation, miscarriage, stillbirth, fetal distress, and neonatal withdrawal.

3. Nursing Implications

a. Educate patient regarding the adverse effects of alcohol consumption and tobacco usage.

b. Provide information on support groups and support all efforts to decrease or cease usage.

VI. COMPLICATIONS OF PREGNANCY

A. Infectious Diseases

1. Human Immunodeficiency Virus

a. Etiology and incidence

(1) Thirty percent maternal–fetal transmission rate.

(2) Maternal and neonatal use of azidothymidine (AZT) decreases the transmission rate by approximately 8 percent.

b. Nursing implications

(1) Blood and body fluid precautions.

(2) Educate regarding use of latex condoms during any sexual contact and encourage a monogamous relationship.

2. Beta-Hemolytic Streptococci

a. Etiology and incidence

(1) High fetal mortality rate with infected fetus.

(2) Time of screening and treatment highly controversial.

(3) Reinfection following third-trimester treatment problematic.

b. Nursing implications: identification (and treatment with antibiotics) to prevent neonatal compromise.

3. Herpes Simplex Virus Type 2

a. Etiology and incidence: increased transmission rate with vaginal delivery and active infection.

b. Nursing implications: educate that cesarean section will be indicated if patient goes into labor with active infection.

4. Hepatitis B Virus

a. Etiology and incidence: treating infant at birth reduces transmission and complications.

b. Nursing implications

(1) Identify hepatitis B carriers during prenatal screening to allow treatment of infant at birth.

(2) Blood and body fluid precautions.

B. Blood Disorders

1. Isoimmunization: Rh Antigen

a. Etiology and incidence

(1) Most common cause of maternal isoimmunization.

(2) An Rh-negative woman carrying an Rh-positive fetus has the potential to develop fetal immune hemolytic disease or erythroblastosis fetalis.

(3) High levels of bilirubin can cause kernicterus, a newborn condition marked by severe neural symptoms.

b. Treatment

(1) Monitor fetal status frequently to establish continued well-being and prevent fetal loss.

(2) Neonate may require phototherapy and transfusion due to inability of immature liver to conjugate bilirubin effectively.

c. Nursing implications

(1) Assess maternal Rh status and whether or not sensitized to identify level of care required.

(2) Educate regarding the need to receive prophylactic Rh immunoglobin (RhIG) or before 28 weeks of gestational age (protection for approximately 12 weeks), and within 72 h of delivery, abortion, amniocentesis, antepartum hemorrhage, abdominal trauma, fetal death, or fetomaternal hemorrhage.

2. Isoimmunization: ABO Hemolytic Disease

a. Etiology and incidence

(1) ABO incompatibility may occur in A or B infants of group O mothers.

(2) This type of isoimmunization generally causes milder hemolytic disease.

(3) The first day after birth the infant will show signs of hyperbilirubinemia and may have hepatosplenomegaly.

b. Treatment: may require phototherapy and, rarely, an exchange transfusion.

c. Nursing implications

(1) Assess newborn for jaundice and notify physician.

(2) Educate parents to the cause of jaundice and discuss treatment plan.

3. Isoimmunization: Other Blood Groups: Kell, Duffy, Kidd, MNS, Diego, P Factors, Lutheran, and Xg Groups

a. Etiology and incidence: listed blood groups have the potential for varying degrees of fetal hemolytic disease.

b. Treatment

(1) Monitor fetal status frequently to establish continued well-being and prevent fetal loss.

(2) Neonate may require phototherapy and transfusion.

c. Nursing implications

(1) Identify antibody at initial prenatal screening.

(2) Educate parents to the need for frequent fetal assessment, possible preterm delivery, and treatment plan.

4. Sickle Cell Disease

a. Etiology and incidence

(1) Autosomal recessive disorder in which the homozygous individual has a significant number of Hgb S where the erythrocytes sickle or deform at low oxygen saturation (<85 percent) or low pH.

(2) Blockage of blood flow from sickled cells causes pain and edema, especially in joints.

(3) Sickle cell crises may be triggered by fever, infection, dehydration, low oxygen intake, or exposure to cold and may last for hours or days.

b. Treatment

(1) Maintain high hemoglobin and less than 50 percent Hgb S to avoid crisis.

(2) Administer antibiotics (prophylactic) and fluids as indicated.

(3) Erythrocytapheresis and transfusion of packed red blood cells are often required.

c. Nursing implications

(1) Educate patient regarding signs and symptoms of fever, fatigue, dyspnea, jaundice, joint swelling, ischemic leg ulcers, susceptibility to infection, and dehydration, and encourage her to seek medical attention if signs and symptoms occur.

(2) Assess for fetal well-being.

5. Anemia

a. Etiology and incidence: may be due to iron deficiency, folic acid deficiency, or drug-induced hemolytic anemia (in individuals with glucose-6-phosphate dehydrogenase [G6PD] deficiency in erythrocytes).

b. Treatment

(1) The first priority of treatment is to determine the underling cause of anemia once this is determined, iron replacement therapy can begin. Treatment of choice is an oral preparation of iron or a combination of iron and ascorbic acid (which enhances iron absorption). In some cases iron may have to be administered parenterally-for instance when a patient can not take any thing by mouth (NPO) or if malabsorption prevents adequate iron absorption in the gastrointestinal tract.

(2) Discontinue drug or toxic substance as indicated.

c. Nursing implications

(1) Educate regarding importance of complying with prescribed iron or folic acid supplements. Educate the patient regarding the need to increase folic acid intake during pregnancy. Folic acid deficiency early in pregnancy can result in spontaneous abortion or birth defects (e.g., neural tube defects), premature birth, low

birth weight, and premature separation of the placenta (abruptio placentae).

(2) Educate those at risk for induced hemolytic anemia (3 percent of black women and whites of Mediterranean or Middle Eastern origin).

6. Thromboembolization: Thrombophlebitis and Phlebothrombosis

a. Etiology and incidence

(1) Pulmonary embolism occurs in approximately half of those with documented deep venous thrombosis (DVT).

(2) Predisposing factors include previous thromboembolization, major vein varicosities, severe thrombophlebitis, vascular damage, hypercoagulability, difficult or prolonged labor, anemia, hemorrhage, heart disease, obesity, heavy smoking, bed rest, severe infection, and cancer.

b. Treatment

(1) Heparin, protamine will counteract heparin's effects, if needed.

(2) Monitor partial thromboplastin time (PTT) (goal is 1.5–2 times control).

(3) Coumadin is generally contraindicated in pregnancy due to possible teratogenic effects.

c. Nursing implications

(1) Identify those at risk.

(2) Educate regarding use of support stockings and heparin for prophylaxis.

C. Obstetric Complications

1. Spontaneous Abortion (Miscarriage)

a. Etiology and incidence

(1) Termination of pregnancy prior to completion of gestational week 20, including any fetus weighing 500 g or less.

(2) Major cause is abnormal products of conception (e.g., chromosomal abnormalities).

(3) Complications include infection and hemorrhage.

b. Treatment

(1) Most require intravenous fluids for fluid replacement and oxytocin to contract the uterus.

(2) Some require blood replacement.

(3) Dilation and curettage (D&C) may be performed to remove retained tissue.

(4) The major complication of D&C is uterine perforation, which may require exploratory laparotomy and broad-spectrum antibiotic therapy.

c. Nursing implications

(1) Assess for uterine cramping and amount of vaginal bleeding.

(2) Provide emotional support.

2. Ectopic Pregnancy

a. Etiology and incidence

(1) Implantation of fertilized ovum outside the uterine cavity (most commonly in the fallopian tube due to inflammatory changes).

(2) Uncontrolled hemorrhage and shock.

(3) Major cause of maternal mortality.

b. Treatment

(1) May include culdocentesis (transvaginal passage of a needle to assess for blood in the abdominal cavity) or laparoscopy for diagnosis.

(2) Laparotomy is best procedure for this surgical emergency to control hemorrhage, remove products of conception, and repair involved organ.

(3) Broad-spectrum antibiotics for infection.

c. Nursing implications: assess for last menstrual period, irregular bleeding, sharp unilateral lower abdominal or pelvic pain, and backache.

3. Abruptio Placentae

a. Etiology and incidence

(1) Placenta separation prior to delivery of the fetus.

(2) Varying degrees of placental separation can occur.

(3) Most present with vaginal bleeding, increased uterine tone, boardlike abdomen, and abdominal or back pain.

(4) Bleeding may be concealed within the uterus.

(5) Fetal stress or distress is present in greater than 50 percent of cases.

b. Treatment

(1) Stabilize with intravenous fluids and blood products as indicated.

(2) Cesarean section for critical hemorrhage, fetal distress, or both.

c. Nursing implications

(1) Prepare for possible cesarean section.

(2) Assess maternal hemodynamic status and fetal status.

(3) Provide emotional support.

(4) Defer vaginal examination.

4. Placenta Previa

a. Etiology and incidence

(1) Development of the placenta in the lower uterine segment within the dilation-effacement zone.

(2) Complete, partial, or low-lying placenta previa presents with *painless vaginal bleeding*.

(3) Diagnostic tests include ultrasound and Kleihauer-Betke test (for fetal blood).

(4) Preterm delivery is a common complication.

(5) Previa should be suspected whenever vaginal bleeding occurs after 24 weeks of gestation. This bleeding is associated with stretching and thinning of the lower uterine segment that occur during the third trimester. Placenta attachment is gradually disrupted and bleeding occurs when the uterus is not able to adequately contract and stop blood flow from open vessels. The initial bleeding usually is small and stops as clots form.

b. Treatment

(1) Most patients require a cesarean delivery.

(2) Close fetal assessment is imperative.

c. Nursing implications

(1) Assess maternal hemodynamic status and fetal status.

(2) Educate regarding the importance of bed rest to increase fetal maturity; provide emotional support.

(3) Defer vaginal examinations.

5. Uterine Rupture

a. Etiology and incidence

(1) Complete or partial rupture occurs in approximately 1 in 1500 deliveries.

(2) Complete rupture may occur in late pregnancy or during labor in patients with previous classic cesarean section or extensive uterine surgery.

(3) Other causes include oxytocin overstimulation of labor, obstructed labor, and operative delivery.

(4) May cause vaginal bleeding, but most will be concealed.

b. Treatment

(1) Operative delivery immediately.

(2) Prevent maternal and neonatal hypovolemic shock with intravenous fluids and blood products.

c. Nursing implications

(1) Identify individuals at risk.

(2) Assess maternal hemodynamic status and fetal status.

(3) Prepare for emergency cesarean section.

(4) Provide emotional support.

6. Puerperal Sepsis

a. Etiology and incidence

(1) Any genital tract infection that occurs as a result of abortion or childbirth.

(2) Genital tract infections may progress to peritonitis, pelvic thrombophlebitis, pulmonary embolism, septicemia, septic shock, and death.

b. Treatment

(1) Antibiotics in large doses.

(2) Surgery may be required for drainage or debridement of serious infections.

c. Nursing implications

(1) Strict aseptic technique for prevention.

(2) Assess for symptoms of infections and septic shock.

7. Pregnancy-Induced Hypertension or Preeclampsia

a. Etiology and incidence

(1) Terminology frequently used interchangeably.

(2) Occurs after week 20 of pregnancy.

(3) Mildest form presents with hypertension only.

(4) Classic triad for preeclampsia includes hypertension, proteinuria, and generalized edema.

(5) Eclampsia is the most severe form of PIH and is characterized by seizures, in addition to the listed conditions.

(6) Incidence of PIH is significantly increased in primigravidas or patients with diabetes, hydramnios, multiple pregnancy, or hydatidiform mole (gestational trophoblastic neoplasia that attaches to the fertilized ovum).

(7) Individuals with chronic hypertension may develop (superimposed) preeclampsia.

(8) PIH is marked by vasospasm and can affect all organs, including the placenta.

b. Treatment

(1) Deliver if 37 weeks of gestation, severe preeclampsia, eclampsia, or HELLP syndrome develops.

(2) Magnesium sulfate to prevent seizures.

(3) Antihypertensives.

(4) Avoid diuretics.

c. Nursing implications

(1) Assess baseline blood pressure (BP) for a systolic increase of 30 mm Hg or more, diastolic increase 15 mm Hg or more, or BP 140/90 or greater at two consecutive readings at least 6 h apart.

(2) Evaluate for generalized edema ($>1+$ pitting edema after 1 h of bed rest) and proteinuria ($1+$ to $2+$ by dipstick method).

(3) Identify any cerebral (headache, confusion) or visual disturbances (scotoma), epigastric pain (liver involvement with potential for rupture), pulmonary edema, cyanosis, hyperreflexia, or clonus (involuntary muscular contraction and relaxation in rapid succession).

(4) Assess for fetal well-being.

(5) Provide for quiet environment.

(6) Observe for signs of HELLP syndrome.

D. Other Complications

1. Diabetes Mellitus

a. Etiology and incidence

(1) Metabolic disorder affecting carbohydrate, protein, and fats, with the potential for long-term degenerative alterations.

(2) Pregnancy is diabetogenic; patients may develop gestational diabetes (type II, which is usually controlled by diet), or overt diabetes may intensify (type I, insulin-dependent).

(3) Poorly controlled diabetics have an increased incidence of fetal anomalies and fetal death.

(4) Macrosomia is common in White's diabetic classification A–C and growth retardation is common in classes D–G.

b. Treatment

(1) Diet consisting of 50 percent carbohydrate, 25 percent protein, and 25 percent fat.

(2) Insulin.

c. Nursing implications

(1) Educate regarding diet, signs of hyperglycemia and hypoglycemia, importance of euglycemia, and compliance with treatment plan.

(2) Assess for glucose variations, infection, ketoacidosis, and fetal well-being.

2. Fetal Death

a. Etiology and incidence

(1) Loss of fetus secondary to maternal or fetal conditions after 20 weeks of gestational age or with weight greater than 500 g.

(2) Sometimes the cause of death cannot be determined.

(3) The mother may feel guilty because she was unable to prevent the outcome.

b. Treatment

(1) Delivery.

(2) Autopsy if indicated (e.g., previous fetal loss) and desired.

(3) Consult social services if available.

c. Nursing implications

(1) Provide emotional support to mother and her significant other.

(2) Dispel any misconceptions.

(3) Provide keepsakes, related literature, and information about local support groups.

3. Adolescent Pregnancy

a. Etiology and incidence

(1) Obstetric hazards for an adolescent include increased mortality rate, incidence of anemia, vaginitis, PIH, and low-birth-weight or small-for-gestational-age (SGA) newborns.

(2) Increased maternal and neonatal morbidity and mortality.

b. Nursing implications

(1) Complete nutritional assessment.

(2) Educate regarding nutritional needs of pregnancy and signs and symptoms of PIH.

(3) Instruct to seek medical care if symptoms occur.

VII. LABOR, DELIVERY, AND RECOVERY: UNCOMPLICATED LABOR OCCURS AT 40 WEEKS OF GESTATION

A. Stages of Labor

Cervical change with regular uterine contractions (may have some bloody show).

B. Oxytocin Challenge Test

Test may be done in late pregnancy to judge the fetal response to induced uterine contractions. Labor is simulated by giving a dilute concentration of IV oxytocin and simultaneously monitoring uterine contractions and FHR. The character of the response is assessed by the physician in order to determine whether or not the fetus can withstand the stress of labor.

1. Stage of Dilation

Onset of labor to complete cervical dilation takes approximately 8 to 12 h for primigravidas and 6 to 8 h for multiparas.

a. Nursing implications

(1) Promote comfort.

(2) Provide emotional support.

b. Latent phase

(1) Begins with the onset of regular contractions and lasts until 3- to 4-cm dilation.

(2) Contractions are generally mild to moderate intensity.

(3) *Note*: False labor will not change the cervix.

c. Active phase

(1) From 3- to 4-cm up to 7-cm dilation.

(2) Contractions are moderately intense, occurring every 2 to 5 min.

(3) Medication is administered intravenously for induction or enhancement of labor. Pitocin is diluted in 1000 mL lactated Ringer's solution to 10 mU/L. This is added as a secondary IV line to a control IV. The initial dose is 0.5 mU/min titrated at a rate of 0.2 to 2.5 mU every 15 to 30 min until contractions are approximately 3 min apart and of acceptable quality.

For prevention and control of hemorrhage due to uterine atony, 10 U oxytocin is added to a 1-L electrolyte solution. Then 10 mU/L is infused at a rate to control atony. Oxytocin 10 U is administered intramuscularly after delivery of the placenta.

d. Transition phase

(1) From 8- to 10-cm dilation.

(2) Contractions are intense, occurring every 2 to 3 min.

(3) May experience nausea and vomiting and the feeling of being out of control.

2. Stage of Expulsion

a. Lasts from complete dilation until delivery of the infant.

b. Lasts from a few minutes to 2 h.

c. Associated rectal pressure is noted as fetus approaches the perineal floor.

d. An incision may be made into the perineum (episiotomy) to prevent tearing and promote delivery.

e. Forceps or a vacuum extractor may be used to assist delivery.

f. Nursing implications

(1) Support maternal pushing efforts.

(2) Prepare for delivery and neonatal resuscitation as indicated.

3. Placental Stage

a. Placenta and membranes separate and are expelled, usually within 5 min postdelivery.

b. Nursing interventions

(1) Assess placenta and document time of delivery.

(2) Administer oxytocin, assess fundal height and consistency, massage uterus to maintain firm consistency.

(3) Evaluate vaginal bleeding.

4. Recovery Stage

a. Two to four days post delivery of placenta.

b. Nursing implications

(1) Assess uterine fundus, bleeding, bladder, and vital signs.

(2) Fundus will rise and may displace to the left or right when the bladder is full.

(3) If unable to void, may need to catheterize until edema decreases.

B. Cardinal Movements in Labor

1. Engagement, descent, and flexion

2. Internal rotation

3. Extension

4. Restitution

5. External rotation (shoulder rotation)

6. Total Expulsion

C. Nursing Implications

1. Identify stage of labor (via cervical dilation and effacement and uterine activity)

2. Identify status of fetal position, fetal membranes (via Leopold's maneuver and vaginal examination), and maternal and fetal status (via history and physical examination and fetal monitor evaluation)

D. Maternal Fetal Monitoring

1. Electronic

a. External for routine monitoring using tocometer (uterine activity) and ultrasound (fetus).

b. Internal for closer monitoring using an electrode attached to the fetus and an intrauterine pressure catheter (IUPC) for uterine activity.

c. Both require cervical dilation and ruptured membranes to apply.

2. Auscultation: use fetoscope or ultrasound stethoscope to assess FHR in low-risk patients.

E. FHR Patterns

1. Baseline

a. Normal FHR: 120–160 bpm

b. Bradycardia: <120 bpm

(1) Etiology and incidence: hypoxia, arrhythmia, maternal hypotension, prolonged umbilical cord compression, vagal response from prolonged head compression.

c. Tachycardia: >160 bpm

(1) Etiology and incidence: prematurity, maternal fever, beta-sympathomimetics (terbutaline), hypoxia, fetal infection.

d. Nursing implications

(1) Establish baseline and cause for variation.

(2) Correct hypoxia with oxygen and notify physician.

2. Deceleration

a. Early

(1) Descent, nadir (lowest point of deceleration), and recovery of deceleration mirrors the contraction; benign.

(2) Etiology: fetal head compression.

(3) Treatment: none required.

(4) Nursing implications: differentiate early from late deceleration.

b. Late

(1) Deceleration begins approximately 30 seconds after onset of contraction and recovers post contraction.

(2) Indication of fetal stress or distress.

(3) Etiology: uteroplacental insufficiency, uterine hyperactivity, maternal hypotension, maternal supine hypotension syndrome.

(4) Treatment: repetitive late decelerations that do not respond to interventions indicate the need for prompt delivery for possible fetal hypoxia and metabolic acidosis.

(5) Nursing implications

(a) Reposition to side.

(b) Increase IV fluids.

(c) Begin oxygen.

(d) Notify physician.

(e) Assess and correct underlying cause, such as hypotension or uterine frequent contractions (discontinue Pitocin).

(f) Assess for signs of fetal well-being.

c. Variable

(1) Abrupt onset and return, shape varies and may resemble u, v, or w.

(2) FHR commonly decreases to 60 bpm.

(3) May be well tolerated by the fetus.

(4) Assess for signs of fetal well-being (see following).

(5) Etiology: umbilical cord compression.

(6) Treatment: possible amnioinfusion (infusion of normal saline into uterus via IUPC to relieve cord compression).

(7) Nursing implications

(a) Attempt to relieve cord compression by repositioning.

(b) If signs of fetal well-being continue to be present, no further intervention is required.

3. Signs of Fetal Well-Being

a. Antepartum

(1) FHR baseline 120 to 160 bpm, accelerations present (FHR increases to 15 bpm above baseline for 15 seconds).

(2) Reactive nonstress test, negative contraction stress test, reassuring biophysical profile, perceived normal fetal movement via mother, average fetal growth forgestational age per ultrasound (or fundal measurement).

b. Intrapartum

(1) Normal FHR baseline with accelerations.

(2) Beat-to-beat variability present (via fetal electrode) is most accurate sign of fetal status and indicates the fetus is tolerating labor even in the presence of late decelerations.

c. Nursing implications

(1) Assess for fetal well-being.

(2) If absent, communicate to parents that the absence of listed signs of fetal well-being does not indicate a problem, just the need to further evaluate the fetus.

F. Analgesia and Anesthesia for Labor and Delivery

1. Positive Conditioning

a. Types

(1) Lamaze

(2) Bradley

b. Nursing implications

(1) Support parents in their decision to attempt a natural childbirth experience.

(2) Educate regarding the potential need for medical intervention if complications should arise.

2. Sedatives, Tranquilizers, Analgesics

a. Types

(1) Seconal

(2) Vistaril

(3) Demerol

b. Nursing implications

(1) Medications cross the placenta and cause short-term fetal central nervous system (CNS) depression.

(2) If medication is received within a few hours of delivery, prepare for neonatal ventilatory support.

3. Regional Anesthesia

a. Types

(1) Epidural

(2) Local

(3) Pudendal

b. Nursing implications

(1) Ensure that oxygen, suction, and resuscitative drugs and supplies are immediately available.

(2) Assess for known medication allergies.

(3) Monitor for hypotension following epidural dosing secondary to sympathetic block and aortocaval compression.

(4) Treat hypotensive episode with hydration, left uterine displacement, and possibly ephedrine.

4. General Anesthesia

a. More commonly used in *emergencies* because it takes less time.

b. Nursing implications

(1) Ensure that resuscitative drugs and supplies are available, including oxygen and suction.

(2) Identify medication allergies.

(3) Prepare for neonatal resuscitation because a prolonged interval from anesthesia induction to delivery isassociated with short-term CNS depression.

G. Vaginal Birth after Cesarean (VBAC)

1. Etiology: demonstrated to be effective and relatively safe

2. Nursing implications

a. Provide emotional support and encouragement.

b. Assess for adequate labor.

c. Use of oxytocin is appropriate with close monitoring.

d. Observe for uterine rupture.

VIII. COMPLICATIONS OF LABOR AND DELIVERY

A. Precipitate Labor and Delivery

1. Active phase dilation of 5 cm or more per hour in a primipara or 10 cm or more per hour in a multipara

2. Nursing implications

   a. Check for nuchal cord and remove.

   b. Allow delivery, dry baby, position and resuscitate as indicated.

   c. Provide reassurance to mother.

B. Cesarean Section

1. Indications are fetal distress, malpresentation, dystocia, cord prolapse, failure to progress in labor, previous cesarean sections, multiple gestation, severe preeclampsia, placenta previa, abruptio placentae, and specific infections.

2. Types of cesarean sections include lower uterine segment (least blood loss and scar least likely to rupture) and classic.

3. Nursing implications

   a. Prepare for surgical procedure.

   b. Obtain signature for informed consent, educate regarding intraoperative and postoperative plan of care.

   c. Allow support person to attend delivery whenever possible.

C. Preterm Labor (Prior to 37 Completed Gestational Weeks)

1. Treatment

   a. Terbutaline or magnesium sulfate to decrease uterine activity

   b. Betamethasone

     (1) Steroidal agent used to increase fetal lung maturity.

     (2) Administer if prior to 32 weeks of gestation.

2. Nursing implications

   a. Assess for potential maternal cause (dehydration, urinary tract infection, diabetes).

   b. Assess fetal cause (infection, polyhydramnios, multiple pregnancy).

D. Premature Rupture of Membranes (Prior to Labor at Any Gestation)

Premature rupture of membranes (PROM) is a spontaneous break or tear in the amniochorial sac before onset of regular contractions, resulting in progressive cervical dilation. Labor usually starts with in 24 h; more than 80 percent of these neonate are mature.

1. Etiology

   a. The cause of PROM is unknown, but the following are considered contributing factors:

     ◆ Uterine infection incompetent cervix (perhaps as a result of abortions)

     ◆ Poor nutrition and hygiene, and lack of proper prenatal care

     ◆ Defect in tensile strength of amniochorial membranes

     ◆ Increased intrauterine tension due to hydramnios or multiple pregnancies over 20 weeks of gestation

2. Signs and Symptoms

   a. Blood-tinged amniotic fluid gush or leak from the vagina.

   b. Maternal fever, fetal tachycardia, and foul-smelling vaginal discharge indicate infection.

3. Treatment

   a. Treatment depends on fetal age and risk of infection. With preterm pregnancy of 28 to 34 weeks, treatment includes hospitalization and observation for signs for signs of infection, baseline cultures, and sensitivity test. If these tests confirm infection, labor must be induced, followed by IV administration of antibiotics. A culture should made of gastric aspirate or a swabbing from the neonate's ear because antibiotic therapy may be indicated for the neonate as well.

4. Nursing Implications

   a. Teach patients in the early stages of pregnancy how to recognize PROM. Make sure they know that amniotic fluid does not always gush; it may leak slowly.

   b. Stress that the patient must report PROM immediately because prompt treatment may prevent dangerous infection.

   c. Warn the patient not to engage in sexual intercourse or to douche after the membranes rupture.

E. Meconium-Stained Amniotic Fluid

1. Treatment: prevent aspiration by visualizing vocal cords for presence of meconium-stained amniotic fluid and suctioning infant's airway prior to inspiration

2. Nursing implications

   a. Assess for potential cause (fetal stress, postdate pregnancy, or unknown) and for fetal well-being.

   b. Ensure that laryngoscope, endotracheal tubes, suction equipment, and oxygen are available at delivery.

F. Postterm Pregnancy

1. Longer than 42 weeks of gestation

2. Cause unknown

3. Treatment

   a. Induce labor with IV oxytocin.

   b. May use vaginal prostaglandin E_2 (PGE_2) to prepare cervix for labor.

   c. Aspirin is an antidote for PGE_2.

4. Nursing implications

   a. Upon rupture of membranes, assess for meconium-staining and notify physician.

   b. Assess for fetal well-being.

G. Dysfunctional Labor or Failure to Progress

1. Treatment

   a. Pitocin augmentation of labor.

   b. Cesarean section for failure to progress with adequate labor.

c. May use IUPC to assess strength of uterine contractions accurately.

2. Nursing implications

a. Assess for adequate strength and frequency of contractions.

b. Titrate oxytocin (Pitocin) drip to obtain adequate labor (e.g., 180–240 montevideo units in 10 min via IUPC).

c. Terbutaline will reverse oxytocin effects.

d. Notify physician for inadequate labor, failure of cervix to dilate, or fetus to descend.

H. Fetal Stress or Distress

1. Etiology

a. Loss of physiologic reserve mechanisms indicating that pathologic changes are occurring (or are about to occur) that affect vital organ function to the point of temporary or permanent injury or death.

2. Treatment: surgical delivery is indicated if fetal tracing does not improve with interventions and vaginal delivery is not imminent.

3. Nursing implications

a. Identify abnormal baseline, late decelerations, or loss of beat-to-beat variability (via spiral electrode).

b. Attempt to resolve by repositioning, increasing IV fluids, and applying oxygen.

c. Prepare for neonatal resuscitation at delivery.

IX. POSTPARTUM: UNCOMPLICATED

A. Etiology

Period of adjustment after pregnancy when the mother's body returns to the nonpregnant state and lactation is possible.

B. Immediate Nursing Care

1. Promote and assess bonding by allowing stable infant to be held and evaluated by parents.

2. Provide positive feedback to parents related to childbirth experience.

3. Assist mother in breast-feeding (as she desires).

4. Assess and cleanse perineum.

a. Apply ice pack to prevent or decrease edema as indicated.

b. Educate regarding perineum care (rinse with warm water after each void or stool).

C. Nursing Assessment

1. Evaluate amount and characteristics of vaginal bleeding.

2. Assess fundus for consistency and location, bladder for distention, and vital signs for variations.

3. Assess pain and effect of pain medication.

D. Nursing Implications

1. Notify physician regarding increased bleeding, boggy uterus, distended bladder, or unrelieved pain.

2. Promote comfort by providing PRN analgesics and sitz bath or heat lamp to perineum (optional after 24 h).

E. Characteristics

1. Uterus

a. Involutes rapidly after delivery.

b. Returns to prepregnancy state within 6 weeks.

2. Lochia

a. Changes from the bloody discharge following delivery (rubra) after 2 to 3 days, to a more serous and lighter color (serosa) for approximately 1 week, and then mucoid and yellowish (alba) for a couple of weeks.

3. Ovulation and Menstruation

a. Nursing mothers rarely menstruate prior to 6 weeks postpartum, but 50 percent will ovulate on or before that time.

b. In nonlactating women, menstruation generally resumes in 6 to 12 weeks postpartum, and ovulation can occur as early as day 25 to 35 postpartum.

F. Lactation

1. Begins approximately 48 to 72 h after delivery.

2. Colostrum is available immediately after delivery for the infant to begin nursing.

3. Suckling is required for continued milk production; therefore, mothers of premature infants should use a breast pump to stimulate nursing and refrigerate or freeze breast milk for later use.

4. Nursing implications

a. Demonstrate various positions, correct latching-on technique, and method to break suction.

b. Instruct to express a small amount of colostrum, massage into nipple, and allow to dry after each feeding to prevent nipple maceration.

X. POSTPARTUM COMPLICATIONS

A. Postpartum Hemorrhage

1. Etiology: loss of more than 500 mL of blood after delivery due to placental problems, uterine atony, birth canal lacerations, uterine rupture, or blood dyscrasias

2. Treatment

a. Identify cause.

b. Administer oxytocic drugs, replace fluids and blood, and repair lacerations.

c. Administer Ergotrate or Methergine to increase the strength, duration, and frequency of uterine contractions and decrease postpartum uterine bleeding.

3. Nursing implications

　a. Notify physician of trickle or spurts of blood, heavy pooling of blood, or boggy uterus.

　b. Massage fundus, avoid bladder distention, and assess for shock.

B. Hematoma

1. Treatment: notify physician.

2. Nursing implications: assess for perineal edema, complaint of perineal pressure, and inadequate pain relief following administration of analgesics.

C. Puerperal Infection

1. Etiology: temperature of 100.4°F occurring on any 2 successive days during the first 10 days postpartum, exclusive of the first 24 h, frequently due to endometritis (infection of the endometrium).

2. Treatment: antibiotics.

3. Nursing implications: identify potential risk factor (ruptured membranes greater than 24 h prior to delivery, traumatic delivery) and notify physician of fever.

D. Mastitis

1. Etiology: obstruction of milk flow from breast infection during the 6 weeks following childbirth due to sporadic mastitis (uninfected milk) or epidemic mastitis (infected milk).

2. Treatment

　a. Antibiotics.

　b. Therapy usually is not required for the infant.

3. Nursing implications

　a. Educate patient to continue breast-feeding with sporadic mastitis.

　b. Wean infant with epidemic mastitis.

　c. Apply cold packs to suppress lactation.

E. Distended Bladder and Inability to Void

1. Treatment

　a. Ice packs to perineum the first 24 h after delivery.

　b. Warm sitz baths, analgesics, straight catheter, or insert Foley catheter, if needed.

2. Nursing implications

　a. Palpate bladder frequently in the first 12 to 24 h to assess for volume and for displacement of uterine fundus upward and to one side.

　b. Medicate for pain as indicated.

　c. Educate patient that inability is temporary and due to hypotonic bladder and edema following delivery.

F. Other: Anemia, Preeclampsia, Thromboembolism (Positive Homan's Sign), Constipation, or Episiotomy Discomfort

XI. PSYCHOLOGIC ADAPTATION TO PARENTING ROLE

A. Phases

1. Taking-in Phase

　a. Lasts 2 to 3 days (post delivery).

　b. Mother is passive, dependent, and concerned about her own needs.

　c. She begins recognition of baby as an individual.

　d. Verbalizes reactions to delivery in order to integrate the experience.

2. Taking-Hold Phase

　a. Occurs 3 to 10 days post delivery.

　b. Anxious regarding mothering abilities.

　c. Strives for independence.

　d. Interested in caring for self and baby.

3. Letting-Go Phase

　a. Occurs from 10 days to 6 weeks post delivery.

　b. Mother is independent and realistic.

B. Postpartum Depression ("Blues")

1. Etiology: most likely to occur after hospitalization.

2. Treatment

　a. Frequent rest periods.

　b. Amount of psychological support needed varies, depending on degree of depression.

3. Nursing implications: observe for anxiety and fear, insomnia, concern about body, crying, fatigue. Assess for depression and postpartum psychosis.

C. Parent–Infant Bonding

1. Treatment

　a. Identify lack of bonding or inappropriate interaction.

　b. Arrange for a social service consult and a home visit for further evaluation.

2. Nursing implications

　a. Assess interaction, including physical contact, taking into consideration phases already discussed.

　b. Encourage questions and verbalization of concerns.

XII. THE NEWBORN (BIRTH TO 28 DAYS)

A. Immediate Nursing Care

1. Dry and place in preheated radiant warmer to prevent heat loss (convection, evaporation, conduction, radiation)

2. Position

　a. To ensure an open airway.

b. Do not hyperextend head. Place neonate supine with head slightly extended.

3. Resuscitation as needed (CPR)

4. Assign Apgar scores at 1 min and 5 min

a. Ten possible points

b. Two points each for heart rate, respiratory effort, muscle tone, reflex response, and color

5. Apply identification bands

6. Give newborn medications

a. Vitamin K injection to prevent bleeding disorders due to sterile gut and low vitamin K levels.

b. Erythromycin eye ointment to prevent gonococcal ophthalmic infections.

B. Nursing Assessment

1. Gestational age assessment (Ballard or Dubowitz tool)

2. Complete physical assessment and identify any variations

C. General Characteristics of the Average Neonate

1. Length: 19 to 21 inches

2. Weight: 6 to 8.5 lb (will lose 5 to 10 percent of birth weight within 1 week of birth)

3. Head: 13.5 to 14.5 inch circumference

a. Fontanelles palpable.

b. Molding or cephalohematoma may be present.

4. Chest: approximately 0.5 inch smaller than the head

a. Breast tissue present.

b. Small amount of discharge from breast may be noted.

5. Extremities: legs and arms flexed, hands fisted, toes in grasping position

6. Face

a. Breathes easily through nose.

b. Eyes are slate blue.

c. Epstein's pearls (small white or yellow masses) may be present in the mouth (on hard palate).

7. Abdomen

a. Soft and rounded.

b. Umbilical cord falls off 6 to 10 days after birth.

8. Genitalia

a. Enlarged.

b. Discharge (possibly bloody) may be present in females neonates.

c. The testicles descended in male neonates.

D. Nervous System

1. Reflexes: blinking, gagging, coughing, sneezing, yawning, startle (Moro reflex), grasping, sucking, rooting, tonic neck (fencing), stepping (dancing), and Babinski are present

2. Strabismus may be present

3. Pupils respond to light

E. Circulatory System

1. Ductus venosus and ductus arteriosus usually close once breathing is established.

2. Blood returning from the lungs increases, which increases pressure in the left atrium, which initiates closure of the foramen ovale.

3. Respirations typically are abdominal and irregular at 30 to 60 bpm.

4. Heart rate greater than 120 and up to 160 bpm.

5. Systolic blood pressure in term neonate ranges from 60 to 70 mm Hg. *Note*: A discrepancy of less than 10 mm Hg between the arms or upper and lower extremities may indicate a cardiac defect, such as coarctation of the aorta.

6. Hematocrit: 51 to 65 percent.

7. Hemoglobin: 14 to 24 g/dL.

F. Nursing Care of Newborn

1. Vital Signs

a. Assess axillary temperature after taking initial rectal temperature.

b. Elevated temperature may indicate dehydration or infection.

c. Subnormal temperature may indicate sepsis or instability of the hypothalamus.

2. Skin

a. Milia: white epidermal cysts caused by sebaceous gland obstruction are commonly seen on the face.

b. Erythema toxicum neonatorum: pink, papular rash covering the thorax, back, abdomen, and groin, which appears about 24 to 48 h after birth.

c. Nevus flammeus: flat, capillary hemangioma is a permanent birthmark.

d. Telangiectatic nevi, stork bites: flat, deep pink localized areas of capillary dilation typically appear on eyelids, nasal bridges, and neck.

e. Mongolian spots: blue-black macules, which are common over the buttocks in dark-skinned neonates.

f. Slight jaundice: common about day 3 (72 h), due to normal reduction lysis of red blood cells.

g. Jaundice: prior to first 24 h denotes a pathologic condition (Rh or ABO incompatibility).

3. Cord Care

a. Cleanse base of stump with alcohol three times per day.

b. *Note*: Sponge bath until cord falls off from 6 to 10 days.

4. Nutrition

a. Sterile water or dextrose 5% generally offered as first feeding.

b. Observe for forceful, projectile vomiting or any repetitive feeding difficulties.

c. May place on right side following feeding to encourage stomach emptying.

5. Elimination

a. Note stool transition from dark, tarry meconium to yellow.

b. Voiding and stooling occurs within first 24 h.

c. All are recorded.

G. Newborn Testing

Obtain blood for the following tests prior to discharge from the hospital.

1. Newborn Screening Recommendations

a. Currently, parents seeking screening for disorders not currently performed by their state must arrange privately for their newborn to be screened, often with additional out-of-pocket expense.

b. Few parents realize that the extent of newborn testing depends entirely on the state in which their baby is born.

c. The March of Dimes is the first national health organization to recommend that every baby born in the United States receive, at a minimum, screening for the same metabolic disorders; the test can mean the difference between life and death. The following is the recommended list for screening.

(**1**) Phenylketonuria (PKU)

(**2**) Congenital hypothyroidism

(**3**) Congenital adrenal hyperplasia (CAH)

(**4**) Biotinidase deficiency

(**5**) Maple syrup urine disease

(**6**) Galactosemia

(**7**) Homocystinuria

(**8**) Sickle cell anemia

(**9**) Medium-chain acyl-CoA dehydrogenase (MCAD) deficiency

2. Hearing Screening

a. The March of Dimes and the American Academy of Pediatrics advise a test for hearing deficiency for all newborns. Newborn screening is performed by testing a few drops of blood, usually from a newborn's heel, before hospital discharge. If a result is positive, the infant usually is retested and given treatment as soon as possible before becoming seriously ill.

H. Newborn Complications

1. Prematurity (less than 38 weeks of gestation)

a. Nursing implications

(**1**) Assess for hypoglycemia, respiratory distress (hyaline membrane disease), infection, feeding problems (necrotizing enterocolitis, poor suck, which may require

gavage feeding), thermal regulation, intracranial hemorrhage.

(**2**) Notify physician.

2. Respiratory distress

a. Inadequate gas exchange secondary to prematurity or aspiration of meconium-stained amniotic fluid or infection.

b. Nursing implications

(**1**) Assess for grunting on expiration, nasal flaring, retractions, see-saw respirations, apnea, cyanosis.

(**2**) Notify physician to obtain orders for oxygen and antibiotics.

c. Respiratory distress syndrome is caused by insufficient production of surfactant, a phospholipid that lines the alveoli, decreasing surface tension to allow them to remain open when air is exhaled. Synthetic surfactant now is available and is used to treat preterm infants, especially those less than 30 weeks of gestational age and weighing less than 2 lb 10 oz.

3. Postmaturity (more than 42 weeks of gestation)

a. Nursing implications

(**1**) Assess for dry, cracked skin, meconium-staining, hypoxia (cyanosis), hypoglycemia (poor feeding, lethargy, poor tone).

(**2**) Check glucose level.

(**3**) Notify physician.

4. Small-for-gestational age or intrauterine growth retardation

a. Nursing implications: observe for hypoglycemia, hypothermia, and respiratory distress.

5. Large-for-gestational age

a. Nursing implications: assess for birth trauma, hypoglycemia (normal glucose 40–80 percent but varies per laboratory).

6. Addicted neonate

a. Secondary to maternal narcotic abuse.

b. Nursing implications

(**1**) Assess for problems, such as poor feeding habits, irritability, and seizures.

(**2**) Consult with social worker and arrange for a home visit for further evaluation, as these babies are at risk for neglect and abuse by care giver.

7. Hyperbilirubinemia

a. Occurs in 50 percent of newborns.

b. Nursing implications

(**1**) Assess for lethargy, concentrated urine, hepatosplenomegaly, positive direct and indirect Coombs' test, increased bilirubin.

(**2**) Maintain eye protection and reposition frequently while receiving phototherapy.

(**3**) Kernicterus possible in severe cases.

8. Infection

   a. May have fever, subnormal temperature, or normal temperature.

   b. Nursing implications

      (1) Assess for poor feeding, lethargy, elevated white blood cell count, respiratory difficulties, poor perfusion, poor tone.

      (2) Initiate and maintain IV access and antibiotics.

9. Delivery injury

   a. Erb-Duchenne paralysis.

   b. Nursing implications

      (1) Assess for upper arm brachial paralysis following difficult delivery, negative Moro reflex.

      (2) Provide intermittent immobilization, positioning, range of motion.

XIII. DISCHARGE, TEACHING, AND PLANNING

A. Assess Home Situation and Support Mechanisms

B. Assure Knowledge Regarding Mother and Newborn Care

C. Discuss Contraception

D. Tell Patient to Abstain from Sexual Intercourse or Tampon Use Until Follow-up Examination

E. Arrange Follow-up Appointment and Referrals as Indicated

TOPICAL OUTLINE

Gynecologic Disorders

I. HISTORY AND EXAMINATION: NURSING ASSESSMENT

A. Past History

1. Menstrual History

a. Establish the age and character of menarche (initial menstruation, which occurs between ages 9 and 17 years) or menopause (cessation of menstruation, which occurs between ages 45 and 53 years).

b. Identify last menstrual period (LMP), previous menstrual pain (PMP), and last normal menstrual period (LNMP).

c. Assess regularity, duration, amount of bleeding, pain, and intermenstrual spotting.

2. Gynecologic History: record the gravida (G), para (P), abortions (Ab), living children (LC), and any complications (including type of uterine incision if cesarean section)

3. Family History: identify any hereditary abnormalities or occurrences of cancer

4. Sexual History: record past or current contraceptive usage, dyspareunia (painful sexual intercourse), number of sexual partners, vaginal or pelvic infections, and sexually transmitted diseases, including HIV

5. Psychosocial History: establish occupation, level of education, religion, culture, use of tobacco, alcohol, or drugs

6. Medical and Surgical History: record any allergies, operations, injuries, and current medications

7. Systems Review: document any complaints related to head and neck, cardiovascular, respiratory, gastrointestinal (GI), urinary, or neuropsychiatric systems

B. Examination

1. Abdomen

a. Note the size, shape, and contour.

b. Identify masses.

2. Pelvic Examination (with Speculum)

a. Perform or assist.

b. Visually inspect and palpate the external genitalia, Bartholin's glands or vulvovaginal glands (just external to the hymen), Skene's glands or paraurethral glands (on the posterolateral aspect of the urethra), introitus, vagina, and cervix.

3. Bimanual Examination

a. Palpate the uterus, ovaries, and uterine tubal areas; perform a rectovaginal examination.

b. Include palpation of vagina, rectum, and rectovaginal septum.

4. Cytologic Examination (Papanicolaou [Pap] Smear)

a. Cancer screening technique.

b. Educate patient to avoid douching for at least 24 h prior to examination.

c. Schedule procedure for a time when not menstruating.

d. Return annually for repeat test for normal cells (class I smear interpretation).

e. If abnormal cells are identified, retesting is scheduled as follows.

    (1) Slightly abnormal

        (a) Usually inflammation (class II)

    (2) Repeat after treatment or within 6 months.

    (3) Cellular abnormality

        (a) Usually atypia (class III)

        (b) Perform colposcopy

    (4) Distinctly abnormal

        (a) Possibly malignant (class IV)

        (b) Colposcopy and biopsy

    (5) Malignant cells (class V)

        (a) Biopsy

5. Breast Examination

a. Types include manual examination by self or health care provider, and mammogram.

b. Manual examination includes palpation of axillary and supraclavicular regions for enlarged lymph nodes, palpation of breast tissue for masses, and compression of areola and nipple for discharge.

6. Nursing Implications

a. Educate patient to schedule annual gynecology examination and perform monthly breast self-examination (BSE), preferable after each menstrual cycle.

b. Notify health care provider if variations are noted.

II. GYNECOLOGIC DISORDERS

A. Dysmenorrhea

Most common gynecologic complaint is severe, painful cramping in the lower abdomen associated with menstruation.

1. Primary Dysmenorrhea

a. Etiology and incidence

    (1) Occurs near menarche.

    (2) Elevated prostaglandin levels lead to painful uterine contractions.

    (3) Excess prostaglandins in smooth muscles help explain the presence of GI symptoms, such as nausea, vomiting, and diarrhea.

    (4) Generally, dysmenorrhea is less likely to occur in women who have delivered a child or who take birth control pills.

b. Signs and symptoms

Lower abdominal or back pain, headache, sweating, tachycardia, nausea, vomiting, or diarrhea.

c. Treatment

(1) Prostaglandin-synthetase inhibitors (ibuprofen, naproxen, indomethacin) alleviate symptoms in nearly 75 percent of sufferers.

(2) Cyclic administrations of oral contraceptives (usually low dose but with higher estrogen content) help alleviate symptoms.

d. Nursing implications

(1) Educate patient about use of heating pad, hot bath, massage, or distracting activity.

(2) Exercise or sleep may achieve relief from primary dysmenorrhea.

2. Secondary Dysmenorrhea

a. Etiology and treatment

(1) Includes conditions of pelvic pathology that cause the pain.

(2) Treatment is directed toward underlying cause.

(3) Pelvic inflammatory disease (PID).

(a) Infectious process that may involve any portion of the upper genital tract.

(b) Therapy with antibiotics generally provides relief.

(4) Endometriosis.

(a) Condition in which endometrial tissue, which responds to hormonal stimulation, is found outside the uterine cavity.

(b) Surgical intervention may be required if hormonal therapy is not effective.

(5) Adenomyosis.

(a) Benign invasion (growth) of the endometrium into the muscular layer of the uterus.

(b) Treat symptoms.

(c) Curative therapy is hysterectomy.

(6) Pelvic congestion.

(a) Engorgement of the pelvic muscles.

(b) Characterized by burning or throbbing pain that is worse on standing and at night.

(c) Therapy is directed toward relief of tension and psychosomatic problems with hysterectomy as a last resort.

b. Signs and symptoms

(1) Pain is more frequently concentrated in a specific area or only on one side.

(2) Generally occurs after age 30 years.

c. Nursing implications

(1) Assess level of discomfort and types of previous interventions and their effectiveness.

(2) Educate regarding potential cause and treatment options.

(3) Jointly establish plan of care.

B. Premenstrual Syndrome (PMS)

1. Etiology and Incidence

a. The combination of cyclic emotional and physical features that occur before menstruation, which involves the autonomic and central nervous systems.

b. Etiology is unknown, but estrogen–progesterone imbalance, excess aldosterone, hypoglycemia, hyperprolactinemia, abnormal prostaglandin activity, premenstrual decrease in endogenous endorphins, and psychogenic factors are proposed.

c. Peak incidence is late twenties to early thirties.

2. Signs and Symptoms

Edema, weight gain, restlessness, irritability, and increased tension that occurs in the second half of at least three consecutive menstrual cycles

3. Treatment

a. Directed toward relief of symptoms.

b. Controversial.

c. Options include progesterone suppositories (in the second half of the menstrual cycle), oral contraceptives, vitamin B_6, diuretics, nonsteroidal antiinflammatory drugs, sedatives, or antidepressants.

4. Nursing Implications

a. Educate regarding the importance of exercise, rest, a well-balanced high-protein diet, restriction of salt, sugar, caffeine, alcohol, and smoking, and use of relaxation and behavioral techniques.

b. Be empathetic and acknowledge condition.

C. Endometriosis

1. Etiology

a. Extrauterine occurrences of endometrial tissue.

b. It is benign, progressive, tends to recur, and occurs more frequently in involuntarily infertile nulliparous women in their mid thirties who have a familial history of endometriosis.

c. Unknown cause.

d. One theory suggests that menstrual flow regurgitates through the fallopian tubes and deposits particles of viable endometrial tissue outside the uterine cavity.

e. Spread occurs by endometrial tissue reproducing itself.

2. Signs and Symptoms

a. Related more to the location than to the degree of the disease present.

b. Pelvic pain, infertility, and abnormal bleeding.

3. Treatment

a. Varies depending on the desire for fertility, age, severity of symptoms, location of lesions, and stage of disease.

b. Analgesic therapy: purely palliative.

c. Endocrine therapy.

(1) Danazol (Danocrine)

(a) Binds to androgen receptors, progesterone receptors, and sex hormone-binding globulin, resulting in an increase of free testosterone and marked endometrial atrophy.

(b) This medication is expensive, causes amenorrhea and inhibition of ovulation, and has significant side effects, including hirsutism (excessive hair growth or the presence of hair in unusual places), weight gain, hot flashes, decreased breast size, acne, GI disturbances, weakness and dizziness, change in libido, and emotional lability.

(2) GnRH agonists

(a) Suppress the pituitary–ovarian axis, creating low levels of FSH, LH, estrogen, and progesterone by binding to LH-releasing hormone and causing endometrial atrophy.

(b) Due to similar effectiveness and less side effects, this therapy may replace danazol.

(3) Estrogen–progestogen and progestogen therapy.

(a) Continuous daily regimens of estrogen and progestin, oral contraceptives, or progestogen.

(b) Causes endometrial atrophy (whereas cyclic hormones may induce endometrial growth).

d. Surgical therapy.

(1) Indicated for rupture of endometrioma (a surgical emergency), ureteral or bowel obstruction, tubo-ovarian masses (>5 cm), endometriomas (>8 cm), severe incapacitating symptoms, pain worsening with medical treatment, or infertility for more than 1 year despite conventional therapy.

(2) Endocrine therapy is frequently prescribed before and after surgery.

(3) Conservative surgery is generally performed (via laparotomy) to retain and enhance the woman's reproductive capability.

(4) Corticosteroids and prophylactic antibiotic usage are recommended to decrease postoperative inflammation and infection.

4. Nursing Implications

a. Assess severity of symptoms, desire of fertility, and response to previous treatment.

b. Educate regarding risks and benefits of treatment options.

c. Ascertain each individual's desired plan of care.

D. Adenomyosis

1. Etiology

a. Unknown cause

b. Presence of endometrial tissue within the myometrium (muscular layer of the uterus).

c. Benign condition that regresses after menopause

2. Signs and Symptoms

a. Hypermenorrheas (excessive menstrual bleeding), premenstrual and menstrual dysmenorrhea, enlarged uterine fundus.

b. May be asymptomatic.

3. Treatment

a. Directed toward relief of symptoms.

b. Curative therapy is hysterectomy.

c. Adenomyosis regresses after menopause.

4. Nursing Implications

a. Assess amount of blood loss at menstruation, level of discomfort, and effectiveness of previous interventions.

b. Educate patient regarding condition and treatment options.

c. Include patient in plan of care.

E. Amenorrhea

1. Etiology and Incidence

a. Absence of menses during the reproductive years.

b. Most common cause is physiologic, such as pregnancy, nursing, or in the puerperium (42-day period following childbirth).

c. Pathologic amenorrhea may be caused by genetic, anatomic, or endocrine disorders and is classified as primary or secondary.

d. Primary amenorrhea is failure of menses to occur by age 16.5 years or within 2 years of full secondary sexual characteristic development (e.g., breast development).

e. Secondary amenorrhea.

(1) Lack of menses for more than 6 months in a woman who has previously had normal menstruation or lack of menses for three typical intervals in the oligomenorrheic (infrequent or scanty menstrual flow) woman.

(2) Predisposing factors include age younger than 25 years, history of previous menstrual irregularities, and extraordinary physical or emotional stress.

2. Signs and Symptoms
Absence of menses

3. Treatment

a. Depends on the individual's desire to ovulate (menstruation, pregnancy) and the etiology of the amenorrhea.

b. Appropriate hormone replacement reestablishes menstruation. Treatment of amenorrhea not related to hormone deficiency depends on the cause. For example amenorrhea that results from a tumor usually requires surgery.

4. Nursing Implications

   a. Perform a gynecologic history and examination, and identify variations.

   b. Review potential causes and treatments of amenorrhea and establish whether or not the woman desires to ovulate.

   c. Establish a plan of care and provide emotional support.

F. Dysfunctional Uterine Bleeding

1. Etiology and Incidence

   a. Abnormal uterine bleeding occurring when all pathologic causes have been excluded.

   b. Occurs at the extremes of reproductive age.

   c. May be caused by a persistent corpus luteum cyst or a short luteal phase, but most patients are anovulatory.

   d. Anovulation results in continuous estrogen stimulation of the endometrium, resulting in hyperplasia, periodic partial endometrial breakdown, and irregular bleeding.

2. Signs and Symptoms
   Abnormal uterine bleeding

3. Treatment

   a. Rule out pregnancy, fibroids, ovarian cysts, and malignancy.

   b. Control bleeding, stabilize the endometrium, and induce controlled menstruation using cyclic therapy (either oral contraceptives or estrogen–progestin) for three to six cycles.

   c. Spontaneous ovulation and menstruation often occurs after 2 to 3 months of cyclic therapy.

4. Nursing Implications

   a. Assess type of bleeding (e.g., frequency, length, and amount) and any other concurrent symptoms.

   b. Assess effectiveness of previous treatments.

G. Postmenopausal Bleeding (PMB)

1. Etiology and Incidence

   a. Bleeding that occurs after more than 12 months of amenorrhea in a woman of menopausal age (older than 45 years).

   b. Far more likely to be of pathologic origin than is abnormal uterine bleeding during the reproductive years.

2. Treatment
   Treat the cause.

III. MENOPAUSE

A. Etiology and Incidence

1. The span of time during which the menstrual cycle wanes and gradually stops.
2. Also called change of life and climacteric.

3. During this period, ovulation, menstruation, and childbearing cease.

4. Menopause may be induced at any age by surgical removal of the ovaries or by pelvic radiation.

5. *Note*: Hysterectomy is the removal of the uterus and does not include removal of the ovaries or surgical menopause.

B. Signs and Symptoms

1. A wide variety of physical and psychosocial symptoms are attributed to the perimenopausal period.

2. Vasomotor instability, such as hot flashes, night sweats, and occasional palpitations and dizziness associated with menopause, are most likely caused by hormonal imbalances.

3. The vaginal mucous membrane is especially sensitive to decreasing estrogen levels.

   a. The vaginal wall becomes thinner and drier; susceptibility to infection increases.

   b. These changes lead to an increase in vaginitis in menopausal women.

4. Other symptoms may include vaginal irritation, burning, pruritus, leukorrhea, or bleeding.

5. Some women experience backache, joint pain, and other symptoms of osteoporosis because a decrease of estrogen may lead to osteoporosis.

C. Treatment

1. Hormone replacement therapy: progestin–estrogen therapy

   a. Contraindications: undiagnosed vaginal bleeding, acute liver disease, chronic hepatic dysfunction, acute vascular thrombosis, neuro-ophthalmic vascular disease, and endometrial or breast carcinoma.

   b. Recommendation: combine progestin therapy with estrogen therapy because studies show that the risk for endometrial carcinoma is decreased if endometrial tissue exposed to estrogen is periodically opposed by progestin.

   c. Estrogen (Premarin).

      (1) May be given orally and used for 25 days each month or continuously.

      (2) Estrogen can also be administered vaginally or via transdermal patches.

      (3) Long-term estrogen replacement is necessary to prevent osteoporosis, which can be treated by using a patch containing 14 μg of estrogen per day; the patch lasts 7 days (1 week). The patch is changed weekly. If patient has a uterus, she must talk with her doctor about the recommended use of progestin.

      (4) Side effects include headache, intolerance to contact lenses, edema, thromboembolism, and hypertension.

      (5) For some patients, oral estrogen increases secretion of renin (a vasoconstrictor), causing hypertension and increased clotting factors as a result of liver stimulation.

d. Progestin (compounds that have the action of progesterone).

> **(1)** Should be given the last 13 to 15 days of estrogen replacement each month to decrease the risk of endometrial carcinoma.
>
> **(2)** If the woman has no uterus, progestins are not indicated.
>
> **(3)** Side effects of long-term progestin therapy are unknown but appear to be limited to periodic vaginal bleeding.

D. Nursing Implications

1. Educate patient regarding the physiologic changes that cause the symptoms she is experiencing.

2. Discuss the risks and benefits of hormonal replacement therapy.

3. Establish whether or not she desires progestin–estrogen therapy and support her decision.

IV. INFERTILITY

A. Etiology and Incidence

1. Failure to conceive after 1 year of attempting pregnancy.

2. Primary infertility denotes individuals who have never conceived.

3. Secondary infertility applies to individuals who have conceived previously.

4. Most common causes of infertility in women:

> **a.** Cervical factors (10 percent): congenital (diethylstilbestrol [DES] exposure) or acquired (infection, surgical treatment).
>
> **b.** Uterine–tubal factors (35 percent): structural abnormalities (congenital, surgical treatment, infection).
>
> **c.** Ovulatory factors (25 percent): CNS function, metabolic disease, or peripheral defects (e.g., ovarian tumor).
>
> **d.** Unknown (15 percent).

5. Most common causes of infertility in men:

> **a.** Male coital factors (40 percent): abnormal spermatogenesis, abnormal motility, anatomic disorders, endocrine disorders, and sexual dysfunction.

6. Infertility in couples: multiple etiologies are found in 40 percent of infertile couples.

B. Nursing Assessment

1. Medical history

> **a.** Obtain complete gynecologic history and male medical history.
>
> **b.** Include frequency of intercourse, difficulty with erection or ejaculation, prior paternity, history of genital tract infections (e.g., mumps, orchitis), congenital anomalies, surgery or trauma, exposure to toxins (e.g., radiation), diet, exercise, alcohol consumption, smoking more than one pack per day, illicit drug use, in utero exposure to significantly high temperature.

2. Physical examinations of the couple.

3. Tests include semen analysis, Sims-Huhner (evaluate initial interaction of the sperm with cervical mucus), hysterosalpingography (assess patency of fallopian tubes), hysteroscopy or laparoscopy, and basal body temperature and midluteal serum progesterone (to confirm ovulation).

C. Treatment

1. Varies from drug therapy to surgery.

2. Some factors or conditions are irreversible.

D. Fertilization

1. In Vitro Fertilization Embryo Transplant (IVF-ET)

> **a.** Procedure of removing the ovum (egg) from the ovary, fertilizing it in the laboratory, then placing the resulting embryo into the uterus.
>
> **b.** Indications: bilateral fallopian tube abnormality, anti-sperm antibodies, extensive endometriosis, and oligospermia.
>
> **c.** Complications: associated with anesthesia, laparoscopy, and any pregnancy, including ectopic pregnancy and multiple gestation.

2. Gamete Intrafallopian Tube Transfer (GIFT)

> **a.** After superovulation (medication induced) and collection of the ova, ova and sperm are mixed, then immediately placed in the uterine tube where natural fertilization can occur.
>
> **b.** Indications: used in patients with intact fallopian tubes.
>
> **c.** Complications: associated with anesthesia, laparoscopy, and pregnancy.

3. Surrogate Embryo Transfer (SET)

> **a.** Sperm is artificially inseminated into a fertile donor following the woman's normal ovulation.
>
> **b.** If fertilization occurs, several days later the fertilized egg is washed from the donor's uterus, placed in the recipient's uterus, and, if successful, implantation will occur soon after.
>
> **c.** Indications: used in situations where the woman is incapable of producing normal mature follicles and where the partner is fertile.
>
> **d.** Complication: failure to lavage a fertilized ovum from the donor resulting in undesired pregnancy.

4. Surrogate Mothering

> **a.** Semen from the partner is artificially inseminated into the host (surrogate mother).
>
> **b.** After birth, the infant is given to the infertile couple.
>
> **c.** Indication: may be used when a woman is not only unable to conceive but also unable to carry a fetus to viability.
>
> **d.** Complication: surrogate mother may become emotionally involved.

E. Nursing Implications

1. Educate the couple regarding the following:

a. Smoking, alcohol, drug use, and sources of increased scrotal temperature (e.g., saunas, hot tubs) may have an adverse effect on spermatogenesis and should be avoided.

b. Lubricants and douching should be eliminated.

c. Advise coitus every 2 days during the preovulatory interval (days 12 to 16 of a 28-day cycle).

d. Encourage the woman to lie on her back for at least 15 min following intercourse to facilitate semen retention and progression.

2. Provide psychological support

a. Communicate that feelings of anger, frustration, disappointment, or possibly depression are not uncommon.

b. Expense of assessment and therapy may be an additional stress.

c. Encourage couple in all their efforts.

V. FAMILY PLANNING

Contraception (pregnancy avoidance) is practiced for pregnancy planning, limiting the number of children, avoiding medical risks of pregnancy, and controlling world population.

A. Periodic Abstinence (Rhythm)

1. Avoidance of intercourse for 2 days prior to ovulation and 2 to 3 days after ovulation should provide effective contraception.

2. Three methods for identifying the time of ovulation:

a. The calendar method predicts ovulation (14 days prior to the next menstrual cycle) by continuously documenting menstrual cycles.

b. Basal body temperature (BBT) assessment.

  (1) BBT rises 0.4 to 0.8°C with ovulation.

  (2) The temperature of the woman is taken orally or rectally each morning before rising.

  (3) Abstinence begins the first day of menses and continues until the third day when the temperature is elevated.

  (4) Coitus is confined to the postovulatory period, usually approximately 10 days each month.

c. Cervical mucus assessment.

  (1) During ovulation, the cervical mucus becomes clear, slippery (egg white consistency), and increases in quantity in response to high estrogen levels.

  (2) Conception can occur at this time.

  (3) During preovulatory and postovulatory periods, mucus is yellowish, decreased in quantity, and becomes thick and sticky, inhibiting sperm movement.

  (4) Conception will not occur at this time.

3. Advantages and disadvantages

a. The combination of these three techniques for determining the fertile period provides the couple with more information than use of just one method.

b. The advantages of the rhythm method are that it encourages couples to communicate, is inexpensive, has no side effects, and has no religious barriers.

c. The disadvantages are that it requires a great deal of self-control to be effective and an acute awareness of signs and symptoms of fertility, which are not always easily detected.

B. Coitus Interruptus

Withdrawal of the penis from the vagina before ejaculation occurs.

1. Advantage: inexpensive.

2. Disadvantage: requires male self-control and the possibility of pregnancy due to semen escaping prior to ejaculation.

C. Spermicides

Preparations that are used to interfere with the viability of sperm and prevent sperm from entering the cervix.

1. Advantages

a. Available in jelly or cream forms, which are available without prescription.

b. Have no serious side effects.

2. Disadvantages

a. Must be applied 30 min before intercourse and repeated before each subsequent coitus.

b. No douching is allowed for 8 h after intercourse.

D. Condoms

1. Pelvic sheath made of latex, rubber, plastic, or animal membrane that serves as a mechanical barrier to prevent sperm from entering the vagina.

2. Addition of a spermicide increases the effectiveness.

3. Advantage

a. Protection from sexually transmitted diseases (STDs) is significantly improved with use of *latex condoms* and a *water-based lubricant*.

4. Disadvantages

a. An animal membrane condom should not be used. Latex condoms are good but should not be used with petroleum jelly (or oil-based lubricant) because material will destroy the protection of the latex.

b. Condom may be defective or may become dislodged in the vagina.

E. Diaphragm

1. Flexible ring covered with dome-shaped rubber cap that is inserted into the vagina to cover the cervix, acting as a mechanical barrier.

2. Spermicidal jelly or cream must be placed in the center of dome and around the rim.

3. Advantage

　a. Fairly inexpensive.

4. Disadvantages

　a. Must anticipate intercourse.

　b. Patient must insert the diaphragm no more than 2 h before intercourse and leave in place for 6 h after coitus.

　c. Diaphragm may become dislodged.

　d. Additional spermicide is needed if intercourse is repeated, taking care not to dislodge the diaphragm.

　e. Woman must be fitted for diaphragm and refitted following childbirth, pelvic surgery, or significant weight gain.

　f. Side effects and complications include toxic shock syndrome, cystitis, cramps, rectal pressure, and allergic reaction to rubber or spermicide.

F. Contraceptive Sponge

Polyurethane sponge containing nonoxynol 9 is inserted into the vagina, acting as a mechanical barrier.

1. Advantages

　a. Available without prescription.

　b. Is effective for 24 h.

2. Disadvantages

　a. Less effective than diaphragm and spermicide.

　b. A few cases of toxic shock syndrome have been associated with its use.

G. Intrauterine Device (IUD)

Flexible device that is inserted into the uterine cavity where it causes a localized sterile inflammatory reaction.

1. Advantages

　a. Inexpensive.

　b. Once inserted, it requires no attention other than determining that it is still in place.

2. Disadvantages

　a. Dysmenorrhea, increased menstrual flow, spotting between periods.

　b. Complications include uterine infection, uterine perforation, and ectopic pregnancy.

H. Oral Contraceptives

Combination of estrogen and progestin preparation in pill form that inhibits the stimulation of a follicle to develop so that ovulation does not occur.

1. Advantages

　a. Most effective contraceptive method other than sterilization or abstinence.

　b. Decreased incidence of endometrial cancer, osteoporosis, benign breast disease, ectopic pregnancy, ovarian cysts, menstrual irregularities, heavy menstrual bleeding, and iron deficiency anemia.

2. Disadvantages

　a. Must remember to take the pill daily.

　b. Side effects include bleeding, thrombus formation and coronary artery disease (especially in smokers older than 35 years), nausea and vomiting, susceptibility to vaginal infections, edema, weight gain, irritability, or missed periods.

　c. Certain antibiotics decrease the effectiveness of birth control pills (e.g., tetracycline and penicillin) and require a backup contraceptive.

　d. May start 2 weeks postpartum.

　e. Use backup contraceptive for first cycle.

I. Injectable Progestins

1. Prevent ovulation by suppressing anterior pituitary function via hormone injection.

2. Most commonly used is 21-carbon progesterone, depomedroxyprogesterone acetate (Depo Provera), which must be given every 90 days.

3. Advantages

　a. No preparation required prior to coitus.

　b. Contraceptive effect occurs within 24 h.

　c. Can use 5 days postpartum and immediately postabortion.

4. Disadvantages

　a. Delay in reestablishing ovulation after discontinuation of the injections (6–12 months).

　b. Amenorrhea, irregular bleeding, and weight gain common.

J. Interception (Postcoital Pill)

Administration of an adequate dosage of progestin or a combination of progestin and estrogen to suppress ovulation after unprotected intercourse.

1. Advantages

　a. If coitus occurs 2 to 6 days prior to ovulation, pregnancy usually will be prevented.

　b. Useful in emergency situations, such as rape, defective or torn condom, or accidental (unplanned) intercourse if taken within 24 to 72 h of coitus.

2. Disadvantages: failure rate depends on when coitus occurs in relation to ovulation and how soon after coitus the hormones are taken.

K. Surgical Sterilization

1. Permanent prevention of pregnancy.

2. Vasectomy is the surgical ligation of the man's vas deferens to prevent passage of sperm.

3. Tubal ligation is the surgical ligation or cauterization of the woman's fallopian tubes to prevent conception.

4. Advantages

   a. Very effective

   b. Will not alter libido.

5. Disadvantages

   a. Sterilization is not always successful.

   b. Complications include risks from surgical procedure and anesthesia.

L. Nursing Implications

1. Assess religious and cultural implications to contraception.

2. Identify factors important to individual(s) that will optimize acceptance and improve compliance.

3. Factors to consider (in addition to culture and religion) include cost, effectiveness, self-control, preparation, and spontaneity.

4. Educate patient regarding the types of contraception available and the advantages and disadvantages of each option.

VI. SEXUALLY TRANSMITTED DISEASES AND INFECTIONS

A. HIV Infection

1. Etiology and Incidence

   a. DNA viral infection, present in blood and body fluids, that may be transmitted to the fetus.

   b. Manifested by a depressed immune system that makes the individual susceptible to opportunistic infections, such as Kaposi sarcoma (cancer), *Pneumocystic carinii* (pneumonia), toxoplasmosis, cytomegalovirus, herpes, tuberculosis, and cryptosporidia and *Candida albicans* infection.

2. Signs and Symptoms

   a. Asymptomatic (and contagious) during initial infection.

   b. Most patients develop symptoms, such as lymphadenopathy, fever, night sweats, fatigue, and a rash, within a few months that will resolve within a few weeks.

   c. Further progression of the disease may be indicated by weight loss, diarrhea, generalized lymphadenopathy, and early immunosuppression (decreased CD4$^+$ lymphocytes).

   d. Acquired immunodeficiency syndrome (AIDS) may be indicated by opportunistic infections and further immunologic suppression (CD4$^+$ lymphocytes). A DNA test is used to determine if HIV is present in the blood.

3. Treatment

   a. Controversial.

   b. Varies with the stage of illness.

   c. Drug therapy includes a cocktail mixture of antiviral agents [zidovudine (AZT), dideoxyinosine (ddI), and di-

deoxycytidine (ddc) or other antiviral agents], and prophylaxis or treatment for opportunistic infections.

4. Nursing Implications

   a. Assess for swollen lymph nodes, rapid unexplained weight loss, diarrhea, fever, night sweats, unexplained fatigue, cough, dyspnea, thrush, candidiasis, or rash with reddishbrown or bluish spots on the skin.

   b. Ensure confidentiality.

   c. Discuss methods to reduce transmission (blood and body fluid precautions) and prevent opportunistic infections (good hand washing, avoid cat litter boxes, and avoid other persons who may be ill).

B. Herpes Simplex, Type II

1. Etiology: genital primary infection of this DNA virus is followed by recurrent flareups that are triggered by stressors, such as emotion, menstruation, fever, and other infections

2. Signs and Symptoms

   a. Painful vesicles that rupture and then drain, leaving shallow ulcers that crust over and disappear within 7 to 10 days.

   b. May have malaise, anorexia, leukorrhea, vaginal bleeding, and, if bladder or urethra is infected, dysuria and retention.

3. Treatment

   a. Deliver by cesarean section if active herpes is present atthe time of birth to prevent transmission of infection to the infant.

   b. Drug therapy may include acyclovir.

   c. There is no cure.

4. Nursing Implications

   a. Educate patient to avoid sexual contact while lesions are present or to use a condom and contraceptive foam (or cream) to prevent transmission.

   b. Discuss emotional stressors and possible methods to manage them.

   c. Communicate that a hot sitz bath may provide some pain relief.

C. Human Papillomavirus (Warts)

1. Etiology: DNA virus causes raised, papillomatous lesions (condylomata acuminata) on the vulva, vagina, or cervix.

2. Signs and symptoms: genital wartlike lesions; occasionally vaginal discharge or pruritus.

3. Treatment

   a. In nonpregnant women, the following medications may be used:

   ◆ Podophyllum Resin (Podocon-25) applied only by physician. Do not use if wart is inflamed or irritated. Very toxic; use minimum amount possible to avoid absorption.

◆ Podofilox (Condylox) applied q12h for 3 consecutive days. Allow to dry before using area. Dispose of used applicator. May cause burning and discomfort.

b. If unsuccessful, cryosurgery, electrocautery, or laser therapy may be necessary.

c. During pregnancy, cryotherapy may be most helpful.

4. Nursing Implications

a. Educate patient regarding the types of therapy available.

b. Establish a plan of care jointly with patient.

D. Gonorrhea

1. Etiology: infection caused by the *Neisseria gonorrhoeae* organism.

2. Signs and Symptoms

a. Itching, burning, and pain in the vulva due to exudate from infected area.

b. Women may remain asymptomatic and have only a grayish-greenish-yellow discharge from the cervix.

c. Men may remain asymptomatic or may develop dysuria (painful urination) and purulent discharge with redness and swelling at infection site.

3. Treatment

a. For adults and adolescents, the recommended treatment of uncomplicated gonorrhea caused by non–penicillinase-producing *N. gonorrhoeae* is a single dose of ceftriaxone (Rocephin). For presumptive treatment of concurrent *Chlamydia trachomatis* infection, doxycycline (Vibramycin) is used.

◆ Common alternative prescriptions may include ciprofloxacin (Cipro), ofloxacin, (Floxin), or spectinomycin (Trobicin).

4. Nursing Implications

a. Sexual partner(s) must be identified and treated to prevent reinfection.

b. Identify penicillin allergy.

E. Syphilis

1. Etiology: infection caused by *Treponema palladium,* which can be transmitted from mother to fetus causing congenital syphilis.

2. Signs and Symptoms (of Stages)

a. *Primary:* presence of hard chancre, a firm painless papule or ulcer with raised borders that appears approximately 3 weeks following infection and lasts 1 to 5 weeks.

b. *Secondary:*

(1) Generalized cutaneous eruption (macular, maculopapular, papular, or pustular) appears 2 weeks to 6 months after the primary lesion.

(2) Generalized adenopathy is common.

c. *Latent:* secondary symptoms have subsided.

d. *Tertiary:* presence of destructive lesions of skin, bone, cardiovascular system, or nervous system disorders.

3. Treatment

a. Administer either benzathine penicillin IM, tetracycline hydrochloride PO, doxycycline PO, or erythromycin PO.

b. Treatment of maternal syphilis prior to 18 weeks of gestation improves neonatal outcome.

c. Congenital syphilis is treated with benzathine penicillin IM.

4. Nursing Implications

a. Identification and treatment of sexual partner(s) is important.

b. Educate patient regarding the common side effect of fever 4 to 12 h after penicillin injection (Jarisch-Herxheimer reaction).

c. Discuss the significance of completing all antibiotics.

F. Chlamydia Trachomatis

1. Etiology: bacterial infection that is often asymptomatic in women.

2. Signs and symptoms: may have an odorous or pruritic discharge.

3. Treatment: drug therapy with tetracycline or erythromycin PO.

4. Nursing implications: educate patient regarding the importance of completing antibiotics and avoiding tetracycline during pregnancy.

G. Trichomonas

1. Etiology: infection involving the vagina, cervix, vulva, urethra, or bladder.

2. Signs and Symptoms

a. Inflammation, edema, and yellow-green odorous discharge.

b. May be asymptomatic.

3. Treatment: metronidazole (Flagyl) PO.

4. Nursing Implications

a. Treat both partners.

b. Educate both partners not to ingest alcohol while being treated with metronidazole.

H. Gardnerella Vaginalis

1. Etiology: gram-negative bacillus ordinarily found in the presence of anaerobic bacteria

2. Signs and Symptoms

a. Copious, odorous (fishy) gray discharge is characteristic.

b. Minimal pruritus or burning is present.

3. Treatment: drug therapy with metronidazole.

4. Nursing Implications

a. Treatment of sexual partner is desirable.

b. Educate patient to avoid ingesting alcohol while being treated with metronidazole.

I. Candida

1. Etiology

a. A fungal infection that occurs when vaginal flora abnormalities are present.

b. Predisposing factors include diabetes, oral contraceptive usage, recent completion of antibiotic therapy, pregnancy, and HIV infection.

2. Signs and Symptoms

a. Vulvar pruritus, nonodorous white cottage-cheese–appearing discharge, vulvar burning, and dyspareunia (pain during sexual intercourse).

b. May be asymptomatic.

3. Treatment: drug therapy for *C. albicans* is miconazole nitrate (Monistat), clotrimazole (Gyne-Lotrimin), or butoconazole (Gynazole-1) via vaginal suppository or applicator.

4. Nursing Implications

a. Educate patient regarding the correct procedure for intravaginal application.

b. Recommend abstinence from sexual intercourse during therapy.

c. Identify the predisposing factor if recurrence is frequent.

J. Toxic Shock Syndrome (TSS)

1. Etiology: bacterial infection most commonly seen in association with tampon use during menstruation.

2. Signs and Symptoms

a. Abrupt onset of high fever, hypotension, and generalized macular rash.

b. System-wide organ involvement evidencing shock is apparent.

3. Treatment

a. Removal of tampon, fluid and electrolyte replacement, corticosteroid administration, and antistaphylococcal antibiotic therapy.

b. Treatment of complications, which include hemorrhage from disseminated intravascular coagulation, adult respiratory distress syndrome, and intractable hypotension.

4. Nursing Implications: recommend that the patient avoid using tampons at night, leave them in place no longer than 6 h, and change tampons every 2 to 4 h during the day.

K. Bartholin Duct Cyst and Abscess

1. Etiology

a. Occlusion of the duct occurs most frequently due to infectious organisms.

b. Permanent occlusion may occur, causing mucus retention and cyst development (usually unilateral).

2. Signs and Symptoms: pain and edema are noted at site and a unilateral mass usually is palpable.

3. Treatment

a. Drainage of infected cyst or abscess.

b. Consider analgesics and broad-spectrum antibiotics for excessive inflammation caused by infection.

4. Nursing Implications: educate patient that local heat may provide some pain relief.

L. Pelvic Inflammatory Disease

1. Etiology: infection of any portion of the upper genital tract.

2. Signs and Symptoms

a. Lower abdominal pain that is dull and constant.

b. May have abnormal vaginal bleeding, fever, or fatigue.

3. Treatment: early identification of causative organism and treatment decrease complications.

4. Nursing implications: educate patient that limiting the number of sexual partners and using condoms and spermicide can prevent or decrease infections leading to PID.

VII. CANCER OF THE REPRODUCTIVE ORGANS

A. Ovarian Cancer

1. Etiology and Incidence

a. Fifth most common cause of death in women. Occurs most frequently in women 20 to 54 years of age.

b. Predisposing factors include high-fat diet, familial tendency, and celibacy.

2. Signs and Symptoms

a. Symptoms vary with size of tumor.

b. Early symptoms include vague abdominal discomfort and weight loss.

c. As cancer progresses, it may cause urinary frequency, constipation, pelvic discomfort, and weight loss.

3. Treatment

a. According to staging of disease, usually a combination of surgery, chemotherapy, and, in some cases, radiation.

b. Total abdominal hysterectomy, bilateral salpingoooophorectomy, omentectomy (removal of the peritoneum covering the abdominal viscera), and lymphadenectomy (surgical removal of the lymph nodes) are surgical options.

c. Chemotherapy includes melphalan, cyclophosphamide, doxorubicin, vincristine, vinblastine, actinomycin, and cisplatin.

4. Nursing Implications

a. Discuss disease and treatment options.

b. Establish plan of care jointly with patient.

c. Provide emotional support.

B. Endometrial Cancer

1. Etiology and Incidence

   a. Second most common genital malignancy of the reproductive system.

   b. Endometrial cancer is related to the hormone estrogen, which is the primary stimulant of endometrial proliferation.

   c. The greatest risk factor is receiving estrogen replacement therapy without progestin therapy.

   d. Other factors include obesity, diabetes, mellitus, menopause, and family history of the disease.

2. Signs and Symptoms

   a. Abnormal uterine bleeding, especially postmenopausal bleeding.

   b. This symptom occurs relatively late in the disease.

   c. Metastasis to other organs may produce other symptoms.

3. Treatment

   a. Precancerous endometrial changes may be treated with the hormone progesterone.

   b. Chemotherapy and hormonal therapy with tamoxifen (Nolvadex), an estrogen blocker, is used to treat late stages of endometrial cancer.

   c. Endometrial cancer usually is treated with surgery, radiation, or a combination of surgery and radiation.

4. Nursing Implications

   a. Provide emotional support.

   b. Involve family in care.

   c. *Note:* If endometrial cancer is diagnosed early, the prognosis is relatively good.

   d. Educate patient regarding risk factors and encourage reduction of factors that place a woman at risk.

C. Cervical Cancer

1. Etiology and Incidence

   a. Third most common cancer of the female reproductive system.

   b. Classified as either preinvasive or invasive.

   c. Predisposing factors include first coitus at less that 20 years of age, high parity, multiple sexual partners, chronic cervical irritation, smoking, and infection with HIV, HSV-2, or human papillomavirus.

2. Signs and Symptoms

   a. Preinvasive cervical cancer produces *no* symptoms or other clinically apparent changes.

   b. Early symptoms of invasive cervical cancer include abnormal vaginal bleeding and persistent vaginal discharge and bleeding.

   c. Later symptoms include anorexia, weight loss, and anemia.

3. Treatment depends on clinical stage of diseas

   a. Preinvasive lesions: Removal of malignant tissue via conization (removing a cone-shaped section of the cervix with a scalpel), cryosurgery (freezing the involved cervical tissues), or laser therapy.

   b. Therapy for invasive squamous cell carcinoma may include radical hysterectomy and radiation therapy (internal, external, or both).

4. Nursing Implications

   a. Educate patient regarding the importance of follow-up care, including serial pelvic examinations and Pap smears to assess effectiveness of treatment.

   b. Instruct the woman that, following conization, cryosurgery, or laser therapy, some cramping or minor pelvic discomfort, slight bleeding, and discharge for a few days are common.

   c. Provide the surgical patient with preoperative and postoperative teaching.

   d. Identify support mechanisms and provide emotional support.

D. Breast Cancer

1. Etiology

   a. Although the exact cause of breast cancer continues to elude investigators, certain factors that increase a woman's risk for developing a malignancy have been identified. These factors are listed in the Risk Factors for Breast Cancer section.

2. Signs and Symptoms

   Lump or mass in breast, changes in size of breast, changes in skin (thickening of skin, scaly skin around nipple, dimpling, edema, or ulceration), drainage or discharge from nipple.

   a. As a general principle, any breast symptom (i.e., mass, discharge, pain or itching) that is unilateral in nature is a more ominous finding than a symptom found bilaterally. However, all findings must be carefully followed up to avoid missing a serious diagnosis such as cancer. Any delay in treatment may adversely affect the woman's subsequent prognosis and treatment options.

   b. Early detection and diagnosis reduce the mortality rate because cancer is found when it is smaller, lesions are more localized, and there tends to be a lower percentage of positive nodes. Therefore, it is imperative that protocols for assessment and diagnosis be establishe In addition to regular BSE from mid adolescence on, use of clinical examination by a qualified health care provider, screening, and mammography (X-ray film of the breast) are advised.

3. The American Cancer Society's current recommendations for breast cancer screening are as follows:

Age (years)	Examination	Frequency
20–39	Breast self-examination	Monthly
	Clinical breast examination	Every 3 years
40+	Breast self-examination	Monthly
	Clinical breast examination	Yearly
	Mammography	Yearly

4. Risk factors for breast cancer

a. Age is the most important risk factor for breast cancer increases as age increases

b. Previous history of breast cancer

c. Family history of breast cancer, especially in a mother or sister

d. Previous history of ovarian, endometrial, colon, or thyroid cancer

e. Early menarche (before age 12 years)

f. Late menopause (after age 55 years)

g. Nulliparity or first pregnancy after age 30 years

h. Use of estrogen replacement therapy

i. Obesity after menopause

j. Previous history of benign breast disease with epithelial hyperplasia

k. Race (Caucasian women have highest incidence)

5. Treatment

a. Surgery, which may be combined with chemotherapy, includes lumpectomy (excision of the tumor), simple mastectomy (removal of breast but not lymph nodes or pectoral muscles), and modified radical mastectomy (removal of the breast, pectoralis major and minor muscles, and axillary lymph nodes).

b. Practice of performing radical mastectomies has declined.

c. Most commonly used antineoplastic agents are cyclophosphamide, 5-fluorouracil, methotrexate, doxorubicin, vincristine, and prednisone.

d. Radiation therapy before and after tumor is removed may also be used.

6. Nursing Implications

a. Refer patient to support group.

b. Educate patient regarding postmastectomy exercises.

c. Involve family in care.

d. Provide emotional support.

e. Discuss options, such as reconstructive breast surgery or a padded bra, which may help the patient maintain a positive self-image.

f. Instruct women to examine breast for lumps 1 week after menstruation; a good time to examine breast is while taking a shower.

EXAMINATION

1. A 15-year-old primigravida is in week 28 of her pregnancy. She has received no prenatal education and began receiving prenatal care only 2 weeks ago. Which of the following best-describes complications this pregnant adolescent may experience?
   1. Anemia, small-for-gestational-age infant, and pregnancy-induced hypertension.
   2. Depression, suicidal behavior, and gestational diabetes.
   3. Excessive weight gain, increased mortality rate, and large-for-gestational-age infant.
   4. Low self-esteem, preterm labor, and congenital anomalies.

2. A 22-year-old multigravida at 22 weeks of gestation complains during a routine prenatal visit of a 5-lb weight gain and vaginal discharg Her assessment included a normal speculum examination. The nurse examines the patient's abdomen and finds that the tip of the uterus is 20 cm above the symphysis pubis. This upper rounded portion of the uterus is the
   1. Corpus.
   2. Isthmus.
   3. Fundus.
   4. Bladder.

3. A patient is pregnant for the third time. She has a 2-year-old son and had a spontaneous abortion at 10 weeks of gestation. The correct gravida and para for this patient is
   1. Gravida II, para I.
   2. Gravida II, para II.
   3. Gravida III, para I.
   4. Gravida III, para II.

4. Upon pelvic examination, a patient's cervix is noted to be a bluish-purple color. This is known as
   1. Goodell's sign.
   2. Braxton Hicks' sign.
   3. Chadwick's sign.
   4. Homan's sign.

5. A patient asks the nurse when she will most likely gain the most weight in her pregnancy. The nurse's best response is
   1. "Most women gain the majority of weight during the last two trimesters."
   2. "Most women gain the majority of weight during the last trimester."
   3. "Weight is gained equally in each of the three trimesters."
   4. "Many women gain so much weight in the first trimester that they need to decrease fat and caloric intake the last two trimesters."

6. The active and latent phase of labor is stage
   1. One.
   2. Two.

3. Three.

4. Four.

7. The stage that begins after the delivery of the newborn is stage

1. One.

2. Two.

3. Three.

4. Four.

8. A newborn male infant is born vaginally at 3:00 AM. Five minutes later, his heart rate is 110 bpm, his cry is loud, his body has active motion of his extremities, he coughs with suctioning, and he is completely pink. The 5-minute Apgar score for this neonate is

1. Five.

2. Six.

3. Eight.

4. Ten.

9. Which one of the following hormones most likely inhibits uterine contractions throughout pregnancy?

1. Progesterone.

2. Prostaglandin.

3. Estrogen.

4. Oxytocin.

10. Following delivery, a newborn is placed in a radiant warmer to prevent hypothermia. The nurse's *first* action should be to

1. Thoroughly dry the newborn.

2. Place an identification band on the newborn's arm.

3. Administer vitamin K.

4. Administer eye drops.

11. A condition that predisposes a patient to postpartum hemorrhage is

1. Twin pregnancy.

2. Breech position.

3. Premature rupture of membranes.

4. Cesarean birth.

12. When a patient has been in active labor for 12 h with minimal cervical changes and documentation of borderline pelvis on her prenatal exam, the nurse could anticipate the physician requesting

1. A permit for a cesarean section.

2. An ultrasonography.

3. An intrauterine pressure catheter.

4. A pelvimetry.

13. The *most likely* indication for vaginal bleeding during the intrapartum period in a high-risk pregnancy is

1. Ectopic pregnancy.

2. Disseminated intravascular coagulation.

3. Abruptio placentae.

4. Soft fundus.

14. The nurse should determine fetal heart rate (FHR) status during active labor with

1. A Tocotransducer.

2. An intrauterine pressure catheter.

3. An ultrasound transducer or fetal electrode.

4. A stethoscope.

QUESTIONS 15 TO 19: CASE HISTORY

Jo Ann, a 26-year-old multigravida at 32 weeks of gestation, is admitted to the hospital with painless, bright-red bleeding and mild contractions every 8 to 12 min.

15. Upon admitting Jo Ann, the nurse will perform assessment of all of the following *except*

1. Fetal heart rate.

2. Uterine contractions.

3. Cervical dilation.

4. Mother's vital signs.

16. The nurse caring for Jo Ann during labor should include observation for

1. Polyuria.

2. Hemorrhage.

3. Water draining from the vaginal area.

4. Painful contractions.

17. Jo Ann's physician schedules her for a cesarean section. Jo Ann asks the nurse why she has to have the baby by cesarean section. The best response by the nurse is

1. "The placenta is separating from the uterine wall, causing you and your baby to be at risk for a potential significant blood loss."

2. "Ask your physician before you have your cesarean section."

3. "The placenta is covering the opening of the uterus; therefore, the baby cannot be delivered through the vagina."

4. "Your will hemorrhage if you get upset, so don't worry about how your baby will be delivered."

18. During the fourth stage of labor, Jo Ann asks, "Why are you pressing on my uterus? It hurts." The nurse's *best* response is

1. "We massage every mother's uterus after she delivers."

2. "I know it hurts, but it has to be done."

3. "If I don't massage your uterus, you will not pass the placenta, and then you may hemorrhage."

4. "I am checking your uterus frequently to make sure it stays firm, so you won't bleed excessively."

19. Shortly after delivery, the nurse assesses Jo Ann's uterus. It is firm and one finger breadth above the umbilicus and is displaced to the left of the abdomen. The nurse's first priority is to
    1. Encourage Jo Ann to void.
    2. Administer an oxytocic drug.
    3. Administer a tocolytic drug.
    4. Vigorously massage Jo Ann's uterus.

End of Case

20. A patient is at 20 weeks of gestation and has insulin-dependent diabetes mellitus (IDDM). The complications she may experience are
    1. Preeclampsia, eclampsia, hemorrhage, and infection.
    2. Excessive weight gain, generalized edema, and nausea and vomiting.
    3. Ataxia, unsteady gait, headache, and severe malaise.
    4. Polyuria, delirium, chills, sweating, and headache.

21. An 18-year-old patient is diagnosed as having insulin-dependent diabetes mellitus (IDDM). She is in week 34 of her pregnancy. Her insulin and diet have been closely regulated throughout her pregnancy. The physician orders several tests to evaluate fetal well-being. After assessing the results of the test, the nurse would immediately report to the physician
    1. A nonreactive nonstress test.
    2. A negative contraction stress test.
    3. If the patient perceived 15 fetal movements in 4 h.
    4. Decreased bilirubin on amniocentesis.

22. A diabetic patient is in gestational week 38. Following a series of tests for fetal well-being, Agnes' physician tells her that she should be induced early because
    1. The pregnant diabetic at term tends to be at high risk for infection.
    2. The placenta of a diabetic mother tends to degenerate early, causing decreased utero–placental circulation.
    3. Hypoglycemic crisis increases for the diabetic mother when she is near term.
    4. The postterm newborn of a diabetic mother will be too large for vaginal delivery.

23. A patient is admitted to the obstetric floor with a diagnosis of abruptio placent With this complication, blood loss usually is
    1. Seldom present.
    2. Minimal.
    3. Less than observed.
    4. Greater than observed.

24. Which of the following values would be considered normal for the mother during the first 10 to 12 days after delivery?

    1. A hematocrit value of 20 to 30 percent.
    2. A sodium value of 120 to 130 mEq/L
    3. A red blood cell (RBC) count of 2.8 to 3.5 million/mm^3
    4. A white blood cell (WBC) count of 30,000 to 35,000/mm^3

25. Which one of the following conditions would indicate to the nurse the possibility of postpartum hemorrhage?
    1. Cesarean birth.
    2. Long labor (19 h) and delivery of twins.
    3. Premature delivery.
    4. Induced labor.

26. A patient's membranes rupture 24 h before she delivers a 7-lb girl. Of the following complications, the nurse would assess for
    1. Endometritis.
    2. Endometriosis.
    3. Pelvic thrombophlebitis.
    4. Ruptured uterus.

27. Which one of the following neonates would be at *lowest* risk for developing hypoglycemia?
    1. A 2-hour-old neonate weighing 9 lbs whose mother's blood glucose was 350 mg/100 mL during labor.
    2. A 7 lbs neonate 10 h after birth whose mother's glucose was 120 mg during labor.
    3. A 35-week gestational neonate weighing 4 lb, 2 h after birth.
    4. A preterm neonate 12 h after birth who is nothing by mouth (NPO) because of respiratory distress.

28. Immediately after delivery, the nurse should be able to feel the top of the uterus
    1. Firm, to the right of the midline, above the umbilicus.
    2. Soft, in the midline, at the umbilicus.
    3. Firm, in the midline, below the umbilicus.
    4. Soft, to the right of the midline, above the umbilicus.

29. Which one of the following would indicate to the nurse that the patient's bladder is full, the uterus has relaxed, and blood clots need to be expressed?
    1. Soft, in the midline, at the umbilicus.
    2. Firm, in the midline, below the umbilicus.
    3. Soft, to the right of the midline, above the umbilicus.
    4. Firm, to the right of the midline, above the umbilicus.

30. To promote an open airway and allow for suctioning, the nurse would place the neonate in
    1. Semi-Fowler's position.
    2. Trendelenburg position, head turned to the side.
    3. Supine, head slightly extended.
    4. Supine, head hyperextended.

31. Which one of the following behaviors will a woman with postpartum transitory depression exhibit?
  1. Anxiety, tearfulness, despondency, and disinterest in her baby.
  2. Frequent requests for pain medication and demands for attention.
  3. Multiple physical complaints in the early postpartum period; desiring to stay longer in the hospital.
  4. Demonstrating nervousness when holding and learning to care for her infant.

32. A 16-year-old primigravida delivered a 7 lb 3 oz boy 6 h ago. Which assessment would require immediate nursing interventions?
  1. Perineal pads spotted with bright-red blood.
  2. Perineal pads soaked with blood and blood cots every 30 min.
  3. Temperature of 100.1°F.
  4. Pulse rate of 95 bpm.

33. A newborn of a narcotic-addicted mother may exhibit
  1. Poor feeding, hypersensitivity to noise, and irritability.
  2. Tremors, dyskinesia, and dyspne
  3. Dystocia, ataxia, and hallucinations.
  4. Diaphoresis, dyspnea, and decreased reflex irritability.

34. The main reason for abstaining from sexual intercourse for 4 weeks following vaginal delivery (or until the first checkup) are to prevent
  1. Painful intercourse.
  2. Bladder infection.
  3. Tearing at the episiotomy site.
  4. Vaginal and cervical infection.

35. A diabetic mother at 37 weeks of gestation delivers an 11-lb newborn. Apgar scores were 8 at 1 min and 9 at 5 min. The problem the nurse would be most alert for in this newborn is
  1. Generalized sepsis.
  2. Anemia.
  3. Hyperglycemia.
  4. Hypoglycemia.

36. Mrs. Adams is brought to the emergency room following an automobile accident. She is in her third trimester of pregnancy. Her abdomen is enlarging, is rigid on palpation, and her pain is severe. Fetal monitoring indicates acute fetal distress. Which of the following complications is Mrs. Adams experiencing?
  1. Abruptio placenta.
  2. Placenta previa.
  3. Hydramnios.
  4. Labor.

37. A 33-week gestational aged neonate is in an isolette and experiences sudden apnea. The nurse should first
  1. Call the pediatrician.
  2. Gently shake the neonate.
  3. Increase the humidity in the incubator.
  4. Administer oxygen with positive pressure.

38. What is the most appropriate stimuli for the nurse to recommend for the first time parent–infant activity?
  1. Rattle and pacifier.
  2. Books and pictures.
  3. Human faces and black and white objects.
  4. Swing and a mobile over the bed.

39. With any malpresentation, the nurse must be particularly alert for
  1. Polyhydramnios.
  2. Prolapsed umbilical cord.
  3. Fetal distress.
  4. Meconium-stained amniotic fluid.

40. Following rupture of membranes, fetal distress may be indicated by
  1. Hydramnios.
  2. Meconium.
  3. Pica.
  4. Bloody show.

41. A 38-year-old, gravida III, para II smokes one package of cigarettes each day. Which one of the following contraceptive methods will she most likely be advised not to use?
  1. Birth control pills.
  2. Intrauterine device (IUD).
  3. Sponge method.
  4. Sterilization.

42. The nurse would advise a woman using a diaphragm to leave it in place after intercourse for
  1. One hour.
  2. Three hours.
  3. Six hours.
  4. Twenty-four hours.

43. Which of the following situations would warrant remeasurement and possible refitting of a diaphragm?
  1. Abdominal surgery.
  2. Childbirth.
  3. Weight gain or loss of 7 lb.
  4. An automobile accident.

44. Phototherapy is used for treatment of hyperbilirubinemia. Which one of the following interventions is the *most inappropriate*?
  1. Turn the newborn every 2 h.
  2. Rub an oil-based lotion on the newborn's skin.
  3. Cover the newborn's eyes with protective patches.
  4. Place the newborn in an isolette without clothes and 18 inches from the phototherapy light.

45. A patient is given methylergonovine (Methergine) 2 mg IM, 4 h post delivery because she is experiencing postpartum bleeding. The nurse should assess for

1. Blood pressure variations.
2. Severe fluid retention.
3. Severe hyperglycemia.
4. Uterine rupture.

46. Sara Johnson is diagnosed with preeclampsia and started on continuous magnesium sulfate drip. Assessment for signs of worsening preeclampsia is necessary for at least

1. Eight hours postpartum.
2. Twelve hours postpartum.
3. Twenty-four hours postpartum.
4. Forty-eight hours postpartum.

47. The nurse's *first* intervention in managing postpartum hemorrhage is

1. To call for blood type and cross-match and have IV equipment ready.
2. To take the patient's vital signs and check urinary output.
3. To massage the uterus firmly until it remains firm and repeat as needed.
4. To explain to the patient that she is hemorrhaging and tell her to stay in bed.

48. During a pelvic examination, the physician notes a definite softening of the lower uterine segment, discoloration of the mucous membranes of the vagina, and softening of the cervix. These signs are referred to respectively as

1. Hegar's, Chadwick's, Goodell's.
2. Goodell's, Chadwick's, Hegar's.
3. Chadwick's, Goodell's, Hegar's.
4. None of the above.

49. A patient at 9 weeks of gestation is admitted to the emergency room complaining of a sharp pain in her right side with some vaginal spotting and nausea and vomiting. The nurse would expect

1. Ectopic pregnancy.
2. Abruptio placentae.
3. Placenta previa.
4. Threatening abortion.

50. An oxytocin contraction stress test shows late decelerations (decrease in FHR that continues after the contraction). This test would be read as

1. Negative.
2. Positive.
3. Active.
4. True.

51. The first sign of preeclampsia *usually* is

1. Hypertension.
2. Epigastric pain.
3. Pedal edema.
4. Proteinuria.

52. A patient is pregnant now, has had one abortion, one stillborn, and one set of twins. She is designated as

1. Gravida II, para I.
2. Gravida III, para III.
3. Gravida IV, para II.
4. Gravida V, para V.

53. On examination, the nurse palpated the fetal occiput toward the back and to the left of the maternal pelvis. The fetal position is

1. Left occipitoanterior (LOA).
2. Left occipitoposterior (LOP).
3. Right occipitoanterior (ROA).
4. Right occipitoposterior (ROP).

54. A patient is 37 gestational weeks, in active labor, and has active herpes simplex virus type 2. This means that she

1. Should plan for a cesarean section.
2. Can delivery vaginally, if she is treated with antibiotics.
3. Has oral lesions.
4. Has vaginal lesions and bleeding.

55. Signs and symptoms of preeclampsia are

1. Hyperreflexia, tachycardia, facial edema, and sudden weight loss.
2. Fever, weight gain, fluid retention, and proteinuria.
3. Tachycardia, hyperglycemia, and generalized edema.
4. Hypertension, proteinuria, generalized edema, and weight gain.

QUESTIONS 56 TO 57: CASE HISTORY

Jerry and Martha Homer have just had their second child. Martha's blood type is O, Rh-negative, and Jerry's blood type is AB, Rh-positive.

56. Their newborn is admitted to the nursery at 10:00 PM. The next morning, the nurse observes that the newborn's skin and sclera of its eyes have become yellow. The nurse should first

1. Place the neonate in phototherapy.
2. Observe for clay-colored meconium.
3. Observe for decreased urine output.
4. Notify the physician.

57. Rh incompatibility was once a leading cause of kernicterus and a significant cause of neonatal death. Incidence of Rh incompatibility has been greatly reduced by the administration of RhoD immune globulin (RhoGam) to

1. All Rh-negative mothers during pregnancy and within 72 h of delivery or abortion of an Rh-positive infant or fetus.

2. All Rh-positive neonates immediately after birth.

3. All Rh-negative mothers within 72 h after delivery.

4. All Rh-negative mothers every trimester and following delivery, if the fetus is Rh-positive.

End of Case

58. When examining the inside of a newborn's mouth, the nurse notices small, raised, white bumps on the palate and gingiva. They do not come off, nor do they bleed when touched. The most likely diagnosis is

    1. Milk curds.
    2. Candidiasis.
    3. Epstein's pearls.
    4. Herpes simplex virus type 1.

59. The sexually transmitted infectious disease that can cause permanent injury to the baby's eyes at the time of delivery is

    1. Syphilis.
    2. Gonorrhea.
    3. Genital herpes (HSV-2).
    4. *Trichomonas vaginalis.*

60. Which one of the following diseases cannot effectively be treated?

    1. Gonorrhea.
    2. Syphilis.
    3. Genital herpes (HSV-2).
    4. *Trichomonas vaginalis.*

61. Diagnoses of venereal disease must be reported to the health department. The *main* reason for this requirement is that

    1. It is the only way of keeping accurate statistics needed to determine the prevalence of venereal disease.
    2. Required reporting helps the individuals involved to think about limiting their sexual contacts.
    3. Persons having sexual contact with the infectious person may need treatment.
    4. To treat a person with venereal disease adequately, a number of services are provided by the health department.

62. A patient, age 16 years, is 22 gestational weeks pregnant and confides to the nurse that she has genital herpes. She asks if her baby will also have the virus. The nurse should respond

    1. "This is one of the few vaginal diseases that does not affect the baby before, during, or after delivery."
    2. "If treatment is started during pregnancy, the baby will not be affected."
    3. "The baby will be treated with several different medications immediately after delivery, and this will protect it."

4. "If you have an active infection at term, a cesarean section will be performed, and the baby probably will not have the virus."

63. When a patient comes into the emergency room after being raped, the first action the nurse should implement for the patient is

    1. To call the patient's family.
    2. To assist the physician in suturing and cleaning lacerations.
    3. To reassure the patient that the patient is safe.
    4. To obtain a specimen of semen.

64. Symptoms women with gonorrhea may have include

    1. Vaginal discharge; a red, swollen, cervix or vulva; dysuria and urinary frequency.
    2. Fever, chills, muscle aches, dysuria, mucopurulent vaginal discharge, and chancre sores in the primary stage.
    3. Malaise, urethral discharge, fever, dysuria, and painless chancre in vaginal area.
    4. Purulent discharge, dysuria, pelvic pain, painful chancre in vaginal area, and vaginal bleeding.

65. The most common complication of gonorrhea in women is ____ and can progress to ____.

    1. Genital herpes; vaginitis.
    2. Mites (scabies); vaginitis.
    3. Salpingitis; pelvic inflammatory disease.
    4. Patchy hair loss; generalized skin rash.

66. Gonorrhea is treated aggressively by one large dose IM of ____ followed by ____.

    1. Rocephin; Vibramycin Hyclate or tetracycline orally for 7 days.
    2. Penicillin; ampicillin or Ancef orally for 7 days.
    3. Penicillin; streptomycin or moxalactam orally for 10 days.
    4. Neomycin; penicillin one dose IM and then orally for 7 days.

67. The most commonly occurring sexually transmitted diseases are

    1. Syphilis, bacterial vaginosis, and chancroid.
    2. Herpes simplex type 2, syphilis, and hepatitis B.
    3. Pubic lice, scabies, and syphilis.
    4. Chlamydia, gonorrhea, and genital herpes.

68. Genital herpes is a(n)

    1. Chronic disease with no known cure.
    2. Acute, curable disease.
    3. Contagious but curable disease.
    4. Chronic disease, if not cured in the early stages.

69. Symptoms in the primary stage of syphilis are

    1. General flulike symptoms and mucous patches.
    2. Generalized lymphadenopathy and patchy hair loss.

3. Condylomata lata and generalized skin rash.

4. Chancre, painless oval ulcer, and lymphadenopathy.

70. Which of the following are sexually transmitted enteric infections?

1. Dysenteries and hepatitis.

2. Chancroid and pubic lice.

3. Chlamydial infections and gonorrhea.

4. Syphilis and genital herpes.

71. In emergency care of patients who are victims of "alleged sexual assault" it is important to

1. First assure the patient that the patient is safe; offer emotional support and privacy, and then gather vital information and evidence that usually is legally evaluated.

2. First give thorough physical care, empathetic psychosocial support, and ensure privacy.

3. Expedite the registration process and place the patient in a private examination room and leave the patient to have some time alone.

4. Obtain a detailed history and physical examination after explaining the need to detail and then gather vital information and evidence that usually is legally evaluated.

72. A drug that may increase male sperm is

1. Clonidine (Catapres).

2. Clomiphene citrate (Clomid).

3. Thioridazine (Mellaril).

4. Spironolactone (Aldactone).

73. A drug that may decrease spermatogenesis and reproductive functioning is

1. Amitriptyline (Elavil).

2. Imipramine (Tofranil).

3. Diazepam (Valium).

4. Phenytoin (Dilantin).

74. Drugs that may cause male impotence are

1. Aramine, Dobutamine, Dilaudid, and Mandol.

2. Aldactone, Lopressor, Aldomet, and Catapres.

3. Minipress, Persantine, Pitressin, and Sectral.

4. Apresoline, Capoten, Codeine, and Corgard.

75. Drugs that may lead to impaired ejaculation are

1. Thorazine and Mellaril.

2. Urecholine and mannitol.

3. Tapazole and Cytomel.

4. Prostigmin and Mestinon.

76. Drugs that lead to decreased libido are

1. Nardil, Parnate, Valium, and Librium.

2. Adriamycin, Ancef, Cytoxan, and Mandol.

3. Antabuse, Bronkosol, Brethine, and Ventolin.

4. Pilocar, Diamox, Propine, and Timoptic.

77. When working with an "alleged sexual assault" patient's clothing, the number one priority is

1. To send the clothing to a laboratory immediately.

2. To note the condition of patient's clothing.

3. To give the clothes to the police immediately.

4. To place the patient's clothing in a paper bag, not a plastic bag.

78. The American Cancer Society recommends that all women over the age of ___ years perform monthly breast self-examinations.

1. Fifteen.

2. Sixteen.

3. Eighteen.

4. Twenty.

79. The nurse teaches patients that they should examine their breasts for lumps

1. One week after menstrual period.

2. One week before menstrual period begins.

3. Each month on the same date.

4. Two weeks after menstrual period.

80. The American Cancer Society recommends annual mammography for asymptomatic women over age___years.

1. Forty.

2. Fifty.

3. Sixty.

4. Sixty-Five.

81. The American Cancer Society recommends a baseline mammography for all women between the

1. Ages of 13 and 16 years.

2. Ages of 18 and 20 years.

3. Ages of 20 and 30 years.

4. Ages of 35 and 40 years.

82. The American Cancer Society recommends mammography screening at intervals of 1 to 2 years of asymptomatic women between

1. Ages 18 and 30 years.

2. Ages 30 and 40 years.

3. Ages 40 and 49 years.

4. Ages 50 and 59 years.

83. Ultrasonography of the breast is useful in determining

1. Cystic (fluid-filled) from solid lesions.

2. Benign from solid cancerous lesions.

3. Lymph node enlargement from malignant tumors.

4. Deep solid lesions and small cancerous cells.

84. The American Cancer Society recommends that women who are or have been sexually active or reached the age of 18 years should have a Pap test and pelvic examination

1. Every 6 months.

2. Every other year.

3. Annually for 3 to 4 years.

4. Annually for the rest of their lives.

85. Which of the following is considered essential to diagnosing breast cancer?

1. Ultrasonography.

2. Core-needle biopsy.

3. Mammography.

4. X-ray film.

86. The Pap test is performed to determine

1. Preinvasive and invasive ureteral cancer.

2. Urinary carcinoma.

3. Only vaginal and noninvasive ureteral cancer.

4. Preinvasive and invasive cervical cancer.

87. With age, the prostatic tissue undergoes benign hypertrophy and hyperplasi This will impede urinary flow, and urinary retention may be precipitated by

1. Sexual intercourse, Valium, and caffeine.

2. Caffeine, constipation, or aspirin therapy.

3. Alcoholic beverages, infection, or repeated delay in voiding.

4. Coke, coffee, and sexual intercourse.

88. Prostate cancer is the most common cancer among men. The diagnostic tests include

1. Serum level of prostate-specific antigen (PSA).

2. Cystoscopy digital rectal examination and ultrasonography.

3. Semen excretion analysis and scrotum biopsy.

4. Scrotum biopsy and digital rectal examination.

89. After a mastectomy with axillary node dissection, patient teaching regarding the effected arm should include

1. No blood pressure can be taken for 6 months.

2. Limited exercise for 4 months.

3. Avoid cuts, pinpricks, and burns, and no blood pressure taken on the affected arm.

4. Keep arm in a dependent position; blood pressure can be taken on the affected arm 1 year after surgery.

90. Early clinical manifestations of breast cancer are

1. Single painless, nontender, hard, irregular, nonmobile mass.

2. Multiple lumps, tender, soft movable mass.

3. One large nodule, tender, soft movable mass.

4. Very small, painless, multiple, movable soft mass.

91. Women most at risk for breast cancer are

1. Over age 65 years, married, younger than 16 years at first pregnancy.

2. Over age 55 years, never married, with a family history of cancer.

3. Over age 65 years, married, multiple sexual partners at a young age.

4. Over age 40 years, never married, with a family history of lung cancer.

92. Radiation to the breast causes the skin to be

1. Dry, tender, red, swollen, and itchy.

2. Pale, moist, painful, and rash over area treated.

3. Cyanotic, dry, pigmented, and painful.

4. Jaundiced, itchy, ulcerated, and painful.

93. Side effects of chemotherapy are

1. Ptosis, diaphoresis, hypoxia, and nausea and vomiting.

2. Photosensitivity, peripheral neuropathy, and stomatitis.

3. Tremor, dizziness, diaphoresis, and severe headaches.

4. Weight loss, irritability, diarrhea and ataxia, and severe headache.

94. A standard radical mastectomy involves the removal of

1. Cancerous mass and all normal tissue for clean margin.

2. The breast, axillary lymph nodes, and pectoral muscles.

3. Axillary lymph nodes, removal of breast, and overlying skin.

4. Resection of breast tissue and some skin from clavicle to costal margin.

95. Medicines used to treat dysmenorrhea include

1. Atarax, Azulfidine, and Dilaudid.

2. Dilantin, codeine, and Ismelin.

3. Midol, Motrin, and aspirin.

4. Aspirin, Mandol, and Macrodantin.

96. Endometriosis is

1. Abnormal location of endometrial tissue that is hormone dependent.

2. Abnormal growth of endometrial tissue within the uterus.

3. Small endometrial abscesses with bleeding outside the uterine cavity causing severe pain.

4. Excessive endometrial tissue in the uterus causing pain, bloating, and premenstrual tension.

97. It is generally accepted that estrogen should not be given to women

1. After a surgical procedure to enlarge the breast or intestinal disorders.

2. Mastitis or when breast-feeding an infant.

3. With bone cancer, osteoporosis, or mastitis.

4. With known or suspected breast or uterine cancer.

98. Treatment for endometriosis includes

1. Premarin and dexamethasone.

2. Pronestyl and dextran.

3. Oral contraceptives and Danocrine.

4. Diazepam and Miltown.

99. Side effects of oral contraceptives are
    1. Pulmonary embolism, pulmonary edema, and hypertension.
    2. Anemia, mental depression, and hypotension.
    3. Syncope, diaphoresis, and hemorrhage.
    4. Iron loss, mental depression, and hypotension.

100. Oral contraceptives decrease effects of
    1. Prednisone, hydrocortisone, and Medrol.
    2. Anticoagulants, insulin, and antihypertensive agents.
    3. Calcium gluconate, Medrol, and Dilantin.
    4. Robitussin, Dilaudid, and Sudafed.

ANSWERS AND RATIONALES

1. **①** The obstetric hazards for an adolescent include an increased mortality rate, anemia, pregnancy-induced hypertension, and low-birth-weight newborns.
    (2, 3, 4) These options are incorrect as seen in rationale (1).

2. **③** A nurse examines a patient at 22 weeks of gestation and finds that the tip of the uterus is 20 cm above the symphysis pubis. The upper rounded portion of the uterus is the fundus.
    (1, 2, 4) These options are incorrect as seen in rationale (3).

3. **③** A patient is pregnant for the third time; therefore, she is gravida III. Having a 2-year-old son counts as a para. Having had a spontaneous or elective abortion (less than 24 weeks) does not count as a para; therefore, she is para I.
    (1, 2, 4) These options are incorrect as seen in rationale (3).

4. **③** When the nurse performed a pelvic examination on the patient, the nurse noted that the cervix was bluish-purple color, which is known as Chadwick's sign. This occurs from about week 4 of pregnancy and is caused by increased vascularity of the vagina.
    (1) Goodell's sign (softening of the cervix), a probable sign of pregnancy, occurs during the second month.
    (2) Braxton Hicks' contractions (sign) are mild, irregular, painless uterine contractions that occur more frequently in late pregnancy. These contractions do not represent true labor.
    (4) Homan's sign is an early sign of phlebothrombosis of the deep veins of the calf in which the patient complains of pain when the leg is extended and the foot is dorsiflexed.

5. **②** Most women gain the majority of weight during the last trimester of pregnancy. It is during the last trimester that babies gain most of their weight.
    (1, 3, 4) These options are incorrect as seen in rationale (2).

6. **①** The latent and active phase of labor, as well as the transitional phase, occur in stage one.
    During the latent phase, the cervix dilates to 3 cm and effaces to 40 percent. During the active phase, the cervix dilates to 10 cm (complete) with 100 percent effacement, and the station increases to approximately 0 to +1. *Note:* Stage one lasts from the onset of regular uterine contractions to the full dilation of the cervix.
    (2, 3, 4) These options are incorrect as seen in rationale (1).

7. **③** The stage that begins after the delivery of the newborn is stage three of labor. The third stage of labor lasts from delivery of the fetus to the delivery of the placenta.
    (1) Stage one is explained in answer 6, rationale (1).
    (2) The second stage of labor lasts from full dilation of the cervix to delivery of the fetus and is generally shorter in multiparous women.
    (4) The fourth stage of labor arbitrarily lasts approximately 2 h after delivery of the placenta, when the mother's hemodynamic status is observed closely.

8. **④** A neonate 5 min after birth has a *heart rate*: >100 bpm (2 points); *respiratory effort*: cry is loud and strong (2 points); *muscle tone*: the body is well flexed and has active motion of extremities (2 points); *reflex*: coughs or cries with suctioning (2 points); and *color*: is completely pink (2 points). This newborn would have an Apgar score of 10, which is the maximum possible.
    (1, 2, 3) These options are incorrect as seen in rationale (4).

9. **①** Progesterone inhibits uterine contractions throughout pregnancy.
    (2) Prostaglandin plays a role in ovulation, formation of corpus luteum, uterine contractility, and milk ejection. Prostaglandins are used to induce labor in second-trimester abortions and may be used to "ripen" (or prepare) a cervix for Pitocin (oxytocin) induction of labor.
    (3) Estrogen is produced by the ovary and adrenal cortex in a prepregnant state; however, the principal source during pregnancy is the placent Estrogen increases from the onset of pregnancy to term.
    (4) Oxytocin is produced by the posterior lobe of the pituitary gland and causes uterine contractions.

10. **①** After placing the newborn in a radiant warmer, the nurse's first action is to dry it thoroughly. Drying the newborn prevents a sudden drop in the newborn's body temperature, called cold stress, which uses significant amounts of glucose. The temperature-regulating mechanism of the hypothalamus is not well developed in the neonate.
    (2) After stabilization, place the identification band on the neonate. Nursing actions should be in this order with some actions overlapping the other: warmth (drying neonate), cardiopulmonary resuscitation (CPR) if needed, Apgar scoring, identification, measurement of weight and length, and newborn medications (IM vitamin K and antibiotic eye prophylaxis).
    (3) Vitamin K is administered to a neonate for prevention of hemorrhagic disease, but this is not the first action.
    (4) This is not the first action. The agent used for prophylaxis varies according to hospital protocols. Ophthalmic erythromycin is frequently used. The ointment is instilled prophylactically into the conjunctival sac for prophylaxis of ophthalmic neonatorum (neonatal blindness) secondary to maternal *N. gonorrhoeae* infection.

11. ❶ Twin pregnancy or any condition that overdistends the uterus predisposes a patient to postpartum hemorrhage. Overdistention of the uterus causes poor uterine muscle tone, which in turn causes poor postpartum uterine contractions, leading to an increased risk of postpartum hemorrhage.

(2) Breech presentation, in which the buttocks, feet, or both are nearest the cervical opening and are delivered first, is the most common example of malpresentation. The major concern in breech presentation is cord prolapse and head entrapment.

(3) Premature or preterm rupture of the membranes will not cause postpartum hemorrhage. With preterm or prolonged rupture of membranes, there may be a danger of infection.

(4) Cesarean birth does not increase the incidence of postpartum hemorrhage.

12. ❶ When a patient has been in active labor 12 h with minimal cervical changes and documentation of borderline pelvis on her prenatal examination, the nurse could anticipate the physician requesting a cesarean permit.

(2, 3, 4) These options are not as likely. The need for additional diagnostic tests may compromise the mother's and fetus's condition if delivery is postponed. An IUPC may be used to assess uterine activity if there was minimal change after a few hours of labor.

13. ❸ Vaginal bleeding during the intrapartum period in a high-risk pregnancy may indicate abruptio placentae, especially if associated with a hard, boardlike abdomen, increased uterine activity, and pain.

(1) Ectopic pregnancy occurs when the fertilized ovum implants outside of its normal place (e.g., in the abdomen, fallopian tubes, or ovaries) and is a complication identified very early in pregnancy.

(2) Disseminated intravascular coagulation is abnormal clotting throughout the entire vascular system causing obstruction and tissue ischemia. It is sometimes seen in preeclamptic patients with the experiencing hemolysis, elevated liver enzymes, low platelets (HELLP) syndrome.

(4) The fundus is the upper rounded prominence of the uterus. If the fundus is soft after delivery, bleeding could occur. The fundus is massaged gently after delivery to keep it firm, decrease blood loss, and expel any clots.

14. ❸ The nurse should determine FHR status during active labor with an ultrasound transducer or a fetal electroe. Ultrasound transducers have high-frequency sound waves that reflect mechanical action of the fetal heart and are used during the antepartum and intrapartum periods for intermittent, as well as continuous, fetal monitoring. Fetal electrodes usually are placed on the fetal scalp to monitor the fetus directly. Variability can be determined (assessment of fetal well-being) with this type of monitoring. *Note*: Intermittent auscultation using a Doppler or fetoscope may be used on patients without identified risk factors.

(1) The tocotransducer monitors frequency and duration of uterine contractions by means of pressure, not intensity. This sensing device is applied to the maternal abdomen and may be used during the antepartum and intrapartum periods.

(2) An IUPC accurately measures frequency, duration, and intensity of contractions. It can be used only when membranes have ruptured and the cervix is sufficiently dilated (during the intrapartum period).

(4) Intermittent auscultation using a Doppler or fetoscope examination may be used to assess FHR in patients with *no* identified risk factors. The fetal monitor (ultrasound transducer or fetal electrode) is more commonly used to assess the fetus during labor.

15. ❸ The nurse would not assess for cervical dilation in a patient with painless bright-red bleeding, with or without contractions, because this procedure may cause the patient to dislodge the placenta. Painless vaginal bleeding is a sign of placenta previa.

(1, 2, 4) FHR, uterine contractions, and the mother's vital signs should be assessed and monitored.

16. ❷ During labor, the nurse caring for a patient showing signs of placenta previa should observe the amount of bleeding and assess for signs and symptoms of hemorrhage.

(1) Polyuria would indicate that she is getting rid of excess fluid.

(3) Water draining from the vaginal area would indicate that the membranes have broken. This is a normal part of labor.

(4) Painful contractions are a normal part of labor.

17. ❸ The primary indication for scheduling this patient for a cesarean section is because the placenta is covering the opening of the uterus; therefore, the baby cannot be delivered through the vagina.

(1) There is a risk for abruptio placentae or separation of part or all of the placenta from the implantation site, especially if cervical dilation occurs. Symptoms include small to moderate amounts of bright-red vaginal bleeding (in 80–85 percent of cases), mild to severe pain that may be localized or diffused, and a rigid (or hard) abdomen (uterus).

(2) When a patient asks the nurse a question, the nurse should be knowledgeable and be able to answer the patient and not have to refer to the physician.

(4) A nurse should acknowledge the patient's anxiety and never tell a patient that if the patient gets upset, she will hemorrhage. This will only increase her anxiety.

18. ❹ After the baby is born, the nurse needs to massage the patient's uterus gently to encourage it to contract and to check it frequently to be sure the uterus stays firm to decrease blood loss.

(1) Telling a patient that "We massage every mother's uterus after she delivers" does not indicate to the patient the rationale for why the massage must be done.

(2) Telling the patient "I know it hurts, but it has to be done" is not the reason it is done. The patient will more readily accept the uncomfortable feeling of having her uterus massaged if she knows it may prevent her from hemorrhaging.

(3) The physician makes sure the placenta is passed or delivered.

19. **①** If, shortly after delivery, the patient's uterus is firm and one finger breadth above the umbilicus and is displaced slightly to the left of the abdomen, the nurse needs to encourage the patient to void. A full bladder is most likely causing displacement of the uterus.

(2, 3, 4) These options are incorrect as seen in rationale (1).

20. **①** Possible complications of a patient with IDDM are preeclampsia, eclampsia, hemorrhage, and infection.

Newborns of patients who are either class A, B, or C diabetics are often macrosomic (very large), which may cause an overdistended uterus, resulting in hemorrhage.

Monilial infection (of the vagina or nipples) and other infections are more likely to occur in women with IDDM.

Preeclampsia occurs in one third of all diabetic new mothers.

(2, 3, 4) These are *not* complications a pregnant IDDM woman would have.

21. **①** A nonreactive nonstress test is not reassuring and must be reported to the physician. This indicates that the fetus may be experiencing stress or distress. A reactive nonstress test is a reassuring sign of fetal well-being (not in distress).

In a reactive nonstress test, the FHR must increase 15 beats for 15 seconds above the baseline and do this at least twice in 20 min. If the FHR fails to do this, it is considered a nonreactive nonstress test, and other tests should be conducted to determine if there is fetal compromise. For example, a contraction stress test may be performed. This is done using spontaneous contractions or oxytocin-induced contractions and evaluating the response of the FHR. If a contraction stress test is negative, there are no decelerations, and this would be reassuring.

(2, 3, 4) These options are incorrect as seen in rationale (1). Fetal movement perception varies per individual and pregnancy considerably. Perception of decreased fetal movement indicates the need for further assessment. Perception of continued fetal movement is reassuring, as is decreasing bilirubin levels.

22. **②** The placenta of a diabetic mother is more prone to undergo degenerative changes late in pregnancy (due to vascular changes), causing uteroplacental deficiency.

(1) A diabetic has been at risk for infection her entire life and is no more at risk when she is pregnant at full term than she was early in her pregnancy.

(3) A diabetic woman who is pregnant is not any more at risk for hypoglycemic crisis when she nears term than she was early in her pregnancy.

(4) Women who have more progressive diabetes mellitus (associated vascular involvement) generally have newborns that are small for gestational age.

23. **④** Blood loss with abruptio placenta is greater than observed because some blood remains in the uterus.

(1, 2, 3) These options are incorrect as seen in rationale (4).

24. **②** The nonpregnant sodium values (135–145) are being approached during the postpartum period; 120–30 mEq/L is within normal postpartum limits. This is the only normal value given.

(1) Normal female hematocrit is 37 to 47 percent. A value of 20 to 30 percent would be very low.

(3) Normal RBC count for women is 4.2 to 5.4 million/mm^3. A value of 2.8 to 3.5 million/mm^3 would be very low.

(4) Normal leukocytosis (low WBC count) of pregnancy averages approximately 12,000 mm^3. During the first 10 to 12 days after delivery, values between 20,000 to 25,000/mm^3 are not uncommon, but 30,000 to 35,000 mm^3 would be very abnormal.

25. **②** A long labor (19 h) and delivery of twins would increase the possibility of postpartum hemorrhage. Both of these factors may cause decreased uterine contractility and hemorrhage.

(1) Cesarean birth does not increase the chances for hemorrhage because the physician can see the blood vessels that are bleeding and tie them off or cauterize them. In vaginal delivery, it may be more difficult to find the source of bleeding.

(3, 4) Neither premature delivery nor induced labor is associated with hemorrhage.

26. **①** If the membranes rupture 24 h before delivery of the fetus, the nurse would assess the patient for endometritis (infection of the endometrium). Membranes provide a barrier from ascending bacteria. Endometritis should not be confused with endometriosis, where endometrium develops outside the uterus in various sites throughout the pelvis or in the abdominal wall. The cause of endometriosis is unknown.

(2, 3, 4) These options are incorrect as seen in rationale (1).

27. **②** Appropriate-for-gestational-age neonate will have the lowest risk for developing hypoglycemia; this neonate will have a normal blood glucose level because the mother's glucose level is normal. All other neonates in the other options are at higher risk for hypoglycemia.

(1) The neonate exposed to high blood glucose levels in utero may experience rapid and profound hypoglycemia 2 h after birth because of the abrupt cessation of a high in utero glucose intake and a slower decrease in insulin production in the neonate.

(3) A 2-hour-old, 35-week-gestational-age neonate, weighing only 4 lb, has minimal fat and glycogen stores due to intrauterine malnutrition and prematurity.

(4) A preterm neonate at 12 h after birth, NPO because of respiratory distress, has not been in utero a sufficient period to store glycogen and fat. The neonate is rapidly using up glucose stores because of respiratory distress. The neonate is NPO and, therefore, is not replacing the glycogen.

28. **③** Immediately after delivery, the nurse should be able to feel that the top of the uterus is firm, in the midline, and below the umbilicus.

(1, 2, 4) These options are incorrect as seen in rationale (3).

29. **③** A soft uterus displaced to one side, or above the midline, 2 h after delivery would be an indication that the uterus has relaxed, and blood clots need to be expressed with gentle massage of the uterus. The uterus should remain firm, midline, and located at or below the umbilicus 2 h after delivery.

(1, 2, 4) These options are incorrect as seen in rationale (3).

30. **③** To open the airway and allow for suctioning of the mouth and nose, the nurse would place the neonate in a supine position with the head slightly extended.

(1, 2, 4) These options are incorrect as seen in rationale (3).

(4) *Note*: Hyperextension of the neonates head will occlude the airway.

31. **①** Postpartum transitory depression begins the second or third day after delivery. Symptoms include anxiety, poor concentration, tearfulness, and despondency. The symptoms usually subside within the first week.

(2) Asking for pain medication more than usual may indicate increased pain, poor pain relief, or an addiction. It does not indicate postpartum transitory depression.

(3) Multiple physical complaints in the early postpartum period may indicate inadequate pain relief or some other physical problem, not depression.

(4) Demonstrating nervousness when holding a first-born child is normal behavior.

32. **②** Immediate nursing intervention is needed if a patient's perineal pads are soaked with blood and the blood clots every 30 min within 6 h after delivery. This is a sign of hemorrhage, and the physician needs to be notified immediately.

(1) The perineal pad may be spotted with bright-red blood 6 h after delivery due to placental blood loss at the placental implantation site, from breaking of small blood vessels in the vaginal area, or from an episiotomy.

(3) The mother will normally have some increase in body temperature during the first 24 h after delivery due to prostaglandin release, but a temperature of 100.4°F or greater should be monitored. If the temperature continues to increase, then the physician should be notified.

(4) A pulse rate of 95 bpm may be due to slight temperature increase, pain, anxiety, or excitement.

33. **①** A newborn of a narcotic-addicted mother may exhibit poor feeding, hypersensitivity to noise, and irritability.

(2, 3, 4) These are not symptoms of a newborn of a narcotic-addicted mother.

34. **④** The major reason for a 4-week waiting period (or until after the first checkup) before resumption of sexual intercourse is to prevent vaginal and cervical infection. The vaginal area is very susceptible to infections after the trauma of childbirth.

(1) It is unlikely that the woman will have intercourse if it is painful.

(2) Intercourse after vaginal delivery will not cause a bladder infection.

(3) If the episiotomy site is not healed, intercourse will be too painful.

35. **④** A diabetic mother's glucose crosses the placenta barrier and stimulates the fetal pancreas to produce large amounts of insulin. At birth, the source of high glucose (the mother) is abruptly removed, but the pancreas temporarily continues to produce large amounts of insulin, causing hypoglycemia.

(1, 2, 3) These options are incorrect as seen in rationale (4). Infants of diabetic mothers are not at higher risk for sepsis or anemia.

36. **①** A pregnant woman in her third trimester of pregnancy who is involved in an automobile accident is at increased risk for abruptio placenta. A sign of abruptio placenta is an enlarged abdomen that is painful and rigid on palpations. Fetal hypoxia or anoxia with possible fetal death can occur.

(2) Signs and symptoms of placenta previa include painless uterine bleeding, which may be intermittent, may occur in gushes, or, more rarely, may be continuous.

(3) Hydramnios (increased amounts of amniotic fluid) usually has unclear pathogenesis. It is associated with fetal GI obstruction or atresias, gestational diabetes or IDDM, and Rh-sensitized pregnancies.

(4) An enlarged abdomen that is painful and rigid on palpation and fetal monitoring indicating fetal distress are all abnormal signs and are not indicative of labor.

37. **②** Periodic apnea is common in preterm newborns. Usually, gentle stimulation is sufficient to initiate breathing.

(1, 3, 4) These options are incorrect as seen in rationale (2). If the neonate's apnea does not respond to gentle stimulation, the next step would be administration of positive-pressure ventilation with 100 percent oxygen, and then notification of the physician. Increasing the humidity of the isolette will have no effect on apnea.

38. **③** Neonates respond well to human faces and black and white objects. Black and white objects offer the best visual contrast. Newborns learn to associate gratification of need with their parent's faces. Newborns may fixate on visual stimuli for periods of 4 to 10 seconds.

(1, 2, 4) These options are incorrect as seen in rationale (3).

39. **②** With a breech presentation, the nurse must be particularly alert for a prolapsed umbilical cord. A prolapsed umbilical cord could partially or completely occlude fetal circulation, causing hypoxia, increased infant mortality, and morbidity.

(1) Hydramnios is not caused by breech presentation [see answer 36, rationale (3)].

(3) Increased FHR is not associated with breech presentation, although acceleration with contractions may be.

(4) Bloody show is normal before birth and is not associated with breech presentation.

40. **②** Following rupture of membranes, fetal distress may be indicated by meconium. The passage of meconium from the fetal bowel before birth may indicate fetal distress. Although the presence of meconium-stained amniotic fluid is not always an indication of fetal distress, the presence of thick particulate of meconium requires visualization of the fetal cord with a laryngoscope and suctioning to prevent meconium aspiration.

(1, 3, 4) These options are incorrect as seen in rationale (2).

41. **①** The contraceptive method that should not be used by a patient 35 years or older who smokes one package of cigarettes each day is birth control pills. The combination of cigarette smoking and use of birth control pills increases the risk of hypertension and the potential for formation of blood clots. Cigarette smoking causes vasoconstriction, which encourages clot formation and hypertension.

(2, 3) The intrauterine device (IUD) and the sponge contraceptive method can be used by those who smoke cigarettes. Neither method promotes hypertension or blood clot formation.

(4) Surgical sterilization is an effective method used for permanent contraception. Smoking would not increase risk factors for this type of contraceptive technique.

42. ❸ A woman using a diaphragm for contraception must leave it in place in the vagina for 6 h after intercourse.

(1, 2, 4) These options are incorrect as seen in rationale (3).

43. ❷ A diaphragm must be remeasured after childbirth and after pelvic surgery. A loose-fitting diaphragm may result in pregnancy.

(1, 3, 4) These options are incorrect as seen in rationale (2).

44. ❷ It would be inappropriate to use an oil-based lotion on a newborn's skin to prevent drying and cracking. Use of a lotion is not recommended because of the sensitivity of the newborn's skin.

(1, 3, 4) A newborn undergoing phototherapy for hyperbilirubinemia should be turned every 2 h, should have the eyes covered with protective patches, and should be placed in an isolette 18 inches from the phototherapy light without clothing.

45. ❶ A patient receiving Methergine for postpartum bleeding should be assessed for hypertension. Methergine causes vasoconstriction and stimulates uterine contractions, which decreases bleeding. Side effects include headache, dizziness, chest pain, and hypertension. A drop in blood pressure may indicate hypovolemia.

(2, 3, 4) These are not side effects of Methergine.

46. ❹ Assessment for signs and symptoms of worsening preeclampsia or eclampsia is necessary for at least 48 h postpartum. These classic signs and symptoms include increasing proteinuria, hypertension, generalized edema [accumulation of interstitial fluid in the face, hands, abdomen, sacrum, tibia, and ankles, as well as excessive weight gain (2–4.5 lb/week)]. Epigastric pain may indicate liver involvement and the risk of liver rupture. Decreased urinary output and an increase in deep tendon reflexes, headache, and scotoma are common. The diagnosis of eclampsia occurs when tonic–clonic seizures occur.

(1, 2, 3) Delivery is the treatment for preeclampsia/eclampsia. Intravenous magnesium sulfate is administered to prevent seizures. Patient's symptoms usually begin to improve within 48 h following delivery.

47. ❸ The nurse's first intervention in managing postpartum hemorrhage is massaging the uterus firmly until it remains firm, and repeat as needed. If the uterus is allowed to relax, hemorrhage may occur. Prevention of postpartum hemorrhage is the nurse's number one responsibility. If it occurs, reducing the amount of hemorrhage becomes the nurse's number one responsibility. *Note*: A distended bladder can displace the uterus and cause an increase in vaginal bleeding.

(1) A physician's order is required to call for blood type and cross-match.

(2) Taking the vital signs is very important in any crisis but not as important as preventing or controlling hemorrhage.

(4) The patient will know that she is hemorrhaging and will know that she must remain in bed.

48. ❶ A definite softening of the lower uterine segment is called Hegar's sign. Discoloration of mucous membranes of the vagina is called Chadwick's sign. Softening of the cervix is called Goodell's sign.

(2, 3, 4) These options are incorrect as seen in rationale (1).

49. ❶ A 9-week pregnant mother with sharp right-sided pain, some vaginal spotting, and nausea and vomiting may be experiencing ectopic pregnancy.

(2) Abruptio placenta will demonstrate enlarged abdomen, which is painful and rigid on palpation (and occurs much later in pregnancy).

(3) Signs and symptoms of placenta previa are painless uterine bleeding. The bright-red blood may be intermittent, occur in gushes, or, more rarely, may be continuous. Abdominal examination reveals a soft (relaxed), nontender uterus.

(4) Signs and symptoms of threatening abortion would be abdominal cramping, uterine irritability, or contractions, usually associated with minimal to moderate vaginal bleeding.

50. ❷ A positive contraction stress test (oxytocin, spontaneous, or nipple stimulation contraction stress test) shows late decelerations (decrease of the FHR, which returns to its baseline following the contractions), indicating uteroplacental insufficiency. A negative test suggests fetal well-being.

(1, 3, 4) These options are incorrect as seen in rationale (2).

51. ❶ The earliest sign of preeclampsia most commonly is hypertension, followed by proteinuria and generalized edema. All of these signs and symptoms may not be present and may not present in this order.

(2) Epigastric pain is generally a late sign of preeclampsia and indicates liver involvement.

(3) Pedal edema is a normal occurrence in pregnancy.

(4) Slight (trace) proteinuria is not uncommon in pregnancy. An increase in proteinuria indicates kidney involvement and generally follows hypertension.

52. ❸ If the patient is pregnant now and has had one abortion, one stillbirth, and one set of twins, she is gravida IV, para II. Gravida is the number of times pregnant without regard to outcome. Para is the number of pregnancies in which the fetus or fetuses have reached the age of viability (approximately 24 weeks), not the number of fetuses delivered. Whether the fetus is born alive or is stillborn after viability is reached does not affect parity.

(1, 2, 4) These options are incorrect as seen in rationale (3).

53. ❷ On examination, the nurse palpated the fetal fontanelles and sagittal suture to identify the presenting part and the relation of the fetal occiput to the mother's right or left side. Fetal presentation was left occipital posterior (LOP). Presentation is determined in the following manner: left of the maternal pelvis (left, L), fetal occipital (occipital, O), toward the back (posterior, P).

(1, 3, 4) These options are incorrect as seen in rationale (2).

54. ❶ A patient with active HSV-2 in active labor should plan to have a cesarean section, preferably within 4 h of membranes rupturing. A fetus that is delivered vaginally may acquire HSV-2 because the virus is located in the vaginal area or may ascend once the protective membranes are gone.

(2) The patient cannot deliver vaginally if she is treated with antibiotics. There is no cure for HSV-2. Acyclovir has been used for treatment of HSV-2, but it is not a cure (and not an antibiotic). The neonate could suffer serious sequelae if it contracts the disease.

(3) HSV-1 is characterized by vesicles that tend to occur where the mucous membrane joins the skin, lips, gingiva, and conjunctiva.

(4) Signs and symptoms of HSV-2 are itching and soreness, which usually are present before a small patch of erythema develops. Then the vesicular lesions erode and disappear. Lesions are painful and usually heal in approximately 10 days, but they will recur possibly in any part of the genitalia.

55. ❹ Signs and symptoms of preeclampsia are hypertension, proteinuria, generalized edema, and weight gain.

(1, 2, 3) These options are incorrect as seen in rationale (4).

56. ❹ The mother's blood type is O, Rh negative, and the husband's blood type is AB, Rh positive. The day after delivery, the nurse observes that the newborn's skin and sclera of the eyes have become yellow, causing jaundice within 24 h of birth. Jaundice this early is abnormal, and the physician should be immediately notified.

The physician will determine what blood work must be done and probably will give an order to place the newborn in phototherapy. When the mother's and the fetus's blood are incompatible and some of the fetal blood comes in contact with the mother's blood, the mother produces antibodies against the baby's blood, causing destruction of the fetal red blood cells.

This destruction produces hyperbilirubinemia and anemia in the newborn. If the anemia is severe, heart failure may result in an edematous hydropic newborn and possible stillbirth.

(1, 2, 3) These options are incorrect as seen in rationale (4).

57. ❶ The incidence of kernicterus has been greatly reduced by the administration of Rho (4) immune globulin (RhoGam) to all Rh-negative mothers during pregnancy and to all unsensitized Rh-negative mothers within 72 h after the delivery or abortion of Rh-positive newborns or fetuses. Kernicterus is a high level of bilirubin in the blood causing severe neurologic symptoms. Rh incompatibility was a leading cause of kernicterus and a significant cause of neonatal death before RhoGam was developed.

(2, 3, 4) These options are incorrect as seen in rationale (1).

58. ❸ When the nurse examines the inside of a newborn's mouth, she observes small, raised, white bumps (Epstein's pearls). They are small, white cysts on the hard palate or gingiva of the newborn. They are normal and will disappear shortly after birth.

(1) Milk curd is milk that has curdled in the baby's mouth and can be removed easily.

(2) Candidiasis (thrush) is a fungal infection characterized by white patches that appear to be milk curds on the oral mucosa. They will bleed if removed.

(4) HSV-1 is characterized by multiple vesicles that progress to shallow ulceration and are most often seen on oral mucous membranes.

59. ❷ The sexually transmitted infectious disease that is the major cause of permanent injury to the neonate's eyes is gonorrhea. Prophylactic treatment (e.g., erythromycin ointment) to both eyes within 1 h of birth is required for all newborns.

(1) Congenital syphilis occurs when the spirochetes cross the placenta after gestational weeks 16 to 18. The following sequelae occur: rhinitis (syphilitic snuffles), cracks and fissures around the mouth, hepatosplenomegaly, anemia, jaundice, hydrocephaly, and corneal opacity. Later, saddle nose, notched-tapered teeth (canines), and diabetes develop in untreated children. None of these problems occur if the mother is treated adequately before week 18.

(3) When genital herpes is active, the fetus can be infected with the disease as it comes down the birth canal. This disease can cause serious eye or nerve damage to the fetus or possibly death, but it is not the major cause of eye disease. It is only a problem when the disease is active and the fetus is then delivered by cesarean section.

(4) *Trichomonas vaginalis* produces a profuse, foamy, grayish-yellowish-greenish discharge, causing irritation, edema of the vulva, and painful intercourse. Urinary frequency and dysuria may occur. Flagyl (metronidazole) is the drug of choice and can be administered orally or vaginally. It does not cause injury to the fetus's eye at the time of birth.

60. ❸ There is no effective treatment for genital herpes.

(1, 2, 4) Syphilis, gonorrhea, and *T. vaginalis* can be treated with penicillin, tetracycline, erythromycin, or metronidazole.

61. ❸ To try and stop the spread of sexually transmitted disease, it is necessary for the health department to notify the individuals who have had sexual relations with the infectious person so that they can seek treatment.

(1) This is not a method established to determine the prevalence of venereal disease. When an individual is notified that a person with whom they had sexual contact has the disease, there is no way of knowing if that person has the disease.

(2) The individual is not required to report to the health department that he or she has had a venereal disease. It is the clinic and the hospital personnel who are required to notify the health department.

(4) Venereal disease can be treated by the physician. There is no need for other health services.

62. ❹ Although genital herpes can be contracted by the fetus through the placenta, it is most commonly contracted when the fetus passes through the infected vagina. A woman who has genital herpes *may* be tested weekly or assessed for signs of viral activity, beginning approximately 6 weeks before her due date. If a culture is positive or symptoms are present, a cesarean section is performed. If the culture is negative, a vaginal delivery imposes no danger to the fetus. There is no cure for genital herpes (HSV-2). Genital herpes can cause spontaneous abortion in the first trimester.

(1) This disease does affect the baby, as seen in rationale (4).

(2, 3) Genital herpes has no cure; therefore, there is no treatment for a newborn with the virus. Cesarean section when the mother has an active virus is the only way to prevent the newborn from contracting HSV-2.

63. ❸ When a patient comes to the emergency room after being raped, the nurse should first reassure her that she is safe and will not be harmed further. A woman who has just been raped is frightened and needs to feel that she is in a safe environment. The patient's major need is psychological support, although she will need some medical attention.

(1, 2, 4) These options are incorrect as seen in rationale (3).

64. ❶ Symptoms women with gonorrhea infection may have include vaginal discharge, a red, swollen cervix or vulva, dysuria, and urinary frequency.

Common lay terms for gonorrhea include white and clap. The disease may be asymptomatic in women. The first actual symptoms of gonorrhea in women may arise from PID.

In men with gonorrhea, symptoms usually are evident earlier than in women. The infection produces a urethra purulent discharge, dysuria, and frequency. All other options have chancre sores, which occur in syphilis, not gonorrhea.

(2, 3, 4) These options are incorrect as seen in rationale (1).

65. ❸ The most common complication of gonorrhea in women is salpingitis, which can progress to PID.

(1) Genital herpes (HSV-2) is a recurrent, systemic infection and is the most common cause of genital ulcerations. This infection is closely related to other herpes infections, such as "cold sores" (HSV-1).

Type 2 herpes is a sexually transmitted genital infection. It is a chronic disease with no known cure.

(2) Mites are parasitic and are the cause of scabies. Vaginitis is the inflammation of the vagina.

(4) Patchy hair loss from eyebrows and scalp may occur in the second stage of syphilis. Generalized skin rash may also occur in the second stage of syphilis.

66. ❶ Gonorrhea is treated aggressively by one large dose of Rocephin IM followed by Vibramycin Hyclate or tetracycline orally for 7 days. After completion of therapy, a follow-up examination and culture should be done.

(2, 3, 4) These options are incorrect as seen in rationale (1).

67. ❹ The most commonly occurring sexually transmitted diseases are chlamydia, gonorrhea, and genital herpes.

Chlamydia infection is known as "the great sterilizer." Undetected and untreated cases can progress to serious, irreversible consequences. Salpingitis (inflammation of the fallopian tubes) will cause scarring and obstruction of the fallopian tubes.

(1, 2, 3) These options are incorrect as seen in rationale (4).

68. ❶ Genital herpes is a chronic disease with no known cure.

(2, 3, 4) These options are incorrect as seen in rationale (1).

69. ❹ Symptoms in the primary stage of syphilis are chancre, a painless oval ulcer, and lymphadenopathy. Lymphadenopathy occurs as local lymph glands near the chancre swell painlessly. If untreated, a chancre disappears after 4 to 6 weeks. The infected patient then is often asymptomatic for a time.

(1, 2, 3) These clinical manifestations occur in the second stage of syphilis.

70. ❶ Dysenteries and hepatitis are caused by enteric (intestine) pathogens. They are acquired from food or water contaminated with fecal matter. These pathogens can also be transmitted by oral and sexual contact.

(2, 3, 4) These are not enteric infections.

71. ❶ The first priority when caring for a patient who is a victim of alleged sexual assault is to first assure the patient that the patient is safe, to offer emotional support and privacy, and then to gather vital information and evidence that usually is legally evaluated and to ensure privacy.

(2, 3, 4) These options are incorrect as seen in rationale (1).

72. ❷ Clomiphene citrate (Clomid) may enhance sexual and reproductive functioning by increasing the sperm count.

(1, 4) Catapres and Aldactone may cause impotence.

(3) Mellaril may cause prolonged, persistent erection without ejaculation.

73. ❹ Dilantin may depress male sexual and reproductive function.

(1, 2, 3) Elavil and Tofranil may lead to decreased libido. Valium does not affect sexual reproduction or function.

74. ❷ Use of Aldactone, Lopressor, Aldomet, Catapres, Reserpine, and Ismelin may cause male impotence.

(1) Aramine is a vasopressor used to manage hypotension. Dobutamine is used to increase cardiac output. Dilaudid is an analgesic used in the management of moderate to severe pain; Mandol is an antiinfective agent. Do not confuse Mandol drug with mannitol, which is an osmotic diuretic used to treat acute renal failure and to reduce intracranial or intraocular pressure.

(3) Minipress is an antihypertensive agent-vasodilator: it dilates both arteries and veins. Persantine is an antiplatelet agent used in combination with warfarin (Coumadin). Pitressin is an antidiuretic used to treat diabetes insipidus and abdominal distention. Sectral is an antihypertensive and antiarrhythmic agent.

(4) Apresoline is an antihypertensive-vasodilator used in combination with a diuretic in the management of moderate to severe hypertension. Capoten is an antihypertensive agent.

Codeine is an analgesic. Corgard is a beta-adrenergic blocker used to treat hypertension.

75. ❶ Use of Thorazine and Mellaril may lead to impaired ejaculation. None of the other drugs will cause impaired ejaculation.

(2) Urecholine is a cholinergic agent used to treat urinary retention, which causes contraction of the urinary bladder.

Mannitol is an osmotic diuretic used to treat acute renal failure and to reduce intracranial or intraocular pressure.

(3) Tapazole is an antithyroid agent used to treat hyperthyroidism and is used in preparation for a thyroidectomy. Tapazole inhibits the synthesis of thyroid hormone.

Cytomel is a thyroid hormone used in replacement or substitution therapy in diminished or absent thyroid function.

(4) Prostigmin is a cholinergic-anticholinesterase agent used to increase muscle strength in symptomatic treatment of myasthenia gravis. It is also used in the prevention and treatment of bladder distention and urinary retention.

Mestinon is a cholinergic-anticholinesterase agent used to increase muscle strength in the symptomatic treatment of myasthenia gravis.

Anticholinesterase is an agent that stops cholinesterase from destroying acetylcholine. Acetylcholine is a neuromuscular transmitter. Patients with myasthenia gravis do not have enough acetylcholine, so they have symptoms of muscle weakness.

Mestinon and Prostigmin agents will increase muscle strength by stopping the breakdown of acetylcholine.

76. ❶ Use of Nardil, Parnate, Valium, and Librium may lead to decreased libido.

(2) Adriamycin is an antibioti Ancef is an antibiotic. Cytoxan is a chemotherapeutic agent. Mandol is an antibiotic.

(3) Antabuse is an alcohol abuse deterrent. Bronkosol, Ventolin, and Brethine are bronchodilators.

(4) Pilocar, Diamox, and Propine are antiglaucoma agents that decrease aqueous humor production. Timoptic is also an antiglaucoma agent that decreases the production of aqueous humor.

77. ❹ When working with an "alleged sexual assault" patient's clothing, the number one priority is to place the patient's clothing in a paper, not a plastic, bag. A plastic bag may destroy evidence needed for police investigation because plastic is airtight and may not allow for proper ventilation, resulting in mold or mildew formation.

(1) Clothing would not be sent to the laboratory, but specimens taken from the patient's body will be sent, but not immediately. The patient needs time to feel that she is in a safe environment and be allowed to talk about her feelings.

(2) Noting the condition of the clothing is not as important as allowing the patient to talk about how she feels.

(3) Clothing is not given to the police immediately because the patient is not asked to remove the clothing immediately.

78. ❹ The American Cancer Society recommends that all women over the age of 20 years perform monthly breast examinations. This examination should be performed 1 week after menstruation in front of a mirror or while taking a shower. The patient should raise her arm up behind her head while she examines the breast on the same side as the arm she has raised.

(1, 2, 3) These options are incorrect as seen in rationale (4).

79. ❶ The nurse teaches patients that all women over age 20 years should examine their breasts for lumps 1 week after the menstrual period.

(2, 3, 4) These options are incorrect as seen in rationale (1).

80. ❷ The American Cancer Society recommends annual mammography for asymptomatic women over age 50 years.

(1, 3, 4) These options are incorrect as seen in rationale (2).

81. ❹ The American Cancer Society recommends a baseline mammography for all women between the ages of 35 and 40 years.

(1, 2, 3) These options are incorrect as seen in rationale (4).

82. ❸ The American Cancer Society recommends mammography screening at intervals of 1 to 2 years for asymptomatic women between the ages of 40 to 49 years.

Mammography is recommended annually for asymptomatic women over age 50 years; at intervals of 1 to 2 years for asymptomatic women between the ages of 40 to 49 years; and a baseline mammography for all women between the ages of 35 to 40 years.

(1, 2, 4) These options are incorrect as seen in rationale (3).

83. ❶ Ultrasonography of the breast is useful for differentiating cystic (fluid-filled) from solid lesions. This is helpful in determining if the lump is a fluid-filled cyst. If the lump is a cyst, there is very little chance it is malignant. If the lump is a solid mass, a biopsy sample will taken and the cells examined to determine if they are malignant.

(2, 3, 4) All of these options state that the ultrasonography will determine if the tissue mass examined is malignant. The ultrasonography cannot determine this. Only a biopsy of the cells can determine malignancy.

84. ❸ The American Cancer Society recommends that women who are or have been sexually active or reached the age of 18 years should have a Pap test and pelvic examination annually for 3 to 4 years. After a woman has had three or more consecutive satisfactory normal annual examinations, the Pap test may be performed less frequently at the discretion of her physician. The Pap test consists of a small amount of secretion taken from the vagina and cervix. After a hysterectomy, a vaginal smear is obtained because the cervix has been removed.

(1, 2, 4) These options are incorrect as seen in rationale (3).

85. ❷ Core-needle biopsy is considered essential for diagnosing breast cancer. An ultrasonography mammography or X-ray film are used to determine clinical manifestation of cancer of the breast but are not considered essential to diagnose malignancy.

(1, 3, 4) These options are incorrect as seen in rationale (2).

86. ❹ A Pap test is performed to determine preinvasive and invasive cervical cancer. Obtaining a Pap smear usually is uncomfortable but not painful. Lubricant is not used on the vaginal speculum because cells may be destroyed.

(1, 2, 3) A Pap test cannot determine cancer of the uterus. Ureteral cancer is rare, and diagnosis is made through urine cytology, intravenous pyelogram (IVP) cystoscopy, ultrasonography, computed tomography, and needle biopsy.

87. ❸ With age, the prostatic tissue undergoes benign hypertrophy and hyperplasia, which will impede urinary flow. Likewise, alcoholic beverages, infection, and repeated delay in voiding may precipitate urinary retention.

(1, 2, 4) These options are incorrect as seen in rationale (3).

88. ❶ Serum level of prostate-specific antigen (PSA) is used to diagnosis prostate cancer in men.

(2, 3, 4) These options are incorrect as seen in rationale . A cystoscope is the examination of the bladder, not the prostate. Ultrasonography may be used to diagnose and locate a renal cyst, to differentiate renal cysts from solid renal tumors, to demonstrate renal or pelvic calculi, or to document hydronephrosis (collection of urine in the renal pelvis due to obstruction outflow). It also is used to guide a percutaneously inserted needle for cyst aspiration of biopsy. One advantage of a kidney sonogram over IVP is that it can be performed on patients who have impaired renal function or an iodine allergy. Ultrasonography and sonogram are the same thing.

89. ❸ After a mastectomy with axillary node dissection, the patient should avoid cuts, pinpricks, burns, and blood pressure in the affected arm.

(1, 2, 4) These options are incorrect as seen in rationale (3).

90. ❶ Early clinical manifestations of breast cancer are single painless, nontender, hard irregular nonmobile masses.

(2) Multiple lumps would not be an early sign of breast cancer but may be a late sign. The lump would not be a tender, soft movable mass. This may indicate a breast cyst.

(3) There may be one large nodule. This would be a late sign, but it would not be a tender, soft movable mass.

(4) Very small, painless, multiple, movable, soft masses may be cysts.

91. ❷ Women older than 55 years, who have never married, and who have a family history of cancer are at the greatest risk for breast cancer.

(1, 3, 4) These options are incorrect as seen in rationale (2).

92. ❶ Radiation will cause skin to become tender, red, swollen, and itchy.

(2, 3, 4) These options are incorrect as seen in rationale (1). The skin does not become pale, cyanotic, jaundiced, painful, ulcerated, or have a rash over the treated area.

93. ❷ Side effects of chemotherapy are photosensitivity; peripheral neuropathy; stomatitis; alopecia (hair loss); depressed red blood cells, white blood cells, and platelets; diarrhea; fatigue; menopausal symptoms; nausea; vomiting; peripheral neuropathy; sterility; and weight loss.

(1, 3, 4) These options are incorrect as seen in rationale (2).

94. ❷ A standard radical mastectomy involves removal of the breast, axillary lymph nodes, and pectoral muscles.

(1) The whole breast, not just the cancerous mass, is removed in a standard radical mastectomy. Some normal tissue for a clean margin will be removed but not all normal tissu When you see "all," it usually is not the right answer.

(3) The removal of axillary lymph nodes, removal of breast, and overlying skin is a modified radical mastectomy. The difference between a modified radical and standard radical mastectomy is that, in the standard radical mastectomy, the pectoral muscles are removed. The modified radical mastectomy is the most commonly performed procedure.

(4) Resection of breast tissue does not tell you how much breast tissue is being resected or if it is cancerous or normal tissue. Skin would not be removed from the clavicle in any of the mastectomies.

95. ❸ Treatment of dysmenorrhea (pain associated with menstruation) includes Midol, Motrin (ibuprofen), and aspirin. Dysmenorrhea is believed to be caused by an excess or an increased sensitivity to prostaglandins. Prostaglandins cause severe muscle spasms, which constrict blood vessels supplying the uterus, causing ischemia and pain.

(1) Atarax is a sedative-hypnotic agent used to treat anxiety. Azulfidine is an antiinfective and GI antiinflammatory used to treat ulcerative colitis. Dilaudid is a narcotic analgesic.

(2) Phenytoin (Dilantin) is an anticonvulsant, antiarrhythmic agent used to treat seizures and digitalis-induced arrhythmias. Codeine is a narcotic analgesic. Ismelin is an antihypertensive agent.

(4) Aspirin, an analgesic and antiinflammatory agent, is used to treat dysmenorrhea. The other two options are not used to treat dysmenorrhea, so this option is wrong. Mandol is an antibiotic.

Macrodantin and Furadantin are both antiinfective agents used to treat urinary tract infections.

96. ❶ Endometriosis is the abnormal location of endometrial tissue that is hormone dependent. Endometriosis is the extrauterine occurrence of endometrial tissue. Although benign, endometriosis is progressive and may have widespread dissemination. The etiology is unknown. It has an inherited predisposition. It causes pelvic pain and infertility.

(2) It is not abnormal for endometrial tissue to grow in the uterus. This is normal.

(3) Endometriosis is not associated with abscesses or bleeding outside the uterine cavity.

(4) Excessive endometrial tissue in the uterus is not endometriosis.

97. ❹ Estrogen should not be given to women with known or suspected breast or uterine cancer, previous or present thrombophlebitis, acute liver disease, cerebrovascular disease, or combined risks, such as obesity, varicosities, high blood pressure, and heavy smoking.

(1, 2, 3) These options are incorrect as seen in rationale (4).

98. ❸ Treatment for endometriosis includes oral contraceptives and Danocrine, a hormone that suppresses ovarian function.

(1) Premarin is a hormone used to treat various estrogen-deficiency stages. Dexamethasone is a glucocorticoid, long-acting, antiinflammatory agent.

(2) Pronestyl is an antiarrhythmic agent used to treat a wide variety of ventricular and atrial arrhythmias. Dextran is a volume expander–anticoagulant used in the emergency treatment of hypovolemic shock.

(4) Diazepam (Valium) is a sedative-hypnotic, anticonvulsant, and skeletal muscle relaxant used in the management of anxiety to provide preoperative sedation and light anesthesia and to relax skeletal muscles. Miltown is a sedative-hypnotic used as a sedative in the management of anxiety disorders.

99. ❶ Side effects of oral contraceptives are pulmonary embolism, pulmonary edema, and hypertension.

(2) Anemia is a condition in which there is a reduction in the number of circulating red blood cells per cubic millimeter, the amount of hemoglobin per 100 mL; or the volume of packed red cells per 100 mL of blood. It exists when hemoglobin content is less than that required to provide the oxygen demands of the body. Anemia may result from excessive blood loss, excessive blood cell destruction (as in sickle cell anemia or with the use of chemotherapy), or in decreased blood cell formation, which is caused by drugs, ionizing radiation, deficiencies of vitamins (vitamin B_{12} deficiency, as in pernicious anemia), deficiency of iron, and folic acid.

(3, 4) These options are incorrect as seen in rationale (1).

100. ❷ Oral contraceptives decrease the effects of anticoagulants, insulin, and antihypertensive agents. Oral contraceptives are considered safest when given to nonsmoking women younger than 35 years age who do not have a history of thromboembolic problems, diabetes mellitus, hypertension, or migraine headaches.

(1) Contraceptives do not decrease the effects of these drugs. Prednisone, hydrocortisone, and Medrol are steroids used to treat inflammation.

(3) Calcium gluconate is an electrolyte used in the treatment and prevention of calcium depletion in diseases associated with hypocalcemia (e.g., hypoparathyroidism). Medrol is a steroid. Dilantin is an anticonvulsant drug.

(4) Robitussin is used in the management of the cough associated with upper respiratory infections. Dilaudid, an analgesic, is used in the treatment of moderate to severe pain. Sudafed is a decongestant used in the symptomatic management of nasal congestion

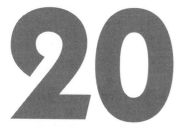

Chapter 20

Growth, Development, and Early Childhood Diseases

TOPICAL OUTLINE

I. GROWTH AND DEVELOPMENT OF CHILDREN

A. Terminology

Title	Age
Neonate (newborn):	Birth to 28 days
Infant:	28 days to 1 year
Toddler:	12 months to 3 years
Preschool:	3 to 5 years

B. Late Infancy: 6 Months to 2 Years: Physiologic Development

1. Birth weight is generally doubled by age 4 to 6 months and tripled by age 1 year.

2. Height increases approximately 50 percent in the first year of life. At 2 years, a toddler's height represents approximately 50 percent of his or her eventual adult height.

3. From age 2 years through the preschool years, growth remains relatively stable.

4. A toddler gains 5.5 lb per year and usually quadruples his or her birth weight by age 2.5 years.

5. Head circumference reflects the growth of the brain and is an important parameter to be assessed until at least age 2 years. At age 2 years, the brain attains approximately 90 percent of adult size.

6. The posterior fontanelle usually closes at age 2 months and the anterior fontanelle by 18 months.

7. When toddlers first begin to walk, the trunk is long, legs and arms are short, and the head is proportionately large, giving them a top-heavy appearance.

    a. They walk with their feet spread apart to create a broad base (toddling gait) that helps to compensate for their weight distribution and immature musculoskeletal system.

    b. During the toddler years, muscle tissue begins to replace the high proportion of adipose tissue characteristic of an infant, and bone ossification takes place.

    c. The legs that were slightly bowed straighten and the pot-bellied appearance disappears.

C. Motor Skills

◆ Knowledge of developmental milestones will help parents promote an environment appropriate to their child's needs.

◆ Knowledge of the motor development of preschoolers can assist the nurse in assessing and intervening to promote developmentally appropriate motor activities and preventing injury by being able to anticipate motor activity.

1. Nursing Assessment of Growth and Development

    a. Roll from side to back 4 to 6 months of age.

    b. Roll from abdomen to side 5 to 6 months of age.

    c. Roll from back to abdomen 6 to 7 months of age.

    d. Palmer grasp 5 to 6 months of age.

e. Pincer grasp 8 to 9 months of age.

f. Sit alone 6 to 8 months of age.

g. Learns to chew at approximately 6 to 7 months of age.

h. Uses spoon and drinks from cup at approximately 16 to 18 months of age.

i. Visual depth perception begins to develop by 7 to 9 months of age. Some investigators have found that even 4- to 6-month-old infants can distinguish depth.

j. Language development; can say "ma-da" at 9 to 10 months of age.

k. At approximately 15 months of age, toddler can build a tower of three to four blocks.

l. Eighteen-month-old toddlers can assist in undressing.

m. Most children are able to stand alone by 12 months and walk alone by approximately 15 months.

n. At 2 years of age, toddlers have acquired a more steady gait and generally run well with fewer falls but are not able to stop quickly.

o. Toddlers are involved in parallel play; child plays independently alongside another child.

p. Two-year-olds can assist in self-care by putting on simple garments, but they are not able to differentiate front from back. They are now able to zip and unzip zippers.

q. Two-year-olds can put on shoes but cannot buckle or tie them.

r. Three-year-olds can dress themselves almost completely but still do not know front from back and cannot tie shoes; can tie shoes between 4 and 5 years of age.

s. Between 15 and 18 months of age, one- to two-word utterances are commonly used to communicate (e.g., bye-bye). Between 18 and 24 months of age, children should know at least 10 words.

t. Between 24 and 30 months of age, three-word sentences are uttered.

D. Anticipatory Guidance: Introduction to Solids

1. The nurse can assist the parent by relaying information about the nutritional requirements of infants and developmental skills that aid feeding, and the rationale for current recommendations about introduction of solids.

2. Infants learn to chew at approximately 6 to 7 months and, therefore, are developmentally ready to consume some solid food.

3. Infants have the Palmer grasp ability by age 5 to 6 months and, therefore, are ready to handle solid foods, including finger foods.

4. Infants can feed themselves items such as melba toast and graham crackers.

5. As the infants gain skill chewing, other bite-sized finger foods may be gradually added, including cheese, canned fruit, and cooked vegetables.

6. Foods that are hard, small, and easily aspirated, such as kernel corn, chunks of meat, popcorn, and nuts, should not be given to infants.

7. Infants will need some practice as they learn the new skill of eating solids, changing gradually from a sucking to a chewing motion.

8. One new food should be introduced at a time, and a number of days (3–6) should intervene before another new food is introduced so that any allergic responses can be more easily identified.

9. It has been generally recommended that the first food offered to the infant be rice cereal, as it is considered to be the least allergenic of the cereal grains and because most cereals are fortified with iron.

10. Parents are instructed to introduce cereal by spoon rather than by adding it to the bottle. Research found that low-income mothers introduced cereal to their infants through bottle feeding (Solemn and coworkers, 1992). They lack the understanding that by feeding their infants cereal in the bottle, they are really introducing solids too early.

   a. Fruits are often the next solid food introduced.

   b. Vegetables are introduced next, followed by meats and eggs.

E. Dental Care

1. Dental development during childhood involves the eruption of two sets of teeth—deciduous and permanent.

2. There are 20 deciduous teeth, also called "primary" or "baby teeth." These are gradually replaced by 32 permanent teeth.

3. Deciduous tooth eruption begins at approximately 4 to 6 months of age.

4. At 1 year of age, a child usually has six to eight teeth. Usually, one tooth erupts for each month of age past 6 months, up to 25 to 30 months of age.

5. Most dentists agree that the first visit to the dentist should be made by 2 years of age, preferably before any dental work needs to be done.

6. In communities where water is not fluoridated, a daily supplemental of sodium fluoride should be given to ensure healthy development of the permanent teeth buds and gums.

7. To protect the first teeth, the gums and teeth can be massaged with a soft, moist, clean cloth after each feeding.

8. Tooth brushing is recommended by 18 months of age when gingival tissue is no longer so easily damaged and when a considerable number of teeth are usually present.

9. The nurse should discuss the general pattern of tooth eruption with the family when the infant is approximately 3 months old.

10. Saliva is now being produced, but the infant has not yet learned to swallow without the sucking reflex.

11. This drooling at 3 months is not directly associated with teething.

12. Many symptoms are associated with eruption of teeth, such as fever, vomiting, and diarrhea. A cause-and-effect relationship between teething and these symptoms has not been established.

13. Teething causes discomfort; the child may be irritable and may chew on fingers and teething rings or rubber toys to find some relief.

14. Teething lotions containing alcohol should be avoided; these products are potentially dangerous and could have systemic effects.

15. A bottle of milk or other sweetened fluid should not be given to infants or toddlers while they are falling asleep.

16. These fluids pool in oral cavity and run down the side of the face into the infant's ears, contributing to ear infections.

17. Frequent bottle feedings at night of fermentable carbohydrates, especially sucrose, have been documented as a caries-producing practice.

18. These carbohydrates are acted on by mouth bacteria (particularly streptococci), and metabolic acids are produced. These acids decalcify the tooth enamel and destroy protein structures, resulting in total destruction of the tooth.

19. Early severe dental caries of the deciduous teeth result from this practice.

F. Toilet Training: 18 to 24 Months of Age

1. Bowel training usually occurs before bladder training.

2. Nighttime toilet training may not be accomplished until 3 to 4 years of age.

3. Avoid making an issue of toilet training or implementing punishment for failure.

4. The average urinary output in a 24-h period for preschoolers is 500 to 780 mL.

G. Discipline

1. Discipline is not punishment but instead is teaching the child desirable behavior.

2. Good discipline protects the child from dangerous situations and is based on love and consistency, which will provide a self-reliant, self-controlled child.

3. If the child has temper tantrums, ignore them.

II. SAFETY DURING PRESCHOOL YEARS

The most frequently occurring accidents during preschool years are motor vehicle accidents, drowning, burns, poisonings, and falls.

A. Motor Vehicle Accidents

Children ages 1 to 4 years die in automobile accidents. The use of seat belts is a very important way to reduce this morbidity and mortality.

B. Poisoning

Most common causes of death in boys, with the highest occurring at 2 years of age. The major reason for accidents with poison is improper storage of the containers. (For more information,

see *Core Review Handbook Of Medications for the NCLEX-RN*, Chapter 16.)

C. Pedestrian Accidents

Children age 3 years are often involved in pedestrian accidents because they have good motor skills but poor judgment.

D. Falls

Occur often between the ages of 1 and 2 years because gross and fine motor skills are being developed. At this age, children have no fear of danger and have a lot of curiosity.

E. Drowning

Second highest cause of death for preschool-aged boys and the third highest for preschool-aged girls.

III. BURNS

A. Pediatric Burn Patients

Burns occur most often in preschool-aged girls and rank as the third most important cause of accidental death in children.

1. Size of burns is expressed as percentage of total body surface area burned.

2. Depth of injury

    a. The severity of the injury and the rate of healing are directly related to the amount of undamaged corium from which new tissue can regenerate. The deeper a burn, the more often it will blister. Blisters do not occur in superficial burns. Testing the skin next to the burn area by blanching and refilling indicates whether circulation in the area is intact.

    b. First-degree burns are now called partial-thickness burns.

    c. Second-degree burns are now called deep thermal burns.

    d. Third-degree burns are now called full-thickness burns. These are associated with flames and grease; age affects how deeply the skin is damaged. The elderly (70 years and older) and the very young (neonates and preschool clients) are most affected.

B. Fluid Loss

1. Without protective skin, fluid loss is very high; with maximum loss approximately 48 h after the burn occurs.

2. Fluid is also lost to third spacing (edema). Third spacing is fluid outside the vascular system.

3. Blood volume decreases and the heart is depressed, causing a state of shock. IV fluid replacement is administered carefully because there will be a shift of some fluid back into the vascular system as capillary permeability returns to normal.

4. When the patient is a child and IV fluid is administered at 50 mL/h but only 25 mL/h has been infused, the nurse must notify the physician for new orders. Children, especially burned children, can develop fluid overload easily.

C. Anemia and Burns

1. Anemia results from the loss of red blood cells (RBCs; hemolysis) and bleeding from wounds.

2. Bone marrow depression will occur if sepsis develops.

D. Effect of Burns on the Kidney

1. Third spacing causes poor kidney perfusion and decreased glomerular filtration.

2. Renal vasoconstriction due to hypovolemic shock also causes poor kidney perfusion.

3. Normally, it takes approximately 3 to 4 days to eliminate edema.

E. Nitrogen Loss

1. Increased nitrogen loss in burn patients far exceeds that seen in other injuries.

2. Nitrogen, a component of protein, is necessary for tissue life.

3. Healing will not occur if there is a negative nitrogen balance.

F. Gastric Ulcers

1. The extraordinary stress on the body causes gastric ulcers (Curling's ulcer).

2. Routine use of antacids such as Zantac, Tagamet, or Pepcid slows the production of hydrochloric acid (HCl acid); antacids neutralize HCl and sucralfate (Carafate) coats the stomach lining.

G. Care and Treatment of Burns

1. Nursing priorities include monitoring patient airways if burns are on the upper body, monitoring and maintaining fluid and electrolyte balance, and nursing care of the wound (burned skin).

2. Method of Care

    a. Dressings usually are not used; instead, Telfa sheets are used to prevent the burned skin from sticking to the sheets. No tape is used; elastic knitting is used if the wound is wrapped.

    b. Routine daily hydrotherapy with whirlpool for debridement of wounds. The patient soaks in a Hubert tank for 20 to 30 min to facilitate removal of exudate and medication from the skin.

    c. Topical medications include silver nitrates, sulfonamides, and Silvadene cream. All are very effective.

        (1) Antiinfective agents are applied directly to the wound, using sterile gloves. Children can apply Silvadene cream on the burn because their own bacteria are endogenous to them.

        (2) Broad-spectrum antimicrobial agents are effective against the microorganism *Pseudomonas,* a common cause of burn (wound) infection.

3. Debridement of Wounds

    a. Natural debridement occurs daily with removal of dressings and hydrotherapy.

    b. Sharp debridement is done by a physician using scissors and tweezers daily during "tubing," or with a scalpel under anesthesia in the operating room or in the patient's room. The nurse will give the patient an analgesic prescribed by physician before debridement.

    c. Enzymatic debridement involves the use of enzymes, such as Travase, which destroy dead tissue and can be safe and effective when used with topical agents.

4. Skin Grafting

    a. Temporary wound coverage

        (1) When the full-thickness burn is large, temporary skin coverage is used.

        (2) Temporary skin covers are rejected by the body and are left in place only until grafting can occur.

        (3) Homografts (skin from another donor of the same species) or heterografts (pigskin) are two common forms of temporary grafts.

        (4) The temporary grafts are observed daily for signs of infection, and areas that slough are routinely replaced.

    b. Permanent skin grafts

        (1) Autografting is a surgical procedure that involves transferring a split-thickness skin graft on the patient's own skin to cover a full-thickness wound.

        (2) The patient usually is immobilized for a period after grafting to prevent loss of the graft.

        (3) The graft is assessed for percentage of take and for signs of infection.

    c. Cultured epithelial autografts

        (1) Cultured epithelial autografts are sheets of skin that are grown from a skin biopsy in a laboratory in a special medium, similar to a Petri dish.

        (2) Cultured epithelial autografts have been relatively successful in providing a permanent skin coverage for patients with burns covering at least 80 percent of total body surface area. For permanent coverage, however, epithelial cultures are fragile, extremely expensive, and not desirable; autografts are preferred.

    d. General information

        (1) The *recipient site* is where the physician puts the graft. The *donor site* is where skin is removed to be used for grafting. Do not wash it.

        (2) Isograft is tissue obtained from a genetically identical individual (e.g., an identical twin).

IV. COMPARISON OF THEORIES OF HUMAN GROWTH AND DEVELOPMENT

A. Theorists: Erikson and Freud

1. The stages of development have been studied and described by several noted psychoanalysts; one of the most accomplished is Erik H. Erikson.

TABLE 20–1 ◆ Comparison of Freud's and Erikson's Stages of Development

Age	Freud's Psychosexual Stages	Erikson's Psychosocial Stages
Birth to 18 months	Oral	Trust vs mistrust
1½ to 3 years	Anal	Autonomy vs shame and doubt
3 to 5½ years	Phallic	Initiative vs guilt
5½ to 12 years	Latency	Industry vs inferiority
Adolescence	Genital	Identify vs role confusion
Young adulthood		Intimacy vs isolation
Middle age		Generatively vs self-absorption

2. Erikson's phases of development are based on Freudian theory, but they differ in several important aspects.

3. Erikson emphasizes the ego, rather than the id, and by doing so de-emphasizes many of the bisexual connotations of Freud's theory.

4. Erikson's basic premise supporting the ego assumes that the individual has an innate ability to cope with a usual, predictable environment.

5. Erikson does not stress Freud's philosophy of instinctual motivation, such as a death wish.

6. Erikson believed that play provides the best vehicle for exploring a child's ego; in contrast to Freud, who believed that dreams were the doorway to the unconscious.

7. Another crucial difference between these two theorists is that Erikson stresses the relationship of the individual to his family, community, and world. This broader framework of interpersonal relationships replaced the Freudian mother–child–father triangle.

8. Freud attempted to prove the existence of the unconscious and devoted his research to the study of its development in humans.

9. Erikson, on the other hand, endeavored to study the phases or stage of human psychological development and stressed the solutions to the potential hazards inherent in each phase.

10. Erikson is one of the few theorists who attempted to study the entire lifespan, although the greatest emphasis has been placed on the first and fifth stages: developing a sense of trust and a sense of identity.

11. Erikson's phase I is concerned with acquiring a sense of basic trust while overcoming a sense of mistrust. The trust acquired in infancy is the foundation for all the succeeding phases.

12. Freud's oral stage during infancy involves id gratification through oral satisfaction.

B. Theorist: Piaget

Piaget developed five major stages of cognitive development.

1. Sensorimotor period—first 2 years of life: During the sensorimotor period, the child moves from neonatal birth reflexes to the construction of symbolic images.

2. Preconceptual stage—2 to 4 years: Children can now form mental images to stand for things they cannot see (symbolic thought), including their various properties.

3. Preoperational period—2 to 7 years: The major qualitative change in cognitive function from the sensorimotor period to the preoperational period involves the ability to use symbols. The child's task is to use language and memory to begin to understand the past, present, and immediate future and to steadily move away from egocentric thought.

4. Concrete operational period—7 to 11 years: At the beginning of this stage, the child thinks and reasons with inductive logic but, by the end of this stage, the thinking is deductive and the child's world shifts from "one of mythology to one of science," in which objects and events have explanations. These children can mentally perform tasks that previously they actually had to carry out. They learn to comprehend conservation and reversibility.

5. Formal operational period—11 years and on: This stage is characterized by logical reasoning and the ability to think about the hypothetical and abstract. It is no longer necessary for mental problems to involve concrete objects. Children in this stage can systematically analyze abstract problems and arrive at their possible solutions.

6. Explanation of Piaget's five major stages

　a. At each stage of development, the individual has mental representation of cognitive structure of her or his world, each of which is called a *schema* (plural schemata).

　b. Each schema becomes more complex, more realistic, and more abstract as development progresses.

　c. Each schema involves a mental representation of some facet of the world and observable behavior.

　d. Schemata become more highly developed through the process of assimilation and accommodation.

　e. Piaget believed that adaptation involves continuous twin processes: assimilation and accommodation.

　f. *Assimilation* is the process of incorporating new information into one's current activity or way of thinking (making the unfamiliar seem familiar).

　g. *Accommodation* is a process involving the changing of mental representations in order to include new information that does not fit the existing schema.

C. Theorists: Skinner and Pavlov

1. *Classic conditioning,* a method of using environmental stimuli to bring about a change in behavior, was demonstrated by the Russian psychologist Ivan Pavlov.

2. Classic conditioning involves a process of stimulus substitution in which a new, previously neutral stimulus is substituted for the stimulus that originally elicited the response. In classic conditioning, the stimulus elicits the response.

3. Pavlov rang a bell whenever food was presented to a dog. Soon the stimulus of ringing the bell was all that was needed to elicit the response of salivation.

4. Benjamin F. Skinner extends the concept of classic conditioning to *operant conditioning,* a type of conditioning in which a behavior or response is altered by the stimuli or consequences that follow the response (behavior modification).

5. There are two types of consequences: reinforcers and punishers. A *punisher* is a consequence that follows a response that has the effect of decreasing the frequency of the response it follows.

6. Behavior modification involves the use of reinforcement and punishment to alter behavior.

V. PSYCHOLOGICAL DEVELOPMENT

A. Late Infancy: 6 Months to 2 Years

1. Psychological Development

    a. Preoccupation with self. Major task is to differentiate self from environment (learns that parents exist when physically absent).

    b. Infants at approximately 6 to 8 months of age recognize parents as persons separate from themselves; may develop separation anxiety at this time, particularly from the mother.

    c. Fear of strangers.

    d. At 2 years of age, infant can venture away from parents for brief periods of time; secure in knowing they will return.

B. (Pre)school Child: 3 to 8 Years

1. Psychological Development

    a. Age of fantasy (monsters).

    b. When the child is hospitalized, use dolls to demonstrate to the child any procedure that may be performed on the child. Allow the child to act out and play out his or her feelings.

    c. Children ages 3 to 5 years are afraid of mutilation of the body.

    d. Children ages 1 to 8 years believe death is reversible. After age 8, they believe death is not reversible (final).

    e. School age: Fear of pain and bodily injury, fear of loss of love (e.g., parents), and anxiety related to guilt.

C. Adolescent

1. Psychological Development

    a. Struggle with independence, self-assurance, and self-confidence are major adjustments for adolescents.

    b. Extreme peer pressure is a major problem.

D. Separation Anxiety

1. Hospitalization causes separation anxiety. In the first stage, the child protests, is angry, and throws toys. In the second stage, the child stops crying, shows no interest in people or food, and is very sad. In the third stage, the child is denial, showing no interest in the surroundings.

2. Infants will regress in motor skills (although all children regress to some degree while hospitalized).

E. Anticipatory Guidance

1. Teach the parent or caregiver about expectations from a child at different ages and in different situations. A parent who knows is better prepared to deal with special situations.

2. Anticipatory guidance is knowing what to expect before it happens; for instance, learning how to prevent poisoning is an example of anticipatory guidance.

VI. VITAL SIGNS VALUES FOR CHILDREN

A. Pulse Rate (bpm)

TABLE 20–2

Age	Range (bpm)
Newborn	70 to 170
2 years	80 to 130
10 years	70 to 110

B. Blood Pressure

TABLE 20–3

Age	Average Systolic and Diastolic Pressure
6 years	100/60
14 years	118/60

C. Respirations

TABLE 20–4

Age	Breaths/min
1 year	40 to 90
5 years	20 to 25

Note: Vital signs are used to determine the need for some medications.

VII. HEALTH SCREENING

A. Assessment

Monitoring the infant's growth and development is the foremost concern of health screening.

1. Infants born at home will need to be screened for phenylketonuria and hypothyroidism.

2. Infants from at-risk populations should be screened for inborn errors of metabolism, such as Tay-Sachs disease (see section 24, unit III).

3. Between 9 and 12 months of age, infants are screened for iron deficiency anemia, as this coincides with the depletion of fetal iron stores.

4. Research data suggest that lead intoxication in infants may be more common than previously believed, warranting lead screening beginning at 6 months of age. Venous blood is the most accurate measure of lead content.

VIII. IMMUNIZATION SCHEDULE

A. Recommended Schedule for Active Immunization of Normal Infants, Children, and Preadolescents

1. *Hepatitis B (HepB) vaccine.* All infants should receive the first dose of hepatitis B vaccine soon after birth and before hospital discharge. The first dose may also be given by age 2 months if the infant's mother is hepatitis B surface antigen (HBsAg) negative. Only monovalent HepB can be used for the birth dose. If the mother is infected with hepatitis, hepatitis B immunoglobulin (HBIG) is given with the first dose of hepatitis B vaccine (HBV1).

2. *Diphtheria and tetanus toxoids with acellular pertussis (DTaP) vaccine.* The fourth dose of DTaP may be administered as early as age 12 months.

3. *Haemophilus influenzae type B (HIB) conjugate vaccine.* Three HIB conjugate vaccines are licensed for infant use. Do not administer to patients with sensitivity to eggs, chicken, chicken feathers, or chicken dander. If an allergic condition is suspected, administer a scratch test or an intradermal injection (0.05–0.1 mL) of vaccine diluted 1:100 in sterile saline. A wheal larger than 5 mm justifies withholding immunization.

4. *Inactivated poliovirus (IPV).* Not administered to patients with known hypersensitivity to streptomycin or neomycin. Inactivated, attenuated sterile suspension of three types of polio virus used to produce antibody response against poliomyelitis infection.

5. *Measles, mumps, and rubella (MMR) vaccine.* Should not be administered to patients with a history of anaphylactic hypersensitivity to neomycin or to patients with immune deficiency conditions. Do not administer to pregnant women.

6. *Varicella vaccine.* Recommended at any visit at or after age 12 months for susceptible children (i.e., those who lack a reliable history of chickenpox). Susceptible persons older than 13 years should receive two doses, given at least 4 weeks apart.

7. *Pneumococcal vaccine.* The heptavalent pneumococcal conjugate vaccine (PCV) is recommended for all children age 2 to 24 months. It is also recommended for certain children age 24 to 59 months.

8. *Hepatitis A vaccine.* Recommended for children and adolescents in selected states and regions and for certain high-risk groups; consult your local public health authority.

9. *Influenza vaccine.* Recommended annually for children age 6 months with certain risk factors (including but not limited to children with asthma, cardiac disease, sickle cell disease, human immunodeficiency virus infection, and diabetes) and for household members of persons in high-risk groups.

B. Other Vaccination Information

1. Smallpox Vaccination

   a. Smallpox vaccination has been discontinued since 1971 except for individuals at special risk (i.e., travelers to certain countries where smallpox is present and for individuals in health-related fields).

   b. Health service personnel, which includes nurses, should be revaccinated every 3 years because of their susceptibility due to potential contact with a smallpox victim.

   c. When smallpox vaccination is administered, it should not be given to the following: children younger than 1 year, individuals with eczema, anyone with an altered immune state, pregnant women, and patients with burns, poison ivy, impetigo, or other acute skin lesions, until completely healed.

2. Hepatitis B Immunization

   a. Universal immunization of infants for hepatitis B (HB) has been endorsed by the American Academy of Pediatrics (AAP) and the Immunization Practices Advisory Committee of the US Public Health Services since 1991 to be given within 12 h of birth and again between the ages of 4 to 6 months after the first dose.

   b. Those who are at high risk for infection with HB virus should also be vaccinated.

   c. Groups at risk for contracting hepatitis include the following:

      (1) Clients and staff of institutions for the developmentally disabled

      (2) Recipients of frequent blood transfusions, and blood products, and dialysis patients

      (3) Close contacts with HB virus carriers and/or those with an acute HB virus infection (e.g., sexual, household, especially mother–child contact)

      (4) Children from countries and localities of high HB virus endemicity

      (5) Heterosexually active persons with multiple partners

      (6) Homosexually active men

      (7) IV drug abusers

      (8) International travelers

TABLE 20–5 ◆ Recommended Schedule for Active Immunization of Normal Infants, Childern, and Preadolescents

Age →	Range of Recommended Ages					Catchup Immunizations				Preadolescent		
	Birth	1 mo	2 mo	4 mo	6 mo	12 mo	15 mo	18 mo	24 mo	4–6 Yr	11–12 Yr	13–18 Yr
NOTE	The HBIG vaccine provides prophylaxis against infection in infants born of HBsAg-positive mothers:											
Hepatitis B[1]	HepB 1	HepB 2			HepB 3	HepB 3	HepB 3					
Diphtheria, tetanus, pertussis[2]			DTaP 1	DTaP 2	DTaP 3	DTaP4				DTaP	Td	
Haemophilus influenzae Type B[3]			Hib	Hib	Hib	Hib	Hib					
Inactivated poliovirus[4]			IPV	IPV	IPV	IPV	IPV	IPV		IPV		
Measles, mumps, rubella[5]						MMR 1	MMR 1			MMR 2		
Varicella[6]						Varicella	Varicella	Varicella	Varicella			
Pneumococcal[7]			PCV	PCV	PCV	PCV	PCV	PCV				
Vaccines below this line are for selected populations (susceptible persons)												
Pneumococcal varicella								PCV	PCV	PCV	PCV	
Hepatitis A[8]										Hepatitis A series		
Influenza[9]								Influenza (Yearly)				

Note: Tetanus and diphtheria toxoids (td) are recommended at age 11 to 12 years if at least 5 years have elapsed since the last dose of tetanus and diphtheria toxoid containing vaccine.

[1] **Hepatitis B (HepB) vaccine.** All infants should receive the first dose of hepatitis B Vaccine soon after birth and before hospital discharge; the first dose may also be given by age 2 months if the infant's mother is hepatitis B surface antigen (HBs) negative. Only monovalent HepB can be used for the birth dose.

[2] **Diphtheria and tetanus toxoids with acellular pertussis (DTaP) vaccine.** The fourth dose of DTaP may be administered as early as age 12 months.

[3] **Haemophilus influenzae type B (HIB) conjugates vaccine.** Three HIB conjugate vaccines are licensed for infant use.

[4] **Inactivated Poliovirus (IPV).** Do not administer to patients with known hypersensitivity to streptomycin.

[5] **Measles, mumps, and rubella vaccine (MMR).** Do not administer to patients with history of anaphylactic hypersensitivity to neomycin or to patients with immune deficiency conditions.

[6] **Varicella Vaccine.** Recommended at any visit or after age 12 months for susceptible children (i.e., those who lack a reliable history of chickenpox). Susceptible persons age >13 years should receive two doses, given at least 4 weeks apart.

[7] **Pneumococcal vaccine.** The heptavalent pneumococcal conjugate vaccine (PCV) is recommended for all children age 2 to 24 months. It is also recommended for certain children age 24 to 59 months.

[8] **Hepatitis A Vaccine.** Recommended for children and adolescents in selected states and regions and certain high-risk groups; consult your local public health authority.

[9] **Influenza vaccine.** Recommended annually for children age 6 months with certain risk factors, including but not limited to children with asthma, cardiac disease, human immunodeficiency virus infection, and diabetes, and for household members of persons in high-risk groups.

(9) Infants born to mothers who are HbsAg positive

(10) Health care workers who are exposed to blood (e.g., those in operating rooms, intensive care units, emergency rooms, laboratories, and those who care for dental patients)

(11) Possible transmission of HB virus in the child care setting is an increasing concern to public health authorities.

(12) Children who are HB virus carriers can transmit the virus if they have generalized dermatitis, bleeding, problems and scratches, or if they bite others.

IX. DEFECTIVE ABSORPTION OF NUTRIENTS

A. Gastroenteritis

Inflammation of the stomach, intestinal tract, or both, can cause defective absorption of nutrients.

1. Cause

    a. An enteric pathogen, such as *Shigella, Salmonella, Staphylococcus aureus, Escherichia coli,* or *Clostridium botulinum* (a species that grows in improperly processed foods).

B. Dysentery

Term applied to a number of intestinal disorders characterized by intestinal inflammation, especially of the colon. It is accompanied by cramping, abdominal pain, and watery stools containing blood and mucus.

1. Cause

    a. Usually a bacteria or virus.

2. Signs and Symptoms for Defective Absorption of Nutrients

    a. Diarrhea, abdominal discomfort (cramping), and nausea and vomiting.

    b. Other symptoms include fever and malaise.

3. Treatment for Gastroenteritis and Dysentery

    a. Antimicrobial agents (IV)

    b. Fluids (IV)

    c. Electrolyte replacement

    d. Antiemetics [orally (PO), intramuscularly (IM), rectal suppository]

    e. Steroids

    f. Watch for dehydration

    g. Avoid milk, which may provoke recurrence

    h. Record intake and output (I&O)

4. Nursing Implications

    a. Administer medications as ordered; give antiemetics 30 to 40 min before meals.

    b. If client can eat, replace lost fluids and electrolytes with ginger ale or broth, as tolerated.

    c. Record I&O carefully.

    d. Observe for signs of dehydration by assessing laboratory values. For example, increased hematocrit may be an indication of dehydration. Also observe urinary output for quantity and concentration.

C. Hirschsprung's Disease (Megacolon)

1. Incidence

    a. Disease is identified and treated in infancy; occurs in 1 of 5000 people.

    b. Occurs almost entirely in white males (seven times more common in males than females).

2. Cause

    a. Congenital disorder consists of the absence of parasympathetic nerve cells in the large bowel.

    b. Normal bowel becomes hypertrophied and greatly dilated because of lack of peristaltic waves in the affected bowel; therefore, fecal mass accumulates and impedes reabsorption of vitamins and minerals.

    Note: Need large amount of water for enema.

3. Signs and Symptoms

    a. Neonate delays passage of meconium or shows other signs of intestinal obstruction.

4. Treatment

    a. Surgical treatment involves pulling the normal ganglionic segment through the anus.

    b. This corrective surgery usually is delayed until the infant is at least 10 to 12 months old and can undergo the surgery with less risk.

    c. Management of an infant until the time of surgery includes daily colonic lavages to empty the bowel.

    d. If total obstruction is present in the newborn, a temporary colostomy or ileostomy is necessary to decompress the bowel.

5. Nursing Implications

    a. A preliminary bowel prep with an antibiotic such as neomycin or nystatin is necessary before surgery.

    b. Prior to surgery, colonic lavage with normal saline solution is necessary to evacuate the intestine.

    c. After corrective surgery, do not use a rectal thermometer or suppository until the wound has healed.

    d. After 3 to 4 days, infant will have first bowel movement; even a liquid stool will create discomfort. Administer stool softener as ordered by physician. Record number of stools.

    e. Instruct parents to avoid foods that increase the number of stools.

    f. Reassure parents that their child probably will gain sphincter control and be able to eat a normal diet, but educate them that complete continence may take several years to develop.

g. To promote bonding after hospitalization, encourage parents to participate in their child's care as much as possible.

h. Measure and record nasogastric (NG) drainage, and replace fluid and electrolytes as ordered.

i. Teach parents to recognize the signs of fluid loss and dehydration (decreased urinary output, increase in specific gravity, sunken eyes, and poor skin turgor).

D. Celiac Disease

1. Cause and Incidence

a. Etiology is unknown, but it is believed to be an inborn error of metabolism or an immunologic response causing sensitivity to and an inability to utilize glutens.

b. The disease is relatively uncommon, although it is one of the two most common malabsorptive disorders in children (cystic fibrosis is the most common). It affects twice as many females as males.

2. Signs

Insidious and chronic symptoms begin when the child begins to ingest grains, the chief source of glutens (rice cereal has a small amount of gluten).

a. Steatorrhea (fat, foul, frothy, bulky stools)

b. General malnutrition, abdominal distention

c. Dry skin, eczema, and psoriasis may occur

d. Peripheral neuropathy caused by lack of vitamin B_6 resulting in convulsions or paresthesia

e. Loss of fat-soluble vitamins (A, D, E, and K)

f. Loss of fluids, electrolytes, and essential minerals

g. Pernicious anemia from poor absorption of vitamin B_6

h. Loss of folic acid and iron may cause iron deficiency anemia

i. Osteoporosis, tetany, and bone pain are due to loss of calcium caused by vitamin D deficiency

3. Symptoms

a. Clinical manifestations: insidious and chronic symptoms do not begin until the child is ingesting grains, the chief source of glutens; rice cereal has small amounts of gluten

b. Weakness and anorexia

c. Stomach cramps

4. Treatment

a. Treatment requires lifelong elimination of gluten from the client's diet. Even with this exclusion, full to normal absorption may not occur for months or at all.

b. Gluten is found in grains of wheat and rye and in smaller quantities in barley and oats. Eliminate these grains and substitute corn and rice.

c. Supportive treatment includes supplemental vitamins, iron, folic acid, vitamin B_6, and reversal of electrolyte imbalance (by IV infusion if necessary). The IV fluid replacement is necessary for dehydration.

d. Medications include corticosteroids (prednisone, hydrocortisone) to treat accompanying adrenal insufficiency, and vitamin K for hypoprothrombin.

e. Celiac crisis is life threatening. Treat with NG tube attached to intermittent suction to decrease abdominal distention. IV fluids with supplements of potassium chloride (KCl), calcium, and magnesium; albumin infusion to prevent shock, if hypoproteinemia is severe; and IV steroids to decrease bowl inflammation.

5. Nursing Implications

a. Explain to parents the necessity for a gluten-free diet.

b. Advise elimination of barley, rye, wheat, and oats and food made from them, such as bread and baked goods; suggest substitution of corn or rice.

c. Advise parents to consult a dietitian for a gluten-free diet, which is high in protein and low in carbohydrates and fats.

d. Instruct parents on recording I&O and number of stools (may exceed 12 per day).

e. Educate parents on signs of dehydration, such as dry skin and poor skin turgor.

f. Explain the need for frequent medical checkups to monitor hemoglobin, prothrombin time, and hematocrit.

g. Advise parents on administration of medications, iron, folic acid, vitamin B_6, and steroids and the need for adequate fluid intake.

E. Failure to Thrive

Failure to thrive (FTT) is also known as maternal deprivation, or it may be called parent deprivation. FTT is a common disorder of infancy.

1. Etiology and Incidence

a. Children are below the third percentile in growth but demonstrate no organic cause.

b. Lack of physical growth is secondary to the lack of emotional and sensory stimulation from the mother or caregiver.

c. The child tends to be stiff and rigid; is uncomforted and unyielding to cuddling or holding; and is very slow to smile or respond socially to others. Or the child may be a floppy infant who feels like a rag doll when held. Neither child molds to the holder's body.

d. Although FTT is believed to be caused by maternal deprivation (caregiver deprivation), it may be caused by organic disorders such as malabsorption syndrome, renal insufficiency, congenital heart defects, or neurologic lesions.

2. Treatment

a. Good nutritional intake and loving care, demonstrated by rocking and holding the infant (or child) when feeding, and comforting them when they cry

b. Meeting emotional needs of infant (child)

3. Nursing Implications

a. Data collection should include the prenatal history (including the circumstances of the pregnancy), prenatal course, feeding history, and the child's growth and development.

b. Assessment of family functioning, including communications patterns, is essential. Because parents of FTT infants often feel inadequate, the nurse must use sensitivity and empathetic interviewing skills to elicit the assessment data.

c. Infant should be observed interacting with his or her primary caregiver in feeding situations and in play situations.

d. Observe the way the child is held and fed and how eye contact is initiated by primary caregiver(s); also note the facial expressions of the child and caregiver during interactions.

X. DEFECTIVE UTILIZATION OF NUTRIENTS

A. Idiopathic Nephrotic Syndrome

1. Incidence

a. Predominantly a disease of preschool-aged children, with a peak of onset between 2 and 3 years of age.

b. Uncommon in infants younger than 1 year.

2. Cause

a. Unknown; it occurs in the absence of systemic disease or preexisting renal disease.

3. Signs and Symptoms

a. The glomerular membrane, which is impermeable to albumin (protein) and other large proteins, becomes permeable to protein, especially albumin, which leaks through the membrane and is lost in the urine (proteinuria).

b. This reduces the serum albumin level (hypoalbuminemia), which decreases the colloidal osmotic pressure in the vascular system. As a result, fluid cannot be held within the vascular system and will shift to the interstitial spaces and body cavities, particularly the abdominal cavity (ascites).

c. The shift of fluid from the vascular system to the interstitial spaces reduces the vascular fluid volume, causing hypovolemia and hypotension.

d. Severe dependent edema of the ankles and periorbital edema and ascites may occur.

4. Diagnosis

a. Massive proteinuria occurs, and the total serum protein level is reduced.

5. Treatment

a. Bed rest

b. High-protein diet

c. Corticosteroid therapy [children who require steroid therapy for a long period of time, 1 year or more, are highly susceptible to complications such as growth retardation, hypertension, gastrointestinal (GI) bleeding, Cushing's syndrome, bone demineralization, infection, and diabetes mellitus]

6. Nursing Implications

a. Maintain child on bed rest during acute phase of disorder.

b. Encourage high protein intake (e.g., meats, eggs, and beans).

c. Administer steroids as ordered by physician.

d. Monitor I&O.

XI. DEFECTS IN THE GASTROINTESTINAL TRACT THAT INTERFERE WITH NUTRITIONAL INTAKE

A. Esophageal Atresia and Tracheoesophageal Fistula

The infant has an esophageal atresia (a pouch) that will not allow food down the esophagus and a fistula (hole) into the trachea that can cause aspiration.

1. Signs and Symptoms

a. Excess amount of mucus (bubbling out)

b. Choking, sneezing, and coughing, especially when being fed

c. The feeding often is expelled out immediately through the nostrils and mouth

d. Cyanosis

2. Diagnosis is confirmed by x-ray film.

3. Treatment

a. Suction of esophageal pocket with NG tube and immediate surgery.

4. Nursing Implications

a. Prevent aspiration. Preoperatively, position the infant with head and chest elevated 45 to 60 degrees. This accomplishes two goals:

(1) Secretions are pooled in the bottom of the esophageal pouch, facilitating withdrawal by constant suctioning

(2) Gravity counteracts gastric reflux into trachea and lungs when the head is elevated.

b. Keeping infant quiet by stroking and gentle handling will reduce crying, which causes gastric regurgitation.

c. The nurse supports the parents before surgery by keeping them informed on the status of their infant.

d. Use pacifier when sump pump is in esophageal pouch to diminish crying and satisfy the infant's need to suck.

e. Postoperatively, two of the nurse's most important goals are to maintain a patent airway and to prevent trauma to the anastomoses.

(1) To meet both of these goals, a suction catheter is marked by the surgeon to the maximum length that can be inserted when suctioning through the nares to ensure that the catheter is not passed farther than a point just above the anastomosis.

(2) The nurse carefully observes the infant for early signs of airway obstruction. An anxious expression on the infant's face is often the first sign, followed by increased respiratory rate.

f. When there is serious airway obstruction, the onset of chest muscle retractions will occur.

g. Postoperatively, the infant usually is positioned with the head slightly elevated, in a warm humidified environment.

h. Hyperextension of the neck must be avoided to prevent pull on the sutured esophagus.

i. Infant's position should be changed from back to side at least every 2 h to prevent pneumonia and to provide comfort.

j. Percussion and postural drainage are also used as preventive measures; for the first 3 to 4 days, only vibration on the back is performed while suture lines heal.

k. Oral feeding can be started by the third day; if infant must remain NPO for 8 days or longer, total parenteral nutrition (TPN) may be administered.

l. If infant has a gastrostomy, it is placed on gravity drainage for 2 to 3 days to prevent aspiration.

m. The infant's head and chest are elevated 45 to 60 degrees using an infant's seat. Gastrostomy feeding of formula or expressed breast milk is administered on approximately postoperative day 4, cautiously increasing volume and strength.

B. Intussusception

Telescoping of intestines (invagination or telescoping of part of the intestine into an adjacent portion of the intestine)

1. Incidence and Etiology

a. Intussusception occurs most commonly in healthy well-nourished male infants approximately 6 months of age.

b. It can occur in children of any age but is rare before 3 months and occurs with decreased frequency after age 3 years.

c. The cause of intussusception is unknown in most cases. Etiologic factors are Meckel's diverticulum or a tumor near the ileocecal valve and are present in fewer than 10 percent of afflicted children.

2. Signs and Symptoms

a. Red currant jelly–like stool (appearance due to the presence of blood and mucus as a result of intestinal irritation), colicky pain, and distended abdomen with sausage-shaped abdominal mass.

b. Infant draws their legs up sharply with a piercing cry.

c. The infant usually vomits, becomes extremely restless, and may appear diaphoretic and pale.

3. Diagnosis and Treatment

a. Barium enema study confirms the diagnosis and, in many cases, can successfully treat the intussusception through hydrostatic reduction.

b. The infant must be prepared for a barium enema as though surgery will follow, because if reduction by barium enema is unsuccessful, the infant undergoes an operation immediately to correct the intussusception.

4. Nursing Implications

a. The nurse must be able to give accurate guidance when parents initially report symptoms. Because the infant may sleep and be comfortable between attacks, the seriousness of the symptoms may be overlooked by a nurse who is not familiar with the signs and symptoms of intussusception.

b. The nurse must advise the family to seek immediate medical attention.

c. Postoperatively, the nurse must help the family cope with the stress of caring for the infant, who is not allowed to eat, requires frequent position changes, and must be restrained to prevent dislodging of the NG tube and IV needle.

C. Pyloric Stenosis

◆ Overgrowth (hypertrophy and hyperplasia) of the circular muscle of the pylorus, which results in obstruction of the pyloric sphincter.

◆ The pylorus is the opening through which food passes from the stomach to the intestines.

1. Incidence and Etiology

Although the cause of pyloric stenosis is unknown, there seems to be a hereditary component or at least a familial tendency.

2. Signs and Symptoms

a. At approximately 3 weeks of age, the infant begins to regurgitate small amounts of milk immediately after feeding.

b. Within 1 week, the vomitus can be propelled distances of several feet and occur with almost every feeding.

c. The vomiting usually occurs during the feeding or shortly thereafter, but in some instances it occurs several hours later.

d. The infant is hungry after vomiting and will take milk again.

e. The vomitus contains no bile because the obstruction is proximal to the ampulla of water, the site at which the common bile duct enters the duodenum.

f. If untreated, the infant will lose weight, show signs of dehydration, and become alkalotic (vomiting HCl acid).

g. With excessive loss of gastric juices, the electrolytes potassium, sodium, and chloride are lost.

3. Diagnosis

a. Symptoms of vomiting after each feeding and peristaltic waves may be noted, moving from left to right toward pylorus. This will be the first indication of pyloric stenosis.

b. The hypertrophied pylorus can be palpated in the right epigastrium under the edge of the liver.

c. If pyloric stenosis is present, barium contrast studies reveal delayed gastric emptying and an elongated, narrow pyloric canal.

d. Frequently, the pyloric mass can also be identified on ultrasonographic examination of the abdomen.

4. Treatment and Nursing Implications

a. If an infant is dehydrated and experiencing an electrolyte imbalance, surgery may be delayed from 24 to 36 h while the infant receives IV fluids containing potassium and other electrolytes as needed.

b. Parents are taught how to protect the IV site while holding their infant and are encouraged to be present during this period to hold, comfort, and talk to the infant.

c. Parents are prepared for the surgery and the postoperative period by being told what to expect.

d. Parents are warned about the potential for vomiting in the immediate postoperative period and the need for gradual reintroduction of fluids (bottle or breast milk).

XII. NEUROLOGIC DISEASES

A. Viral Meningitis (Aseptic Meningitis)

1. Etiology

a. Viral meningitis often follows mumps, measles, herpes, and herpes simplex virus.

b. *Haemophilus influenzae* type B (HIB) is the leading cause of bacterial meningitis and septic arthritis in infants. Approximately 75 percent of all serious HIB infections occur in children younger than 18 months. (HIB vaccine may be given simultaneously with DTP and MMR vaccine if different injection sites are used. For more information on bacterial meningitis, see Chapter 9.)

2. Signs and Symptoms

a. Headache, fever, malaise, GI symptoms, nausea and vomiting, sore throat.

b. Symptoms usually subside spontaneously and rapidly; the child is well in 3 to 10 days, with no residual effects.

3. Diagnosis

Diagnosis is made based on concurrent or recent viral illness and examination of cerebrospinal fluid (CSF) to differentiate this condition from bacterial meningitis.

4. Treatment

a. Treatment is supportive. The child is hospitalized for close monitoring of neurologic status.

b. Severely ill children may need placement in the intensive care unit for intubation, mechanical ventilation, and increased intracranial pressure (ICP) monitoring.

c. Persistent seizures may be common.

d. Hydration is closely monitored because overhydration increases cerebral edema.

e. Anticonvulsant drugs (e.g., phenytoin [Dilantin]) are crucial.

f. The prognosis for outcome and sequelae of encephalitis (inflammation of the brain) is guarded. Young infants have the poorest prognosis.

5. Nursing Implications

a. Nursing care for an infant with acute viral meningitis follows the care for a child with increased ICP. Nursing care includes the following:

(1) Surveillance to allow prompts recognition of signs and symptoms leading to early treatment (e.g., perform neurologic check every 1–2 h).

(2) Administration of medication (e.g., mannitol, Dilantin).

(3) Elevate head of bed 30 degrees to facilitate venous outflow from brain by gravity.

(4) Maintain fluid restrictions as ordered to decrease cerebral blood volume.

(5) Provide psychosocial comfort measures.

b. Families may feel frightened and frustrated at having no definitive treatment for what can be a severe illness.

c. Nursing diagnosis of powerlessness is often appropriate for the families.

d. Interventions include allowing the patient frequent opportunities to express feelings, and support for spiritual and emotional needs.

B. Spinal Cord Defects

1. Spina Bifida Cystica or Occulta

a. Spina bifida cystica is the incomplete fusion of one or more of the vertebral laminae, resulting in external protrusion of the spinal tissue.

b. This open type of defect occurs most commonly in the lumbosacral area.

c. If the anomaly is not visible externally, it is termed *spina bifida occulta.*

d. If there is an external saccular protrusion, the defect is termed *spina bifida cystica.*

2. Types of Spinal Cord Defects

a. *Myelomeningocele:* More severe and most common open "neural tube defect" (NTD) involving a protruding saclike structure that contains meninges, spinal fluid, and neural tissue. The spinal nerve roots may terminate in the sac, significantly affecting motor and sensory function below that point. Can cause neurogenic bladder; predisposes infant to infection and renal failure, bladder bowel incontinence, and total paralysis of the legs.

b. *Meningocele:* Less common open NTD containing only meninges and CSF. Neurologic complications can occur but are less severe than myelomeningocele.

c. *Spina bifida occulta:* Incomplete closure of one or more vertebrae without protrusion of the spinal cord or meninges. It often is accompanied by a depression with a tuft of hair or soft fatty deposits. Rarely causes neurologic deficit.

3. Incidence and Etiology

   a. Myelomeningocele is the most common open NTD, affecting 0.2 to 4.2 of every 1000 live births.

   b. The cause is defective embryonic spinal cord development (neural tube fails).

4. Signs and Symptoms

   a. Spina bifida may be overlooked, but occasionally it is palpable.

   b. Meningocele and myelomeningocele are visible; protrusion on the spine can be seen and any neurologic defects are observable.

5. Treatment

   a. Spina bifida: No surgery necessary.

   b. Meningocele: Surgical closure necessary.

   c. Myelomeningocele: Surgical closure, but does not reverse neurologic deficits.

6. Prognosis

   a. Varies, depending on the degree of neurologic defect.

   b. Prognosis is poor when large spinal cord area is open, as with myelomeningocele, where meninges, CSF, and a portion of spinal cord protrude out of the spine.

   c. Prognosis is better for those with spina bifida occulta and meningocele than those with other spinal cord defects.

C. Hydrocephalus

Congenital hydrocephalus is caused by abnormal enlargement of cerebral ventricles and skull.

1. Etiology

   a. Excessive accumulation of CSF within the ventricular space.

   b. Blockage of outflow of CSF from the cerebral ventricles.

2. Incidence

   a. Congenital hydrocephalus is encountered in approximately 1 in 2000 fetuses.

3. Diagnosis by CT scan.

4. Treatment

   a. Surgical placement of a ventriculoatrial shunt is the most effective treatment and allows fluid to drain from the lateral ventricle of the brain into the right atrium of the heart. This shunt is rarely used and is chosen only if a concurrent abdominal problem exists or for use in neonates.

   b. Generally, the ventriculoperitoneal bypass procedure is used in older children with blockage of outflow (noncommunicating hydrocephalus). Technical difficulties can preclude its use in neonates because these spaces are poorly developed; the procedure is performed as soon as possible to prevent brain damage.

   c. Correction of CSF obstruction is accomplished by direct removal of the obstruction, for example, resection of neoplasm, cyst, or hematoma.

   d. Medical therapy is directed toward reducing production of CSF but has proved to be ineffective in some cases of hydrocephalus involving overproduction of CSF. In these instances, acetazolamide (Diamox) has been only modestly successful in reestablishing equilibrium between CSF production and absorption.

5. Nursing Implications

   a. The infant's head must be balanced carefully and must be supported. The head is edematous and susceptible to decubitus ulcer; change position and turn every 1 to 2 h.

   b. Measure circumference of head once during each shift.

   c. Observe fontanelle for bulging, fullness, and tension.

   d. I&O important; feed frequently because of tendency to vomit.

   e. Help parents cope.

6. Postoperative Care

   a. Place infant on nonoperative side, with head level with body.

   b. Infant should be kept flat in bed and not held in an upright position immediately after surgery and postoperatively for 10 to 15 days. An upright position will cause the CSF to drain too rapidly out of the ventricles. (CSF drainage stabilizes after approximately 15 days.)

   c. If fluid drains too rapidly out of the lateral ventricle, it can pull the brain into the spinal cord, causing death.

7. Prognosis: Untreated hydrocephalus has a 50 to 60 percent mortality rate.

   a. Of the treated surviving children, approximately one third are intellectually normal.

   b. A large majority of these children have physical handicaps.

   c. c. Half have neurologic handicaps such as ataxia, poor fine motor coordination, perceptual deficits, and spastic diplegia (paralysis similar on both sides of the body).

   d. The prognosis of children with treated hydrocephalus depends mainly on the cause of the condition.

D. Microcephaly

1. Infants are born with very small heads and probably total brain damage, for which there is no treatment (the brain never had a chance to expand).

2. If the fontanelles are closed, it indicates microcephaly.

3. If the fontanelles are open, there is a chance that the head may grow normally, with no brain damage.

E. Craniosynostosis

1. Premature closing of the sutures of the skull, producing deformity of the head; frequently with damage to the brain and eyes.

2. If the fontanelles close prematurely, they can be surgically opened.

3. If the fontanelles close too quickly, the brain cannot expand, causing brain damage.

XIII. RESPIRATORY DISEASES

A. Sudden Infant Death Syndrome (SIDS)

1. Incidence

a. SIDS is the number one cause of death in infants aged 2 weeks to 1 year.

b. It outranks death from all types of congenital abnormalities, and it kills more than twice the number of children that die of cancer each year.

c. SIDS deaths number 8000 to 10,000 per year.

d. Autopsies often reveal pulmonary edema.

2. Characteristics of Death from SIDS

a. Conclusive evidence points to an occluded airway as the cause of death.

b. There are four characteristics of every death (occurs unexpectedly).

    (1) Infant is asleep.

    (2) Apnea occurs.

    (3) Death is silent.

    (4) Death usually occurs between the ages of 4 weeks to 7 months.

c. The known fact that the infant could not (did not) cry out supports the conclusion that the airway was blocked at the area of the vocal cord from laryngeal spasm.

d. The infant is often found in a corner of a disheveled bed with blankets over the head and frothy, blood-tinged sputum in the mouth and nose. The diaper is filled with stool, and a hand still clutches the sheet (as if the infant died in distress).

3. Nursing Implications

a. Encourage parents to participate in support groups. Help parents understand that the infant's death was not their fault.

b. Give the parents time with the deceased infant.

B. Croup

1. Incidence

a. Croup usually results from a viral infection and is seen more often in children aged 3 months to 3 years.

b. Bacterial infections are most common in children aged 3 to 7 years.

c. It occurs more often in males than in females.

2. Signs and Symptoms

a. Signs indicate an inspiratory stridor (a harsh sound due to varying degrees of laryngeal obstruction), respiratory distress, and characteristic sharp, barklike cough.

b. These symptoms can last only a few hours or can persist for 1 to 2 days.

3. Treatment

a. If a viral infection, humid atmosphere is necessary. If croup occurs at home, suggest to the parents that they take the child with them in the shower, which is a moist atmosphere.

b. If bacterial infection, antibiotics are used in conjunction with moist air.

4. Assessment

a. Carefully monitor cough and breath sounds.

b. Observe for severity of retractions, cyanosis, respiratory rate, fever, and cardiac rate.

c. Avoid sedation because it may depress respiration.

C. Respiratory Distress Syndrome (RDS) or Hyaline Membrane Disease

1. Etiology

a. The preterm newborn is born before the lungs are fully developed.

b. Prior to birth, there is evidence of respiratory activity. The lungs make a feeble respiratory movement, and fluid is brought into the lungs.

c. At the time of birth, the newborn must initiate breathing and then keep the previously fluid-filled lungs inflated with air. Most full-term newborns successfully accomplish these adjustments, but the preterm newborn with RDS is unable to.

d. Several factors are involved. Most authorities believe that the lack of surfactant is the major cause of RDS. Without surfactant, the newborn is unable to keep the lungs inflated.

2. Incidence

a. RDS is the most common cause of neonatal mortality.

b. RDS is seen almost exclusively in preterm newborns, in newborns of diabetic mothers, and in newborns born by Cesarean section (usually premature in both cases).

3. Signs and Symptoms

a. RDS occurs within 30 min to 2 h after birth; breathing gradually becomes more difficult, and the infant displays substernal retraction.

b. Retractions are a prominent feature of pulmonary difficulties in preterm newborns because they have a compliant chest wall.

c. Within a few hours, respiratory distress becomes more obvious. The respiratory rate increases (from 80 to 120 breaths/min), and breathing becomes more labored. The newborn becomes cyanotic, flaccid, and unresponsive.

d. Auscultation of the chest reveals diminished breath sounds. Assisted ventilation is necessary or the newborn will die.

4. Treatment

a. Assist ventilation.

b. General supportive measures include minimal handling of neonate, maintaining a constant thermal environment, and providing adequate caloric intake and hydration.

c. Oral feedings are contraindicated in any situation that creates a marked increase in respiratory rate because of the hazards of aspiration.

d. Synthetic surfactant has been developed and is beginning to be used in research hospitals.

XIV. COMMONLY OCCURRING BRAIN TUMORS IN CHILDREN

A. Neuroblastoma

Brain tumors are classified according to histology and location.

1. Etiology and Incidence

    a. Brain tumors are the most common solid tumors in children, accounting for approximately 20 percent of childhood malignancies, and are the second most common type of cancer in children and adolescents.

    b. They occur most often in children between the ages of 5 and 10 but can occur at any age from infancy to adulthood.

2. Signs and Symptoms

    a. The signs and symptoms of brain tumors in children are diverse and related to the location of the tumor in the brain and child's age.

    b. Symptoms are most often associated with signs of ICP. Early signs and symptoms may be headache or change in behavior and personality.

    c. Because many early symptoms of intracranial tumors are similar to those of common childhood illnesses, early diagnosis is often difficult. Changes in behavior in school, such as irritability and fatigue, may be attributed to the child's dislike for school.

    d. It may not be diagnosed until physical changes become significant enough to require medical assistance.

3. Clinical Manifestations of Elevated ICP

    a. Infants: Bulging anterior fontanelle; full tense, bulging above bone. Bulging should be checked when infant is not crying because crying will cause temporary bulging of the fontanelle.

    b. Normal increase in head circumference: more than 2 cm per month in first 3 months of life, more than 1 cm per month in the second 3 months, and more than 0.5 cm per month for the next 6 months.

    c. All children may have headaches that are generalized or localized; often present on awakening and standing up in the morning; pain is increased by Valsalva maneuver, coughing, straining at stool, holding breath. Other symptoms include the following:

        (1) Irritability, fatigue, altered consciousness, memory loss, confusion

        (2) Vomiting in the absence of nausea, especially on arising in the morning; may be projectile

        (3) Altered vision, diplopia (double vision); strabismus (deviation of the eye, may be crossed), results from pressure on one or both abducens nerves and child will have restricted visual field

    d. Late Signs (Immediate Intervention Required)

        (1) Altered vital signs; elevated systolic blood pressure caused by an attempt to bring more blood to injured ischemic brain tissue causes a widening pulse pressure.

        (2) Bradycardia caused by pressure on cranial nerve X (vagus nerve) nucleus, which is in the lower brainstem and on the vasomotor center in the medulla.

        (3) Altered respiratory pattern caused by pressure on the respiratory center in the medulla can result in ataxia (defective respiratory muscle coordination) and apnea.

XV. CLASSIFICATION OF MALIGNANT BRAIN TUMORS

A. Medulloblastoma

1. Incidence

    a. Occurs twice as often in boys as in girls.

    b. Peak incidence is between 5 to 10 years of age.

2. Signs and Symptoms

    Clinical manifestations are a 1- to 3-month history of headache, vomiting, ataxia, and nuchal rigidity.

3. Treatment

    a. Surgical resection using microsurgery aided by precise delineation on CT or MRI scan.

    b. Chemotherapy may be administered before and after surgery.

B. Cerebella Astrocytoma

1. Incidence

    Cerebella astrocytoma is the most common childhood brain tumor.

2. Signs and Symptoms

    a. Clinical manifestations include 3- to 6-month history of headache, vomiting, and visual disturbance.

    b. Ataxia and poor hand coordination; child gradually becomes irritable and lethargic.

3. Treatment

    a. Extensive surgical resection; radiation may be used after surgery.

C. Brainstem Tumor

1. Incidence

    a. Peak incidence from 6 to 10 years of age.

2. Signs and Symptoms

   a. Rapid 1- to 3-month onset of cranial nerve deficits.

   b. Upper and lower extremity weakness is common.

3. Treatment

   a. Surgery rarely performed because of involvement of brain's vital center.

   b. Radiotherapy is used palliatively to extend survival from several months to 1 year.

D. Cerebellar Astrocytoma

1. Incidence

   a. Peak incidence from 8 to 12 years of age.

2. Signs and Symptoms

   a. Clinical manifestations include headache, vomiting, visual disturbance, seizures, weakness, and sensory abnormalities.

3. Treatment

   a. Complete surgical resection often is not possible; radiation is used in high doses.

   b. Chemotherapy may be beneficial when combined with radiation.

E. Optic Pathway Tumor

Slow-growing tumor occurring in optic nerve.

1. Incidence

Peak incidence approximately 5 years of age or younger.

2. Signs and Symptoms

   a. Clinical manifestations include visual deficits (decreased acuity), which can cause blindness.

3. Treatment

   a. Surgical excision sometimes possible when only one optic nerve is involved.

   b. Radiation therapy may be curative or palliative, depending on the extent of tumor invasion.

   c. Chemotherapy may be beneficial for children younger than 5 years and is preferable because radiation is very destructive to the tissue of very young children.

4. Diagnostic Assessment

   a. If a brain tumor is suspected, one or more studies can be done. A CT scan is a noninvasive, radiologic procedure that produces multiple serial pictures of a cross-section of the brain.

   b. If a contrast-enhancing isotope is given IV at the time of CT scan, most tumors will take up the isotope at the site of the tumor if it is magnified, providing more information of the tumor's size.

   c. CT scans have become the single most important study for diagnosing brain tumors.

   d. MRI may also be used; it is a noninvasive, nuclear procedure that has proved effective for early diagnosis of many types of brain tumors and for monitoring tumor growth.

   e. Other studies used to evaluate the extent of malignancy include bone marrow aspiration and biopsy and lumbar puncture.

5. Nursing Implications

   a. Nurse will assess for signs of increased ICP, such as change in alertness, elevated systolic blood pressure, decreased pulse and respiration, change in pupil reaction, and vomiting.

   b. Assess the parent's need for information about diagnostic studies and give information as needed.

   c. During diagnostic phase, the family usually is anxious and distraught once they recognize the possibility that their child may have a brain tumor.

   d. The nurse must assist the family during this phase by continually reassessing the family's ability to cope with medical information and necessary procedures.

   e. The child undergoing radiation therapy has unique needs that must be addressed in terms of nursing management.

     (1) Short-term goal involves assisting the child and family in understanding to what degree this treatment will be successful.

     (2) The nurse must assess the level of fear and anxiety associated with the treatment.

     (3) Children may experience side effects of radiation therapy involving the tissues and organs that lie within the radiotherapy treatment field.

     (4) The family must be told that the side effects of radiation therapy can occur acutely, during treatment, or shortly after treatment is completed, and that late effects can occur in future years.

       (a) Children receiving radiotherapy to the head and neck region likely will experience oral ulceration, decreased salivation, and loss of taste sensation.

       (b) Oral ulcers and loss of taste sensation can lead to dehydration and poor nutritional intake.

       (c) Long-term dental, hearing, vision, learning, and growth problems may require specialized management.

       (d) It usually is frightening for children to begin radiation therapy treatment because they are left alone in rooms with large machines.

       (e) Because children must lie perfectly still on a flat bare table while alone in a room during radiotherapy treatment, sedation usually is required.

       (f) Even general anesthesia and use of immobilization devices to allow for safe and precise administration of radiotherapy may be necessary.

       (g) Because the terminology of treatment can confuse the family, the nurse should explain that cancer chemotherapy drugs are also called "antineoplastic agents," with "anti" meaning against and neoplastic meaning "new, abnormal cell growth."

(i) Most antineoplastic agents affect cells in the process of dividing into new cells.

(ii) Normal, rapidly growing cells, such as bone marrow, hair follicle cells, cells in the oral cavity and rectum, and cells of gonads, re affected to varying degrees.

(iii) Understanding these concepts helps the nurse to explain the side effects of chemotherapy to the family.

(iv) Chemotherapy causes bone marrow depression, resulting in

- Decreased RBCs (anemia)
- Decreased white blood cells (WBCs; neutropenia/leukopenia)
- Decreased platelets (thrombocytopenia)

(v) The nurse would establish patient goals to include the following:

- The child will remain as free as possible of infections associated with leukopenia/neutropenia.
- The child will remain as free as possible of serious bleeding episodes related to thrombocytopenia.
- The child will remain as free as possible of anemia associated with decreased RBCs.

(vi) The nurse will carry out the following nursing interventions:

- Encourage verbalization of feeling (ventilation of emotion is often preliminary to problem solving activity).
- Assist the child to identify strength.
- Encourage supportive peer contact when appropriate.
- Prepare the child and family for hair loss, reassuring that it will not be permanent.
- Encourage good oral care to reduce ulcers caused by radiotherapy or cancer chemotherapy.
- Explain to the child and family why rectal temperature should not be taken. (Chemotherapy causes destruction of cells in rectum; bleeding can occur).
- Allow the child to have control over pain medication, as appropriate to developmental age.

- When planning and teaching new coping strategies, keep in mind that a child may use motor and emotional strategies (pound with hands on table, or bed, cry and scream). These are extremely useful for children who have poorly developed cognitive coping abilities.
- Refer to social workers, psychologists, child life specialists, hospice as appropriate to deal with concerns.

XVI. CONGENITAL DEFECTS

A. Cleft Lip and Cleft Palate

- Cleft lip and cleft palate are hereditary defects.
- Slight indentation is called a *harelip*.
- Wide defect is called an *open cleft*.

1. Etiology and Incidence

   a. Cleft lip, cleft palate, and combinations of these are the most common of all facial anomalies.

   b. Cleft lip with or without cleft palate is more common in boys.

   c. Cleft palate is more common in girls.

   d. Boys more commonly have a combined cleft lip and cleft palate, and usually of more severe degree than in girls.

   e. Cleft palate occurs in 1 per 1000 births and cleft palate alone in 1 per 2500 births.

   f. Higher incidence rate in the Japanese population (twice that of the white population) and a lower incidence rate in the African-American population (less than half as many as the white population).

   g. Cleft lip and cleft palate have a strong genetic component.

2. Types: Unilateral or Bilateral

3. Severity of Defects: Cleft Lip and Cleft Palate

   a. A complete cleft lip involves roots of the teeth and the floor of the nose; the upper gums may also be deformed.

   b. A cleft palate may involve the soft palate (back) of the mouth, the hard palate (front) of the mouth, or both. It opens a passage from the nasopharynx and the nose, causing feeding and respiratory difficulties. A cleft palate can occur with or without a cleft lip.

4. Feeding of Infant with Cleft Lip or Cleft Palate

   a. If the newborn has an open cleft and is unable to develop suction using a bottle, use a large nipple with a large hole.

   b. The newborn with a cleft lip and cleft palate may be able to be breast fed.

   c. An infant with a cleft lip and cleft palate is held in an upright position at a 60- to 80-degree angle, with the head rested in the bend of the parent's elbow. This position decreases the likelihood of aspiration because the natural cough reflex can more readily clear the airway.

d. The nipple should be positioned firmly in the baby's mouth in a normal position. Observation of the infant's face is important because it provides clues as to how the infant is tolerating the feeding. Before gagging or choking, the infant elevates eyebrows and wrinkles the forehead. The nipple can be removed.

e. The local La Leche League Chapter may be able to help a new mother who would like to breast-feed her infant or express breast milk to save and feed her baby later.

5. Pathophysiology, Etiology, and Incidence

a. Ear infections, speech difficulties, and hearing problems are common in children with cleft palate.

b. Under normal conditions, the muscles of the soft palate aid in proper functioning of the eustachian tube.

c. In the presence of a cleft palate, these muscles do not function efficiently, resulting in inefficient drainage of the middle ear, causing a greater susceptibility to ear infections.

6. Nursing Implications

a. The infant should not be fed in a lying-down position or confined to a supine position for long periods.

b. Good mouth care is important for reducing infections.

c. Milk feeding should be followed by a small amount of clear water to rinse the mouth.

d. The nurse needs to educate the parents that when a child has a cleft palate, language acquisition can be hampered by an inability to hear, particularly if careful attention is not given to early treatment of middle ear infections.

e. In many cases, myringotomy and placement of ventilation tubes may be necessary.

f. Discuss with the family the use of a prosthesis to occlude the cleft palate. Explain that the prosthesis has some benefit in facilitating language acquisition, but there is no evidence that it assists in feeding.

7. Medical Management

a. Surgery on cleft lip is completed as early as possible, usually when the infant weighs 10 lb.

b. Cleft palate surgery can be performed to prevent a speech deficit if the gums (gingiva) are not involved. If the gums are involved, surgery will be performed after the permanent teeth are in place.

c. Postoperative cleft lip surgery.

(1) Infant cannot sleep face down (place on back).

(2) If the infant is left alone, the infant's hands must be restrained to prevent the infant from pulling on the suture line. The infant should be held as much as possible.

(3) To clean around the suture line, use only a swab and hydrogen peroxide (cotton will stick to wound).

8. Parents Coping with Child's Surgery

To ease the psychological effect, allow the parents to look at before-and-after surgery pictures of another child with a similar, surgically repaired cleft lip.

B. Congenital Cardiac Defects

1. Transposition of great vessels

a. The aorta is located in the right ventricle instead of the left ventricle, and the pulmonary aorta is located in the left ventricle instead of the right ventricle.

b. More common in males than in females.

c. Surgery must be performed immediately after birth, and the mortality rate is very high.

2. Tetralogy of Fallot

a. Most common cyanotic congenital heart disease. (Almost all other congenital heart diseases are acyanotic.) For cyanosis to occur, there must be more pressure in the right ventricle than in the left ventricle, which seldom occurs. Pulmonary stenosis and the overriding aorta increase right ventricular pressure. Symptoms depend on the severity of the defects.

b. Tetralogy of Fallot has the following features: pulmonary stenosis, ventricular septal defect (VSD), overriding aorta, and right ventricular hypertrophy. The severity of these problems dictate the severity of the cyanosis.

c. It is correctable by surgery.

3. Coarctation of the Aorta

a. Blood pressure is higher than normal in the upper part of the body and lower in the lower part of the body, resulting in headaches, dizziness, faintness, and cool extremities. The child will be acyanotic.

b. Stroke volume is decreased.

4. Patent Ductus Arteriosus (PDA)

a. Most common cardiac anomaly (acyanotic).

b. Occurs twice as often in females as in males.

c. Many infants are asymptomatic.

d. Often diagnosed by "machinery murmur" sounds (like gears grinding).

5. Persistence of Fetal Circulation (PFC)

a. Syndrome most often seen in full-term infants.

b. Characterized by cyanosis that does not respond to administration of 100% oxygen.

c. In PFC, right-to-left-shunting through the foramen ovale and ductus arteriosus appears to result from persistent elevation of pulmonary vascular resistance after birth.

d. The neonate will be cyanotic for the first 24 h after birth. Provide 100% oxygen, which usually will achieve closure of the ductus arteriosus and foramen ovale, and a decrease in pulmonary resistance will occur within 24 h. If PFC persists after 24 h, surgery will be needed to close the foramen ovale and ductus arteriosus.

6. Atrial Septal Defect (ASD)

    a. Shunting from left to right; child is acyanotic.

    b. If the ASD is large, surgery will be performed to repair defect.

7. Ventricular Septal Defect (VSD)

    a. Shunting from left to right; child is acyanotic.

    b. If the VSD is large, surgery will be performed to repair the defect.

8. Pulmonary Stenosis

    a. Right ventricle hypertrophies.

    b. The pulmonary artery can be replaced or repaired in the area that is stenosed.

XVII. VASCULITIS

A. Kawasaki Disease (KD)

1. Kawasaki disease is a febrile, multisystem disorder in which vasculitis is the most potentially dangerous characteristic.

2. Generally considered a self-limiting disease, KD can be fatal if aneurysms or myocardial infarction occurs.

1. Etiology, Incidence, and Pathophysiology

    a. KD may be seen in a child of any age but is virtually restricted to prepubertal children.

    b. It is most common in boys younger than 2 years and in persons of Japanese ancestry.

    c. Genetics has been suggested as a possible explanation for the higher incidence among Japanese children, but the evidence supporting this is inconclusive.

    d. KD has a seasonal pattern, with a significantly greater number of cases in the winter and spring months.

    e. Although the cause of KD remains unknown, several possible causes have been proposed. Environmental factors (e.g., rug shampoo) have been implicated but remain unconfirmed. This suggests that hypersensitivity or an altered immune system plays a role.

    f. Studies have shown a sharp rise in antibody production in the first 4 weeks of the disease.

    g. The most common and potentially dangerous effect of the KD process is vasculitis, which can result in occlusive or ischemic manifestations during the acute disease process or at a later period in life.

    h. Over the course of the illness, any or all parts of the vascular system can be involved, beginning with the microvessels (arterioles, capillaries, and venules) and progressing to involve small- and medium-sized vessels.

    i. The vascular changes in the cardiac muscle and coronary arteries are of the most concern because they can lead to lifelong morbidity or mortality.

2. Signs and Symptoms

    a. Typically, the child with acute KD has an unexplained fever of 102° to 106°F that does not remit with administration of antipyretics.

    b. Additionally, a pruritic, polymorphic rash; a marked cervical lymphadenopathy; dry, red, cracked lips; a "strawberry" tongue; and bilateral conjunctivitis are observed.

    c. The child is likely to be irritable and lethargic.

    d. The clinical course of the disease occurs in three phases. Symptoms appear and resolve in a typical pattern.

    e. In the acute phase (the first 6–12 days), fever, strawberry tongue, cracked fissured lips, rash, erythema and edema of the palms and soles, and lymphadenopathy are seen.

    f. In the subacute period (10–35 days), desquamation of the toes, feet, fingers, and palms occurs.

    g. The child likely will continue to be irritable and anorectic and have conjunctival injections.

    h. During this period, arthritis, thrombocytosis, and cardiac and vascular manifestations will occur.

    i. The recovery phase is said to continue until the erythrocyte sedimentation rate (ESR) becomes normal (perhaps as long as 10 weeks after onset).

3. Therapeutic Management

    a. Therapy for KD continues to be controversial. Aspirin has been the primary means of therapy for both antiinflammatory and antiplatelet effects (e.g., to counteract thrombocytosis).

    b. In the acute period, dosages up to 100 mg/kg/day of aspirin are prescribed for the antiinflammatory effect.

    c. For unexplained reasons, therapeutic aspirin levels are difficult to achieve in the acute period.

    d. The most widely accepted explanation for this finding is a markedly impaired absorption of aspirin.

    e. Because of the potential of side effects from aspirin and gastritis, other antiinflammatory preparations may be prescribed.

    f. Studies indicate that aspirin does not reduce the occurrence of coronary artery abnormalities.

    g. High-dose IV gamma-globulin given in conjunction with aspirin, however, appears to be effective in rapidly reducing fever, as well as having a rapid, generalized antiinflammatory effect.

4. Nursing Implications

    a. Assessment of cardiac status is critical. A cardiopulmonary monitor is indicated if there are signs of myocarditis. Tachycardia, gallop rhythm, chest pain, and ECG changes (depressed ST segment) suggest myocarditis.

    b. Tachypnea or dyspnea, rales or other noisy respirations, costal retractions, nasal flaring, orthopnea, distended neck veins, and edema are all signs and symptoms of congestive heart failure.

    c. Promote skin integrity by noting the presence of any rash and edema.

d. Keeping the skin clean, dry, free of irritation from linens and clothing, and well lubricated helps preserve the integumentary system, which is the barrier to infection and makes the child more comfortable as well.

e. Protect edematous areas from friction and prolonged pressure.

f. Monitor temperature because the fever associated with KD tends to be high and not relieved by medication; careful monitoring is indicated.

g. Because the etiology of the hyperthermia cannot be changed by the nurse, management is symptomatic and includes increased fluid intake and removal of clothing and blankets.

h. Adequate nutritional status may be difficult to maintain, and ongoing assessment of I&O (both fluids and solids) is important.

i. IV fluids are administered to maintain hydration during the acute stage.

j. The discomfort of the mucous membranes may be one deterrent to adequate nutrition. Pain that results from gastritis or other organ involvement can decrease appetite and willingness to eat and drink, requiring nursing intervention.

k. Reduce family fear and anxiety by keeping them informed of the child's prognosis and encouraging them to assist with the child's care.

l. The vascular and potential cardiac involvement associated with KD often arouses fear regarding the child's prognosis.

m. Some children have coronary artery aneurysms, experience infarctions (which may occur in any organ system or part of body), or die in the acute, subacute, or recuperative phase of the disease process, but families should be reassured that only 3 percent of clients with KD develop fatal complications and that recovery is uneventful in 97 percent of cases.

EXAMINATION

1. A 4-year-old boy is admitted to the hospital with a 3-week history of fever, fatigue, and pallor. A bone marrow examination shows 85 percent blast cells and a WBC count of 18,000/mm^3; his RBC count is within normal limits. A diagnosis of acute lymphocytic leukemia (ALL) is made. The laboratory finding *most likely* to explain the patient's fatigue and pallor is

   1. Hemoglobin 6 gm/dL.
   2. Platelet count 30,000/mm^3.
   3. WBC count 18,000/mm^3.
   4. Potassium 3.5 mEq/L.

2. Following a course of chemotherapy, a child's WBC count is 1200/mm^3. With this in mind, a specific nursing intervention will include

   1. No special precautions; this count is within normal limits.
   2. Restricting the patient to a private room and protecting him from infection.
   3. Monitoring the patient's respirations closely.
   4. Administering oxygen for dyspnea and maintaining bed rest.

3. A child has a platelet count of 30,000/mm^3. An appropriate nursing intervention related to this finding would be

   1. Keeping child isolated to avoid infection.
   2. Encouraging a diet high in iron.
   3. Providing frequent periods of rest.
   4. Discouraging active play to avoid getting hurt.

4. Keeping in mind that leukemia is an opportunistic disease and the major cause of cancer death in children, the priority nursing measures for the child would include

   1. Frequent neurologic assessments.
   2. Ensuring correct administration of supplemental iron.
   3. Careful washing of hands prior to caring for the client.
   4. Monitoring platelet infusion for signs of reaction.

5. A client is being observed for a possible infection related to acute lymphocytic leukemia. All of the following are appropriate nursing measures *except*

   1. Frequently monitoring vital signs and taking rectal temperatures.
   2. Increasing fluid intake and keeping child quiet.
   3. Keeping child on bed rest during fever.
   4. Administering glycerin suppositories for constipation.

6. The greatest threat to a child recovering from a bone marrow transplant is

   1. Hypovolemic shock.
   2. Hemorrhage.
   3. Infection.
   4. Renal failure.

7. Preoperative care for the child suspected of having a Wilms' tumor includes

   1. Measuring abdominal circumferences once during every shift.
   2. Avoiding palpating the abdomen.
   3. Monitoring for intestinal obstruction.
   4. Assessing for signs of infection.

8. Children with retinoblastoma exhibit "cat's-eye reflex," meaning that shining a light into the eye produces a

   1. Red appearance on the lens.
   2. Dark red spot on the pupil.
   3. White appearance on the lens.
   4. Upward deviation of the retina.

QUESTIONS 9 TO 12: CASE HISTORY

Roy, a 4-year-old boy, is admitted to the hospital with weight loss, anorexia, and fatigue. Roy is diagnosed with a medulloblastoma, the most common brain tumor in children.

9. At the time of surgery, the tumor is assessed at stage IV. The *best* description of this stage is
   1. Presence of metastasis.
   2. Lymph node involvement.
   3. Single tumor with regional involvement.
   4. Involvement of the central nervous system.

10. Which of the following is a clinical manifestation of an intracranial tumor?
   1. Urinary retention and anemia.
   2. Diarrhea, weight loss, dizziness, and anemia.
   3. Decreased urinary catecholamines, hypotension, and headache.
   4. Headache, vomiting, papilledema, seizure activity, and ataxia.

11. What is the primary reason Roy is scheduled for surgery?
   1. Excise the entire tumor if possible.
   2. Biopsy the tumor and assess for brain damage.
   3. Remove metastatic nodes on the liver.
   4. All of the above.

12. Roy is started on chemotherapy with the drug vincristine. A priority nursing intervention related to early identification of possible toxic effects of this drug is
   1. Dipstick each urine for blood; frequent assessment of guaiac of stools; rash and pruritus.
   2. Assess for level of consciousness (LOC) and for urinary retention.
   3. Monitor nausea and vomiting, anorexia, urinary retention, neurotoxicity, and alopecia.
   4. Examine for presence of rash on skin, irritation of oral cavity, frequency of stools, and acidosis.

End of Case

13. An important nursing goal for the child experiencing idiopathic thrombocytopenia purpura is to avoid
   1. Trauma.
   2. Loud sounds.
   3. Fatigue.
   4. Sunlight.

14. The most characteristic finding in an infant with hearing deficit is
   1. Hyperactivity.
   2. Delayed speech.
   3. Excessive fears.
   4. Behavioral problems.

15. A chemotherapeutic agent that will cross the blood–brain barrier is
   1. Cytarabine (Cytosar-U).
   2. Vincristine (Oncovin).
   3. Methotrexate (Amethopterin).
   4. Cyclophosphamide (Cytoxan).

16. A patient, age 14 years, is diagnosed as having vaginal herpes simplex virus type 2 (HSV-2). Signs and symptoms and treatment of this condition are
   1. Pruritus and edema of the vagina, fever, lethargy, and fatigue; treatment with oral metronidazole.
   2. Intense burning and itching at the site of outbreak and raised vesicles that rupture in 24 h, and pain; treatment with acyclovir.
   3. Solitary clusters of red pimples causing itching, vaginal discharge, foul-smelling discharge; treatment with penicillin.
   4. Gray-white, nonirritating vaginal discharge; white, cottage-cheese–like discharge, and red, edematous mucous membranes; treatment with clotrimazole vaginal suppository.

17. Parents of toddlers with delayed language skills are encouraged to
   1. Enroll them in special preschool classes.
   2. Have them play with older children.
   3. Read to them.
   4. Encourage them to use proper words.

18. A 3-year-old child suspected of having the spastic form of cerebral palsy (CP) would most likely
   1. Walk on his toes with a scissors gait, crossing one foot in front of the other.
   2. Exhibit frequent episodes or seizure activity characterized by brief (<30 seconds) loss of consciousness.
   3. Have visual deficits, such as diplopia, with decreased visual acuity.
   4. Have frequent respiratory infections with acute spasmodic laryngitis.

19. The parents of an infant diagnosed with CP ask the nurse about the severity of their child's handicap. The best response the nurse can give is
   1. With early and vigorous therapy, he may have only mild problems.
   2. It's hard to tell so early, but no mental retardation is expected.
   3. Children with CP vary in symptoms and severity, but they can be helped with treatment.
   4. No one can really tell how much disability there will be until the child starts school.

20. Children with CP are often at risk for nutritional deficits because they have

1. Difficulty controlling the muscles of chewing and swallowing
2. A restricted sense of taste and are finicky eaters.
3. GI impairment that decreases absorption of nutrients.
4. Frequent episodes of vomiting related to muscle spasticity.

21. When a child with CP is admitted to the hospital, it is important that the nurse obtain from the parents
   1. Special permission for use of restraints.
   2. Utensils used for feeding.
   3. Assurance that someone will stay with the child continually.
   4. Special instructions related to skin care.

22. Vitamin K deficiency may be seen in newborns because the
   1. Body storage of vitamin K is depleted within 2 weeks after birth.
   2. Newborn's GI tract cannot absorb vitamin K.
   3. Large amount of milk intake interferes with absorption.
   4. Newborn has a sterile GI tract and cannot synthesize vitamin K.

23. A 10-year-old boy with asthma is discharged from the hospital and is on a daily dosage of terbutaline (Brethine) and cortisone (Cortone). The client and parents should be taught to
   1. Test his urine to determine if it contains glucose.
   2. Continue to restrict fluid intake.
   3. Keep the client away from sources of infection.
   4. Encourage a high-calorie, low-sodium diet.

24. A child, age 5 years, is admitted to the hospital with a 2-week history of puffy eyes and decreased urinary output. The child is diagnosed with idiopathic nephrotic syndrome (NS). In reviewing the child's laboratory findings, the nurse would most likely find
   1. Low urine specific gravity of 1.001.
   2. Urinalysis reveals a 4+ protein.
   3. Anemia.
   4. Decreased serum sodium.

25. Nursing care for a child with nephrotic syndrome would include
   1. Maintenance of a low-protein diet.
   2. Severe restriction of sodium fluids.
   3. Frequent skin care and changes of position.
   4. Use of nonallergenic tape over puncture sites.

26. A neonate's failure to pass meconium within the first 24 h after birth could indicate
   1. Intussusception.
   2. Dehydration.
   3. Celiac disease.
   4. Hirschsprung's disease.

27. A 3-week-old patient is admitted to the hospital with a history of "spitting up" since he was 1 week old. Billy's mother says, "Billy's spitting has now increased to what I would call forceful vomiting." The most likely diagnosis for Billy would be
   1. Hirschsprung's disease.
   2. Celiac disease.
   3. Pyloric stenosis.
   4. Intussusception.

28. A 10-year-old female client is diagnosed with insulin-dependent diabetes mellitus (IDDM). She asks the nurse why she cannot take a pill like her Aunt Jessie does, rather than insulin shots. The most correct response by the nurse would be
   1. The pill stimulates cells in the pancreas to produce insulin, and your cells are not able to produce insulin.
   2. The pills will stimulate insulin production in the adult pancreas but will not in the child's pancreas.
   3. When you are able to cut down on the amount of sweets you eat, then maybe you can start taking the pill.
   4. Your doctor makes that decision; ask him.

29. A 2-year-old female client is brought to the emergency room (ER) after waking up with a barklike cough and stridor. On arrival to the ER, she has respiratory distress and is afebrile. The diagnosis is croup. The nurse instructs the parents to
   1. Perform percussion and postural drainage before putting the patient to bed and before meals.
   2. Encourage frequent coughing and deep breathing.
   3. Run a cool-mist vaporizer in patient's room during the day.
   4. Follow a schedule of postural drainage and increase fluid intake.

30. The symptoms *most* commonly seen in croup are
   1. Wheezing, colicky pain, and vomiting.
   2. Stridor, rapid pulse, and barklike cough.
   3. Drooling, rapid pulse, and occasional hoarse cry.
   4. Fever, vomiting, and abdominal retractions on inspiration.

31. Which of the following is the *most* threatening to a hospitalized toddler's autonomy?
   1. Frequent visits by parents and friends of the family.
   2. Participation in playroom activities with other children.
   3. Complete bed rest.
   4. Riding to the x-ray department in a wheelchair in a hospital gown.

32. Which one of the following phrases *most accurately* describes myelomeningocele?
   1. The incomplete fusion of the vertebrae at one level that may have an overlying dimple or tuft of hair.

2. Herniation of a portion of the spinal cord and meninges into a cyst.

3. Incomplete fusion of one or more of the vertebral laminae.

4. Cyst formation containing CSF, blood, and meninges.

33. When explaining how to correctly collect specimens for identification of pin worms, the nurse should tell the mother to

1. Bring in a fresh stool specimen.

2. Administer a laxative the night prior to collection of a specimen.

3. Place a tongue blade covered with tape over the child's anus.

4. Have the child defecate and then smear a small amount of stool on a slide.

34. Activated charcoal is administered to the child who has ingested a poison substance in order to

1. Induce vomiting.

2. Increase the effectiveness of ipecac.

3. Increase movement through the GI tract.

4. Absorb the compound.

35. When giving parents anticipatory guidance about accident prevention for toddlers, the nurse tells the parents

1. If the toddler feels the heat, she learns that a stove is hot.

2. Falls are not as great a danger now as they were during infancy.

3. Areas previously childproofed may now be accessible to the toddler.

4. Toddlers understand the word "no" and will listen to parental rules.

36. A mother brings her 3-year-old son and 8-month-old daughter to the health center. She states that her son enjoys pouring and playing with water. The water safety rule for the bathroom is reviewed with the mother. The only correct rule given here is

1. Never leave children alone in the bathtub.

2. Never leave a child in the bathtub unless an older child is in with them.

3. Have the child test the water temperature with his hand.

4. It is safe to leave children alone in a bathtub if there is only 12 inches of water.

37. The nursing diagnosis appropriate for health promotion of a well toddler is

1. Potential for injury related to increased mobility.

2. Activity intolerance related to rapid growth.

3. Alteration in growth and development related to rapid growth.

4. Alteration in bowel elimination related to interest in playing, not drinking.

38. A mother brings her 2-year-old son to the clinic for his measles, mumps, and rubella (MMR) vaccine. Prior to giving the vaccine, it is important for the nurse to ask if he has

1. Recently been checked for anemia.

2. Ever experienced an allergic reaction to eggs.

3. Been in contact with anyone with rubella (German measles).

4. Been in close contact with a pregnant relative or baby-sitter.

39. In explaining the use of "time out" as a form of discipline for a 2-year-old child, the nurse tells the parents

1. To send the child to his or her bedroom for 20 min.

2. To allow the child to take his or her own favorite toy to the room.

3. The total time out should be no more than 2 to 3 min.

4. To explain to the child why the behavior was bad (after the "time out").

40. The behavior that would indicate to parents that a toddler is ready to begin toilet training is

1. Showing interest in flushing the toilet.

2. Staying dry throughout the night.

3. Spending time in the bathroom with parents.

4. Pulling at wet diapers or taking off wet diapers.

41. A mother of an 18-month-old child tells the nurse that her child is a finicky eater. The best advice that the nurse can give to the mother is

1. Give small amounts and cut food into small pieces to allow for finger feeding.

2. Don't force the child to eat food but make sure that the child drinks all of his milk.

3. Serve small portions and make the child sit at the table until he eats all of his food.

4. Serve the child in front of the TV to keep his attention.

42. When toddlers say "no" to eating food, they may be

1. Saying they do not like the food, be testing their parents, be practicing independence.

2. Deciding the types of foods they like and dislike.

3. Trying to impress on their parents that they have the right to choose their own food.

4. Saying no because they like the word; it has no meaning at all and is just a habit that children develop.

43. When a doctor is having a consent form signed for a surgical procedure on a child, the nurse knows that

1. Only a parent or legal guardian can sign the consent form.

2. The person giving consent must be at least 18 years old.

3. The risk and benefits of procedures are part of the consent process.

4. The mental age of 7 years or older is required for consent to be considered "informed."

44. The nurse is planning how to prepare a 4-year-old child for a diagnostic procedure. Guidelines for preparing this preschooler should include

   1. A plan for a short teaching session of approximately 35 min each day.
   2. Telling the child that the procedure is not a form of punishment.
   3. Keeping equipment out of the child's view.
   4. Telling the child that the procedure will be simple.

45. The nurse is preparing a 6-year-old child before obtaining a blood specimen by venipuncture. The child tells the nurse that he does not want to lose his blood. The appropriate approach by the nurse would be to

   1. Explain that the process will not be painful and that it will be over quickly.
   2. Discuss with the child how the body is always in the process of making blood.
   3. Suggest to the child that he does not have to worry about losing a little bit of blood because he is old enough now not to be afraid.
   4. Tell the child that he will not need a Band-Aid afterward because it is such a simple procedure. If he does not watch the nurse draw the blood, it will not hurt.

46. When administering a gavage feeding or medication to an infant through an NG tube, the nurse should

   1. Lubricate the tip of the feeding tube with petroleum to facilitate passage.
   2. Check the placement of the tube by inserting 20 mL of sterile water.
   3. Administer feedings over a period of 15 to 30 min.
   4. Place the infant on its right side or abdomen for 1 h after feeding.

47. In preparing to give "enemas until clear" (colonic lavage) to an 18-month-old child before surgery for Hirschsprung's disease, the nurse would anticipate that the physician would order

   1. Tap water (120 mL).
   2. Fleet solution (200 mL).
   3. Saline (300 mL).
   4. Oil retention (300 mL).

48. In relation to growth, the parents of a toddler can expect

   1. A growth spurt at approximately 18 months of age.
   2. A 4- to 6-lb weight gain between ages 3 and 4 years.
   3. Small weight losses and larger gains related to changing appetite.
   4. Little increase in height before age 3 years.

49. An 18-month-old child is seen in the clinic for a well-child checkup. While completing the assessment, the nurse notes a protruding abdomen. The nurse's assessment is that

   1. The child may be constipated.
   2. Further evaluation is warranted.
   3. An abdominal tumor must be ruled out.
   4. This is a normal finding.

50. A premature infant's dietary intake needs to be particularly sufficient in

   1. Glucose.
   2. Iron.
   3. Zinc.
   4. Vitamin C.

51. Visual development in an 18-month-old is directly related to parental need for anticipatory guidance related to

   1. Prevention of falls.
   2. Selection of a dentist.
   3. Signs of eye infections and need for glasses.
   4. High dietary intake of vitamin A.

52. Toddlers are most interested in play that involves

   1. Watching TV, especially cartoons, and playing Nintendo.
   2. Interaction with other toddlers and playing games with them.
   3. Active use of small and large muscle groups for climbing and running.
   4. Adults telling or reading stories for 30 min at a time.

53. The mother of a 2-year-old boy tells the nurse that the child insists on taking a favorite blanket to bed with him at night and at nap time. The mother asks the nurse if she should send the blanket to nursery school with him. The best response by the nurse is

   1. No, this is a good time for him to give it up and grow up.
   2. No, he doesn't need it away from home; he will be too busy playing.
   3. Yes, it will help him feel secure in his new place.
   4. Yes, it may cause severe emotional problems to take it away now.

54. Sigmund Freud believed that the major task of the toddler period is

   1. Anxiety over separation from mother.
   2. Toilet training.
   3. Development of the superego.
   4. Developing gender identity.

55. A mother tells the nurse that at 2 years of age, her daughter is speaking new words almost daily. For the past month, the child has shown little interest in new vocabulary. The nurse should

   1. Explain that the child's energies now are focused on developing motor skills.
   2. Suggest that the mother spend 1 h per day reading to the toddler.

3. Evaluate the possibility of hearing loss and refer for testing.

4. Perform a Denver developmental screening test to check for delays in vocabulary development.

56. The *most* appropriate group lay activity for a toddler's developmental level is

1. Board games, such as checkers; each child has a turn, and this allows the child to begin sharing and playing together.

2. Coloring in books with children their own age; encourages finger coordination.

3. Playing in a sand box with other children using lots of toys for digging and pouring.

4. Games where each child has a turn with a toy and then gives the toy to the child next to them in the group.

57. A 2-year-old child has three dolls. When another toddler attempts to play with one, the child grabs it and yells "it's mine." The best way to deal with this situation is to

1. Explain to child about sharing with other children.

2. Take one of the dolls and give it to the other child.

3. Wait until child is distracted and take one of the dolls.

4. Find another doll for the other child to play with.

58. A 20-month-old child is hospitalized with pneumonia. Her parents both work but visit daily. Each time they prepare to leave, the child cries and clings to them. While they are gone, she constantly watches and calls for them. The parents are distressed by this child's behavior and ask the nurse what to do when leaving. The best response by the nurse is to tell the parents to

1. Stay with the child until she falls asleep, and then leave.

2. Give the child kisses and hugs, then tell her they are leaving but will be back.

3. Tell the child they are going to get her ice cream and will be back soon.

4. Ask the nurse to take the child for a walk, then leave.

59. A 20-month-old child in the hospital who cries and clings to her or his parents when they leave is most likely in the stage of separation anxiety called

1. Protest.

2. Despair.

3. Denial.

4. Detachment.

60. Which one of the following ways can parents helps toddlers develop autonomy?

1. Offering them reasonable choices.

2. Limiting the amount of direct supervision.

3. Encouraging independent decision making.

4. Setting firm limits.

61. An 18-month-old child is admitted to the hospital after falling down the stairs. After giving information to the nurse, her mother leaves. The child does not cry when her mother leaves and sits quietly on the nurse's lap. This behavior is indicative of

1. Experience with hospitals in the child's past.

2. Good preparation of the child for a stay in the hospital.

3. Questionable disturbance in the parent–child relationship.

4. Early development of autonomy.

62. The most important teaching needs for a 15-year-old boy admitted with transitional cell carcinoma of the bladder would include information on

1. Side effects of chemotherapeutic drugs.

2. Available entertainment for teenagers.

3. Outreach programs for children.

4. Discharge procedures.

63. During a well-baby visit to the clinic, the nurse would expect the mother of a normal 7-month-old to report that he is

1. Walking nearly unassisted.

2. Creeping up and down four steps.

3. Sitting alone for brief periods.

4. Beginning to hold his head erect.

64. The mother of an 18-month-old child asks the nurse for advice regarding control of temper tantrums. The best response is

1. He is too old to act like that.

2. Consult a child psychologist.

3. Identify when he is getting frustrated and redirect his activities.

4. Physically restrain him until he has regained control.

65. Which of the following actions taken by the mother of a 6-month-old infant who is experiencing discomfort associated with teething indicates that the nurse's teaching plan has been successful?

1. She provides the infant with a hard rubber toy to bite on.

2. She reports that the baby was less irritable after placing an aspirin against the erupting tooth.

3. She gives the baby an ice cube to suck on.

4. She puts whiskey and sugar solution on the baby's gum.

66. Herpes zoster is caused by the varicella virus and causes

1. Ringworm and smallpox.

2. Shingles and chickenpox.

3. Measles and mumps.

4. Impetigo and measles.

67. Ringworm, an infection frequently found in school children, is caused by

1. Bacterial infection.

2. Virus.

3. Fungus.

4. Allergic reaction.

68. A nurse should explain that ringworm is

1. Not contagious.

2. Expected to resolve spontaneously.

3. Spread by direct and indirect contact.

4. A sign of uncleanliness.

69. Therapeutic management of the child with ringworm infection would include

1. Applying Burow's solution compresses to affected area.

2. Administering oral griseofulvin.

3. Administering topical or oral antibiotics.

4. Applying topical sulfonamides.

70. An important nursing intervention for the care of a child with acute bacterial conjunctivitis is

1. Warm, moist compresses to remove crust from the eyes.

2. Continuous warm compresses to relieve discomfort.

3. An oral antihistamine to minimize itching.

4. Application of optic corticosteroids to reduce inflammation.

71. The Denver Developmental Screening Test (DDST) is a device for

1. Measuring the intelligence quotient of adolescents.

2. Detecting developmental delays in infancy and the preschool-aged child.

3. Assessing the genetic intelligence of the school-aged child.

4. Screening children for tuberculosis.

72. A 9-year-old child has been complaining of a stomach ache and abdominal pain and has been vomiting. The child's mother tells the community health nurse that the child has been unable to attend school because of these symptoms. Questioning by the nurse reveals that the pain started at McBurney's point and shifted to the right lower quadrant; the patient has abdominal rigidity. The nurse advises the parents to

1. Give the child a soapsuds enema and take him to the ER.

2. Take his temperature and keep him in bed; if pain persists, call the physician.

3. Give him an acetaminophen for pain and ginger ale to drink, and take him to the ER.

4. Take him to the local hospital ER immediately.

QUESTIONS 73 TO 81: CASE HISTORY

Ann, a 14-year-old girl, was admitted to the hospital with insulin-dependent diabetes mellitus (IDDM) and is diagnosed as being in a diabetic coma.

73. What substance found in excess in Ann's blood would account for the sweet, fruity odor that the nurse notes on her breath?

1. Urea.

2. Glycogen.

3. Amino acids.

4. Ketone bodies.

74. The sign and symptoms *least* likely to appear in Ann's nursing history is

1. Having had a recent rapid weight gain.

2. Feeling more hungry and thirsty than usual.

3. Feeling more tired after exercise than usual.

4. Having to urinate several times during the night.

75. The test *most* likely to determine the amount of insulin Ann needs is a

1. Urine sample to determine the level of pH and specific gravity.

2. Urine sample to determine the amount of glucose.

3. Blood sample to determine the amount of glucose.

4. Blood sample to determine the amount of albumin and globulin present.

76. The physician places Ann on a sliding scale using the chemstick procedure with a glucose meter. To determine the amount of insulin Ann needs at different times of the day, she should do the tests

1. Shortly before meals and at bedtime.

2. Approximately halfway between meals.

3. Immediately after meals and at bedtime.

4. Upon awakening in the morning and again at bedtime.

77. Ann should be taught that all of the following factors increase the body's requirement of insulin *except*

1. Overeating.

2. Acute infections.

3. Increased emotional strain.

4. Increased physical exercise.

78. The *first* action Ann should be taught to take when it appears that she may be going into diabetic acidosis is that

1. She should drink a cup of warm water, eat some fruit, and call the physician if she continues to feel like she is going into a diabetic coma.

2. Insulin should be withheld until she sees her physician or until she eats some candy, and then test her blood sugar level.

3. She should go to the nearest ER for IV therapy to prevent coma and eat a candy bar on the way.

4. She should check her blood to determine the sugar level and then give herself insulin, per her physician's orders.

79. If Ann develops diabetic acidosis, the nurse should know that the typical signs and symptoms are

1. Dilated pupils and polyuria with protein and sugar.
2. Slow pulse rate and rapid respirations.
3. Excessive perspiration and shallow rapid breathing.
4. Deep, rapid respirations, polyuria, and nausea and vomiting.

80. Ann's condition becomes critical and she has a myocardial infarction (MI) resulting in metabolic acidosis. Signs and symptoms of metabolic acidosis are
   1. Shallow rapid respirations, tachycardia, and decrease in level of consciousness. (LOC)
   2. Rapid deep respirations, bradycardia, and decrease in level of consciousness. (LOC)
   3. Increased urinary output, tachycardia, arrhythmias, and decreased level of consciousness. (LOC)
   4. Shallow respirations, Cheyne–Stokes respiration, and decreased level of consciousness.

81. Ann's condition deteriorates and she develops pulmonary insufficiency, causing respiratory acidosis. Signs and symptoms of respiratory acidosis caused by pulmonary insufficiency are
   1. Deep, rapid respirations and increase in carbon dioxide level.
   2. Shallow respirations, change in level of consciousness, (LOC), and decrease in pH.
   3. Tachycardia, tachypnea, polyuria, and increase in pH.
   4. Shallow respirations, increased urinary output, and tachypnea.

End of Case

82. A 2-day-old child is diagnosed with a large tracheoesophageal fistula with esophageal atresia. The *first* signs and symptoms of tracheoesophageal fistula with esophageal atresia include
   1. Immediately after the patient is fed, she has projectile vomiting and becomes cyanotic.
   2. Immediately after eating, the patient vomits, has diarrhea, and develops tachypnea.
   3. The patient drools excessively, vomits, and has diarrhea.
   4. Immediately after the child is fed, the child struggles, becomes cyanotic, and stops breathing.

83. Which one of the following signs is the first indication to the nurse that a child is in need of tracheal suctioning?
   1. Hyperinflation of the lungs.
   2. Drooling and coughing.
   3. Substernal retractions.
   4. Apnea.

84. Following surgical repair of a child's tracheoesophageal fistula, the nursing measures that will *best* help meet the child's psychological needs while giving her formula through a gastrostomy tube are

   1. Hold and rock her in a rocking chair for 3 h each shift.
   2. Talk or sing to her and bottle-feed her.
   3. Give her a pacifier and hold her as often as possible.
   4. Lightly stroke her abdomen.

85. Which of the following values are normal for a neonate?
   1. Pulse (P) 70 to 170; respirations ® 40 to 90; fasting glucose level 30 to 80 mg/dL.
   2. P 100 to 180; R 50 to 100; fasting glucose 50 to 90 mg/dL.
   3. P 110 to 190; R 52 to 110; fasting glucose 60 to 110 mg/dL.
   4. P 110 to 200; R 54 to 115; fasting glucose 70 to 120 mg/dL.

86. The major stress from middle infancy throughout the preschool years is caused by
   1. Denial.
   2. Despair.
   3. Separation anxiety.
   4. Toilet training anxiety.

87. According to Erikson's psychosocial phases, children between the ages of $5\frac{1}{2}$ and 12 years are in which phase?
   1. Trust vs mistrust.
   2. Autonomy vs shame and doubt.
   3. Initiative vs guilt.
   4. Industry vs inferiority.

88. More children die in automobile accidents between the ages of
   1. 1 month to 1 year.
   2. 1 to 4 years.
   3. 2 to 6 years.
   4. 5 to 10 years.

89. The second highest ranking cause of accidental death of preschool boys is
   1. Burns.
   2. Automobile accidents.
   3. Poisoning.
   4. Drowning.

90. The second highest ranking cause of accidental death of preschool girls is
   1. Burns.
   2. Drowning
   3. Poisoning.
   4. Automobile accidents.

91. At what age does the highest incidence of poisoning occur in children?
   1. 9 months.
   2. 1 year.

3. 2 years.

4. 3 years.

92. The type of fluid replacement a doctor will use if a child is burned depends on

1. The degree of burns.

2. Blood volume.

3. Hematocrit.

4. Skin turgor.

93. If a blood transfusion is to be given to a 2-year-old who has acute lymphocytic leukemia (ALL), the physician would order

1. Whole blood; start with normal saline.

2. Packed cells; start with normal saline.

3. Packed blood cells; start with Ringer's lactate solution.

4. whole blood; start with Ringer's lactate solution.

94. After leukemia, the most second common disease that causes death in children is

1. Wilms' tumor.

2. Reye's syndrome.

3. Sickle cell anemia.

4. Brain tumor.

95. A child with a ventricular septal defect (VSD) will have

1. Shunting of blood from the left side of the heart to the right.

2. Shunting of blood from the right side of the heart to the left.

3. Shunting of blood from patent ductus arteriosus to left ventricle.

4. Shunting of blood from superior vena cava to inferior vena cava.

96. A child with cyanotic heart disease will have

1. Passage of blood from the left side of the heart to the right side of the heart.

2. Passage of blood from the right side of the heart to the left side of the heart.

3. Left ventricular hypertrophy.

4. An overload of the right atrium.

97. A 2-year-old boy is admitted to the hospital for an appendectomy. Compared to older children and adults, infants and toddlers have a higher incidence of perforation of the appendix and peritonitis because they

1. Have a greater pain tolerance.

2. Describe their symptoms poorly.

3. Have a weaker appendiceal wall.

4. Have less resistance to infection.

98. A child is ordered to have ear drops instilled after discharge from the hospital, and the nurse must teach the procedure

to the parents. Instill the drops by pulling the earlobe in a direction that is

1. Up and forward.

2. Up and backward.

3. Down and forward.

4. Down and backward.

99. A practice that is often recommended to help prevent the recurrence of otitis media is

1. Cleanse the ears thoroughly and often.

2. Use continuous, low-dose antibiotic therapy.

3. Have the child blow the nose well and regularly.

4. Eliminate a bedtime bottle offered when the child is in bed.

100. A complication commonly associated with extensive and infected burns is

1. Curling's ulcers.

2. Cushing's disease.

3. Diabetes insipidus.

4. Chronic hypertension.

ANSWERS AND RATIONALES

1. **❶** The laboratory finding most likely to explain fatigue in a child with acute lymphocytic leukemia (ALL) is a hemoglobin of 6 g/dL. Normal hemoglobin for a child is 11 to 16 g/dL. Hemoglobin carries oxygen from the lungs to the tissue. The first symptoms of ALL in children usually are pallor, low-grade fever, and lethargy (signs of decreased RBC production). A child can have petechiae and bleeding from oral mucous membranes and bruise easily because of low platelet count. As the spleen and liver begin to enlarge from infiltration with WBCs, abdominal pain, vomiting, and anorexia occur. As abnormal lymphocytes begin to invade the bone periosteum, the patient experiences bone pain and joint pain. CNS invasion leads to symptoms such as headache or unsteady gait.

2. A platelet count of 30,000/mm^3 is very low (normal for a child is 150,000–400,000/mm^3). A low platelet count will cause spontaneous bleeding, petechiae, and ecchymosis.

3. A WBC count of 18,000 mm^3 is very high (normal for a child is 6000/mm^3 to 17,000/mm^3). A high WBC will reduce the child's ability to fight infections in ALL because so many white cells are immature and nonfunctioning.

4. A potassium of 3.5 is within normal range (normal for children is 3.5–5.0 mEq/L).

2. **❷** If after chemotherapy a client's WBC count is 1200/mm^3, it will be important to protect the child from infection by restricting him to a private room because many of the mature WBC are destroyed with the immature cells.

1. This option is incorrect as seen in rationale (2). The platelet and WBC counts are very low; special precautions are necessary.

3. Monitoring respiratory breathing is an incorrect option; the client does not have a respiratory problem.

4. Administering oxygen for dyspnea and maintaining bed rest are necessary if there is a low RBC count because the RBCs carry oxygen. The child's RBC count is within normal limits. (It is almost impossible to maintain a 4-year-old on bed rest).

3. ④ A child's platelet count of 30,000/mm^3 is very low (normal is 150,000–400,000/mm^3), and the child will have a tendency to bleed. Therefore, active play should be discouraged because the child may injure himself and hemorrhage may occur.

1. There is no need to keep a patient with a low platelet count in isolation. The question asks for intervention related to low platelet count, not a low WBC count.

2. A diet high in iron would be necessary for a child with a low RBC count. Iron is necessary for the production of RBCs, including hemoglobin. Hemoglobin is the oxygen-carrying pigment of the erythrocytes (RBCs).

3. Frequent periods of rest would be most important if the RBC count were low. A client with ALL should have frequent periods of rest; however, the question was related to the platelet count.

4. ❸ The major cause of death from leukemia is infection, so careful hand washing prior to caring for the child with ALL is most important.

1. Leukemia is not a disease of the CNS, so frequent neurologic assessment is not a priority. ALL can invade the nervous system as the disease progresses, but it is not the major cause of death.

2. Ensuring the correct administration of iron will help to correct the low RBC count, but this is not a major cause of death for children with ALL.

4. Monitoring of platelet infusion for signs of reaction is important, but this is not the major cause of death.

5. ❶ It is important to monitor vital signs, but the temperature cannot be taken rectally. Chemotherapy works by destroying rapidly multiplying cells; therefore, it destroys cancer cells because they multiply rapidly. Oral and rectal mucosa cells also multiply rapidly, and the chemotherapy destroys these normal cells. This causes irritation and bleeding in the oral cavity and in the rectum.

A side effect of chemotherapy is constipation, and the child's rectum is already irritated from chemotherapy; using glycerin suppositories is important. Increasing the child's fluid intake will help to keep the kidney and bladder flushed out and reduce the chance of kidney or urinary tract infection. Keeping the child quiet and relatively inactive will allow the child to conserve energy and fight off infections.

(2, 3, 4) If a child with ALL is being observed for possible infection, it is important to increase fluid intake, keep the child quiet and somewhat inactive during the fever, and give glycerin suppositories for constipation.

6. ❸ The greatest threat to a child recovering from a bone marrow transplant is infection because of nonfunctioning

WBCs. Before a bone marrow transplant, cyclophosphamide (Cytoxan) is given to suppress bone marrow and T lymphocyte production so that the T lymphocytes do not reject the transplant marrow.

(1, 2, 4) These options are incorrect as seen in rationale (3).

7. ❷ If a child is suspected of having a Wilms' tumor, the abdomen should not be palpated; this may cause the spread of cancer from the tumor throughout the body.

(1, 3, 4) These options are incorrect as seen in rationale (2). There is no reason to measure the abdominal circumference, monitor for intestinal obstruction, or assess for signs of infection, although all clients are monitored for infections before surgery.

8. ❸ Children with retinoblastoma exhibit "cat's-eye reflex," such that shining a light into the eye produces a white appearance on the pupil. It eventually causes retinal detachment. Retinoblastoma is a malignant tumor of the retina of the eye and is the most common eye tumor in children.

(1, 2, 4) These options are incorrect as seen in rationale (3).

9. ❶ Medulloblastoma is the most common brain tumor seen in children. When assessed at stage IV, it has metastasized.

2. When cancer metastasizes, the lymph nodes may or may not be involved; in time, the cancer will metastasize to the lymph nodes.

3. A single tumor with regional involvement would be stage I.

4. Involvement of the CNS may or may not be involved when cancer metastasizes.

10. ❹ Clinical manifestation of intracranial tumor includes headache, vomiting, papilledema, and seizure activity. Papilledema is edema of the optic papilla.

(1, 2, 3) These options are incorrect as seen in rationale (1). The patient would lose weight and develop anemia, but these make only part of the options right.

11. ❶ When possible, the entire medulloblastoma is removed. It is more difficult to remove all of the tumor when it is in the brain because the removal of vital brain tissue could leave the patient with multiple neurologic problems. Medulloblastomas are fast-growing malignant tumors that are found most often in the cerebellum. These tumors occur between the ages of 3 to 5 years, occur more frequently in males than in females, and metastasize through the CSF. Signs of increased ICP become apparent after only approximately 2 months of tumor growth. Both the head and the spinal cord areas of children are radiated to discourage CSF metastasis. Intrathecal chemotherapy with vincristine or methotrexate may be used. A catheter is inserted through the skull, and the chemotherapy agent is administered directly to the tumor.

2. Biopsy of a brain tumor usually is a "last resort." The diagnosis usually is made by skull radiograph or CT scan. A biopsy will be obtained during surgery to remove the tumor. Brain damage will not be assessed. Surgery will provide information concerning the tumor.

3. If the cancer has metastasized to the liver, the child will be considered terminal because of the rapid growth of this tumor. Because liver cancer usually is diagnosed in the late stage of cancer and because symptoms are slow to develop, the tumor probably would have metastasized throughout the body.

4. All of the above is an incorrect choice because (1) is the only correct option.

12. ❸ Toxic effects of vincristine are nausea and vomiting, anorexia, urinary retention, neurotoxicity, and alopecia.

(1, 2, 4) These options are incorrect as seen in rationale (3).

13. ❶ An important nursing goal for the child experiencing thrombocytopenia purpura is to prevent trauma. In this disease, the platelet count may be as low as $20,000/mm^3$. Laboratory studies reveal marked thrombocytopenia. The cause of the illness is unknown, but it most likely results from an increased rate of destruction of platelets by an antiplatelet antibody, making this an immunologic illness. A nursing diagnosis used with thrombocytopenic purpura may be "potential for injury related to the possibility of easy bleeding." Therefore, trauma must be avoided.

(2, 3, 4) These options are incorrect as seen in rationale (1).

14. ❷ The most characteristic finding in infants with hearing deficit is delayed speech. An infant must be able to hear the spoken word to learn to speak.

(1, 3, 4) A hearing deficit will not cause behavioral problems, excessive fear, or hyperactivity. The infant with a hearing deficit has never heard voices and noise, so the infant does not realize there is anything wrong.

15. ❶ A chemotherapeutic agent that will cross the blood–brain barrier is cytarabine (Cytosar-U).

(2, 3, 4) These chemotherapy drugs do not pass the blood–stain barrier. Very few chemotherapeutic drugs pass the blood–brain barrier, which is the reason why chemotherapy may be administered through the skull, directly into the tumor using a Hickman catheter or any other catheter designed to deliver chemotherapy directly to the tumor.

16. ❷ Signs and symptoms of vaginal HSV-2 are intense burning and itching at the site of outbreak, raised vesicles that rupture in 24 h, and pain. Treatment for vaginal herpes includes acyclovir (Zovirax), an antiviral agent. Psychological supportive measures are important because there is no cure. Warm or cold sitz baths, pain medication, and antibiotics for secondary infection may be used.

(1, 3, 4) These options are incorrect as seen in rationale (2).

17. ❸ Parents of toddlers with delayed language skills are encouraged to read to their children. Children enjoy being read to and listen intently, which helps them to learn to speak more words (build vocabulary) and pronounce the words more clearly.

(1, 2) Enrolling a child with delayed language in special preschool classes or having them play with older children can cause the child to lose self-confidence. Other children may laugh at them when they are unable to speak clearly and communicate effectively, which can cause the child to have an increased language deficit.

4. Encouraging the child to use proper words causes the child to focus on the problem and puts pressure on the child, which can increase the child's language deficit.

18. ❶ A 3-year-old child suspected of having cerebral palsy (CP) would most likely walk on his or her toes with a scissors gait, crossing one foot in front of the other. CP is the most common cause of crippling in children. It is a neuromuscular disorder, and early diagnosis is essential for effective treatment. It requires careful clinical observations during infancy and precise neurologic assessment.

CP is suspected when the infant has difficulty sucking; seldom moves voluntarily or has leg or arm tremors with voluntary movement; crosses his or her legs when lifted from behind, rather than pulling them up or "bicycling" like a normal infant; or has legs that are hard to separate, making diaper changing difficult.

CP cannot be cured, but proper treatment can help affected children reach their full potential within the limits set by the disorder.

(2, 3, 4) These options are incorrect as seen in rationale (1).

19. ❸ When the parents of an infant diagnosed with CP ask the nurse how severe a handicap their child will have, the nurse's best response would be, "Children with CP vary in symptoms and severity, but they can be helped with treatment." This is a realistic statement that does not offer the parents false reassurance.

(1, 2) The statements "With early and vigorous therapy, he may have only mild problems" and "It's hard to tell so early, but no mental retardation is expected" are not true statements. A child with CP will have some very serious problems such as mental retardation, speech disorder, and seizures. No amount of vigorous therapy can eliminate these problems.

4. The statement "No one can readily tell how much disability there will be until the child starts school" is not true. Most of the child's disabilities will be present at preschool age.

20. ❶ Children with CP are often at risk for nutritional deficits because they have difficulty controlling the muscles of chewing and swallowing. Because of impaired motor function, eating, especially swallowing is difficult.

(2, 3, 4) These options are incorrect as seen in rationale (1).

21. ❷ When a child with CP is admitted to the hospital, it is important that the nurse obtain the utensils that the child uses at home. Because of impaired motor function, muscle weakness, and tendency toward muscle contraction, the child needs special utensils in order to feed themselves.

1. A child with CP should not be restrained. He or she is not combative and does not need restraints.

3. There is no reason for someone to stay with a child with CP continually.

4. The child with CP does not have any special skin care needs.

22. **4** Vitamin K deficiency may be seen in newborns because they have a sterile GI tract and cannot synthesize vitamin K. Certain bacteria (normal flora) must be present in the GI tract for vitamin K to be synthesized.

(1, 3) The infant's body does not store vitamin K, so it is not depleted within 2 weeks after birth. The infant takes in vitamin K through breast milk or formula. Vitamin K is needed for the synthesis of prothrombin, which is necessary for coagulation of blood.

2. The GI tract is not impaired, but the bacteria necessary for synthesis of vitamin K are not present.

23. **3** A child taking a daily dosage of prednisone should be kept away from sources of infection because prednisone suppresses the normal immune response.

(1, 2) Prednisone may increase blood glucose, and some sugar may spill into the urine. Prednisone also increases fluid retention. Normally, if a child is on prednisone for a short period of time and the dosage is not unusually large, there will be no problem with increased blood glucose or fluid retention. The child would not be on fluid restrictions.

4. There is no reason to encourage a high-calorie or low-sodium diet. Protein is necessary for healing and normal development. If the child is on a large dosage of prednisone, then the child may need to be on a sodium-restricted diet to reduce fluid retention.

24. **2** A child with idiopathic NS will spill large quantities of protein in the urine. NS is a condition characterized by hypoalbuminemia, hyperlipidemia, and edema. Prognosis is highly variable, depending on the underlying cause. The diagnosis of NS is made based on various laboratory tests. A urinalysis usually reveals a 3+ or 4+ proteinuria.

Approximately 70 percent of NS cases result from primary (idiopathic) glomerulonephritis. The dominant clinical feature of NS is mild to severe dependent edema of the ankles and sacrum and periorbital edema, especially in children. Such edema may lead to ascites, pleural effusion, and swollen external genitals. Accompanying symptoms can include orthostatic hypotension (because fluid is outside of the vascular system), lethargy, anorexia, and depression. Major complications are malnutrition, infection, and coagulation disorders.

Treatment of NS necessitates correction of the underlying cause, if possible. Supportive treatment consists of protein replacement with a nutritional protein diet. Some clients respond to an 8-week course of corticosteroid therapy (such as prednisone), followed by a maintenance diet. Others respond better to a combination of prednisone or cyclophosphamide (Cytoxan).

1. Urine specific gravity would be very high because of all protein molecules in the urine. Normal specific gravity is 1001 to 1025.

(3, 4) Loss of proteins will not cause anemia or elevated serum sodium.

25. **3** Nursing care of a client with NS includes frequent skin care and changes of position. Edema causes rapid breakdown of skin; decubitus ulcers will develop in children with NS if they do not receive good skin care and frequent changes of position.

1. A child with NS needs a high-protein diet because he or she is losing large quantities of protein in the urine.

2. The child with NS may be on a sodium-restricted diet but not on a severe sodium restriction, and most likely would not be on a fluid-restricted diet. An increase in sodium or fluid is not causing the edema; it is caused by lack of protein that reduces the osmotic pressure in the vascular system. Fluids move out of the vascular system and into interstitial spaces (edema).

4. Use of nonallergenic tape over puncture sites would only be necessary if the child with NS was allergic to other tape.

26. **4** A newborn's failure to pass meconium within the first 24 h after birth may indicate Hirschsprung's disease, a congenital disorder of the large intestine. It is characterized by absence or marked reduction of parasympathetic ganglion cells in the intestinal wall. This impairs the intestinal motility and causes severe constipation. Without prompt treatment, a neonate will develop bowel obstruction and may die within 24 h. Hirschsprung's disease is believed to be a familial congenital defect, occurring more often in males than in females.

Clinical manifestations usually appear shortly after birth, but mild symptoms may not be recognized until later in childhood or during adolescence. The newborn with Hirschsprung's disease commonly fails to pass meconium within 24 to 48 h, shows signs of bowel obstruction, abdominal distention, irritability, poor sucking reflex, refusal to take feedings, failure to thrive, dehydration, and liquid stools.

Surgical treatment is necessary but is delayed until the infant is at least 10 months old. Management until surgery consists of daily colonic lavages to empty the bowel. If total obstruction is represent in the newborn, a temporary colostomy or ileostomy is necessary to decompress the bowel.

1. In intussusception, the bowel turns back into itself (telescoping). Intussusception is most common in infants and occurs three times more often in males than in females.
Signs and symptoms of intussusception are intermittent attacks of colicky pain; vomiting of stomach content; "currant jelly" stools, which contain a mixture of blood and mucus; and tender distended abdomen, with a palpable, sausage-shaped abdominal mass.

2. Dehydration will not cause a failure to pass meconium.

3. Celiac disease is characterized by poor food absorption and intolerance for gluten, a protein in wheat and wheat products. With treatment, such as eliminating gluten from the client's diet, prognosis is good.

The cause is unknown, but females are affected more often than males. This disorder produces the following clinical manifestations: recurrent attacks of diarrhea, steatorrhea (fat in stool), abdominal distention, stomach cramps, weakness, anorexia, and increased appetite without weight gain. Symptoms develop during the first year of life when gluten is introduced into the child's diet as cereal.

Treatment requires permanent elimination or reduction of gluten from the client's diet. Supportive treatment may include supplemental iron, vitamin B_{12}, folic acid, reversal of electrolyte imbalances (by IV infusion, if necessary), corticosteroids (prednisone or hydrocortisone), and vitamin K for hypoprothrombinemia.

27. ❸ When a 3-week-old baby continues to spit up large amounts of formula and then has forceful vomiting, pyloric stenosis may be indicated. Obstruction of the pyloric sphincter is one of the most common surgical disorders of early infancy. This disorder usually is seen soon after birth, with vomiting becoming progressively more severe and projectile. It is five times more common in male infants than in female infants. The cause of pyloric stenosis is unknown. Diagnosis is made by upper GI x-ray studies. Treatment is surgical repair of the pyloric sphincter.

(1, 2, 4) Hirschsprung's disease is discussed in answer 26, rationale (4). Celiac disease is discussed in answer 26, rationale (3). Intussusception is discussed in answer 26, rationale (1).

28. ❶ When a child has IDDM, the beta cells of the pancreas can no longer produce insulin. The patient must take insulin by subcutaneous (SC) injection and will have to take insulin for the rest of his or her life. A patient with non–insulin-dependent diabetes mellitus (NIDDM) will have some active beta cells; an oral hypoglycemic medication will stimulate these beta cells to produce insulin.

2. The statement "The pills will stimulate insulin production in the adult pancreas but will not in the child's pancreas" is incorrect. Oral hypoglycemic medication will stimulate live beta cells to produce insulin in a child's pancreas as well as in an adult pancreas.

(3, 4) These options are incorrect as seen in rationale (1).

29. ❸ The nurse should instruct the parents of a child with croup to run a cool-mist vaporizer in the child's room at night and during the day and to take the child into the shower with them in an acute care situation.

Croup is a severe inflammation and obstruction of the upper airway, occurring as laryngotracheobronchitis (most common), laryngitis, and acute spasmodic laryngitis. Croup is a childhood disease affecting males more often than females (typically between 3 months and 3 years), usually during the winter months.

Croup usually results from a viral infection, but it can be caused by bacteria. Most children are cared for at home with rest, cool humidification during sleep, and antipyretics (e.g., acetaminophen) to relieve symptoms. In an acute case, taking the child into a shower will provide a more humid atmosphere.

(1, 2, 4) These options are incorrect as seen in rationale (3).

30. ❷ The symptoms most commonly seen in croup are stridor (labored breathing with retractions), rapid pulse, and a barklike cough.

(1, 3, 4) These options are incorrect as seen in rationale (2).

31. ❸ One of the most threatening things to a hospitalized toddler's autonomy is complete bed rest. The toddler is just beginning to assert independence, is very active, and does not want to be kept in bed. Bed rest is very threatening to a toddler who does not understand the reason for it.

1. Frequent visits by parents and friends help the child feel safe and not abandoned. This is not a threat to the child's autonomy.

2. Toddlers love to play with other children, even if they do not know them. This encourages autonomy (not threatens it); normally, toddlers make friends easily.

3. Riding to the x-ray department in a wheelchair could be fun for a child, not a threat to autonomy.

32. ❷ Myelomeningocele is the most severe "neural tube defect" (NTD), involving a protruding saclike structure that contains meninges, spinal fluid, and neural tissue. The spinal nerve roots may terminate in the sac, significantly affecting motor and sensory function below that point.

1. The incomplete fusion of the vertebrae at one level with an overlying dimple of turf hair is called spina bifida occulta. It is the most common NTS and usually occurs without any evidence of dermatologic, neurologic, or musculoskeletal disorders.

3. The incomplete fusion of one or more of the vertebral laminae, resulting in an external protrusion of the spinal tissue, is called spina bifida cystica. This type of defect usually occurs in the lumbosacral area. There are two classifications of spinal bifida cystica: myelomeningocele and meningocele. Spina bifida cystica is a general classification for these disorders; therefore, this is an incorrect option.

4. Meningocele is the formation of a saclike cyst containing meninges and spinal fluid that protrudes through a defect in the bony spine.

33. ❸ To collect a specimen for the identification of pin worms, a tongue blade covered with tape is placed over the child's anus during the night. The sticky side of the tape is placed on the rectum. During the night, the worms crawl into the anus and lay their eggs. The eggs will stick to the tape on the tongue blade.

1. A fresh stool specimen may not have any pin worms in it, but the child may still have pin worms. Fresh specimens are best for revealing parasites or larvae; therefore, a collected specimen should be taken directly to the laboratory for examination.

(2, 4) These options are incorrect as seen in rationales (3) and (1).

34. ❹ Activated charcoal is administered to the child who has ingested a poisonous substance to absorb the compound. Activated charcoal effectively absorbs most poisons, with the exception of cyanide. It also absorbs syrup of ipecac; therefore, the emetic should be given and allowed to exert its effect before the activated charcoal is given. Activated charcoal, however, is most effective if administered within 30 min of ingesting the poison.

(1, 2, 3) These options are incorrect as seen in rationale (4).

35. ❸ When giving parents anticipatory guidance for toddlers, the nurse tells the parent that "Areas previously child-proofed may now be accessible to the toddler." Anticipatory guidance is the ideal way to handle a problem. Prevent it—deal with it before it becomes a problem. Parents who know what to expect will be prepared for a problem when it appears.

1. The statement "If the toddler feels the heat, she learns that a stove is hot" is incorrect. The child does not have to experience every danger to prevent it from happening. If a parent waits for a child to be burned, the burn could be fatal.

2. The statement "Falls are not as great a danger now as they were during infancy" is not true. Falls continue to be a great danger throughout life.

4. The statement "Toddlers understand the word 'no' and will listen to parental rules" is a false statement. Toddlers tend to ignore the word "no" and find it very difficult to obey their parents. They are interested in establishing their autonomy.

36. ❶ A water safety rule given to parents should be to *never* leave children alone in the bathtub.

2. A 3-year-old child is too young to take care of any child in a bathtub; this is not a safety rule.

3. It is the adult's responsibility to check the temperature of the water, not the child's responsibility. The water may be too hot and burn them.

4. It is not safe to leave children alone in the bathtub if there is only 12 inches of water; they can turn on the faucet and fill the tub or drown in 12 inches of water.

Note: The safety rules are many but the only one given in this situation is option (1).

37. ❶ The nursing diagnosis appropriate to health promotion of the well toddler is potential for injury related to increased mobility.

2. A well toddler does not have intolerance to activity; he or she loves activity. This nursing diagnosis is incorrect.

3. A well toddler normally does not have an alteration in growth and development. This nursing diagnosis is incorrect.

4. A well toddler normally does not have an alteration in bowel elimination. This nursing diagnosis is incorrect.

38. ❷ Prior to giving a child a vaccine for measles, mumps, and rubella (MMR), the nurse should ask the parents if the child is allergic to eggs because they are used in the development of the vaccine.

1. It is not necessary to know if the child has anemia; if the child has anemia, he or she can be vaccinated for MMR.

3. If the child has been in contact with someone who had rubella (German measles), he or she can still get an MMR vaccine. Being exposed to measles would not affect the MMR vaccine given to the child unless the child was exposed 10 to 14 days before scheduled for his or her first MMR vaccine. Then the child would be given gamma-globulin and MMR vaccine at a later date.

4. The child being in contact with a pregnant relative or babysitter has no effect on the MMR vaccine given to the child. If the child has rubella (German measles), then he or she should not be around a pregnant woman. If the pregnant woman gets German measles while she is pregnant, the chances of her child having a birth defect are high.

Congenital rubella is by far the most serious form of the disease. Intrauterine rubella infection, especially during the first trimester, can lead to spontaneous abortion or stillbirth, as well as single and multiple birth defects. As a rule, the earlier the infection occurs during pregnancy, the greater the damage to the fetus.

39. ❸ In explaining the use of "time out" as a form of discipline for a 2-year-old child, the nurse tells the parents that the total time out should be no more than 2 to 3 min. A 2-year-old child will forget why he or she has to remain in a room after a few minutes and will become upset if he or she is left in the room.

1. This option is incorrect as seen in rationale (3).

2. Allowing a child a favorite toy in "time out" is not disciplinary action; the child may believe he or she is put in time out just to play for a little while.

4. The parent needs to explain to the child before "time out" why his or her behavior was not acceptable. A child should not be told that what his or her behavior was bad because the child may then think of himself or herself as bad.

40. ❹ The behavior that would indicate to parents that a toddler is ready to begin toilet training is when the toddler pulls off wet diapers. The child is uncomfortable wearing a wet diaper and can recognize that he or she is the one who is wetting the diaper. The parent can tell the child, "If you do not like your diaper wet, then you can go ("pee") in the toilet." The child may pull off the wet diaper and ask the mother to take him or her to the toilet.

1. Flushing the toilet indicates that the toddler likes to hear the water run and has nothing to do with being ready to be toilet trained.

2. Many children stay dry throughout the night long before they are ready to be toilet trained. If they do not wet their diapers at night, it is probably because they did not drink much fluid before going to bed.

3. Spending time in the bathroom with parents does not indicate that they are ready to begin toilet training. They may just want to be near their parents.

41. ❶ When an 18-month-old toddler is a finicky eater, the best advice the nurse can give the mother is, "Give small amounts and cut food into small pieces that allow for finger feeding." A toddler is interested in autonomy; allowing the child to feed himself gives the child the autonomy that he is seeking.

2. Children should never be forced to eat all of their food or drink all of their milk because they might aspirate the food or the milk. This method will not encourage them to eat the food.

3. Making a toddler sit at the table until they eat all of their food will make the child hate eating. The child may be at the table for an hour and still not have eaten all of his food. This is punishment that is associated with eating and certainly will not encourage the child to eat.

4. If a toddler who is a finicky eater is served food in front of the TV, the toddler will watch TV and not eat.

42. ❶ When toddlers say "no" to eating a food, they may not like the food, may be testing the parents, or may be practicing independence.

2. Toddlers know what foods they like and dislike, but this is not always the reason they say no to eating a food.

3. Toddlers do not have the cognition to think about impressing people.

4. Toddlers say no for many reasons; option (1) covers some of them.

43. ❶ When the doctor is having a consent form signed for a surgical procedure on a child, the nurse knows that only a parent or legal guardian can sign the consent form.

(2, 3, 4) These options are incorrect as seen in rationale (1).

44. ❷ The nurse knows that the guidelines for preparing a preschooler for a diagnostic procedure is to tell the child that the procedure is not a form of punishment. Preschool children believe that diagnostic procedures and treatments are punishments for something they have done.

1. This answer calls for a short teaching session; 35 min is not a short teaching session. A preschool child will lose interest in a teaching session that lasts more than a few minutes; dolls or stuffed animals must be used to explain procedures and keep the child's attention.

3. The child needs to see the equipment that will be used for diagnostic purposes or for treatment the day before so that he or she will be familiar and not be afraid of it.

4. The nurse should not tell the child that the procedure will be simple because the procedure may not be simple to the child. The child will be more afraid when the procedure hurts or causes some discomfort. The child will not trust the nurse and will be more fearful of the hospital's treatments and its personnel.

45. ❷ When a nurse is preparing a child for a venipuncture, the nurse needs to understand that a 6-year-old child has a great fear of bodily injury. Because children have an inadequate comprehension of medical events, they have a fear of invasive and/or painful procedures. The nurse should discuss with the child how the body is always in the process of making blood. Discussing the procedure with the child and allowing the child to express his or her feelings will help to reduce anxiety.

(1, 4) If the nurse tells the child that the procedure is not painful and he or she will not even need a Band-Aid, the nurse is not being honest with the child. Then when the child then experiences pain, he or she will no longer trust nurses and will fear every procedure.

3. A nurse should never tell a child or an adult not to worry; this does not help them cope with their fears and it makes the patient feel as if the nurse is not concerned.

46. ❹ When administering a gavage feeding or medication through an NG tube to an infant, the nurse should place the infant on the right side or abdomen for 1 h after the feeding. The stomach is on the left side; therefore, the infant should not be placed on the left side because the pressure on the stomach can cause the infant to vomit. If the infant is placed on the right side or on the abdomen and vomits, the vomit will come out of the mouth and not be aspirated. Being in this position for 1 h will allow time for the food or medication to leave the stomach.

1. The question is when administering a gavage feeding, not when putting an NG tube into the stomach. Read your stem carefully.

2. The placement of the NG tube should not be done with water, because the tube might be in the lungs. The correct procedure for checking NG placement is to push air through the NG tubing with a large syringe while listening over the stomach with a stethoscope. If a bubbling sound (air) is heard, then the nurse knows the NG tube is in the stomach; withdraw stomach content and check acidity.

3. There is no reason to administer tube feedings over a period of 15 to 30 min. If there is an order for continuous tube feeding, then the tube feeding is continuous—not over 15 to 30 min.

47. ❸ When giving "enemas until clear" to an 18-month-old child before surgery for megacolon (Hirschsprung's disease), the nurse would anticipate that the physician would order 300 mL of saline enema.

Hirschsprung's disease is a congenital disorder of the large intestine, characterized by the absence or marked reduction of parasympathetic ganglion cells. The disorder impairs intestinal motility and causes severe constipation. Before surgery, at least once per day, a large amount of saline is given as an enema (colonic lavage). Enemas given with the standard amount of fluid are not sufficient because the colon is so large and laxatives will not clear the colon adequately. Saline (salt) is used to draw as much fluid as possible into the intestines.

(1, 2, 4) These options are incorrect as seen in rationale (3).

48. ❷ In relation to growth, the parents of a toddler can expect a 4- to 6-lb weight gain between the ages 3 and 4 years.

(1, 3, 4) These options are incorrect as seen in rationale (2).

49. ❹ An 18-month-old child seen in a clinic for a well-child assessment will have a protruding abdomen, which is normal for this age. The abdominal muscles are not yet strong enough to keep the abdomen pulled in, but this will change as the child grows older.

(1, 2, 3) These options are incorrect as seen in rationale (4).

50. ❷ Maternal iron stores are adequate for the first 4 to 5 months of age in the full-term infant but are reduced considerably in premature infants or infants of multiple births. When exogenous sources of iron are not supplied to meet the infant's growth demands following depletion of fetal iron store, iron deficiency anemia results. Iron is necessary for hemoglobin synthesis. Hemoglobin is the oxygen-carrying molecule on the RBCs.

(1, 3, 4) These options are incorrect as seen in rationale (2).

51. ❶ Visual development in a toddler (18-month-old) is directly related to parental need for anticipatory guidance related to prevention of falls because the child's depth perception is not fully developed.

(2, 3, 4) These options are incorrect as seen in rationale (1).

52. ❸ Toddlers are most interested in play that involves the active use of small and large muscle groups for climbing and running. At this age, the toddler is very active and very curious.

It is a dangerous age because toddlers can climb and get into things.

1. A toddler may enjoy cartoons but will not sit still for very long. The toddler is not old enough to play Nintendo.

2. Toddlers are not interested in playing games with other children. They like to sit beside each other and play, but not to share.

4. Toddlers enjoy having adults read to them, but only for 3 to 5 min at a time; their attention span is very short.

53. ❸ If a mother tells the nurse that her 2-year-old son insists on taking a favorite blanket to nursery school with him and wants to know if she should allow this, the nurse's best response is, "Yes, it will help him feel secure in his new place."

1. Telling a toddler he needs to grow up and removing his security blanket will make the child insecure and afraid.

2. Telling the mother that the child does not need the blanket away from home and that he will be too busy playing to want his blanket is not true. Many toddlers have blankets or toys they sleep with and carry around all of the time because the object offers them security. Taking this security away when they are away from home would cause the child to feel insecure and cause emotional upset.

4. To tell a mother that it would cause severe emotional problems if the blanket was taken away is not true; it may seriously upset the child emotionally but it would not cause severe emotional problems. If something happened to the blanket (it might get lost), then the mother may believe that the child will have severe emotional problems.

54. ❷ Sigmund Freud believed that the major task of the toddler period is toilet training, and he described this stage as the genital stage. Bowel training may be accomplished between the ages of 18 and 24 months. Bladder training may not be accomplished until the ages of 3 to 5 years, especially nighttime control.

Erikson's phase 1 is concerned with acquiring a sense of basic trust while overcoming a sense of mistrust. The trust acquired in infancy is the foundation for all the succeeding phases. Erikson's phases are sense of trust (birth to 1 year); sense of autonomy (toddler, 1–3 years); sense of initiative (preschool, 3–6 years); sense of industry (school age, 6–12 years); sense of identity (12–18 years); sense of intimacy, sense of generactivity (young and middle-aged adults); and sense of ego integrity vs despair (elderly).

1. Separation anxiety is prominent during the latter half of infancy (8 months) and is still present to some degree when toddlers are 1 to 3 years old; it is even seen in preschool children. Toddlers are more willing to meet strangers and will tolerate longer periods of separation. There is less of the extreme fear of separation that was prominent during the latter half of infancy.

3. Development of superego, or conscience, has its beginning toward the end of the toddler years (age 3 years) and is a major task for the 3- to 5-year-old preschool-aged child. Learning right from wrong and good from bad is the beginning of morality.

4. Most children are aware of their gender and the expected set of related behaviors by 1½ to 2½ years of age. This is called developing gender identity. Although toddlers might be aware of their particular sex, they do not possess the language and cognitive skills to investigate sexual identity as fully as preschool-aged children. Freud has long recognized this task by describing this period as the genital stage.

55. ❶ A mother tells the nurse that at 2 years of age her daughter was speaking new words almost daily. For the past month, however, her daughter she shows little interest in new vocabulary. The nurse should explain that the child's energies are now focused on developing motor skills.

(2, 3, 4) These options are incorrect as seen in rationale (1).

56. ❹ The most important group play activity for a toddler's developmental level is games where each child has a turn with a toy, and then the child gives the toy to the child next in the group. Because toddlers (age 12 months to 3 years) are experimenting with self-control and independence, they will not share toys with other children. They will pass a toy from one child to another when an adult is supervising group play. Toddlers will play alongside, not with, other children. They have gradually progressed from solitary play in infancy to parallel play. Preschool-aged children (3–5 years) will become involved in associative play; for example, two children playing with dolls may share doll clothing.

1. These games are too advanced for toddlers; toddlers will not play games with each other.

(2, 3) These options are incorrect; the question asks for the most appropriate group play, and these options are solitary play. Coloring books or playing in a sandbox with other children does not change the activity; it is still solitary play.

57. ❹ When a 2-year-old child has three dolls and another child grabs one and yells, "it's mine," the best way to deal with this situation is to find another doll for the other child to play with. The 2-year-old child is still self-centered and is not able to share. Forcing a 2-year-old child to share will only upset them. By the time the child is 3 years old, he or she can begin to share toys and engage in associative play.

(1, 2, 3) These options are incorrect as seen in rationale (4).

58. ❷ When parents must leave a 20-month-old child in the hospital, they should play peek-a-boo, kiss and hug the child, and tell the child that they will come back. Peek-a-boo helps the child to learn that when the parents disappear, they will come back. Telling the child that they are leaving is being honest with the child, so the child can believe the parents and feel secure.

(1, 3, 4) These options are incorrect as seen in rationale (2).

59. ❶ When a 20-month-old child cries and clings to her parents while they are trying to leave, it is because the child is in the stage of separation anxiety called protest.

(2, 3, 4) These options are incorrect as seen in rationale (1).

60. ❶ A way in which parents can help toddlers develop autonomy includes offering them reasonable choices. This allows the child to learn how to make independent decisions. Giving a toddler a choice between two different dresses to wear is a reasonable choice for a toddler.

2. Limiting the amount of direct supervision of a toddler could be very dangerous.

3. Encouraging independent decision making is only appropriate if these decisions are not too difficult for a toddler to make.

4. Setting firm limits might mean not allowing the toddler to make decisions. The toddler has to be allowed to make some decisions if he or she is to develop autonomy.

61. ❸ If the child sits quietly on the nurse's lap and does not cry when the mother leaves the hospital, this behavior may indicate a questionable disturbance in the parent–child relationship.

1. Even if an 18-month-old child had experience staying in the hospital, she would still cry when her mother left her. If the hospital experience was a bad one, the child would be even more upset when the mother left.

2. Good preparation of an 18-month-old child for hospitalization would not stop the child from crying when the mother leaves. The child at this age finds it difficult to be separated from his or her mother. The toddler is not sure if the mother is coming back.

4. An 18-month-old child is not ready to begin developing autonomy.

62. ❶ Teaching needs for a patient with transitional cell carcinoma of the bladder would include information about the side effects of chemotherapy, information related to surgery and biopsy, and effects of radiation therapy on skin and other symptoms.

(2, 3, 4) These options may be of some interest to a teenager but not as important as the information in option (1).

63. ❸ The nurse would expect the mother to report that the 7-month-old child is sitting alone for brief periods.

1. Walking does not occur until 12 to 21 months of age.

2. Creeping up and down stairs occurs between 10 and 12 months.

4. Holding the head erect occurs at 2 to 3 months.

64. ❸ Temper tantrums are best controlled by identifying when the child is getting frustrated and redirecting his or her activities. Almost every toddler has temper tantrums.

1. If an 18-month-old child is having temper tantrums, it would be an untrue statement to tell a mother that her child is too old to act like that. The mother needs to be given information that will help to reduce the temper tantrums. Before a nurse can help a parent manage a toddler's temper tantrums, the mother must explore the reason for the behavior.

2. Temper tantrums are usually a normal part of a child's development; there is no need to consult with a child psychologist.

4. A child having a temper tantrum should not be restrained. Restraint would only draw more attention to the child and may cause him or her to increase the temper tantrums. The toddler needs to be shown a better way to express his or her feelings.

65. ❶ Providing the infant with a hard rubber toy is safe and helps to relieve the discomfort and the need to chew on something while cutting teeth.

2. The practice of placing an aspirin tablet against the erupting gum area should be avoided. An aspirin can erode gingival (gum) tissues and can be easily aspirated.

3. Ice cube can erode the gingival tissues and can easily be aspirated.

4. Whiskey (alcohol) products are potentially toxic to infants.

66. ❷ Herpes zoster is caused by the varicella virus and causes shingles and chickenpox.

(1, 3, 4) These options are incorrect as seen in rationale (2).

67. ❸ Ringworm is caused by fungus.

(1, 2, 4) These options are incorrect as seen in rationale (3).

68. ❸ A nurse should explain that ringworm is spread by direct and indirect contact.

(1, 2, 4) These options are incorrect as seen in rationale (3).

69. ❷ Therapeutic management of the child with ringworm infection would include administration of oral griseofulvin.

(1, 3, 4) These options are incorrect as seen in rationale (2).

70. ❶ An important nursing intervention in the care of a child with acute bacterial conjunctivitis (pink eye) is to apply warm, moist compresses to remove crust. It is benign and self-limiting but extremely contagious, particularly among children. Discharge from the eye is moderate to copious and can cause the eyelids to stick together.

2. Continuous compresses are unnecessary; it would be extremely difficult to maintain continuous compresses.

3. Oral antihistamines are not used to minimize itching.

4. Corticosteroids are contraindicated in the presence of infectious conjunctivitis because they reduce ocular resistance to bacteria. A specific antibacterial medication (local and systemic) is used in conjunction with eye irrigations and warm compresses to remove crust from the eye.

71. ❷ The Denver Developmental Screening Test (DDST) is used to detect developmental delays in infancy and in the preschool-aged child.

(1, 3, 4) These options are incorrect as seen in rationale (2).

72. ❹ When a mother tells the home health nurse that her child has been vomiting, complains of a "stomach ache," and has abdominal pain, the nurse will ask the mother if the child's pain started at the umbilicus (McBurney's point) and then shifted to the right lower quadrant. It would be important to take the child to the hospital because these can be symptoms of appendicitis.

1. An enema may cause the appendix to rupture.

2. Taking the child's temperature, keeping him in bed, and, if the pain persists, calling the physician is incorrect because the child needs to be seen by a physician immediately. The child may have appendicitis, and the appendix may rupture.

3. The child should have nothing by mouth; if the child has appendicitis, he may have surgery immediately.

73. **④** An above-normal amount of glucose outside the cells is called hyperglycemia. A person in a hyperglycemic state can develop ketone metabolic acidosis and go into a diabetic coma. A normal blood glucose for an adult is 70 to 120 mg/dL. Ann is 14 years old; therefore, she has the same blood glucose levels as an adult. When a diabetic client does not have enough insulin, the body must burn fat for energy. When fat is broken down and used for energy, it releases ketone bodies into the urine, causing a sweet, fruity odor on the person's breath and a low blood pH (acetic).

(1, 2, 3) These options are incorrect as seen in rationale (4).

74. **①** A person with insulin-dependent diabetes mellitus (IDDM) will have weight loss, not weight gain. Other signs are polyuria, polydipsia, hyperglycemia, dehydration, and hypovolemia. The wasting of glucose in the urine will cause weight loss.

(2, 3, 4) These options are incorrect as seen in rationale (1).

75. **③** The test used to determine the amount of insulin a person needs is a simple blood sample to determine the amount of glucose in the blood. Formerly, urine samples were used to determine the person's blood glucose level. This procedure definitely is not as accurate as using blood (chemstick) with a glucose meter.

(1, 2, 4) These options are incorrect as seen in rationale (3).

76. **①** A person on a sliding scale should have his or her blood sugar checked by the chemstick procedure (using a glucose meter) shortly before meals and at bedtime. It reading is obtained at this time because it would be more accurate than after the person has eaten. With a sliding insulin scale, the physician writes an order stating how much regular insulin is to be given for various levels of blood glucose. For example, if the blood glucose level is 200 to 250 mg/dL, then 10 U of regular insulin may be administered. Always remember that regular insulin is used on a sliding insulin scale, peaking in 2 to 4 h. Normal adult blood glucose is 70 to 120 mg/dL.

(2, 3, 4) These options are incorrect as seen in rationale (1).

77. **④** Remember, this is an *except*-type question. Look for the option that is not true. Increased physical exercise will increase the use of glucose and, therefore, decrease the body's requirement for insulin. This is the only option that will decrease the body's requirement for insulin.

1. Overeating will increase the body's glucose supply and, therefore, increase the need for insulin.

2. Acute infection causes stress on the body, and stress increases the release of corticosteroids; this will increase the production of glucose. With more glucose, the body will need more insulin.

3. Increased emotional strain is a stress on the body. Corti steroid levels will increase, which will increase glucose; therefore, more insulin is needed.

78. **④** If Ann feels she is going into diabetic acidosis, she should check her blood sugar level, then give herself insulin per physician's orders.

(1, 2, 3) These options are incorrect as seen in rationale (4). All of these options suggest that she eat foods high in sugar, which would put her deeper into a diabetic coma.

79. **④** Typical signs and symptoms of diabetic acidosis are deep rapid Kussmaul's respirations (very deep, gasping type), polyuria, nausea and vomiting, hypotension, and abdominal rigidity. Late signs are coma or stupor.

(1, 2, 3) These options are incorrect as seen in rationale (4).

80. **②** Signs and symptoms of metabolic acidosis are rapid, deep respiration as a compensatory mechanism to rid the lungs of carbon dioxide (CO_2), which is at a very high level in metabolic acidosis; bradycardia is caused by acidosis because of the acetic effect on the heart muscle; decreased level of consciousness (LOC) is caused by electrolyte imbalance; profound shock occurs.

1. Shallow respirations do not occur because there is a need for the respiratory system to compensate and exhale carbon dioxide. Bradycardia occurs as a result of acidosis, not tachycardia. Decreased LOC would occur.

3. An increased urinary output would not occur because the heart would be unable to perfuse the kidneys. Bradycardia would occur because of the low pH and its effect on the heart; tachycardia would not occur; decreased LOC would occur.

4. Deep, rapid respirations, not shallow respirations, would occur in an attempt to rid the lungs of carbon dioxide. Cheyne-Stokes respiration is a breathing pattern of several breaths and then apnea; it is a sign of impending death.

81. **①** Signs and symptoms of respiratory acidosis include increase in CO_2 level; deep, rapid respirations; and change in LOC.

(2, 3, 4) These options are incorrect as seen in rationale (1).

82. **④** The first signs and symptoms of tracheoesophageal fistula with esophageal atresia occur immediately after the infant is fed. The infant will struggle, become cyanotic, and stop breathing. Esophageal atresia is the congenital closure of the esophageal tube. Tracheoesophageal fistula is a break between the trachea and the esophagus, allowing food to enter the trachea. Surgery must be performed immediately to correct the problem or else the infant will die.

1. Projectile vomiting by an infant is a sign of pyloric stenosis.

2. If an infant vomits and has diarrhea and tachypnea immediately after eating, an intestinal bacterial infection or a viral infection may be involved.

3. Vomiting and diarrhea may be a sign of infection or intolerance to infant formula.

83. **③** The first indication to the nurse that an infant with tracheoesophageal fistula and esophageal atresia needs tracheal suctioning is substernal retraction.

1. Hyperinflation of the lungs is seen in lung diseases such as emphysema and asthma.

2. Drooling and coughing are normal behaviors for an infant.

4. Apnea may indicate tracheal obstruction or lung disease.

84. ❸ For the first week or more after a tracheoesophageal repair, the infant cannot swallow milk and cannot have an NG tube for feeding. The best way to meet the psychological needs of an infant who must be fed by a gastrostomy tube or TPN intravenously is to give the infant a pacifier and hold the infant as often as possible. The pacifier satisfies the need to suck, and holding the infant helps him or her to associate pleasure with eating.

1. Holding the infant and rocking in a rocking chair for 3 h each shift may not meet the infant's needs. During some shifts, the infant may have to be held more than during other shifts.

2. Talking and singing to the infant is okay, but an infant with a tracheoesophageal fistula cannot be bottle-fed; the infant will aspirate.

4. Lightly stroking the infant's abdomen will not offer the infant the psychological support he or she needs.

85. ❶ The following are normal values for newborns: pulse 70 to 170; respirations 40 to 90; and fasting glucose level 30 to 80 mg/dL.

(2, 3, 4) These options are incorrect; correct values are given in rationale (1).

86. ❸ The major stress occurring during the period from middle infancy throughout preschool years is caused by separation anxiety.

1. Denial is a defense mechanism.

2. According to Erikson's psychosocial phases, integrity vs despair occurs in the elderly.

4. Toilet training occurs between the ages of 1 and 3 years. Anxiety should not be associated with toilet training, unless the parents are demanding and lack understanding.

87. ❹ Children between the ages of 5½ and 12 years are going through the phase of industry vs inferiority. These children are in school and if they are industrious and get good grades, then they will develop some self-confidence; if they get poor grades, they will feel inferior.

1. The trust vs mistrust phase is from birth to 18 months. The child learns to trust or mistrust the caregiver. If the child is loved and cared for, she or he will grow up to trust. She or he will usually be unafraid to love or trust anyone.

2. The autonomy vs shame and doubt phase is from 18 months to 3 years of age. This is the age when the child demands independence. The parents can help the child establish autonomy, or they can abuse them mentally or physically when the child is trying to be independent, which will cause the child to have feelings of shame and doubt.

3. The initiative vs. guilt phase is from 3½ to 5½ years. This is the age when the child is learning right from wrong and is trying to learn new skills. If the parents encourage the child even when the child fails to accomplish tasks, the child will develop initiative. If the parents are negative about the child's accomplishments, the child will feel guilty about not pleasing his or her parents.

88. ❷ More children die in motor vehicle accidents during the period from of 1 to 4 years of age than at any other time of life. Failure to use child restraint devices (infant carriers or car seats) often results in death because children are thrown around or ejected from the automobile.

(1, 3, 4) These options are incorrect as seen in rationale (2).

89. ❹ The second most common cause of accidental death of preschool boys is drowning, most likely because boys spend a great deal of time outdoors and are interested in exploring their surroundings.

(1, 2, 3) These options are incorrect; the ages at which these accidents occur most often are given in rationales for questions 88, 90, and 91.

90. ❶ The second most common cause of accidental death of preschool girls is burns, most likely because girls spend more time indoors, watching and helping in the kitchen.

(2, 3, 4) These options are incorrect; the ages at which these accidents occur most often are given in rationales for questions 88, 89, 90, and 91.

91. ❸ The highest incidence of poisoning occurs in children 2 years old. At this age, a child is very curious, is very mobile, and has no fears.

(1, 2, 4) These options are incorrect as seen in rationale (3).

92. ❸ The type of fluid replacement a doctor will use if a child is burned depends on the hematocrit (the amount of erythrocytes [RBCs] packed by centrifugation in a given volume of blood). Erythrocytes carry oxygen, which is necessary for life. The physician will determine if packed cells are to be given by reviewing the laboratory workup. If the hematocrit is low, packed cells may be given. If the hematocrit is high, as it would be in cases of severe burns, then IV fluids would be administered. A high hematocrit can cause the blood to clot.

1. The degree of burn would be an estimate of depth of the burn.

2. Blood volume does not give information about the number of RBCs. If the blood volume was very high, the hematocrit probably would be low.

4. Skin turgor can give some indication of hydration, but it would not be as accurate as the hematocrit.

93. ❷ If a blood transfusion is to be given to a 2-year-old child with acute lymphocytic leukemia (ALL), the nurse would expect the physician to order packed cells started with normal saline. A child with ALL has an abnormal decrease in the number of blood platelets (thrombocytopenia). The packed cells will help replace the platelets with WBCs destroyed by the disease and help replace the RBCs destroyed by chemotherapy. Chemotherapy depresses bone marrow and will depress the production of all cells. Only normal saline can be used to start blood.

(1, 3, 4) These options are incorrect as seen in rationale (2).

94. ❹ After leukemia, brain tumors cause the most deaths in children.

1. Wilms' tumor is a malignant tumor on the kidneys that occurs primarily in children. Signs and symptoms are painless, intermittent hematuria and a palpable abdominal mass. Pain and

hypertension will occur in the later stages. The tumor should not be palpated because it can spread cancer cells throughout the body.

2. Reye's syndrome almost always follows within 1 to 3 days of an acute viral infection, such as an upper respiratory infection or type B influenza, and may be linked to aspirin use. It is an acute childhood illness that causes fatty infiltration of the liver with concurrent hyperammonemia, encephalopathy, and increased ICP. Prognosis depends on the severity of CNS depression.

3. Sickle cell anemia is a congenital hemolytic anemia that occurs primarily in the black population. RBC become sickle shaped and break easily. Such cells impair circulation, resulting in chronic ill health (fatigue, dyspnea or exertion, and swollen joints), periodic crises, long-term complications, and premature death. Penicillin prophylaxis can decrease diseases caused by infections. Fifty percent of these clients die by their early twenties; few live to middle age (45–55 years).

95. ❶ A child with a ventricular septal defect will have shunting of blood from the left side of the heart to the right; the pressure in the left side of the heart is greater during systole, and the blood is pushed to the right (to the pulmonary artery and the lungs). Therefore, the blood is oxygenated, and the child will not be cyanotic.

(2, 3, 4) These options are incorrect as seen in rationale (1).

96. ❷ A child with cyanotic heart disease will have passage of blood from the right side of the heart to the left side. When blood is shunted from the right side of the heart to the left, this blood never reaches the lungs; rather, it goes out the aorta to the body. An example of cyanotic heart disease is tetralogy of Fallot.

(1, 3, 4) These options are incorrect as seen in rationale (2).

97. ❷ Infants and toddlers have a higher incidence of ruptured appendices because they cannot describe their symptoms properly.

(1, 3, 4) The options are incorrect as seen in rationale (2).

98. ❹ The method of instilling ear drops in children is to pull the earlobe down and back and then to instill the medication.

(1, 2, 3) These options are incorrect as seen in rationale (4).

99. ❹ A practice that is often recommended to help prevent recurrence of otitis media is to eliminate a bedtime bottle offered when the child is in bed. When the child sucks on a bottle lying down, some of the liquid from the baby's mouth runs down the child's face and into the ear. This keeps the ear moist and vulnerable for infection. Bacteria grow rapidly in dark, moist areas.

(1, 2, 3) These options are incorrect as seen in rationale (4).

100. ❶ A complication commonly associated with extensive burns and infected burns is Curling's ulcer, an ulcer in the stomach or duodenum. It is thought to be caused by an increased production of hydrochloric (HCl) acid. The increase in HCl acid is thought to be caused by severe pain from the burns.

Because Curling's ulcer occurs commonly in conjunction with severe burns, clients suffering from burns are given a medication such as Zantac, Tagamet, Pepcid, or Carafate as soon as they are admitted to the hospital, in hopes of preventing ulcers from occurring.

(2, 3, 4) These options are incorrect as seen in rationale (1).

Chapter 21

Psychiatric Disorders

TOPICAL OUTLINE

I. ESTABLISHING A THERAPEUTIC RELATIONSHIP

A. Initial Phase

The admission procedure offers an opportunity for an initial interaction between the patient and the nurse.

1. The nurse should acknowledge the patient by name and should introduce himself or herself. The nurse must demonstrate acceptance of the patient's behavior, establish rapport, and provide an opportunity for the patient to begin to develop trust.

2. During this phase of a therapeutic relationship, the patient may test the nurse's commitment by missing appointments or by some type of acting-out behavior. It is in this phase of the relationship that the patient's problems are identified, nursing diagnosis and patient goals are determined, priorities are set, and plans are formulated to achieve the goals.

3. The nurse strives to care for a patient in such a manner that a sense of trust and confidence develops.

4. Offer the patient unconditional acceptance.

5. The nurse should actively listen to the patient and allow the patient to discuss feelings of anxiety, hostility, guilt, and frustration. Open-ended questions are used, for example, "Tell me more," or "You were saying," which encourages a patient to vent his or her feelings.

6. Stay with the patient and respect his or her personal space. Sit down in the room with the patient, showing him or her that you have time.

B. Working Phase

In the working phase of the relationship, the patient and the nurse are actively involved in meeting the goals established during the initial phase of the relationship.

1. The patient may fluctuate between dependence and independence in an attempt to acknowledge the painful and difficult aspects of his or her life.

2. In this phase, the patient should feel more secure and openly discuss topics that he or she was initially unable to discuss.

3. The nurse needs to encourage a plan of action, implement the plan, and evaluate the results of the plan in order to alter the patient's behavior.

4. Assess the patient's readiness for independent functioning.

C. Termination Phase

Termination means dissolving the relationship between the nurse and the patient.

1. As the termination phase draws near, the nurse reminds the patient of the agreed-upon duration of the relationship and encourages him or her to socialize with others. Tapering off contact with the patient is a helpful way to encourage the patient's independence.

2. The termination phase can be traumatic for the patient. The nurse recognizes this loss and helps the patient adapt to this problem. The nurse recognizes that termination invokes stress and he or she supports the patient's coping behavior.

3. Focusing on the future in a more relaxed, less intense interaction helps the patient to adjust.

4. The nurse needs to provide referrals to others on the health care team as needed.

II. DEFENSE MECHANISMS

A. Denial

1. Denial is a commonly used coping mechanism by which a person denies the existence of some external reality. The person who uses denial as a coping mechanism is unaware that he or she is using it.

2. For example, when a patient is diagnosed with cancer, he or she may deny it by saying, "Oh no, there must be a mistake. I don't have cancer."

3. For a brief or lengthy period of time, denial generally operates as a protective and often healthy mechanism, protecting the patient from the shock of reality until he or she is better able to deal with it. In time, denial usually diminishes, and the patient gradually begins to deal with reality.

B. Regression

1. Regression involves a retreat to a less mature level of thought or action in an attempt to avoid anxiety and to cope with stress.

2. For example, a young child will become frightened when admitted to the hospital and may return to habits such as bed wetting, thumb sucking, or wanting a bottle again.

C. Displacement

1. Displacement is the discharge of pent-up emotions—usually anger—onto objects, animals, or people perceived as less dangerous than those that originally induced the emotions.

2. For example, after an argument with her husband, the wife leaves and slams a door or breaks a dish.

D. Repression

1. A person unconsciously forces unacceptable certain feelings or thoughts into his or her unconscious.

2. For example, a person who was sexually abused may have repressed a large part of his or her formative years into the unconscious mind so he or she cannot remember them. The memories are too painful and are repressed, which occurs at the unconscious level.

Note: Do not confuse repression with *suppression,* which is the conscious rejection of unacceptable thoughts, traits, or wishes by ascribing them to others.

E. Suppression

1. A person consciously excludes from his or her mind certain thoughts or feelings that cause anxiety. Suppression operates at the conscious level.

2. For example, "I'll think about it tomorrow."

F. Rationalization

1. Rationalization is the justification of behavior to conceal one's true feelings.

2. For example, a person who fails an examination may rationalize that the examination was not fair.

G. Fantasy

1. Fantasy is nonrational mental activity that allows a person to escape from the daily pressures of life. The person enters a world where he or she can daydream about whatever brings him or her pleasure.

2. Adults spend time each day daydreaming; it provides an escape from the pressures of life.

3. The excessive use of fantasy by adults or children reduces the person's contact with reality and can render them incapable of dealing with the demands of life.

H. Intellectualization

1. Through intellectualization, a person uses his or her intellectual power of thinking, reasoning, and analyzing to avoid emotional issues; talking directly about how he or she feels is too painful or threatening.

2. For example, an alcoholic patient uses intellectualization when he or she objects to the definition of alcoholism as a way of avoiding his or her problem with excessive use of alcohol.

III. COMMUNICATION TECHNIQUES

Part I: Nurse–Client Interaction

The nurse needs to understand his or her own feelings before he or she can help others understand their feelings.

A. Clarifying Feelings

1. The nurse restates an emotional word or phrase used by the patient. The nurse tries to help the patient label his or her feelings to create a clearer picture of how the patient feels.

2. For example, the patient might say, "I left my children alone on several occasions, but I don't think that I've really ever hurt them." The nurse replies, "You are concerned that you may have hurt your children?"

B. Reflecting Feelings

1. The nurse helps the patient to identify and talk about feelings that he or she is experiencing.

2. For example: Patient: "I thought the man who hurt me was my friend." Nurse: "The man who raped you was a friend before he raped you?"

C. Confronting Feelings

1. The nurse identifies the patient's contradictions by using a questioning tone of voice.

2. For example: Patient: "I know my husband beats me, but he really does love me."
Nurse: "Your husband beats you, and you are telling me he loves you?"

D. Verifying Perceptions

1. The nurse describes his or her perception of the patient's behavior and asks the patient for verification.

2. For example: Patient: "I don't have a drinking problem; all of my problems stem from my divorce."

Nurse: "You are having difficulty accepting the fact that you are an alcoholic?"

E. Self-Disclosure

1. The nurse demonstrates genuine regard for the patient by means of therapeutic use of self.

2. For example: Patient: "I am very frightened to go back to work after being off for so long."

Nurse: "It must be difficult for you. I was off work for several months last year because of an illness, and I was nervous about going back."

IV. COMMUNICATION TECHNIQUES

Part II: Nurse-Directed Communication

A. Giving Information

1. Communicating facts to a patient is a frequent nursing intervention.

2. For example, "You are scheduled for surgery at 8:00 AM. You will receive three enemas this evening; don't eat or drink anything after midnight tonight."

B. Silence

Although silence often is uncomfortable for the nurse, it is an effective way to encourage the patient to communicate. Silence also can be used to slow the pace of the conversation.

C. Summarizing

Summarizing is an effective way to assist the patient in examining the nurse–client interaction. It is also an appropriate technique for terminating a nurse–client counseling session.

D. Directing

Directing encourages the patient to explore and express his or her thoughts and feelings. Expressions from the nurse such as, "You were saying," "Please continue," and "Go on, you were saying" encourage the patient to focus on the subject being discussed.

E. Questioning

Frequently, the nurse uses open-ended questions during the therapeutic communication sessions. Open-ended questions encourage expanding and exploring, for example, "How," "What," "When," "Will you elaborate," and "Will you give me an example." The nurse avoids asking closed-ended questions that can be answered with a "yes" or a "no."

F. Interviewing

Interviewing is a specific type of guided and limited intercommunication with an identified purpose. An interview is conducted to collect a database for analysis and for decision-making purposes.

V. BARRIERS TO THERAPEUTIC COMMUNICATION

A. Preaching to the Client

A barrier to communication is the nurse advising or telling the patient what he or she should do, think, or feel. To advise the patient on these issues impinges on his or her individuality and his or her right to determine how to feel, think, or act.

B. Belittling the Client

A nurse belittles a patient when the nurse treats the patient with indifference or acts if the patient is not important, or defends the patient's doctor, hospital, or nursing staff.

C. Closed-Ended Questions

Closed-ended questions limit the patient's response to one- or two-word answers, such as "yes" or "no." These questions inhibit the patient's freedom to elaborate on his or her thoughts and feelings.

D. False Reassurance

False reassurance is a common barrier to therapeutic communication, for example, telling the client that "Everything will be all right," or "Don't worry, everything will be fine." This reassurance can become a habit, and it tends to terminate communication.

VI. ANXIETY DISORDERS

A. Anxiety

1. Description

   a. Anxiety can be defined as a fear that is not justified by reality or an extreme reaction to a real threat.

   b. Anxiety consists of three major components: behavior, cognition, and autonomic responses.

   c. Behavioral aspects such as avoidance in the case of anxiety is specific to certain situations. For example, not taking a scheduled examination will temporarily reduce anxiety.

   d. The cognitive component of anxiety is related to the thought process. For example, just thinking of a test may produce anxiety.

   e. The behavioral and cognitive components of anxiety cause the autonomic response, which increases heart rate and blood pressure.

2. Effects of Anxiety

   The effects of anxiety include physiologic, perceptual, and cognitive.

   a. Physiologic Effects of Anxiety

   (1) Initially, the neurotransmitters epinephrine and norepinephrine are released from the adrenal medulla, and cortisone is secreted by the adrenal cortex.

(2) Epinephrine increases heart rate and dilates the bronchioles.

(3) Norepinephrine causes peripheral vasoconstriction and increases blood pressure.

(4) Glucocorticoids and epinephrine increase the blood glucose level and urinary frequency because the kidneys are better perfused.

b. Perceptual Effects of Anxiety

(1) Anxiety increases the way an individual perceives and processes sensory input. In mild anxiety, a person is capable of grasping increased sensory input. The five sensory channels—sight, smell, taste, touch, and hearing—are more responsive to sensation.

(2) Moderate anxiety dulls perception; the individual's sensory channels are less responsive to sensory input.

(3) In severe anxiety, the patient's perception becomes increasingly distorted, and sensory input is reduced.

(4) Anxiety that reaches a level of panic causes perception to become grossly distorted. At this point, the individual is incapable of recognizing what is real and what is unreal and is completely out of control.

c. Effects of Anxiety on Cognition

(1) Cognition is the ability to concentrate, learn, and solve problems.

(2) Mild and moderate anxiety levels are more conducive to concentration, learning, and problem solving.

(3) Severe anxiety seriously hinders cognitive function.

(4) The severely anxious individual has difficulty concentrating.

(5) Nonverbal behavior usually reveals both fine and gross motor tremors, facial grimaces, and other purposeless activity, such as pacing and hand wringing.

(6) Panic level anxiety produces even greater emotional pain and behavioral disorganization than the other levels of anxiety.

B. Panic Disorder

1. Description

a. Panic disorders are characterized by recurrent, unpredictable anxiety attacks of panic proportions. Panic attacks usually are manifested by a sudden onset of intense apprehension or terror and often are associated with feelings of doom.

b. The individual experiences dyspnea, chest pain, palpitations, choking or smothering sensation, dizziness, vertigo, paresthesia, sweating, and fainting.

c. During panic attacks, the individual may make extreme efforts to escape from what he or she perceives to be causing the panic.

C. Phobic Disorders

1. Description

a. A phobia is a persistent, irrational fear of an object or situation that, when looked at objectively, does not pose a danger. As a result, the individual experiences a compelling desire to avoid the dreaded object or situation.

b. The phobic person usually recognizes that the fear is unreasonable in proportion to the actual danger presented.

D. Social Phobia

1. Description

a. The individual has a persistent irrational fear and desire to avoid situations in which he or she may be exposed to scrutiny by others, and the fear of humiliating himself or herself.

b. The phobic person perceives others as threatening sources of criticism and considers himself or herself as insignificant and unimportant in comparison to others.

E. Agoraphobia

1. Description

a. Agoraphobia is a marked fear of being alone or in a public place from which escape would be difficult or help would be unavailable in the event the person suddenly becomes disabled.

b. A patient with agoraphobia usually is excessively dependent on others and may become symptomatic for the first time after the loss of a significant relationship.

c. Agoraphobia is most intense when the individual enters enclosed spaces such as airplanes, cars, stores, or churches, or in situations where the person is surrounded by crowds.

d. Complications such as chemical dependence and major depression are common.

F. Nursing Implications

1. Nursing Diagnosis
Nursing diagnoses applicable to patients with anxiety disorders include the following:

a. Disturbed cognitive functioning associated with severe anxiety

b. Impaired verbal communication related to severe anxiety

2. Planning: Goal Setting

a. Planning: Despite the differences among the anxiety disorders, the major goals for nursing care have applicability to each of them.

b. To help the patient reach the planned goals, the nurse needs to establish a supportive relationship with the patient.

c. This relationship is characterized by trust, respect, and empathy on the part of the nurse.

d. Displaying these attributes to the patient on a consistent basis will lay the groundwork for therapy to begin.

e. These goals are concerned primarily with the patient learning about anxiety and how to cope with it.

f. To learn and apply self-help techniques designed to increase problem-solving and coping skills reduces anxiety.

g. The nurse needs to explain the concept of anxiety to the patient in simple terms and emphasize that all people feel anxious from time to time. In doing so, the nurse reduces the patient's anxiety by "normalizing" this experience to a degree.

h. Ask the patient to maintain a diary in which he or she records when he or she feels anxious, what he or she is doing at the time, what he or she is thinking, and who he or she is with.

i. Ask the patient to maintain a graph with anxiety levels on one axis and time measure in 20-min intervals on the other axis. These activities can help the patient to develop an awareness not only of when, but also under what circumstances, his or her anxiety was mild, moderate, severe, or panic proportions.

j. Discussing and analyzing the findings with the patient are crucial in the process of planning and goal setting.

k. Once the patient has identified those factors associated with uncomfortable symptoms of anxiety, the nurse needs to help the patient to identify ways of reducing anxiety to a tolerable level.

3. Relaxation Therapy

    a. Relaxation therapy can be used to help the patient learn how to control his or her anxiety.

    b. The patient learns to perform progressive muscular relaxation and deep breathing exercises to decrease his or her anxiety.

    c. Using this form of therapy, by way of audio tapes each morning and evening, helps the patient to control his or her anxiety.

4. Group Therapy

    Besides involvement in learning self-help skills, patients with anxiety disorders also benefit from individual and group therapies designed to assist them in identifying their emotions and automatic behaviors used to relieve uncomfortable feelings.

5. Treatment

    a. Usually, antianxiety agents are prescribed for anxiety disorders during the initial phase of treatment.

    b. Because many anxiety-disordered individuals are at risk for developing chemical abuse dependence, antianxiety agents—which are, for the most part, addictive—are administered sparingly and on a short-term basis.

    c. Antianxiety agents do not cure anxiety disorders, but they do calm patients sufficiently so that they can engage in and benefit from therapies that may be useful, if not curative.

    d. The extent to which nursing care for patients with anxiety disorders is effective is based on the patient's subjective report of his or her feeling state as well as changes in his or her behavior—such as decreased muscular tension and tremors and increased appetite—which indicate improvement.

VII. ANXIETY DISORDERS OF CHILDHOOD OR ADOLESCENCE

A. Nursing Implications

1. Separation Anxiety Disorder

    a. Separation anxiety, or panic on separation from home and/or parent, is a major problem for the hospitalized child from age 6 months to approximately 3 to 4 years.

    b. Support during separation, for example, by a primary nurse and a minimal number of other nursing staff providing empathy and verbal and physical reassurance can be enormously helpful.

    c. The nurse's respect for the child's normal routine, preferences, and coping style, along with familiar toys from home, help to reduce the trauma of hospitalization.

    d. If the parents cannot be with their child, they or the child's siblings can make tapes of their voices, reading a favorite story or just talking or singing a favorite song.

2. Stages of Separation Anxiety Disorder

    a. Young children usually react to separation from their families by going through stages of protest, despair, and denial, and in that order.

    b. During the protest stage, the child cries and screams for his or her parents (sometimes for hours) and may be inconsolable.

    c. During stage 2 (despair), the child may become passive or withdrawn and ignore his or her parents or act angry when they return to the hospital. During this stage, the parents themselves need reassurance and support because the intensity of their child's despair or anger can add to their own feelings of helplessness and guilt.

    d. During the final stage (denial), the child may appear to be adjusting well to the hospital environment, when, in reality, he or she may be resigning himself or herself to what he or she feels is total abandonment.

        (1) An inexperienced nurse may see the child as a "good patient" (passive and quiet) and that the presence of the parents upsets the child and may discourage them from visiting.

        (2) This perpetuates the problem because the lack of contact with the parents will intensify the child's feelings of abandonment.

        (3) In addition to encouraging and supporting the parents' visits and overnight stays, the nurse should offer the child realistic reassurance.

        (4) This includes telling the child where the parents are and when they will return.

3. Older Child and Adolescent with Separation Anxiety

    a. The older child or adolescent is also vulnerable to separation anxiety.

    b. This includes separation from peers.

c. The older child's distress may not be as obvious or overwhelming as it is for the younger patient.

d. For the older age group, phone calls, tapes, cards, and regular planned visits from family and friends are helpful.

4. Discharge: At discharge, the child who has forged attachments and relationships during his or her hospital stay must be helped to separate from the hospital by a thoughtful plan.

a. This can include calls or visits to the hospital at the time of follow-up appointments or at other times when his or her favorite nurse is available.

b. A referral to a public health or home nursing agency can provide useful backup.

c. It is imperative to have a coordinated discharge and follow-up plan for the chronically, physically, or emotionally ill child.

VIII. DISRUPTIVE BEHAVIOR DISORDERS

A. Attention-Deficit Disorder

1. Incidence and Etiology

a. One of the most extensively studied diagnoses in child psychiatry is attention-deficit disorder (ADD), formerly called hyperactivity.

b. It is a commonly diagnosed problem in the United States, occurring in 5 to 10 percent of school-aged children.

c. The agreed-upon criteria for ADD are those required by the *Diagnostic and Statistical Manual of Mental Disorders, Third Edition* (DSM-III-R).

d. Despite extensive research on the possible biochemical etiology of ADD, none has been found.

e. There is evidence for psychosocial etiology in the responsiveness of the behavioral problems associated with ADD to treatment based on learning theory.

f. Parent and child training methods of delivering positive reinforcement (e.g., token system) and mildly aversive consequences (e.g., time out) as an intervention strategy have been especially useful in the school setting.

2. Behavior Related to Attention-Deficit Disorder
The child with ADD displays, to a degree greater than other children of the same mental age, the following behaviors:

a. Squirming and fidgeting

b. Difficulty remaining seated when requested

c. Difficulty taking turns in games and in classroom settings

d. Difficulty following through on others' instructions

e. Difficulty sustaining attention in tasks or play

f. Frequent shifting from one uncompleted activity to another

g. Excessive talking

h. Frequent interruptions of others

i. Difficulty playing quietly

3. Treatment

a. Methylphenidate (Ritalin) is the drug of choice for adjunct treatment of ADD.

b. The therapeutic effect of Ritalin is the correction of hyperactivity in ADD to increase mental alertness and improve mood.

c. Ritalin has high dependence and abuse potential.

d. The principal adverse effects of treatment are insomnia and suppression of growth.

e. Insomnia results from central nervous system (CNS) stimulation and can be minimized by taking the last dose of the day no later than 6 h before bedtime.

f. Dextroamphetamine (Adderall) is considered a very effective drug for treatment of ADD. It is still being investigated and can be used only in clinical research situations or can be used by children who were taking the drug before it was pulled from the market for further investigation.

4. Prognosis

a. Previously, it was thought that ADD was likely to remit as the child grew older. However, extensive follow-up research has led to the recognition that adolescents and even adults may continue to benefit from treatment.

b. These individuals must continue to develop coping strategies to deal with their impulsiveness in new or changing situations (e.g., the workplace).

5. Nursing Implications

a. The nurse can care for children with ADD in a variety of clinical settings.

b. The nurse should always seek the parents' input regarding their usual management methods for dealing with the child.

c. Prompt and reliable praise for appropriate behavior and consistently implemented familiar negative consequences when undesirable behavior occurs will help the child adjust to his or her new environment.

d. During illness and/or hospitalization, emphatic support of nursing and medical staff is needed for the child to cope adaptively. This is especially true if the child's stimulant medication must be temporarily discontinued.

IX. EATING DISORDERS

A. Anorexia Nervosa

Eating disorder exemplified by self-imposed starvation, with a fear of not being in control of one's own life. It can cause death. Anorexia nervosa occurs primarily in white female adolescents living in middle- to upper-middle–class environments.

1. Psychological and Physiologic Disturbances

a. Body image: The patient feels fat despite being emaciated.

b. The patient misinterprets internal and external stimuli, especially hunger, and may be starving herself to death.

c. The patient has overwhelming feelings of ineffectiveness and inadequacy.

d. The patient usually has not established her own identity.

e. Prolonged starvation has serious medical consequences that usually are secondary to malnutrition, dehydration, and disturbances in electrolyte balance.

f. First, in cases of weight loss of approximately 25 percent of average normal body weight, the patient can develop amenorrhea.

g. The loss of menses can be a particularly hazardous complication, especially if prolonged, because it can cause infertility and estrogen loss.

h. Lack of estrogen over a long period of time (years) contributes to calcium deficiency and skeletal changes resulting in osteoporosis.

i. Weight restoration to at least 90 percent of average normal body weight usually is necessary to ensure return of normal menses.

j. A secondary, potentially dangerous effect of starvation over a prolonged period of time is decreased myocardial muscle mass.

k. Diminished cardiac functioning combined with dehydration leads to decreased heart rate, blood pressure, and cardiac output.

l. Less serious, though debilitating, side effects of starvation include lack of energy, weakness, intolerance to cold, and pain when sitting or lying down due to lack of body fat.

m. Depression, which frequently coexists with anorexia nervosa, causes a decreased ability to concentrate and sleep disturbances.

2. Family Involvement

a. The patient thinks that she cannot live up to her family's expectations.

b. The patient usually is described as being loving, devoted, well behaved, and always obeying her parents. This compliance can conceal the patient's feelings that she is deprived of controlling her own life.

c. As the patient matures and wants to make her own decisions, the feelings she is having are frightening to her. She fears that she will lose her parents' approval.

d. The patient acts out by not eating (being thin), but is in need of love and protection.

B. Bulimia Nervosa

Eating disorder primarily occurring in adolescent girls who have uncontrolled episodes of rapidly eating large amounts of food over a short period of time and then vomiting, ending in exhaustion and guilt.

1. Psychological Disturbances

a. Binge-eating results in feelings of physical and emotional discomfort.

b. The bulimic patient gives in to impulses and then controls body size through purging (vomiting).

c. Severe weight loss usually does not occur in bulimic patients (as it does in anorexic clients).

2. Physiologic Disturbances

a. Esophageal ulcers from vomiting hydrochloric (HCl) acid, which is repeatedly pushed up into the esophagus from episodes of vomiting.

b. Alkalosis from the loss of HCl acid.

c. Hypokalemia (low potassium) and hypochloremia (low chloride) from vomiting and constant use of diuretics.

d. "Lazy bowel syndrome" and malabsorption from abuse of laxatives and diuretics.

e. Tooth decay caused by the almost-constant exposure to the stomach contents (from vomiting).

f. Amenorrhea occurs but seldom in the bulimic patient.

C. Pica

1. Description

Appetite for ingestion of materials not fit for human consumption, such as starch, clay, ashes, plaster or paint chips, crayons, matches, or cigarette butts.

2. Etiology

a. Most children have a particular craving for a few items, which is largely determined by availability of the substance.

b. Although several investigators have tried to associate pica with specific nutritional deficiencies such as iron and magnesium, no evidence of nutritional inadequacy has been found.

3. Behavior Related to Pica

a. Between the ages of 12 and 18 months, children begin ingesting the object as a further extension of their curiosity and exploration.

b. This normal mouthing activity accounts for the high incidence of poisoning in toddlers. Between the ages of 3 and 5 years, this behavior tends to disappear.

4. Theories and Contributing Factors

Oral gratification from sucking on a bottle may be transferred to chewing on a window sill or eating paint chips because of lack of stimulation and attention from the mother.

a. Times of stress, such as birth of another sibling, are frequently associated with commencement of pica activity.

b. The most common maternal pattern seen in these families is dependency.

(1) Such mothers have a history of despair, passivity, and inactivity in everyday life. As a result, they are unable to stimulate or discipline the child to more constructive forms of activity.

(2) Another frequent pattern is the parent who is unaware of the child's pica, either from lack of knowledge that ingestion of such substances is harmful or from lack of supervision.

(3) The passive parent is "mentally" absent from home, but other parents may be "physically" absent to the point of delegation of all parental responsibility to other siblings or other adults.

X. MAJOR AFFECTIVE DISORDERS

According to the *Diagnostic and Statistical Manual of Mental Disorders, Fifth Edition* (DSM-V), the main characteristic of a mood disorder is the presence of a full or partial depressive or manic syndrome. A syndrome is a cluster of symptoms that a person experiences during a mood change that continues for a designated time. In addition to the mood change itself, the cluster of symptoms must include cognitive, motivational, physical, and behavioral changes in the individual.

A. Bipolar Disorder

1. Bipolar disorder consists of one or more manic episodes, followed by a depressive episode. Manic episodes typically begin suddenly, with a rapid escalation over a few days.

2. The first manic episode usually occurs before age 30 years, but it is very prevalent in children and adolescents.

3. Bipolar disorder is equally common in men and women, and it has a strong genetic or familial component.

B. Major Depression

1. Major depression (unipolar) is a disorder where the individual experiences recurrent major depressive episodes without signs of mania.

2. Depression is 10 times more common than schizophrenia and five times more common than major anxiety disorders.

3. Risk factors for depression include gender, age, marital status, social class, life events, personal resources, and personality characteristics.

4. Twice as many women as men are diagnosed with bipolar or major depression. However, men are diagnosed with bipolar (manic-depressive) disorders as often as women.

5. Women in our society generally have less power and are more dependent and passive than men. These characteristics can predispose women to chronically low levels of self-esteem and few personal resources to cope with stress, which may make the development of unipolar depression more likely.

6. Younger people experience unipolar and bipolar disorders more frequently than older people.

7. Unipolar depression appears to be somewhat less prevalent in married persons and in those living in intimate relationships than in the unmarried population.

8. Unipolar disorders have a higher incidence in the lower social classes than do bipolar disorders.

9. Patients with unipolar depression show higher scores than the general population on tests for introversion, neuroticism, obsessions, dependency, and guilt.

C. Signs and Symptoms of the Depressive Period

1. Behavioral

   a. Social withdrawal (social isolation)

   b. Decreased initiative (less involvement in activities)

   c. Irritability (negativism and sensation of being heavily burdened)

   d. Alcohol and drug abuse (the patient may use these substances to decrease anxiety and facilitate sleep)

2. Cognitive

   a. Difficulty concentrating (thought process slows down, short attention span)

   b. Helplessness (negativism permeates most aspects of patient's life)

3. Mood

   a. Sadness (feeling of a dark cloud or black veil hanging over them)

   b. Low self-esteem (negative feelings about self)

   c. Loss of emotional attachment (decreased interest in other people)

   d. Crying spells (constant crying or feeling the desire to cry)

4. Motivational

   a. Passivity (not actively involved in any decision making and prefers to have others care for them)

   b. Suicidal ideation (danger is greatest when they have enough energy to kill themselves or are hallucinating)

5. Physical

   a. Sleep disturbance (insomnia or sleeping 12–14 h at night; some sleep during the day)

   b. Loss of energy (fatigue)

   c. Psychomotor retardation (slowing down in body movement)

   d. Change in appetite (anorexia or increase in food intake)

   e. Weight loss (or gain)

   f. Anxiety (may feel anxious constantly)

D. Signs and Symptoms of the Manic Period

The manic patient's mood is the exact opposite of the patient experiencing depression; that is, happy, self-satisfied, confident, aggressive, feels "on top of the world," decreased need for sleep, talkative, and in total control of his or her life.

E. Major Affective Disorders

   ◆ Nursing Interventions: Should be directed toward the accomplishment of reasonable goals.

1. Knowledge of the patient's personality (likes and dislikes) is helpful in setting goals for the patient.

2. If patients are able to provide appropriate and meaningful information about themselves, they should always be considered the best source of information.

3. Manic and depressed patients usually neglect their appearance and personal hygiene. Therefore, the nurse may need to assist the patient with bathing, dressing, selecting clothes, and performing personal hygiene care. The nurse carrying out these duties should explain to the patient that he or she is being helped because he or she is unable to perform these functions.

4. The patient may have slow movements because of depression. The nurse should not rush the patient in order to save the nurse's time; this will slow the patient's recovery.

5. Because the manic patient sleeps little, rest periods and a calm, soothing atmosphere should be provided.

6. The patient who is manic needs protection from himself or herself. He or she may be too busy to eat or to take care of personal hygiene. Eating problems can be handled in the same manner as with the depressed client.

7. The nurse should praise the patient who takes an interest in cleanliness and appearance.

8. The nurse should set limits and use firm actions in providing physical care and should constantly assess for suicidal ideation and intention.

XI. ORGANIC MENTAL DISORDERS

A. Description

1. The hallmark of an organic mental disorder is that the associated mental changes are cause by a specific lesion in the CNS. This lesion can be structural or chemical.

2. Patients with organic mental disorders have problems with intellectual functions such as comprehension, calculation, general knowledge, abstract reasoning and memory, and language.

3. Typically, long-term memory in the organically impaired patient is spared; clients usually have no difficulty remembering their youth or other past events.

4. As a general rule, the more chronic the organic brain syndrome, the more long-term memory will be impaired.

5. As a group, the organic mental disorders are perhaps the most devastating illnesses. Acute organic brain syndromes are terribly frightening for family members to witness because these syndromes cause behavioral changes in the patient that range from embarrassing to life threatening.

6. The confusion associated with an acute organic brain syndrome can lead to extreme degrees of combativeness or to dangerously impaired judgment.

B. Family Involvement

1. Families are surprised that patients with early dementia will have markedly impaired recent memory but completely intact memory for the past. ("She remembers school as if it were yesterday, but she cannot remember what she had for breakfast.")

2. As memory impairment progresses, the names of people who are important to the patient, such as grandchildren and close friends or business associates, are forgotten.

C. Dementia

Dementia is a term describing clinical behavior that manifests itself in the insidious development of the following.

- ◆ Decreased cognitive functioning
- ◆ Disorientation
- ◆ Memory deficit
- ◆ Intellectual deficit

1. Incidence and Etiology

a. More than one million persons, or 8 percent of the American population over the age of 65 years, are affected significantly enough by the dementia due to organic brain disease that deters independent living.

b. This means that more than 60 percent of the residents of nursing homes manifest organic mental disease.

c. Medical intervention that has prolonged the lives of those requiring critical care and the lives of those with chronic disease has also created a completely new entity of cerebral damage and dysfunction, which results in psychiatric morbidity.

d. There now is an awareness of this psychopathology in the survivors. At this time, however, little has been done in terms of investigation to document the magnitude of the problem.

D. Alzheimer's Disease

1. Etiology and Incidence

a. The most characteristic disease of the senile dementias is Alzheimer's disease, which occurs twice as often in women than in men.

b. This disease has no known etiology, although research has generated several theories.

c. Genetic studies show that an autosomal (chromosomes other than the sex X and Y chromosomes) dominant form of Alzheimer's disease is associated with early onset and early death, accounting for about 100,000 death a year. A family history of Alzheimer's disease and the presence of Down syndrome are two established risk factors.

d. Accounts for more than half of all dementias.

e. An estimated 5 percent of persons older than 65 years have a severe form of this disease, and 12 percent suffer from mild to moderate dementia.

2. Signs and Symptoms

a. Insidious deterioration of personality and hygiene (appearance).

b. Patient is restless, up all night and day, cannot write even simple sentences, and forgets recent events.

c. May occur as early as age 50 years.

d. Prognosis is poor for patients with Alzheimer's disease.

3. Treatment

Treatment includes Donepezil (Aricept), Rivastigmine (Exelon), and Tacrine (Cognex); they are used to elevate acetylcholine, which slows the neuronal degradation that occurs in Alzheimer's disease.

4. Diagnosis

   a. Look at history.

   b. True diagnosis cannot be made until autopsy.

5. Theories

   a. Physiologic studies indicating that degenerative changes in the cholinergic neurons and biochemical changes involving the biosynthetic enzyme for acetylcholine give credence to an etiology of a neurotransmitter deficiency.

   b. Higher than normal amounts of aluminum deposits have been detected in the brains of patients with Alzheimer's disease. These deposits may be a cause or a result of the disease.

   c. Other studies show an abnormally high titer of antibodies present in Alzheimer's patients, giving rise to the question of whether the disease is a result of an immunologic effect.

   d. A higher incidence of Alzheimer's disease has been associated with adult Down syndrome patients, and the disease also appears to be familial.

6. Criteria for Alzheimer's Disease

   a. Amnesia: inability to learn new information or to recall previously learned information.

   b. Agnosia: failure to recognize or identify objects despite intact sensory function.

   c. Aphasia: language disturbance that can manifest in both understanding and expressing the spoken word and can progress to mindless repetition of words.

   d. Apraxia: inability to carry out motor activities despite intact motor function (e.g., ability to grab a doorknob but not knowing what to do with it).

   e. Behavior progress: from indifference to agitation memory dysfunction progresses from recent memory loss/remote memory loss and can reach the point where the patient does not know her or his name.

   f. Wandering: possible causes are confusion, restlessness, boredom, or sensory overload, especially in hospital or nursing home settings.

   g. Nursing Interventions

      (1) Safety first (e.g., removing small floor rugs and other objects the patient can fall over)

      (2) Identification

      (3) Medic Alert bracelets

      (4) Motion or sound detectors (be sure batteries are working)

      (5) Alternative outlet for energy (e.g., give patients small tasks such as putting objects in a basket or folding linens)

      (6) Medications especially helpful in reducing restlessness

7. Nursing Implications

   a. Coordinating Treatment

      (1) The nurse is the pivotal person to provide resources, to call together a team of health care professionals, and to coordinate treatment planning that is meaningful to the patient with Alzheimer's disease and his or her family.

      (2) Nurses join with the patient and his or her family to help them attain some quality of life.

      (3) Care of the patient with Alzheimer's disease is most challenging and requires all of one's knowledge, skill, and ability.

      (4) The multiplicity of issues and the complexity of care encourage a multidisciplinary approach to Alzheimer's disease.

      (5) Treatment plans must be specific and individual.

   b. Family Involvement

      (1) The patient can be variable, unpredictable, and dependent, according to the patient's functional disabilities and degree of brain damage.

      (2) He or she requires increasingly more help; this is difficult, too difficult in fact, for one person to handle. Look around and find others who can help care for the patient and the family.

      (3) Caregivers can be relatives, friends, supporting volunteers, and professional and nonprofessional staff.

      (4) Empathize with the patient and family about what it must feel like to be terrified, out of control, lost, mute, and lonely.

      (5) The nurse must help the family understand that the patient with Alzheimer's disease cannot be left alone. The patient will walk out of his or her house and may be unable to find his or her way back home.

      (6) Their families experience grief, guilt, loneliness, embarrassment, and frustration.

      (7) Patients with Alzheimer's disease are not deliberately stubborn, suspicious, inappropriate, or ungrateful; their behavior is beyond their control.

      (8) Nurses need to interpret this behavior and help the family to understand that the behavior is part of the disease process. Nurses also are the model of appropriate behavior and communication with both the family and the patient.

      (9) Families are members of the multidisciplinary team.

      (10) Invite families to join nurses, physicians, and others in finding the best possible solutions to the dilemmas of caring for a patient with cognitive impairment.

XII. PERSONALITY DISORDERS

A. Paranoid

1. Distinguishing Characteristics

   a. The distinguishing characteristic of patients with paranoid personality disorder is inalterable suspicion of others.

   b. They usually are unable to acknowledge and accept their own negative and angry feelings toward others.

c. To a great extent, the paranoid person perceives the world as being composed of clues hidden or with special meaning.

d. Paranoid individuals generally perceive other persons as dishonest, full of trickery, and out to undo them.

e. These patients usually view themselves as self-sufficient, objective, rational, emotionally balanced, and very important.

f. Paranoid patients are hypercritical of others and prone to collect real and imagined injustices. Often, they use the legal system to seek retribution for such injustices.

g. Although these patients criticize others freely, they regard criticisms directed at themselves as signs of betrayal, jealousy, envy, or persecution.

h. Their cognitive function, thus, deals primarily with making the imagined real and the real invalid.

i. The paranoid patient remains coldly reserved and on the periphery of events, and seldom mixes smoothly with people in social situations.

j. Rather, these individuals remain withdrawn, distant, and secretive in social situations.

k. Most individuals with paranoid personalities experience lifelong effects of the disorder.

l. In some, this disorder may precede the development of schizophrenia.

m. In others, paranoid personality disorder may remit with maturity and reduction of life stressors.

2. Treatment

a. Few individuals with paranoid personalities voluntarily seek mental health services.

b. Individual, rather than group, psychotherapy is indicated for persons with paranoid personalities.

3. Nursing Implications

a. Respect the patient's needs for interpersonal distance by being more "professional" than friendly and more matter-of-fact than warm.

b. The nurse can explain what needs to be done and why in a straightforward and sincere manner.

c. Avoid becoming defensive when challenged or accused of something by paranoid patients.

d. Humor does not work well with these patients because it may threaten them.

e. A nurse should not sit down near a paranoid patient while he or she is in bed because intimacy increases the patient's defensiveness.

B. Schizoid

Schizoid patients are not schizophrenic, although both populations may have significantly impaired relationships.

1. Distinguishing Characteristics

a. Schizoid patients maintain a firm grip on reality.

b. Their major problem is their inability to relate warmly to other people.

c. They are often reclusive and live with parents or in isolation.

d. They seem to have little need for human contact or comfort. This deficiency is compensated for by an active fantasy life.

e. The diagnostic criteria for schizoid personality disorder are designed to separate this disorder from the more disturbed schizophrenia.

f. There have been no conclusive studies implicating genetic or biologic features.

g. Schizoid patients rarely, if ever, appear to experience anger and joy.

h. Patients indicate little, if any, desire to have sexual experiences with another person.

C. Schizoid: Avoidance Personality Disorder

1. Distinguishing Characteristics

a. Patients with schizoid and avoidant personality disorder have much in common; both experience significant difficulty in establishing relationships.

b. Patients with avoidant personality disorder have some ability to trust and invest in relationships but do not handle surprises well, for example, a last minute change in planned surgery.

c. The nurse should let this type of patient know when he or she will be available or unavailable. He or she may need explanations about rotating shifts and why staff are at times unavailable.

d. These patients are easily hurt by criticism or disapproval.

e. They have no close friends, and they avoid social or occupational activities.

D. Borderline Personality Disorder

1. Distinguishing Characteristics

a. The patient with borderline personality disorder exhibits a cross-section of almost all the perceptual, cognitive, affective, and behavioral disturbances presented in other personality disorders.

b. These patients typically cannot tolerate anxiety; as a result, they use all the major maladaptive coping behaviors—avoidance, acting out, withdrawal, and psychosomatization—to defend themselves against anxious feelings.

c. An outstanding feature of the borderline personality patient's perceptual pattern is the tendency to view other people as "all good" or "all bad." In other words, a borderline personality patient may view others as either kind, rewarding, and supporting, or as hateful, distant, and punitive.

d. Patients with borderline personalities often have identity disturbance with regard to their self-image, social, sexual, and occupational role.

e. These patients fail to learn from their mistakes; for this reason, they continuously repeat their mistakes. Their ability to solve problems and to cope adaptively with anxiety is seriously impaired.

f. They shift from a mood of joy to anger or depression and return to a normal mood often within a few hours. This is a cardinal sign of borderline personality disorder.

g. Another striking characteristic of this personality disorder is the intensity of affect (emotions). Anger, depression, loneliness, emptiness, impatience, self-pity, low self-esteem, and deficient self-confidence are some of the emotions experienced intensely and erratically by patients with borderline personality.

h. Nonverbally, these patients display their highly changeable and intense affect through impulsive behavior.

i. Some of these behaviors are extravagant spending, sexual promiscuity, and hyperingestion of food and mood-altering drugs.

j. Verbally, they are self-critical, whining, threatening, manipulative, demanding, argumentative, complaining, and blaming.

k. Getting in and out of difficulty becomes a way of life for these patients.

l. Many individuals with borderline personality disorder seek mental health care services. Usually, they present with symptoms of depression, psychosis, or suicidal crisis.

m. Treatment is aimed at reducing the presenting symptoms. Because personality disorder is a deeply ingrained pattern, it is resistant to treatment. Only the most intensive and prolonged psychotherapy can effect long-term behavioral changes.

2. Behavioral Patterns
The following is a summary of behavioral patterns that commonly occur in individuals with personality disorders, despite their different diagnostic labels.

a. Splitting view of others as either "all good" or "all bad."

b. Projection of one's feelings and experiences onto others; in addition, resorting to fault finding, criticism, and confrontation to reduce their own feelings of inadequacy.

c. Passive-aggression, or the tendency to turn anger against the self with the underlying motive to force others to comply with their wishes and needs; this tendency is behaviorally expressed through such acts as wrist cutting, nonlethal drug overdose, and eating disorders, such as obesity, anorexia nervosa, and bulimia.

d. Narcissism or tendency to perceive the self to be all-powerful and important and, therefore, entitled to criticize or belittle others; this individual often gives the impression of being vain and arrogant.

e. Dependency, expression of unreasonable wishes and wants, in a demanding manner while denying dependent behavior.

f. No-win relationship style or the tendency to seek out relationships that offer a promise of something for nothing; individuals manifesting this behavior feel entitled to take without giving.

3. Nursing Implications

a. Nursing diagnoses include the following:

(1) Ineffective individual coping related to labile affect

(2) Ineffective individual coping related to depression

(3) Ineffective individual coping related to splitting

b. To plan and implement effective care for personality disordered patients, the nurse need to develop a high degree of self-awareness.

c. Because many personality disordered patients tend to mistrust other people, the nurse needs to exercise special care to establish trust.

d. A straightforward, matter-of-fact approach, as opposed to an overly warm approach, is indicated when working with these patients.

e. Punctuality, respect, honesty, and genuineness add significantly to trust formation.

f. The nurse should avoid interpreting the patient's behavior because mistrustful patients tend to view interpretation as intrusive and controlling.

g. The nurse needs to use open-ended questions designed to assist these patients in focusing on their behavior and its consequences.

h. The nurse must maintain congruence between verbal and nonverbal behaviors; incongruent behavior by the nurse causes these patients to become more suspicious of the nurse.

i. Confrontation can be necessary to work effectively with some personality disordered patients who attempt to use manipulation. Pointing out a patient's problematic behavior to him or her is termed confrontation.

4. Confrontation
The purpose of confrontation is to help the patient become more self-aware. The keys to effective confrontation include the following:

a. Pointing out the behavior soon after its occurrence.

b. Being specific in describing the behavior.

c. Using a nonaccusatory, nonjudgmental, matter-of-fact manner.

d. Maintaining a focus on the patient's actual behavior rather than the patient's explanation of it.

5. Manipulative Behavior
Because of the manipulative, dependent, and acting-out behaviors displayed by the personality disordered clients, it may be necessary for the nurses to use limit setting.

6. Limit Setting
Limit setting includes the following:

a. Identifying the behavior that the patient needs to control.

b. Proposing an appropriate, alternative behavior for the patient to pursue.

c. Anticipating that the patient will test the nurse to determine if he or she will withdraw the time out.

d. Remaining unwavering and consistent in the use of limit setting.

e. Limit setting must be sensitively and judiciously applied to ensure effectiveness.

f. Effective limit setting requires both clinical skill and personal maturity.

E. Obsessive-Compulsive Disorder

1. Distinguishing Characteristics

a. Obsessive-compulsive disorder is a psychiatric condition in which the individual experiences recurrent obsessions and/or compulsions.

b. The term *obsession* as used here refers to recurrent, persistent ideas, thoughts, images, or impulses.

c. *Compulsions* are ritualistic behaviors that the individual feels compelled to perform either in accordance with a specific set of rules or in routine manner.

d. Performing the compulsive ritual is designed to prevent or reduce anxiety associated with some future event that the individual wishes to prevent or produce.

e. At the same time, the obsessive-compulsive patient unrealistically believes that the ritualistic behavior magically solves problems or atones for past misdeeds.

f. If the nurse or someone else intervenes to stop the compulsive behavior, severe anxiety results.

g. The obsessive-compulsive client can experience mild to severe symptoms.

h. If symptoms are mild and conducive to occupational productivity, the individual may not feel the need to seek treatment.

i. Severe symptoms that interfere with the quality of life almost always result in the individual seeking help.

2. Treatment

a. If treatment is not sought or is unsuccessful, these individuals may become so overwhelmed that they become depressed and even suicidal.

b. Treatment can be as simple as keeping the patient occupied with other activities to avoid carrying out ritualistic behavior; in time, he or she may not feel a need for this behavior.

c. This treatment would be accompanied by other methods to reduce and cope with anxiety.

F. Passive-Aggressive Personality

1. Distinguishing Characteristics

a. Patients with passive-aggressive personalities tend to perceive the world, and themselves, as negative. For example, these patients search for mistakes, faults, and injustices in almost all situations.

b. Underlying the passive-aggressive personality are characteristics torn between hope and hopelessness, compliance and noncompliance, and independence and dependence.

c. Such ambivalence leads to irritable moodiness, discontent, dissatisfaction, and obstinacy.

d. Low self-confidence and resentment toward authority figures, on whom the passive-aggressive individual depends and whom he or she views as superior, are also associated with this ambivalence. Ambivalence in this situation means having simultaneous good feelings toward and repulsion against the authority figure.

e. Jealousy, hostility, and aggressive strivings occur to a significant degree in this disorder.

f. The content of his or her verbalization usually centers around themes of feeling unappreciated, unloved, overworked, overburdened, and being unfairly treated, misused, and abused.

g. The individual uses indecisiveness, procrastination, delay tactics, inefficiency, obstructionism, and errors of omission to vent hostile envious feelings and aggressive strivings at the same time, permitting the passive-aggressive personality to appear friendly and even submissive.

h. These covertly aggressive tactics manipulate or induce others to behave in a manner that will increase the passive-aggressive person's feelings of safety and security.

i. The passive-aggressive person avoids seeking adaptive solutions through learning and problem solving; therefore, it is not surprising that they often develop anxiety and depressive episodes as well as suicidal crises.

j. If the patient seeks help, behavioral modification, family and group therapies, and crisis intervention techniques are often used.

XIII. SOMATOFORM DISORDERS

◆ Somatoform disorders discussed include somatization disorder, pain disorder, hypochondriasis, and conversion disorder.

A. Somatization Disorder

1. Genetic and environmental factors contribute to the development of somatization disorder. It usually develops before age 30 years and is more common in females than in males.

2. The major characteristic of somatoform disorders is that patients have physical symptoms for which there is no known organic cause or physiologic mechanism. Evidence is present or a presumption exists that the physical symptoms are connected to psychological factors or conflicts. These patients are not in control of their symptoms, which are unconscious and involuntary. Patients express conflicts through bodily symptoms and complaints using the defense of somatization.

3. Patients with these disorders repeatedly seek medical diagnosis and treatment, even though they have been told that there is no known physiologic or organic evidence to explain their symptoms or disability.

4. Current research suggests that genetic, developmental learning, personality, and sociocultural factors predispose, precipitate, and maintain somatoform disorders. Stressful life events also can precipitate bodily concerns and somatization.

When multiple recurrent signs and symptoms of several years' duration suggest that physical disorders exist without a verifiable disease or pathophysiologic condition to account for them, somatization disorder is present. The patient with somatization disorder usually undergoes repeated medical examinations and diagnostic testing that, unlike the symptoms themselves, can make them preoccupied with the belief that they have a specific disease.

5. The main characteristic is that these individuals verbalize, for several years, recurrent, frequent, multiple somatic complaints without physiologic cause. It usually begins before age 30 years.

6. These patients see many physicians through the years and may even have exploratory and unnecessary surgical procedures.

B. Pain Disorder

1. The main characteristic is that these individuals verbalize severe pain in one or more anatomic sites that causes significant distress or impaired functioning.

   a. The location or complaint of the pain does not change, unlike the complaints voiced in somatization disorder. Psychological factors play a role in the development and maintenance of pain disorder. There is no organic basis for this disorder.

   b. Patients with pain disorder are often doctor shoppers and may use analgesics excessively without experiencing any relief from their pain.

   c. These patients are often anxious about their symptoms and depressed about never getting better.

C. Hypochondriasis

1. The main characteristic is that these individuals verbalize worry about having a serious disease based on the misinterpretation of bodily signs and sensations.

2. Medical evaluation and reassurance do not help dispel the fear. These patients displace anxiety onto their bodies and misinterpret bodily symptoms. Hypochondriacs check for reassurance from physicians or friends in ways that are similar to the compulsive behavior of patients with obsessive-compulsive disorder.

3. Hypochondriacs are afraid that they have a disease, whereas patients with obsessive-compulsive disorder fear getting an illness and constantly check for germs.

4. Like patients with obsessive-compulsive disorder, hypochondriacs constantly check for reassurance about their illness.

D. Conversion Disorder

1. The main characteristics are that these individuals verbalize signs and symptoms of neurologic disease, such as paralysis, blindness, or seizures.

2. The primary gain for these patients is the alleviation of anxiety provided by this disorder because conflict is kept out of conscious awareness.

3. A secondary gain is the gratification received as a result of how the people in these patients' environments respond to their illness.

4. Another characteristic of this disorder is that the symptom often is determined by the situation that produced it. For example, a soldier suddenly develops paralysis of his hand. As a result, he can no longer engage in combat because he cannot pull the trigger on his gun.

E. Psychotherapeutic Management of Somatoform Disorders with Nursing Implications

1. The focus of the nurse–patient relationship is to improve patients' overall levels of functioning by building adaptive coping behaviors. Patients with somatoform disorders often are not able to identify and express their feelings, needs, and conflicts. Teaching them how to appropriately verbalize feelings helps to eliminate or diminish the need for physical symptoms.

2. Patients need time to understand their need for physical symptoms. Awareness and insight develop slowly as they begin to verbalize their needs.

3. Assertiveness, decision-making, goal-setting, stress management, and social skills groups often benefit these patients.

4. Outpatient therapy is also necessary for most patients. Because patients with somatoform disorders usually are overusers of medical care, some hospitals and clinics provide psychotherapy groups as part of the medical care. These groups focus on underlying psychosocial needs, not on physical needs.

XIV. ACUTE STRESS DISORDER AND POSTTRAUMATIC STRESS DISORDER

A. Criteria for Acute Stress Disorder (ASD)

1. Exposure to a traumatic event involving threat of death/injury to self or others.

2. Dissociative symptoms during or immediately after the event: absence of emotions, numbing, detachment, decreased awareness of surroundings (in a daze), and amnesia.

3. Increased anxiety, sleep disturbance, hypervigilance, startled response, irritability, restlessness, decreased concentration.

4. Re-experiencing or reliving the traumatic event: distressing thoughts, dreams, flashbacks, illusions, impairment in functioning (occupational, social, or other important areas).

5. Onset occurs within 4 weeks after the event.

6. Duration lasts for 2 days to 4 weeks.

B. Criteria for Posttraumatic Stress Disorder (PTSD)

1. Same criteria as for ASD.

2. Numbing of responsiveness, restricted affect, such as not being able to love, lack of expectation about the future, inability to recall aspects of the event, decreased participation/interest in activities, estrangement and detachment from others, outbursts of anger, and hallucinations.

3. Acute occurs within 6 months after the event.

4. Delayed occurs 6 months or more after the event.

5. Chronic lasts 3 or more months.

C. Nurse–Patient Relationship

1. When the patient is aware of the current influence of the trauma, there is often a tendency for him or her to believe that "no one can understand what I've been through unless they have been through it too." Therefore, the nurse needs to be nonjudgmental, honest, empathic, and supportive. The nurse can convey the message, "I haven't been through what you have, but the more you tell me, the better I will understand what you have been and are experiencing." It is important to acknowledge any unfairness or injustices that were part of the trauma.

2. It may take time for patients to recognize the relationship between current problems and the original traumatic event. When patients are not initially aware of the connection between the original trauma and current feelings and problems, the nurse should gently clarify those connections as they emerge. These patients also need to hear that they are not "crazy" but that they are having typical reactions to a serious trauma.

3. As patients struggle through the sometimes lengthy process of re-experiencing, reintegrating, and processing memories of and feelings about trauma experiences, patients need empathy and reassurance that they will be safe and not overwhelmed with anxiety.

4. Some of the traumatic stressors that may precipitate the development of ASD and PTSD are war, community violence, torture, natural and manmade disasters, bombings, major fires, accidents, catastrophic illness, injury to self or others, chronic abuse, rape, assault, and major personal or business losses.

D. Psychopharmacology

1. Medications for patients experiencing ASD or PTSD are used generally for short-term therapy during the acute crisis or for intensive counseling periods to prevent or reverse neurochemical fear conditioning and sensitization. The choice of medications depends on the primary symptoms. Some of the medications that may be prescribed are as follows:

a. Benzodiazepine, e.g., diazepam (Valium), may be prescribed to reduce levels of fear and symptoms of anxiety.

b. Lithium carbonate is sometimes given to patients who are experiencing explosive outbursts and intense feelings of being out of control. It can also help decrease startle response and nightmares.

c. Antipsychotics are used if patients have psychotic thinking.

E. Community Resources

1. A particularly useful therapeutic aid for patients experiencing ASD and PTSD is group therapy or self-help groups with others who have experienced the same or a similar trauma. A community may have a veterans outreach center as well as groups for victims of rape, incest, or torture and for their family members. The community may hold meetings for victims after a community disaster. There also may be a victim's assistance program for crime victims.

2. Victims of a variety of traumas may benefit from group meetings that focus on the similarities in their reaction and feelings, such as mistrust, helplessness, fear, guilt, numbing, detachment, nightmares, and flashbacks.

XV. PSYCHOACTIVE SUBSTANCE ABUSE DISORDERS

A. Alcohol

1. Incidence and Social Impact

a. Alcohol abuse and dependency is one of the most serious public health problems in the United States.

b. The incidence of alcohol-related accidents resulting in fatalities or in permanent disabilities is enormous.

c. The social impact of the disorder on family members, especially children, is devastating.

d. Many American adolescents suffer from alcoholism; many children are born with abnormalities or suffer from fetal alcohol syndrome.

2. Distinguishing Characteristics

a. Prolonged heavy drinking results in physical and behavioral tolerance.

b. Physical tolerance means that more alcohol is required to achieve the desired effect.

c. The drinking history of alcoholics frequently reveals the ability to increase tolerance and maintain this increase over a long period of time, maybe years.

d. Persistent heavy drinking frequently results in chemically induced alcoholic blackouts. This is not the same as "passing out," which is defined as a loss of consciousness.

e. During a blackout, the individual appears to function while drinking but is later unable to remember what occurred.

f. The patient may awake the next morning and wonder, "How did I get here?" or "Where did I leave my car?"

g. Blackouts may be a symptom of alcohol abuse and dependency.

h. Intoxication occurs after drinking and is evidenced in behaviors such as fighting and impaired judgment. Physiologic signs are slurred speech, unsteady gait, and flushed face.

3. Withdrawal Syndrome

Alcohol withdrawal occurs after reduction in or cessation of prolonged heavy drinking. Signs and symptoms of withdrawal include the following:

a. Coarse tremors of hands, tongue, and eyelids

b. Nausea and vomiting

c. General malaise or weakness

d. Increased blood pressure and pulse

e. Anxiety, depression, or irritable mood

f. Insomnia and nightmares

4. Alcohol Withdrawal Delirium

Alcohol withdrawal delirium occurs within 48 h after cessation of drinking and is referred to as delirium tremens (DTs). The most serious forms of the withdrawal syndrome include the following:

a. Delirium clouding of consciousness (unawareness of environment)

b. Severe tremors that increase body temperature

c. Misinterpretation, illusions, or hallucinations that usually are visual and vivid

d. Incoherent speech, insomnia

e. Decreased psychomotor activity

f. Frequent agitation, increased blood pressure

g. Seizures

h. If untreated, this syndrome can cause serious medical complications, such as fluid and electrolyte imbalance, pneumonia, and dehydration

5. Medical Consequences

The medical consequences of heavy alcohol consumption can adversely affect almost every body system and results in the following:

a. Gastritis or gastric ulcers

b. Acute and chronic pancreatitis

c. Esophagitis and esophageal varices

d. Alcohol cardiomyopathy

e. Cirrhosis of the liver (most serious and irreversible consequence)

f. Portal hypertension

g. Alcohol hepatitis

B. Amphetamines and Cocaine

These drugs are known as *stimulants* because they act directly on the CNS.

1. Distinguishing Characteristics of Stimulants

a. The individual taking stimulants becomes more talkative and active; he or she has an increased sense of well-being, self-confidence, and alertness.

b. Stimulants are frequently used to decrease appetite, reduce fatigue, and combat mild depression. A common stimulant is caffeine, which is found in coffee, tea, and many soft drinks.

c. Cocaine is a stimulant classified as a narcotic and falls under the category of controlled substances.

2. Classification

a. Abusers of amphetamines (e.g., cocaine) can generally be classified into medical abusers and street abusers.

b. *Medical abusers* may use these drugs to aid in weight loss or to treat fatigue.

c. Students may use them to stay awake when studying; others use them to stay awake when driving long distances.

3. Distinguishing Characteristics of Cocaine

a. Cocaine is a white powder that may be taken by sniffing through the nose ("snorting"), where it is rapidly absorbed through the nasal mucous membranes.

b. Cocaine can be injected intravenously ("mainlining") or mixed in the same syringe as heroin (called a "speedball").

c. When cocaine compound is freed from the hydrochloride salt, it is called "free base" and is sold in "crack" or "rock" form for smoking. Crack appears to be the most dangerous and most addictive form of cocaine.

d. Smoking cocaine is a quick and efficient way of delivering the drug in a concentrated form to the brain, taking approximately 6 to 8 seconds to act.

4. Physical Effects of Cocaine

a. Physical symptoms of amphetamine intoxication include increased heart rate and blood pressure, dilated pupils, perspiration, chills, and nausea and vomiting.

5. Psychological Symptoms

a. The psychological symptoms include talkativeness, hypervigilance, grandiosity, and psychomotor agitation.

b. Individuals who are intoxicated with amphetamines display maladaptive behavior, such as fighting and impaired judgment.

6. Delirium

Symptoms of cocaine delirium include labile (unsteady) affect, violent aggressive behavior, and tactile and olfactory hallucinations.

7. Delusional Disorder

a. Symptoms include rapid development of perceived persecution, distortion of body image, and misperception of faces.

b. Persecutory delusions can lead to aggressive or violent behavior.

c. Tactile hallucinations, such as the feeling of insects crawling on the skin (formication), occur.

8. Cocaine Withdrawal

a. Symptoms of withdrawal include depression, irritability, anxiety, fatigue, psychomotor agitation, and sleep disturbance, manifested by insomnia.

b. Paranoid and suicidal thoughts can occur. The symptoms last for more than 48 h after cessation of the drugs.

9. Medical Consequences

    a. During cocaine intoxication, an individual can experience formication. Severe ulceration of the skin can result from the user's attempts to dig out these imaginary "insects."

    b. An overdose of cocaine can produce cardiac arrhythmias, convulsions, and respiratory depression.

    c. Repeated heavy use of "snorting" the "crack" can cause tissue ulcerations in the nasal septum.

    d. Cocaine use may produce a paranoid psychosis similar to paranoid schizophrenia disorder.

C. Cannabis (Marijuana, Hashish)

Marijuana and hashish are derived from cannabis, a hemp plant.

1. Effects

    a. The most predominant effects of cannabis are euphoria and an altered level of consciousness of the individual without hallucinations.

    b. The drug usually is smoked or eaten.

    c. According to federal government estimates, there are an estimated 16 to 20 million regular users of marijuana in the United States.

2. Intoxication

    a. Signs and symptoms include increased heart rate, conjunctival infections, increased appetite, and dry mouth.

    b. Psychological symptoms include euphoria, subjective intensification of perceptions, sensation of slowed time, and apathy.

    c. Maladaptive behavioral effects include impaired judgment, panic attacks, suspicious paranoid ideation, and excessive anxiety.

3. Delusional Disorders

    a. Delusional syndrome can occur with persecutory delusions during an episode of intoxication or immediately following the use of cannabis. It usually does not last more than 7 h after cessation of marijuana use.

4. Medical Consequences

    a. Marijuana inhaled has an irritating effect on the lungs and can result in acute or chronic bronchitis and sinusitis in heavy smokers.

    b. Increased heart rate and decreased strength of cardiac contractions. If client has a cardiac condition, marijuana may cause client to go into congestive heart failure.

    c. There is research controversy concerning a link between marijuana use and brain damage.

    d. There appears to be some possibility that use of this substance leads to abuse of more potent drugs; this fear has not been substantiated.

XVI. SCHIZOPHRENIC DISORDERS

A. Theories Surrounding Schizophrenia

1. Research on schizophrenia has identified genetic and biochemical influences as factors contributing to the course and treatment of schizophrenia.

2. These biochemical differences may be present in the CNS of the person with schizophrenia, causing them to process sensory information in an abnormal manner.

3. An imbalance between the neurotransmitters dopamine and norepinephrine could be the biologic factor that causes schizophrenia.

4. The interpersonal theory is based on the premise that a person learns values, attitudes, and communication patterns through his or her family and culture.

B. Disturbances in Thinking

1. The client has "loose associations," or disconnected thoughts, which are shown in his or her verbal patterns. As the person's anxiety increases, his or her speech becomes increasingly illogical.

2. Evidence of magical thinking is seen in the patient who believes that his or her thoughts or wishes can control other people or events.

3. A schizophrenic patient can have minimal or seemingly no awareness of his or her environment; he or she may act like he or she is living in a dream world.

4. The patient can experience feelings of depersonalization. He or she may feel that his or her body belongs to another person or that he or she is somehow removed from his or her own body.

5. The patient can have illusions. An illusion is a misinterpretation of a real sensory experience, for example, seeing a shadow on the wall at night and immediately calling the police because the patient believes that someone broke into his or her home.

6. A delusion is a fixed, false belief that the client has and he or she cannot be corrected by reasoning with him or her.

7. A patient with paranoid schizophrenia generally has delusions of persecutions. He or she believes that everyone is out to hurt him or her. He or she may believe that his or her phone is "bugged."

8. A patient with delusions of grandeur believes that he or she is someone famous and that he or she has power that others do not have.

9. Hallucinations are false sensory perceptions without an external stimulus. A patient may "hear" the voice of the devil. The voice usually condemns the person for past sins.

    a. Auditory hallucinations are the most common form of hallucinations.

b. Visual hallucinations are the second most common and can manifest as threatening, frightening monsters.

C. Nursing Implications

1. Major Goals for Schizophrenic Patients

   a. Promote trust by establishing a one-on-one therapeutic relationship with the patient in a nonthreatening environment.

   b. Encourage social interaction.

   c. Increase the patient's self-esteem.

   d. Validate the patient's perception and reinforcement of reality.

   e. Encourage independent behavior.

   f. Reduce the patient's anxiety and psychotic symptoms.

   g. Coordinate therapy with family and those involved in the patient's life.

   h. Promote physical safety and help the patient meet his or her physical needs.

   i. Assess the patient's ability to carry out daily living activities, giving special attention to their nutritional status. Monitor their weight if they are not eating. If they think that their food is poisoned, let them fix their own food when possible or offer food in closed containers that they can open and offer them apples, oranges, or bananas. Dive fluid to them in closed containers.

2. Administering Medications and Food to a Schizophrenic Patient

   a. The nurse giving medications to a schizophrenic patient should observe the patient's behavior carefully while the medication is being taken.

   b. A suspicious patient may hide tablets or capsules in the cheek or under the tongue and spit them out as soon as the nurse leaves. If the nurse suspects this behavior, a mouth check should be done.

   c. The nurse should never trick the patient into taking medicine by putting it in food or fluid; if the patient discovers this, it can destroy his or her trust in the staff or cause the patient to stop eating and drinking, leading to malnutrition and dehydration.

   d. Sometimes, patients refuse to take any medications by mouth; in such cases, medications must be given intravenously (IV) or by injection. If given a choice of taking medication by mouth or by injection, however, the patient will sometimes choose taking the medication orally. If the medications are given by injection, it should be done quickly, with as little physical restraint as needed for the patient's safety.

   e. The nurse should not become involved in a lengthy debate to persuade the patient to take oral medicine.

   f. The nurse should be aware of the patient's right to refuse treatment (generally, only lifesaving treatment can be given without permission).

XVII. PSYCHIATRIC PATIENT AND INTERPERSONAL RELATIONSHIPS

A. Establishing the Nurse–Patient Relationship

1. Initially, a one-to-one nurse–patient relationship is most often helpful for the patient who is socially isolated or withdrawn. The goal is to help the patient establish healthy interpersonal relationships with a variety of people.

2. As soon as a trusting relationship has been established and the nurse and patient begin to relate more comfortably, other people should gradually be included in the client's social network. For example, the nurse can invite another patient to join a card game or share in a discussion, or the nurse can use his or her knowledge about other patients to introduce patients who have common interests.

B. Goal Setting

It is difficult to develop a strong relationship with a patient who has difficulty establishing intimacy. In addition, setting goals implies a commitment to change. Patients who have disruptions in personal relationships are reluctant to commit to change.

1. Although it is desirable to have the patient's full participation in goal setting, it can be necessary for the nurse to set initial goals.

2. The long-term nursing goal for nursing care of the patient with disruptions in related to promoting growth toward achieving maximum interpersonal satisfaction. This is achieved by establishing and maintaining self-enhancing relationships with others.

3. Short-term goals are more specific to the individual's problems and focus on modifying specific communication patterns; for example, the patient will use nonverbal communication more congruent with the verbal content of his or her speech. Another example of a goal is for the patient to verbally identify angry feelings when they occur during a one-on-one interaction. These goals need to be developed with the patient's participation.

4. Learning to relate more directly and openly can cause anxiety. Therefore, the patient's ability to tolerate anxiety must be taken into consideration when determining goals. Increasing the patient's anxiety level before he or she has increased coping ability can reinforce the patient's use of dysfunctional coping behavior.

C. Group Therapy

Group therapy can be beneficial for the patient.

1. Knowing that others have ambivalence and share feelings of fear and guilt enables the depressed patient to cope with his or her feelings.

2. The patient can thereby stop his or her maladaptive behavioral patterns and develop more satisfying relationships.

3. The overall aim for this patient is to increase self-worth and self-esteem through identification with the group and awareness of personal strengths.

EXAMINATION

1. Bipolar disorder is characterized by mood swings that range from
   1. Elated to manic-depressive.
   2. Severe depressive to suicidal.
   3. Anxiety to panic.
   4. Elated to hallucination.

2. A male patient has a diagnosis of bipolar disorder, manic type. He is hyperactive and has not slept for 3 days. The most appropriate nursing intervention would be to
   1. Isolate him in his room until he calms down.
   2. Reduce distractions and encourage brief periods of rest.
   3. Ask the physician to prescribe restraints.
   4. Ask the physician to prescribe phenobarbital.

3. A male patient has been in the unit 3 days and is creating chaos on the ward by using dominating and manipulative behavior. The best nursing intervention for this behavior would be to
   1. Inform him that his behavior is unacceptable.
   2. Provide him with alternative behaviors.
   3. Establish specific limits on his behavior.
   4. Have him moved to another ward.

4. A husband and wife have come to the outpatient clinic. The wife says that she is concerned about her husband because she never knows what to expect of him. She says, "He is sometimes happy and sometimes sad, and sometimes he has self-confidence, while at other times he is extremely down on himself and blames me for all his problems." During assessment, the nurse should first gather information about
   1. Psychopathologic problems the husband is experiencing.
   2. The husband and wife's marital relationship.
   3. The husband's symptoms and their frequency and duration.
   4. The husband's physical health.

5. A 17-year-old female patient is admitted to the psychiatric ward from the medical intensive care unit after being treated for a deliberate overdose of a prescribed antidepressant medication. The nurse caring for this patient should be aware that the warning signs for suicide include
   1. Depression after losing her job and home.
   2. Auditory hallucination and low socioeconomic status.
   3. Feelings of failure and depression as a businessperson.
   4. Feelings of hopelessness and previous suicide attempts.

6. Recognizing the dynamics of suicide, the nurse knows that the most appropriate nursing action for a patient who has attempted suicide is to
   1. Let her spend time alone to reflect on her suicide attempt.
   2. Encourage her to verbalize her feelings and pain.
   3. Avoid the topic of suicide.
   4. Discuss with her why it was wrong for her to attempt suicide.

7. A patient tells the nurse that her boyfriend walked out of her apartment, telling her that he never wanted to see her again. She tells the nurse that she would rather be dead than live without him. Based on this information, the nurse's short-term plan for the patient should include the goal that the patient will
   1. Find another boyfriend.
   2. Recognize that she was too dependent on this boyfriend.
   3. State that she feels okay being alive.
   4. Admit that her suicide attempt was wrong.

8. The nursing staff on a medical unit is meeting to discuss the major emotional needs of patients on the unit. To determine major emotional needs of patients, the nursing staff would *first* identify
   1. Which nursing approach has been effective or which approach needs to be changed.
   2. How the nursing staff can meet the dependent needs of their patients.
   3. Which patients need psychiatric help.
   4. Which patients have emotional disequilibrium or increased anxiety.

9. The staff on a medical unit discussed which method of data collection by the nurse would be most helpful in identifying emotional needs of their patients. They have concluded that the *most* effective method is to
   1. Review the patient's charts.
   2. Have the patient's family supply the physical and emotional history.
   3. Interview the patient immediately on admission.
   4. Review the nursing notes of the patient's problems.

10. The nursing staff agrees that the basic principle of planning nursing care is to
    1. Help patients to believe that they will improve.
    2. Accept patients as they are and allow them an active part in planning for their needs.
    3. Meet all of the patients' physical and emotional needs and allow them to take an active part in their care.
    4. Know the patients and understand all of their needs and allow them to take an active part in their care.

11. A patient has been admitted to a drug rehabilitation unit for 3 weeks. She was given a pass to leave and has returned to the psychiatric unit in an agitated state. She is experiencing vivid hallucinations and persecutory delusions. She continues to be agitated and combative for several hours. Blood is drawn for drug screening. The *most* likely substance used by the patient while she was on pass is
    1. Diazepam (Valium).
    2. Opium.
    3. Codeine sulfate.
    4. Phencyclidine (PCP).

QUESTIONS 12 TO 15: CASE HISTORY

Mrs. Davis, who is 75 years old, has been admitted to a nursing care facility. She has been living with her daughter for the past 5 years. Her daughter, who is a registered nurse (RN), states that her mother has progressively lost contact with reality, hallucinates, cannot carry on a conversation, and refuses to eat or sleep.

12. When Mrs. Davis is admitted to the nursing home, the most therapeutic action would be to
    1. Have a flexible treatment of nursing care and an individualized approach for the patient.
    2. Have the daughter stay for the first week to help her mother adjust to her new home.
    3. Restrain the patient to prevent injury.
    4. Put Mrs. Davis in a room with other patients to help her regain her orientation.

13. Mrs. Davis' physician orders haloperidol (Haldol) 10 mg daily. After the fourth day of therapy, she develops a mask-like face, "pill-rolling" motions of the fingers and thumb, and a shuffling gait. The nurse should
    1. Withhold the medication and notify the physician of the patient's symptoms.
    2. Ask the physician to reduce the dosage of Haldol.
    3. Give the medication at the next scheduled time.
    4. Obtain an order for benztropine (Cogentin) from the physician.

14. After 1 month of therapy, Mrs. Davis is talking and is more interested in her surroundings. She will now carry on a conversation with her primary nurse. She tells the nurse that she has been afraid because she has been hearing strange voices and wonders if the nurse can hear them also. The nurse should reply
    1. The voices are only in your thoughts.
    2. I believe you when you say you are hearing voices, but I cannot hear them.
    3. I will move you in with other patients and that will get your mind off of the voices.
    4. I don't hear any strange voice, but that doesn't mean that others can't hear them.

15. Mrs. Davis refuses to take her bath or have her bed changed. The nurse's best therapeutic reply would be
    1. Soap and water and a clean bed will make you feel like a new person, and those strange voices may just go away.
    2. When you're ready for a bath, just let me know.
    3. All clients in this unit must have a bath every day. I will give you your bath now.
    4. Which of your pretty gowns do you want to put on after your bath? I will give you a good back rub after we have finished with your bath.

End of Case

16. A female patient is admitted to the psychiatric unit with a diagnosis of severe depression. She states to the nurse, "God is punishing me for all my sins." The nurse's best response is
    1. Why do you feel that way? God forgives everyone's sins.
    2. You really must feel upset about this.
    3. Are your sins so bad that they are causing you depression?
    4. I think if you feel that way, you should talk with your minister.

QUESTIONS 17 TO 20: CASE HISTORY

Mr. Bill Martin, a 22-year-old man, is admitted to the psychiatric hospital for evaluation after numerous incidents of threatening, angry outbursts, and three episodes of hitting a coworker. Mr. Martin is extremely anxious and tells the admitting nurse, "I didn't mean to hit him. He made me so mad I just couldn't help it. I don't want to hit anyone again."

17. The most therapeutic response for the nurse to make is
    1. I am sure you didn't mean to hit him, and I know you won't do it again. We are going to help you.
    2. Tell me about all of your problems, and we will work with you to solve them.
    3. It sounds like you were really angry. When you feel angry, you need to tell us instead of hitting so that we can help you work through your anger.
    4. It sounds like you were really angry. When you feel angry, go lie down on your bed and don't talk to anyone until you are over your anger.

18. Mr. Martin rushes out of the recreation room where he is watching television with other patients. He is hyperventilating and flushed, and his fists are clenched. He says to his primary nurse, "That dumb bastard, he is just like Mike. I had to leave the room, or I would have knocked him across the floor." The most therapeutic response for the nurse to make is
    1. Even if you are angry, you can't use that language in this hospital.
    2. I can see you are really angry. I will get you some Ativan to help you calm down. After you have calmed down, we will talk about what happened.
    3. I am glad you left the recreation room without hurting anyone. Go to your room and calm down. I will come in soon and talk with you.
    4. I can tell you are very angry, and you did well to leave the situation. Let's walk up and down the hall while you tell me about it.

19. In the first group therapeutic meeting, Mr. Willow, a 60-year-old patient, sits near the nurse and says loudly, "I have heard Mr. Martin goes around hitting everyone. I am afraid

of him. I don't want him hitting me." The most therapeutic response by the nurse is

1. Mr. Martin is new to the group. He doesn't know anyone here, so go around and introduce yourselves.
2. You don't know Mr. Martin yet, Mr. Willow. When you get to know him, I am sure you won't be afraid.
3. It can be frightening to have new people on the unit. One of the purposes of this group is for people to get to know each other and talk together about things like being afraid.
4. Everyone in here is different, and all of you have different problems. Mr. Willow, you know there is nothing to be afraid of. We will keep you from being hurt by anyone.

20. Mrs. Smith tells the group in therapy why she is in the hospital. "My doctor tells me I need to stand up for myself and quit letting people run all over me. Maybe I should be like Mr. Martin. He always stands up for himself." In order to respond to Mrs. Smith, it is most important for the nurse to understand that

1. Denial of anger with passive unassertive behavior is a serious pathophysiologic condition and antipsychotic drugs must be used.
2. Not being able to stand up for yourself is directly related to the excessive use of alcohol.
3. A blaming personality is inherited from parents and therefore is almost impossible to eliminate.
4. Denial of anger with passive unassertive behavior is a maladaptive behavior pattern.

End of Case

QUESTIONS 21 TO 27: CASE HISTORY

Mrs. Ellen Hart, a 28-year-old married homemaker, is referred to the mental health center because she is depressed.

21. During the initial interview with Ellen, the nurse notices bruises on Ellen's upper arm and asks about them. After denying any problems, Ellen starts to cry and says, "He didn't really mean to hurt me. I hate the children seeing their father act so crazy. I am so worried about them." It would be most important during the interview to determine

1. The resources available to the client.
2. Whether Ellen wants a divorce from her husband.
3. The type and extent of abuse in the family.
4. The potential of immediate danger to Ellen and her children.

22. Ellen describes her husband as a "good family man" who works hard to provide for his family. Ellen doesn't work outside the home. She says, "I am proud to be a housewife and mother. My husband tells me that being a mother is

my job." The family pattern that the patient describes best illustrates abusive family characteristics, which are

1. Tight, impermeable boundaries, and good self-esteem.
2. Imbalanced power ratio and dysfunctional feeling tone.
3. Submissive behavior and functional feeling tone.
4. Role stereotyping and submissive behavior.

23. The primary nurse discussed the Hart family in a staff meeting. Of the following statements made by other staff members, the one that would be *most* helpful to the primary nurse as she develops Ellen's nursing care plan is

1. Have you thought about suggesting that Ellen attend the group we have for women in abusive families?
2. Have you thought about calling her physician about how many times Ellen has come to his office because her husband beat her up?
3. I think the police should be notified in case he hits her again.
4. Have you thought about calling the school nurse to find out if the children are being abused?

24. What is the characteristic *least* likely to be true about Mr. Hart?

1. He is a college graduate and has worked at the same job for 15 years.
2. His mother abused him as a child.
3. He has not met his own expectations for career achievement.
4. He has a warm emphatic relationship with his wife between episodes of abuse.

25. Ellen says to the nurse, "My 6-year-old son refuses to go to school because he is afraid I won't be home when he returns." The nurse's most therapeutic response is

1. I am sure he is feeling insecure right now. Allow him to stay home with you for a few days to reassure him.
2. Would you like to have him talk with the child therapist? I think it would really help him.
3. Children often feel responsible for trouble in the family. Have you asked him about what he is afraid might happen?
4. He is too young to come home to an empty house after school. If you can't be there, find someone else to be there with him.

26. The nurse finds herself dreading Ellen's appointments because she feels she is not working effectively with her. The most appropriate action by the nurse would be to

1. Tell Ellen that she has done all she can for her and now Ellen is responsible for herself.
2. Request that Ellen's case be transferred to another staff member.
3. Discuss her feelings with Ellen.
4. Recognize that these are normal feelings when working with abused women.

27. After several months of treatment, Ellen informs the nurse that she has decided to stop treatment because there has been no abuse during this time. Ellen tells the nurse, "I am less depressed, and my husband and I are getting along real well now. I have learned to cope with my problems." In discussing this decision with Ellen, it would be most important for the nurse to

1. Warn the patient that abuse often stops when one partner is in treatment but begins again when the person stops treatment.
2. Tell Ellen that she must do what she is told or she will always have problems.
3. Find out more from Ellen about her decision to stop therapy.
4. Tell Ellen that this is really a bad decision to make at this time.

End of Case

QUESTIONS 28 TO 34: CASE HISTORY

Mr. Joel Augustine, a 23-year-old man, is admitted to the hospital with chronic ulcerative colitis for the fourth time in 11 months. Joel is a familiar patient to the nursing staff caring for him.

28. The most therapeutic statement to this patient from his primary nurse would be

1. I thought we had cured you the last time you were in here, but it is good to see you again.
2. What brings you back this time?
3. It's been 3 months since you were last here. What do you think about being back in the hospital?
4. You got your same room back; I am sure that makes you feel more at home.

29. Joel tells the nurse he would give anything to get rid of his illness. He looks down at the floor and says, "Sometimes I imagine myself to be all powerful, so powerful that I would put other men to shame." When he thinks of himself in this way, the defense mechanism the client is using is

1. Dissociation.
2. Fantasy.
3. Projection.
4. Repression.

30. Joel's physician schedules a partial bowel resection and construction of an ileostomy. After his physician leaves Joel's room, the patient says to the nurse, "That doctor of mine loves cutting on me; the more gut he can cut out, the better he likes it." The most therapeutic response by the nurse would be

1. Are you saying that you don't want to go to surgery again?
2. I thought you liked your physician; what happened to change that?

3. The more he cuts out, the better he likes it. What do you mean by that?
4. You sound like you are really upset; maybe we can talk about it sometime.

31. The nurse feels sympathy for Joel instead of empathy. The best definition of empathy is

1. To experience and perceive the feelings of another person.
2. To identify with another person's feelings.
3. To have parallel feelings with another person.
4. To feel condolence and feel in agreement with the other person.

32. Joel should be involved in suitable activity in his room. When choosing his activity while his illness is being treated, the activity should

1. Include activities with other clients.
2. Enhance improvement of social skills.
3. Involve exercise that will help prevent constipation.
4. Be conducive to rest and relaxation.

33. Joel becomes increasingly morose and irritable after thinking more about his physician's recommendation for an ileostomy. He is rude with his visitors, and he tells the nurses to leave him alone when they attempt to give him medication and treatments. The best nursing intervention when the patient has a hostile outburst is to

1. Encourage Joel to discuss his immediate concerns and feelings with the nurse and not to let his anger build up inside him.
2. Offer Joel positive reinforcement each time he cooperates with the nurse and ask visitors to complement Joel when he is nice to them.
3. Continue with the assigned tasks and ignore his behavior; if he cooperates, reward him with some food he likes.
4. Encourage the patient to direct all of his anger at the nursing staff because they are used to handling angry outbursts by patients.

34. Arrangements are made for a member of the ileostomy club to meet with Joel. The chief purpose for having a representative from the club visit Joel is to

1. Show Joel support and give him realistic information about ileostomy.
2. Convince Joel that he will not be disfigured and can lead a full life.
3. Provide support for the ileostomy team that will be working with Joel.
4. Let Joel know he has resources in the community to help him.

End of Case

35. A female patient receives nursing instructions about lithium before discharge. Learning has occurred in this patient if she notifies her physician that she has experienced
    1. Symptoms of upper respiratory tract infection.
    2. Swollen lymph nodes.
    3. Dry mouth.
    4. Vomiting and diarrhea.

36. A female patient is attending a community group with a central focus on eating disorders such as bulimia and anorexia nervosa. She tells the nurse group leader, "I know my binges of eating and then vomiting are not normal, but I can't do anything about them." The most therapeutic response by the nurse is
    1. Do you feel angry when you cannot stop eating?
    2. The group will help you do something about your problem.
    3. What are your feelings when you go on these eating sprees?
    4. This must be difficult for you; we will help you as much as we can.

37. The nursing action that would best help a female patient with bulimia control the use of laxatives, diuretics, and vomiting is
    1. To have someone with the patient all of the time to supervise her actions until she learns self-discipline.
    2. To make frequent visits to the patient's home to check on all of her behavior.
    3. To have the patient keep a record of when and why she eats.
    4. To make a long-term goal with the patient, putting limits on all of her behavior.

38. The most appropriate intervention for an antisocial male patient using manipulative behavior is to
    1. Provide negative feedback for acting out behavior.
    2. Ignore manipulative behavior rather than confront it.
    3. Encourage the patient to discuss feelings of fear with the nurse and with a psychologist.
    4. Channel all of the patient's requests and questions related to care to the primary nurse.

39. An appropriate short-term goal for an antisocial patient using manipulative behavior is for the
    1. Staff to not allow the patient to use manipulative behavior.
    2. Patient to acknowledge manipulative behavior when called to his or her attention before leaving the hospital.
    3. Patient to demonstrate less impulsive behavior before leaving the hospital.
    4. Patient to use his or her manipulative behavior in situations that are not related to health care needs.

40. An antisocial patient flatters his or her primary nurse, demonstrates dislike for the rest of the nurses, verbally abuses another patient, and lies to the psychiatric physician. The behavior that most clearly warrants limit setting is
    1. Flattering the primary nurse.
    2. Verbal abuse of another patient.
    3. Lying to the psychiatric physician.
    4. Dislike for the rest of the nursing staff.

41. Which of the following statements characterizes the thinking of an individual with antisocial personality?
    1. I really feel bad that I have a bad temper, but I try to keep it under control.
    2. I keep trying to do the right things for my family, but I fail so many times, it really hurts me.
    3. I hit my wife because she nags me all the time, and she deserves it whenever I beat on her.
    4. I really feel bad about the way I hurt my family.

42. The rationale for limit setting as an intervention for the manipulative patient is that
    1. Some external controls must be used until the patient develops internal control.
    2. A provision of an outlet for feelings of guilt and frustration is made by allowing him or her to discuss his or her feelings with others.
    3. The patient's frustration and anger will decrease if nursing staff assumes responsibility for their behavior.
    4. Meeting the patient's need will reduce his or her need for manipulative behavior.

43. As the nursing staff continues to work with a male antisocial patient using manipulative behavior, they will find it most difficult to
    1. Monitor his behavior.
    2. Maintain consistent limits.
    3. Preserve the quality of life for the patient.
    4. Monitor suicidal attempts.

44. Impulsive behavior is characterized by
    1. Rigid moral code driven by impulsive behavior.
    2. Distortion of reality.
    3. Impulsiveness with little time between thoughts and actions.
    4. Manipulative behavior and a need to control their environment.

45. A paranoid personality disorder is described as haughty, aloof, superior acting, and highly suspicious. The nurse working with a male client states, "The client is always verbally putting me down. I would like to tell him to knock if off." The nurse's preceptor would correctly advise the nurse to
    1. Let the patient know how you feel about him.

2. Show your anger; this will help your patient understand his own anger.

3. Stop talking with the patient; listen, but don't reply.

4. Demonstrate respect and honesty or the relationship with the patient will deteriorate.

46. A patient with a paranoid personality tells the nurse that he believes that no one at the hospital likes him, and some wish they could harm him. This thinking is making use of

1. Projection.
2. Hypervigilance.
3. Intellectualization.
4. Introjection.

47. A patient with a paranoid personality disorder is very critical of the nursing staff because the patient is

1. Asking for attention.
2. Seeking sympathy.
3. Projecting self-hate and anger.
4. Manipulating the nurse.

48. A patient with a personality disorder is admitted to the psychiatric unit. Which of the patient's behaviors will have the highest priority and make it necessary for the nurse to schedule frequent team meetings? The client with

1. Auditory hallucinations.
2. Anxiety attacks that occur frequently.
3. Ability to evoke interpersonal conflict.
4. Denial.

49. A 50-year-old school teacher was at work when she was told her husband died in a car accident. She went through the funeral ritual in a state of numbness. Family and friends tried to get her to vent her feelings by crying. Which of the following statements *does not* offer a possible explanation for the patient's lack of crying?

1. The unconscious use of denial is considered normal for several days after the death of a loved one.
2. Every mentally impaired individual usually will show little or no emotion during the time of grief.
3. Culture is a determinant of grief responses. Some cultures are very emotional; others view emotional display as negative.
4. The acute stage of grief involves shock and denial that can last for several days.

50. A patient who started on tricyclic antidepressant therapy should be told

1. That a tyramine-free diet is necessary.
2. To avoid exposure to sunlight.
3. That mood improvement may take 7 to 28 days.
4. That only 1 g of sodium daily is allowed.

51. A nurse working with a severely depressed patient can avoid feelings of frustration by knowing that the patient will

1. Be receptive to the plan for nursing care.

2. Show signs of improvement after several scheduled sessions.

3. Show gratitude for attention.

4. Be withdrawn and disinterested in a relationship.

52. The nurse enters the room and the patient is crying. The patient says, "My husband died without even telling me he was sick." The most appropriate statement for the nurse to make would be

1. Look at it this way, your husband didn't have to suffer.
2. When my time on earth is up, I want to die quickly.
3. You will feel a lot better a year from now.
4. The loss of your husband must be very painful for you.

53. A man's wife died in a car accident, and for the first year after her death, he experienced sensations of somatic distress. Somatic distress is often experienced during the acute stage of grieving. Symptoms include shortness of breath, exhaustion, and pain sensation. Which statement by the patient would indicate successful completion of the grieving process?

1. After 14 months, he remembers realistically both the pleasures and disappointments of his relationship with his wife.
2. Three years after his wife's death, he talks about her as if she were alive, then weeps when others mention her name.
3. For 2 years after his wife's death, he has kept her belongings in their usual place.
4. Twenty months after his wife's death, he states he has never cried or experienced feelings of loss, although they loved each other and were very good friends.

54. A severely depressed patient is admitted to the mental health unit. She tells the nurse, "No one cares about me. I am not worth anything to anyone, not even my family." The most helpful reply by the nurse would be

1. Let me tell you that our nursing staff really cares about you.
2. Your family really cares about you; they are just really busy working.
3. One of us will sit with you for 10 min every 3 h starting at 1 PM today.
4. I would like to stay and listen to how you feel, but I am just too busy.

55. A patient is admitted to the mental health unit. She states that her husband divorced her and married a younger woman, and her children left her to go live with their dad. The nursing diagnosis is self-esteem disturbance related to feelings of abandonment as evidenced by feelings of worthlessness. An appropriate short-term goal is that the client will

1. Take sedatives and antidepressants as needed.
2. Initiate social interaction with another patient and maintain social contact with the patient for 1 week.

3. Identify four personal behaviors that tend to push others away within 3 days.

4. Verbalize three positive qualities about herself each day for 1 week.

56. A severely depressed female patient with a low self-esteem begins to show improvement by wearing a new dress and combing her hair. The nurse wishes to reinforce the patient's improved personal appearance. The most appropriate remark would be

1. I care about you, and I want to try to help you get better, so keep up the good work.

2. Now you are making it easier for the nursing staff to work with you.

3. Your hair is combed, and you are wearing a new dress.

4. You look great. Your hair is pretty, and your dress is beautiful.

57. An appropriate care plan for a severely depressed patient should include the following nursing orders *except*

1. Monitor blood chemistry and observe eating patterns.

2. Provide activities that will involve concentration and use of all fine motor skills.

3. Monitor bowel movement and encourage the use of gross motor skills.

4. Observe and record sleep patterns nightly.

58. A very important planned nursing intervention for a severely depressed patient is

1. Regularly planned, unobtrusive observations around the clock.

2. Allowing the client to remain alone if he or she prefers.

3. An opportunity to assume a role in the therapeutic work on the unit.

4. Encourage the patient to spend as much time sleeping during the day as he or she feels is necessary.

59. A patient with bipolar disease is admitted to the unit in a manic state and demonstrates gross hyperactivity. The physician orders Thorazine qid and lithium bid. The nurse should understand that the Thorazine used at the beginning of the treatment will

1. Potentiate the antimanic action of lithium.

2. Produce long-term control of hyperactivity.

3. Minimize the side effects of lithium.

4. Bring the client's hyperactivity under control rapidly.

60. Which of the following evidence supports the possibility of genetic transmission of bipolar disorder?

1. Creative people are more likely to develop bipolar disorder.

2. Patients with bipolar disorder have a higher rate of relatives with bipolar disorder than the general public.

3. More cases of bipolar disorder are found in higher socioeconomic families.

4. Most families with bipolar disorders come from a low socioeconomic background.

61. After a female manic patient is admitted to a psychiatric unit, the initial nursing intervention should be a plan to

1. Restrain the patient for her own safety during the hyperactivity state.

2. Encourage patient to act out feelings during the manic stage.

3. Work closely with the patient and set limits on her behavior as necessary.

4. Encourage her to socialize with other patients to help reduce her hyperactivity.

62. Which of the following are antipsychotic drugs?

1. Thorazine, Mellaril, and Haldol.

2. Elavil, Prozac, and Tofranil.

3. Cogentin, Artane, and levodopa.

4. Marplan, Nardil, and Parnate.

63. The most common psychosis is

1. Paranoia.

2. Bipolar disorder.

3. Schizophrenia.

4. Maladaptive behavior.

64. Which of the following are monoamine oxidase inhibitors (MAOIs)?

1. Thorazine, Mellaril, and Haldol.

2. Elavil, Prozac, and Tofranil.

3. Cogentin, Artane, and levodopa.

4. Marplan, Nardil, and Parnate.

65. Foods to be avoided during therapy with MAOIs are

1. Organ meats, oranges, and diet sodas.

2. Aged cheese, alcoholic beverages, and caffeine.

3. Potatoes, carrots, and diet sodas.

4. Soups, meat, eggs, and milk.

66. Drugs to be avoided during therapy with MAOIs are

1. Valium, aspirin, and steroids.

2. Lasix, Valium, and lidocaine.

3. Prostigmin, Prozac, and Pamelor.

4. Levodopa, meperidine, and antihistamines.

67. Which of the following are tricyclic antidepressants?

1. Elavil, Tofranil, and Pamelor.

2. Marplan, Nardil, and Parnate.

3. Lithium, Cogentin, and Artane.

4. Haldol, Mellaril, and Navane.

68. A hyperactive manic patient has driven the staff to the end of its tolerance 2 days after admission. The best action to take is to

1. Let the patient know that the nursing staff will not tolerate his or her behavior.

2. Allow the patient more time to express his or her feelings to the nursing staff and physicians.

3. Put the patient in isolation for a day to slow him or her down.

4. Have the nursing staff meet to discuss the need for staff consistency and setting limits on the patient's behavior.

69. A 20-year-old single woman was admitted to the hospital because she was grabbed from behind by a man who put a gun to her head and then raped her. The aspect of the patient's crisis that produced the most psychological trauma is the

1. Memory of the event.

2. Physical pain experienced.

3. Violation of her physical integrity.

4. Fear of being pregnant.

70. The behavior that would indicate that a rape victim is in the acute phase of the rape-trauma syndrome is

1. Fear and flashbacks.

2. Confusion and disbelief.

3. Fear of men and bad dreams.

4. Decreased motor activity and anxiety.

71. A patient in the acute phase of the rape-trauma syndrome tells the nurse she does not remember what happened, cannot talk about it, and needs to forget everything that happened. The coping strategy can be assessed as

1. Temporary attention-deficit disorder.

2. Use of denial.

3. Use of somatization.

4. Reaction formation.

72. An appropriate intervention for the nurse to use during the acute phase of rape-trauma syndrome is

1. Allow the patient's family in the room and involve them in the history-taking process.

2. Put an arm around the patient and reassure her that the nurse is there to help her.

3. Put her in a private room with soft music and tell her that the physician will be with her as soon as he can.

4. Allow the patient time to talk at a comfortable pace. Assure her that she is in a safe place and ask her questions in a nonjudgmental way.

73. What area should the nurse address when taking a history from a patient in the acute phase of the rape-trauma syndrome?

1. Does the patient plan to press charges against the man who raped her?

2. Is the patient taking contraceptive medication?

3. What support system is available for the patient?

4. Did the patient know the man who raped her?

74. The following psychotherapeutic intervention should be used by the nurse working with a patient in the acute phase of the rape-trauma syndrome. The nurse should

1. Make decisions for the patient because she is confused and her anxiety level is very high.

2. Ask the patient to answer many short questions rather than long, drawn-out questions and keep asking them until all of the history is completed.

3. Reassure the patient that her short dress and the way she acted had nothing to do with being raped.

4. Allow the patient to verbalize negative expressions or feelings of self-blame when she feels comfortable enough to talk.

75. If a rape victim states, "I should have known better than to walk home alone at this hour of the night," the nurse's most appropriate reply would be

1. You probably walked home alone many times before. It's just a crazy world.

2. Don't blame yourself; it only increases your anxiety.

3. You are so right. Walking alone at night is a very dangerous thing to do.

4. You believe that this would not have happened if you had not walked home alone tonight.

76. A short-term goal for a patient with acute rape-trauma syndrome that could be achieved by the time she leaves the emergency room is that the patient will state

1. I feel safer and am more relaxed.

2. My physical symptoms of pain and discomfort are no longer present.

3. My memory of the rape is less vivid and less frightening.

4. I will keep the follow-up appointment with the rape crisis counselor.

77. A rape victim attended rape crisis counseling once per week for 5 months. Which of the following behaviors will indicate that the process of reorganization has taken place?

1. Discussing positive feelings about herself with her friends.

2. Experiencing problems returning to school.

3. Asking friends to go with her so she will not be alone.

4. Her family was supportive the first week after the rape.

78. A rape victim tells her crisis counselor that her family is not very supportive. The belief that contributes to the family's response is

1. Any woman is a potential rape victim.

2. Women do not ask to be raped.

3. Nice girls do not get raped.

4. Rape is an act of aggression.

79. A rape victim tells the emergency room nurse, "I feel dirty. I don't want anyone to touch me until I take a bath." The nurse should

1. Give the patient a basin of warm water and a towel.

2. Explain that washing would destroy evidence.

3. Explain to the patient that every person who is raped feels dirty.

4. Take the patient to the shower and stay with her.

80. A female patient with somatoform disorder will

1. Assume all of the responsibilities for her family.

2. Become very involved in others' problems.

3. Exaggerate or misinterpret physical symptoms.

4. Misinterpret her physical surroundings.

81. A patient tells the nurse, "I love coming to this hospital because everyone is so interested in me. I wish people outside the hospital paid that much attention to me, but they don't." Based on this statement, the nurse would continue to gather assessment data to support a nursing diagnosis of

1. Self-esteem disturbance.

2. Social isolation.

3. Self-care deficit.

4. Ineffective family coping.

82. A patient is afraid she has AIDS and goes from physician to physician requesting diagnostic tests and treatment. She tells the nurse, "I know I have AIDS, and I feel sure I may also have lupus, but the doctors have not been able to diagnose any disease. I am getting tired of having to go to doctors every week. If I miss any more work, I may not have a job." Based on these statements, the nurse will want to continue to gather assessment data to support a diagnosis of

1. Somatization.

2. Psychosis.

3. Projection.

4. Hypochondriasis.

83. Which statement is true about patients who have somatoform conversion disorders? The patient will

1. Go from physician to physician for help.

2. Attend psychotherapy sessions.

3. Seek medical advice and psychiatric advice without encouragement.

4. Verbalize emotional needs easily.

84. A female patient with a diagnosis of low self-esteem tells the nurse that her symptoms make her more interesting to people. An appropriate intervention to help the client increase her self-esteem would be to

1. Tell the patient to avoid all negative interactions and to seek psychiatric help.

2. Help the patient to set only long-term goals to help her lose weight.

3. Help the patient to verbalize her negative feelings about herself to her family and friends.

4. Focus attention on the patient as a person rather than on the symptoms.

85. To plan effective care for a patient with somatoform disorders, the nurse must understand that the symptoms displayed

1. Can be voluntarily controlled.

2. Provide relief from anxiety.

3. Have a psychological and physiologic basis.

4. Can be controlled with antipsychotic drugs.

86. An appropriate nursing diagnosis for a patient with a somatoform disorder is

1. Impaired social interaction related to unconscious need to focus on physical symptoms in order to feel more comfortable.

2. Impaired family coping related to psychological and physical problems.

3. Ineffective individual coping related to altered health maintenance.

4. Altered personality disorder related to multiple physical symptoms.

87. A patient has had difficulty holding a job; he accuses a coworker of conspiring to take his job. The patient has had previous admissions to the psychiatric unit. When the nurse meets the patient he states, "You are all trying to kill me, isn't that true?" The most appropriate response by the nurse would be

1. Every nurse on this unit will work with you, and you will end up caring for every one of us.

2. We know you have some problems, but we are used to working with people who have problems.

3. Thinking that people want to kill you must be very frightening.

4. Your comments are not acceptable, and we will not tolerate your remarks.

88. A patient states, "I don't know why I have to be in the hospital. The people who want to destroy me should be here." The patient constantly scans the environment. He tells the nurse that the two patients in the hall are after him and will hurt him if they get a chance. The nurse may correctly assess this behavior as

1. An auditory hallucination.

2. A schizophrenic reaction (an idea of reference).

3. An anxiety reaction caused by mood disturbance.

4. A delusion of fear caused by medications.

89. The etiology of schizophrenia that might explain a patient's fear of their environment is

1. All children from a divorced family will always perceive the world as dangerous.

2. A child raised with hostile inconsistent care, rejection, and ridicule will perceive the world as dangerous.

3. A personality identity disturbance related to a traumatic event.

4. A child raised in foster homes with six other children.

90. A patient taking Thorazine 100 mg PO qid for 2 months tells the nurse that he has stopped taking his Thorazine because of the way it made him feel. The common side effect this client is most likely referring to is
1. Nausea, diarrhea, watery eyes, and unsteady gait.
2. Diarrhea, runny nose, and malaise.
3. Skin rash, mild fever, and sweating.
4. Dry mouth, orthostatic hypotension, and shuffling gait.

91. When a patient continues to demonstrate noncompliance with chlorpromazine (Thorazine), the most appropriate nursing intervention is to
1. Advise the patient to reduce dosage for a day or two and then return to the prescribed order.
2. Teach the patient the side effects of Thorazine and to report severe side effects to the physician.
3. Advise the patient that he will die if he does not take his medication every day per physician's orders.
4. Instruct the patient on how to give his own IM injections, which will decrease the side effects of the medication.

92. A 70-year-old man diagnosed with schizophrenia has a prescription for chlorpromazine (Thorazine) PO qid. He refuses to take his medication daily because he does not like taking pills. His family tells the physician they feel helpless. The physician may prescribe a treatment of
1. Amitriptyline (Elavil) IM qid.
2. Diazepam (Valium) PO qid.
3. Prolixin decanoate IM qid.
4. Alprazolam (Xanax).

93. Side effects of fluoxetine (Prozac) are
1. Leukopenia, GI bleeding, and nausea.
2. Insomnia, drowsiness, and nervousness.
3. Pruritus, nausea, and vomiting.
4. Diarrhea, hypertension, and nausea.

94. When assessing for hallucinating behavior, the nurse would observe for
1. Mumbling or talking to self as though responding conversationally to someone, and looking around the room as though to find the speaker.
2. Aloofness, ambiguous, loner- and very secretive-type personality, and sitting and staring into space as if listening to someone.
3. Haughtiness, suspiciousness, distractibility, irritability, and noncompliance with impaired communication.
4. Paranoid, aloof, loner, suspicious, mumbling or talking to self as though responding conversationally to someone.

95. A male nurse giving a bath to a paranoid male client in the withdrawn phase of catatonic schizophrenia must
1. Increase sensory input by conversation, television, and radio.
2. Move the patient as little as possible and speak softly.

3. Ask the client to squeeze his hand when he understands the message; continue this procedure until the patient responds.
4. Explain all physical care activities in simple explicit terms, working with the patient as if he will respond.

96. A schizophrenic patient is experiencing hallucinations and delusions. What activity would be most appropriate for the patient?
1. Racquetball game.
2. Checkers.
3. Solitary card game.
4. Basketball game.

97. The most appropriate nursing diagnosis for a patient in the withdrawn phase of catatonic schizophrenia would be
1. Self-care deficit.
2. Psychologically impaired.
3. Altered self-image.
4. Noncompliance.

98. A highly suspicious male client who has delusions of persecution has refused all hospital meals for 4 days. The most appropriate nursing intervention would be to
1. Bring the patient his food and allow him to choose between eating the food or having a nasogastric tube put in for feeding.
2. Allow the patient to leave the hospital long enough to secure food he feels is not poisoned.
3. Allow the patient to go to the hospital kitchen and watch the staff prepare his food.
4. Serve the patient foods in sealed containers and allow him access to lobby food machines.

99. To establish a relationship with a severely withdrawn male schizophrenic patient, the nurse should
1. Spend 5 min with the patient every hour, give him directions in a clear, slow manner, and allow time to respond.
2. Sit with the patient for 1 h each day, allowing the patient to discuss how he or she feels.
3. Sit facing the patient for short periods several times per day, accept silence, and state when the nurse will return.
4. Spend at least 2 h every day with the patient, place a hand on the patient's arm, and ask him to tell the nurse when he wants the nurse to leave his room.

100. Two schizophrenic patient asks the nurse, "Can you hear them? They talk with me all the time; I can't get any rest." The most helpful reply by the nurse would be
1. Try to keep yourself busy, and then you won't hear the voices.
2. I can't hear the voices, so you know they are make-believe.
3. I can't hear the voices, but I can tell you are upset.
4. Talk with your doctor about increasing your medication.

ANSWERS AND RATIONALES

1. ❶ Bipolar disorder is characterized by mood swings that range from elated to manic depressive. One day the patient is very happy, and the next day the patient is very depressed. The patient may be so elated for 3 or 4 days that he or she cannot sit or rest. After that period, the patient may be depressed for several days.

3. Severe depression can lead to suicide but this is not a bipolar disorder.

(2, 4) These options are incorrect as seen in rationale (1).

2. ❷ If a male patient with bipolar disorder manic type is so hyperactive that he cannot sleep, the best nursing intervention would be to reduce the amount of distraction and to encourage brief rest periods.

1. Isolating a patient with bipolar disorder who is hyperactive would make him more hyperactive.

3. There is no reason to restrain a patient who is hyperactive; he is no danger to himself or to others.

4. The physician makes the decision concerning ordering phenobarbital for a patient. The nurse should not ask for an order. It is the nurse's responsibility to help the patient to sleep by making the environment less distracting and using relaxation methods. Sleep without the use of sedatives is much more beneficial than sleep induced with a sedative.

3. ❷ A male patient with bipolar disorder can create chaos on the ward by using dominating and manipulative behavior. The nurse working with this patient needs to provide alternative behavior. This will help the patient learn more acceptable behavior, and it will reduce the chaos on the ward.

1. The nurse should not inform a patient with bipolar disorder that his behavior is unacceptable because this will destroy the relationship that the nurse is trying to establish. When working with a psychiatric patient, the nurse must establish a trusting relationship with the patient in order to help him or her.

3. The nursing staff may have to set some limits on a hyperactive patient but this would not reduce the clients use of dominating and manipulative behavior.

4. Moving a patient to another floor is never a correct answer because the nurse is just moving the problem to another floor instead of solving the problem.

4. ❸ When a wife tells the nurse that she is worried about her husband because he is sometimes happy and sometimes sad, sometimes self-confident, and at other times extremely down on himself and blames her for all his problems, the nurse must first get information about the patient's symptoms and their frequency and duration.

1. There is not enough information for a diagnosis of psychopathologic problems in the client's family. A nurse would not make this medical diagnosis.

(2, 4) The nurse does not have enough information to make a diagnosis about the couple's relationship. The physical health is not an issue in this situation.

5. ❹ When a 17-year-old female is admitted to the psychiatric ward for overdose of a prescribed antidepressant, the nurse caring for the patient should be aware that warning signs for suicide include feelings of hopelessness and any previous suicide attempts. The patient may feel hopeless or may believe that she has no reason to live and would be better off dead. She may want to draw attention to herself in order to get her family's love and support.

1. Many people are depressed after losing a job and a home, but they do not plan suicide.

2. Auditory hallucinations are not related to suicide attempts. Low socioeconomic status is not a cause of suicide.

3. Many people have feelings of failure as a businessperson, but they do not attempt suicide; they gradually work through their feelings and move on with life.

6. ❷ In recognizing the dynamics of suicide, the nurse knows that the most appropriate nursing action for a patient recovering from a suicide attempt is to encourage her or him to verbalize feelings and pain. Remember, whenever there is an option such as "allow the client to verbalize his or her feelings," it is most likely the right answer.

1. Letting the patient spend time alone to reflect on his or her suicide attempt can be very dangerous because he or she may commit suicide. Being alone could make him or her more suicidal. The patient needs to be able to talk with a professional so he or she can understand and deal with his or her feelings.

3. Avoiding the topic of suicide does not help the patient verbalize feelings.

4. The nurse should not make the patient feel guilty about attempting suicide.

7. ❸ This 17-year-old has attempted suicide because her boyfriend left her and told her that he never wanted to see her again. The teenager has told the nurse that she would rather be dead than live without him. Based on this information, the nurse's short-term plan for this patient should include the goal that the teenager be able to reach a point where she can say she "feels okay being alive." If the patient feels that being alive is okay, she can progress to long-term goals.

1. Finding another boyfriend will not solve the problem that the patient has of believing that her happiness depends on other people.

2. Recognizing that she was too dependent on her boyfriend may be a long-term goal, and she needs to learn to work toward eliminating her codependency.

4. Making the patient feel guilty about attempting suicide will not help her deal with her feelings. Nurses are not supposed to judge what is right or wrong for a patient; that is the patient's responsibility.

8. ❹ When the nursing staff on a medical unit meets to discuss the major emotional needs of their patients on the unit, the nursing staff would first identify which patients have emotional disequilibrium or increased anxiety.

1. Nursing interventions can be developed once patients with emotional problems have been identified, as well as their specific problems.

2. The daily living needs refer to physical needs of the patient, not emotional needs. Patients may depend on nurses for baths, food, and so on.

3. A patient may have emotional needs that the nursing staff can meet; this does not mean the client needs psychiatric help. Emotional needs are a normal part of every person.

9. ❸ The method most helpful for the nurse to identify the emotional needs of their patients would be to interview them immediately on admission.

1. Reviewing the patients' charts will not help the nurse to identify the emotional needs of patients. In most situations, the patient is considered the best source of information about his or her emotional needs. When the patient is admitted is the best time to discover what emotional need brought him or her to the unit.

2. The physical and emotional history supplied by the patient's family gives the nurse the family's perception of their own emotional needs. The patient is always the best source of information unless he or she has a severe mental disorder.

4. The nurses' notes on the patient problems may only relate to physical needs.

10. ❷ The nursing staff agrees that the basic principle of planning nursing care is to accept patients as they are and allow them an active part in planning for their needs. This shows respect for the patient and gives the patient some control over his or her care.

1. A nurse should not help the patient believe that he or she will improve. If the patient does not improve, he or she will not trust the nurse. The patient may firmly believe that he or she is getting better when, in fact, he or she might be dying of cancer. This is not a basic principle for planning nursing care.

3. The nurse cannot meet all of the patient's emotional and physical needs. This is not a basic principle for planning nursing care.

4. It is difficult for a nurse to really know a patient and to understand his or her needs. The nurse may know what the patient's needs are, but it is difficult to really know the patient and understand all of his or her needs; this is not a basic principle of planning nursing care. When the word "all" is used in an option, it usually is an incorrect option.

11. ❹ Side effects of phencyclidine (PCP) are vivid hallucinations and persecutory delusions. Persons under the influence of PCP are agitated and combative. They are potentially dangerous to self and others, and they are best treated by being placed in isolation in a quiet room, under observation. The client may need to be restrained and medicated.

(1, 2, 3) Diazepam (Valium), opium, and codeine produce a sedative effect; all will produce sleep. Valium is an antianxiety drug; opium works as an analgesic or sedative/hypnotic; and codeine is made from opium and is an analgesic and sedative/hypnotic.

12. ❶ The most therapeutic action by the nurses would be flexible treatment of nursing care with an individualized approach for a 75-year-old woman who has lost contact with reality, hallucinates, cannot carry on a conversation, and refuses to eat or sleep.

2. The daughter may be unable to stay at the nursing home with the patient for the first week (even if the daughter could stay, the mother does not know who she is). It is the nurse's responsibility to ensure that the patient has individualized care.

3. This patient will not harm herself or others; therefore, she should not be restrained.

4. Putting this patient in a room with others will not help her to regain her orientation; it may increase her disorientation.

13. ❶ Side effects of Haldol are pill-rolling motions, drooling, tremors, rigidity, masklike face, and shuffling gait. These are also symptoms of Parkinson's disease. The physician must be notified immediately at the onset of these symptoms. The physician will order Cogentin to treat these side effects. Although Haldol normally takes 2 weeks to be effective, it is possible for an individual to have a hypersensitive reaction.

(2, 3, 4) The nurse does not ask the physician to reduce a dosage or order a medication, or wait to give the medication on the next shift if symptoms are still present. As explained in rationale (1), the physician must be notified immediately.

14. ❷ When a patient states that she is hearing strange voices, the nurse should reply, "I believe you when you say you are hearing voices, but I cannot hear them." This statement lets the patient know that she is the only one hearing the voices.

1. It would be very upsetting for the patient if the nurse told her that the voices are only in her thoughts because she truly believes that she is hearing voices.

3. Telling the patient that the nurse will move her to be with other patients to get her mind off the voices she is hearing will anger her. The nurse will be unable to develop a helpful and trustful relationship with the patient because she will feel threatened and belittled by the nurse.

4. Telling the patient that others might be able to hear the voices reinforces her belief that she is hearing voices.

15. ❹ When a female patient refuses to take a bath or have her bed changed, the nurse's best therapeutic reply would be, "Which of your pretty gowns do you want to put on after your bath? I will give you a good back rub after we are finished with your bath." This allows the patient to focus on the pleasures of having a bath and encourages her to cooperate.

1. Telling the patient that soap and water and a clean bed will make her like a new person is telling her how she will feel. A nurse never tells a patient how he or she should or should not feel. Telling her that a bath will make the voices go away is belittling her.

2. If the nurse tells a patient who has refused a bath to let the nurse know when she is ready for a bath, the patient may never be ready for a bath.

3. Telling a patient that everyone on the unit must have a bath every day and that she is going to have one right now will only upset her. It takes away her right to make a decision and belittles her.

16. **2** This statement focuses on the patient's statement, and it serves to open channels of communication.

1. This response asks the patient to decide why she feels the way she does. It does not reflect on her feelings or stimulate conversation.

3. This statement encourages the patient to think of herself as a sinner and can cause her more depression. It does not encourage communication.

4. This response does not stimulate communication; in fact, it tells the patient to discuss her feelings with someone else.

17. **3** The most therapeutic response for the nurse to make to Mr. Martin is, "It sounds like you were really angry. When you feel angry, you need to tell us instead of hitting so that we can help you work through your anger." The patient needs to learn how to express his anger so that it does not build up to a point where he cannot handle it.

(1, 2, 4) These options are incorrect because they fail to help Mr. Martin learn how to deal with his anger in a more constructive way.

18. **4** After Mr. Martin tells the nurse that he had to leave the TV room because he was so angry with another man in the room that he felt like throwing him across the floor, the most therapeutic response by the nurse is, "I can tell you are very angry, and you did well to leave the situation. Let's walk up and down the hall while you tell me about it."

This response gives positive reinforcement to his constructive control of his anger. By walking with the patient and allowing him to express his anger, he is learning how to better manage his angry feelings.

1. Telling a patient that he or she cannot use "foul" language in the hospital will only make the patient more angry. It does not help the patient to change his behavior.

2. Offering him Ativan (a sedative/hypnotic antianxiety agent) to calm him down does not allow the patient to deal with his feelings of anger or allow him to begin to channel his anger in a more appropriate manner.

3. The statement "I am glad you left the recreation room without hurting anyone" is a therapeutic response, but the nurse telling the patient to go to his room and she will come in soon is not a therapeutic response. The patient needs to deal with his feelings now while he is still very angry so that he can learn to channel his anger in an appropriate manner. If the patient continues to hold his anger inside, he may return to the recreation room and hurt someone before the nurse gets to his room. "Soon" to the nurse may mean a half-hour, but "soon" to the very angry patient may mean 5 min.

19. **3** The most therapeutic response by the nurse to this client is, "It can be frightening to have new people on the unit. One of the purposes of this group is for people to get to know each other and talk together about things like being afraid."

This statement opens the problem up to the group for discussion. It is not the responsibility of the group leader (the nurse) to tell patients how they should feel. It is the nurse's responsibility to offer the group the opportunity to discuss whatever problem is of concern to them and to work on solving them with each other.

(1, 2, 4) These options are incorrect as seen in rationale (3).

20. **4** To respond to Mrs. Smith, it is most important for the nurse to understand that denial of anger with passive unassertive behavior is a maladaptive behavior pattern. This understanding is necessary so that the nurse can help Mrs. Smith learn how to express her anger in an appropriate manner.

(1, 2, 3) These options are incorrect as seen in rationale (4).

21. **4** When a patient has been beaten by her husband and is admitted to the mental health center, it is most important during the interview to determine the potential of immediate danger to the patient and her children. Men who beat their wives usually beat their children and may kill them in a rage of anger. The husband may come to the mental health center and beat his wife or possibly kill her. Safety is always a priority; the other problems do not have to be met immediately.

(1, 2, 3) These options are incorrect as seen in rationale (4).

22. **2** The fact that Ellen's husband beats her and tells her that it is her job to stay home illustrates abusive family characteristics. There is an unbalanced power ratio and a dysfunctional feeling tone.

A major characteristic of an abused family is the unbalanced power ratio. In this case, the husband has all the power and the wife has none. An example of dysfunctional feeling tone is the wife stating that her husband is a "good family man," when the truth is that he is not. The wife has been so "beaten down" physically and emotionally that she is confused about who she is and how she feels. Her anger is all inside her, and she cannot express it because her husband will not allow it.

(1, 3, 4) These options are incorrect as seen in rationale (2).

23. **1** The most helpful plan of care for this patient would be to have her attend a group meeting for women in abusive families. This will give the patient a chance to express her anger and frustrations and to know that she is not alone. Listening to other women tell similar stories of abuse and how these women are working through their emotional problems will help her work through hers. Also, the group will be able to share ideas to meet the special needs of the children.

2. Calling Ellen's physician to find out how many times she was in his office because her husband beat her will not help the patient to solve her problems.

3. Notifying the police because the husband may hit a patient again does not help a patient to solve her problems.

4. Asking the school nurse if she treated the children for abuse does not help the patient to solve her problems. Only the patient can solve her problems.

24. **4** The characteristic that is *least* likely to be true of Mr. Hart is that between episodes of abuse he has a warm empathetic relationship with his wife. Men who abuse their wives have no respect for them and continually belittle them. It is a means of controlling their wives so that the wives will not leave them. Husbands tell abused wives that they are no good and that no one else would want them.

1. Mr. Hart may be a college graduate and may have worked at the same job for 15 years. Wife abuse and child abuse cross all socioeconomic levels.

2. Mr. Hart's mother may have abused him, and he is repeating that learned behavior. Many men who abuse their wives were abused as children. Remember this was an *except* question.

3. Mr. Hart may not have met his own expectations for career achievement. He may be vice-president of a company and still feel he is a failure because he is not president. Whatever he accomplishes will not make him happy. He is insecure and has low self-esteem, and beating his wife gives him a feeling of some control over his life.

25. ❷ When Ellen tells the nurse that her 6-year-old son is afraid to go to school because he is afraid his mother will not be there when he comes home, the nurse should discuss with Ellen that the child "is aware of the fighting going on between her and her husband, and he is worried about what might happen. Would you like to have him talk with a child therapist? I think it would really help him." This statement will help a patient to realize that her child is frightened and afraid that he might be left alone and that her child needs to talk with someone about his fears.

(1, 3, 4) These options are incorrect as seen in rationale (2).

26. ❹ When the nurse finds herself dreading a patient's appointments because she feels she is not working effectively with her, the most appropriate action by the nurse is to realize that these are normal feelings when working with abused women.

Progress can be so slow when working with women in abusive families that the nurse may feel she is making no progress. The abused woman not only has all of her own emotional problems to deal with but also those of her children.

(1, 2, 3) These options are incorrect as seen in rationale (4).

27. ❸ In discussing this situation with the patient, it would be most important for the nurse to find out more from her about her decision to stop therapy.

Many times, the husband will stop abusing the wife so that she will stop her therapy. He does not want to lose control over her, so he will try very hard to get her to stop therapy. The husband may have told her if she did not stop going to therapy, he would really hurt her or the children. The nurse needs more information before she can make an assessment.

1. If the nurse tries to warn the wife that the husband is just being nice until she stops therapy and that it is likely that he will become abusive again, the patient may not believe her. If the nurse allows Ellen to discuss her decision to stop therapy, Ellen may come to realize that it is her husband who wants her to quit. She may admit to the nurse that her husband has threatened to harm her if she does not stop therapy.

It is possible that the husband is trying to change his behavior, and for that reason, the couple is getting along better, which would be a good reason to continue therapy, not stop it.

(2, 4) The nurse should not tell the patient what she should do. The patient needs a support system to help her make the best decisions for herself.

28. ❸ Joel is admitted to the hospital for the fourth time in 11 months with chronic ulcerative colitis, and he is familiar to the nursing staff caring for him. The most therapeutic statement the primary nurse would make is, "It's been 3 months since you were last here. What do you think about being back in the hospital?" This statement allows him to respond with his true feelings. It will help the nurse to know how to meet his emotional and physical needs.

1. To say to a patient who is very ill that "We thought we had cured you the last time you were in here" is cruel. It makes the patient feel like he should be cured and not be back in the hospital.

2. The statement "What brings you back this time?" makes the patient feel like he is not wanted and that he is always coming to the hospital. The nurse should know from the patient's records why he is admitted.

4. Having the same room again may not make the patient happy; the patient is ill and being in the same room may be distressing to him.

29. ❷ A client who has been ill repeatedly says to the nurse, "Sometimes I imagine myself to be all powerful, so powerful that I would put other men to shame," is using the defense mechanism of fantasy. Fantasy is excessive retreat into daydreams to escape problems. Fantasy is the creating of mental images modified by need, wish, or desire.

1. Dissociation is a defense mechanism that operates unconsciously to separate and detach emotional significance from an idea or experience.

3. Projection is a defense mechanism that is the unconscious rejection of unacceptable thoughts, traits, or wishes, and ascribing them to others.

4. Repression is a defense mechanism that excludes from awareness distressing internal feelings, impulses, ideas, or wishes. Repression is unconscious and is not to be confused with suppression, which is conscious.

30. ❸ When a patient makes the statement to the nurse, "That doctor of mine loves cutting on me; the more gut he can cut out, the better he likes it," the most therapeutic response by the nurse would be, "The more he cuts out the better he likes it. What do you mean by that?" This allows the client to express his anger or fears about his surgery, and discussing his anger or fears with the nurse will help him work through these feelings. He may have questions about his surgery that he is afraid to ask because he fears the answer.

(1, 2, 4) The nurse should not guess what the client might mean.

31. ❷ The best definition of empathy is to identify with another person's feelings.

(1, 3, 4) These options are incorrect as seen in rationale (2).

32. ❹ When planning an activity for a patient with ulcerative colitis, the nurse should be sure that the activity will be conducive to rest and relaxation. A person with ulcerative colitis tends to be anxious and nervous, which increases the symptoms of colitis. The patient should not participate in competitive activities.

1. Activities with other clients may not offer the patient the rest and relaxation that he needs to improve.

2. The patient needs to relax and not be under any pressure; learning how to improve his social skills could produce anxiety.

3. The patient has diarrhea (one of the signs of colitis), so he does not have to exercise to prevent constipation.

33. **①** The nurse's best intervention when a patient has a hostile outburst is to encourage him to discuss his immediate concerns and feelings with the nurse and not to let anger build up inside. The only way to work through his feelings of anger is by expressing how he feels and why he feels that way.

2. Offering a client positive reinforcement each time he cooperates will not help him to get rid of his angry feelings.

3. Ignoring the patient's behavior will not help him to express his hostility.

4. Directing the patient's anger at the nursing staff will only increase his inner feeling of anger because he is not dealing with his own; the patient's anger will continue to build.

34. **①** A member of the ileostomy club meets with a patient who has just had an ileostomy to show support and give the patient realistic information about ileostomy. This helps the patient see that he will be able to lead a normal life, and it allows the patient to ask questions and have them answered by someone who has had an ileostomy.

(2, 3, 4) These options are incorrect as seen in rationale (1).

35. **④** Vomiting and diarrhea can be signs of lithium toxicity; there may be some other cause of vomiting and diarrhea, but the loss of fluid will increase the concentration of lithium in the blood and produce toxicity. If a patient is vomiting or has diarrhea, she needs to notify her doctor because she may have or may develop lithium toxicity.

(1, 2) Swollen lymph nodes and upper respiratory infection would be associated with a condition such as infection or cancer.

3. Dryness of the mouth is a side effect of lithium, but it is not serious.

36. **③** When a patient with bulimia tells the nurse that she knows that binges of eating and vomiting are not normal but she is not able to stop, the nurse's best therapeutic response would be, "What are your feelings when you go on these eating sprees?" The nurse is trying to get the patient to determine what it is that makes her overeat. If the she can determine what drives her to eat, she can begin to deal with the problem. She can then begin to cope with the cause and can make progress toward controlling her eating.

(1, 2, 4) These options are incorrect as seen in rationale (3).

37. **③** The nursing action that would best help a patient control the use of laxatives, diuretics, and vomiting is to have the her record when and why she eats.

The patient uses laxatives, diuretics, and vomiting because she overeats and does not want to gain weight. If she can determine why she overeats, then she can begin to have some control

over her eating. Bulimic and anorexic patients feel like they have no control over their lives. These patients believe they are overweight, although they are underweight. Controlling their weight gives them the feeling of having some control over their lives. They need therapy to feel better about themselves.

(1, 2, 4) These options are incorrect as seen in rationale (3).

38. **④** Manipulative patients frequently make requests of many different staff members, hoping one will give them what they want. Having the primary nurse as the decision maker provides consistency and prevents the patient from playing one staff member against another.

1. Acting-out behavior is not specific to manipulative behavior; it could be any behavior.

2. Ignoring manipulative behavior does not change the behavior, it just allows it to continue.

3. There is no relationship between fear and manipulative behavior.

39. **②** Having the patient acknowledge his manipulative behavior will help him to become more aware of his manipulation. This is fundamental to decreasing the use of manipulation.

1. Not allowing the patient to use manipulative behavior is not a goal, it is a nursing intervention.

3. Getting the patient to demonstrate less impulsive behavior is a goal, but the patient is manipulative, not impulsive.

4. If the patient uses his behavior selectively, he will not learn to control it. He can only stop this behavior by a goal that will help him eliminate the behavior.

40. **②** Limits must be set when the patient's behavior impacts the rights of others.

(1, 3, 4) These options are incorrect as seen in rationale (2).

41. **③** The antisocial patient often acts out feelings of anger and experiences no guilt or remorse.

(1, 2, 4) These statements show signs of concern and remorse; this does not reflect the feelings of an antisocial individual.

42. **①** Lack of external controls leads to manipulative behavior such as lying, conning, flattering, begging, and doing whatever they have to do to get what they want. Therefore, to protect the rights of others, external controls must be consistently maintained until the patient is able to behave appropriately.

2. Antisocial patients do not have feelings of guilt; therefore, they have no need to vent their feelings of guilt and frustrations.

3. The nursing staff can never assume the responsibility for a patient's behavior.

4. The nursing staff cannot meet every need of the patient and, even if they could, it would increase, not decrease, manipulative behavior. The patient would believe his behavior was being rewarded.

43. **②** Maintaining consistent limits is the most difficult intervention due to the patient's ability to use manipulation and the many different staff members that work with a patient.

(1, 3, 4) These options are incorrect as seen in rationale (2).

44. ❸ Impulsive behavior is characterized by the individual acting in haste without taking time to consider the consequences of his or her actions.

1. If a patient had a rigid moral code, he or she would think before he or she acted, so this is not a characteristic of impulsive behavior.

2. Individuals can have impulsive behavior but have no distortion of reality; therefore, distortion is not a characteristic of impulsive behavior.

4. Manipulative behavior is not a characteristic of impulsive behavior.

45. ❹ The nurse must understand that respect, honesty, and courtesy are of utmost importance when working with a paranoid patient. The nurse cannot retaliate or the relationship with the patient will deteriorate. The goal is to make the patient feel secure and comfortable.

1. If a nurse lets the patient know how he or she feels about him, the relationship with him would be destroyed. Remember, he is highly suspicious.

(2, 3) These options are incorrect as seen in rationale (4).

46. ❶ The patient with paranoid personality disorder may unconsciously use the defense mechanism projection to control anxiety. The use of projection allows the patient to disown his unacceptable feelings, ideas, or attitudes by attributing them to others.

2. Hypervigilance implies that the individual rigidly observes all that goes on around him or her.

3. Intellectualization is the analysis of personal or social problems using an intellectual basis despite the individual's personal and emotional reactions to those problems.

4. Introjection is an immature, unconscious defense mechanism used in the identification of the self with another or with some object, with the victim assuming the supposed feelings of the other personality.

47. ❸ Projection allows the patient to disown negative feelings about self and see these feelings as being directed at self from an outside source such as the nurse. The patient projects self-hate and anger to the nurse.

(1, 2, 4) These statements are not characteristic of a paranoid personality disorder.

48. ❸ A patient with the ability to invoke interpersonal conflict will require frequent team meetings. The meetings are held to counteract the effects of the patient's attempts to split the staff and set them against one another.

(1, 2, 4) Auditory hallucinations, anxiety attacks, and denial are behaviors that can be handled by an individual nurse. Team meetings will be used to discuss these behaviors, but they are not destructive to the staff unity.

49. ❷ This is the incorrect option because not every mentally impaired individual will show little or no emotion during a time of grief. The option to use all-inclusive words such as "every" usually is the wrong option. Not many things in life are always, ever, and all.

(1, 3, 4) These options are correct statements, so none of these can be the *does not* statement.

50. ❸ It takes 7 to 28 days for a person's mood to improve when taking tricyclic antidepressants. The patient needs to understand that it takes several weeks before he or she will feel less depressed.

1. Foods high in tyramine should not be eaten when a patient is taking monoamine oxidase inhibitor (MAOI) antidepressants. Eating foods high in tyramine while taking MAOIs results in the accumulation of dopamine, epinephrine, and norepinephrine, causing hypertension.

2. Sunlight will not affect a patient taking tricyclic antidepressant medication.

4. Sodium is not restricted when taking tricyclic antidepressants. When a patient is taking lithium, a normal intake of sodium is recommended. Low levels of sodium can predispose the patient to toxicity.

51. ❹ A depressed patient avoids recognizing painful feelings by withdrawing. Patients often reject the attention the nurse gives and appear not to respond to nursing interventions. Understanding this behavior reduces the nurse's frustration.

(1, 2, 3) These options are incorrect as seen in rationale (4).

52. ❹ The statement "The loss of your husband must be very painful for you" validates the bereaver's experience of loss.

(1, 2, 3) These are trite remarks that tend to increase the individual's sense of isolation.

53. ❶ The work of grieving is over when the bereaved can remember the loved one realistically and acknowledges both the pleasure and disappointments associated with the loved one. This does not mean that the bereaved will no longer grieve; for example, a mother will always grieve for her dead child. It does mean that the individual now is free to enter into new relationships and activities.

(2, 3, 4) These statements reflect that the bereaved has not worked through the grieving process.

54. ❸ The statement "One of us will sit with you for 10 min every 3 h starting at 1 PM today" lets the client know the nurses will take that time to be with her. The time spent with a depressed client can be very meaningful and helpful. Spending short, frequent periods minimizes both the patient's and the nurse's anxiety. Sitting with the patient demonstrates that the nurses have the time to spend and are not in a hurry. Scheduling time gives structure and purpose to the meetings.

(1, 2, 4) These are trite remarks that say nothing meaningful to the patient.

55. ❹ To be able to verbalize something positive about herself indicates some improvement in self-esteem. Using this as a short-term goal will help the patient to overcome her feelings of worthlessness.

1. Taking sedatives will cause the patient to sleep and escape from her problems, which is no way to solve her feelings of worthlessness. Taking antidepressants will decrease her depression but will not improve her self-image.

2. A person with low self-esteem needs to work on improving her own feelings. She is not ready to interact with other patients.

3. This patient is not antisocial; she does not push others away. Her problem is low self-esteem.

56. ❸ Depressed patients often see the negative side of things. They find it hard to believe that a compliment given to them is really true. Therefore, it is most appropriate to use neutral comments such as, "Your hair is combed, and you are wearing a new dress."

1. Telling a depressed patient to keep up the good work would really depress them. A depressed patient does not feel like she has done any good work.

2. Telling a depressed patient that she is easier to work with because she combed her hair and put on a new dress is placing importance on the nursing staff. Nursing care must always be patient focused.

4. This complimentary statement will not be believed by a severely depressed person. Therefore, it will not serve any purpose other than to depress her.

57. ❷ The activities that should be provided for a severely depressed patient call for minimal concentration and involve the use of gross motor skills, not fine motor skills. Remember, this was an *except* question.

(1, 3, 4) These three nursing interventions are very appropriate when caring for a severely depressed client.

58. ❶ An important planned nursing intervention for a severely depressed patient is regularly planned, unobtrusive observation around the clock because a patient can kill himself or herself at any time.

2. Allowing a suicidal patient to remain alone, if that is his or her preference, would be very dangerous. The patient may prefer to be alone so he or she can kill himself or herself.

3. A suicidal patient could not possibly assume therapeutic work when he or she is in need of therapeutic help.

4. Encouraging the patient to sleep as much as possible would be to encourage the patient to escape from his or her problems. Sleep is one way that depressed patients try to escape from their problems.

59. ❹ A patient with bipolar disease admitted to the unit with gross hyperactivity will be administered Thorazine, which will bring the patient's hyperactivity under control rapidly. Lithium is not used to reduce hyperactivity.

(1, 2, 3) These options are incorrect as seen in rationale (4).

60. ❷ Evidence of genetic transmission is supported when a twin or relatives of patients with a particular disorder have an incidence of the disorder greater than the incidence in the general public.

(1, 3, 4) These options are incorrect as seen in rationale (2).

61. ❸ The most important initial nursing intervention for a hyperactive manic patient would be to work closely with the

patient and set limits on behavior as needed. A hyperactive manic patient has poor judgment and can injure self or accidentally injure others.

(1, 2, 4) These options are incorrect as seen in rationale (3).

62. ❶ Thorazine, Mellaril, and Haldol are antipsychotic drugs.

2. Elavil, Prozac, and Tofranil are tricyclic antidepressants.

3. Cogentin, Artane, and levodopa are antiparkinson agents.

4. Marplan, Nardil, and Parnate are monoamine oxidase inhibitors.

63. ❸ The most common functional psychosis is schizophrenia. Psychosis is a mental disorder of such magnitude that there is personality disintegration and loss of contact with reality. It usually is characterized by delusions and hallucinations, and hospitalization is generally required.

1. Paranoid condition can be cause by drugs or alcohol. There is also a paranoid schizophrenic disorder.

2. Bipolar disorder is a psychosis, but it is not the most common.

4. Maladaptive behavior occurs in many mental disorders and is not a psychosis.

64. ❹ Marplan, Nardil, and Parnate are (MAOI) monoamine oxidase inhibitors.

1. Thorazine, Mellaril, and Haldol are antipsychotic agents.

2. Elavil, Prozac, and Tofranil are tricyclic antidepressants.

3. Cogentin, Artane, and levodopa are antiparkinson agents.

65. ❷ Foods to be avoided during therapy with MAOIs include aged cheese, alcoholic beverages, caffeine, chocolate, raisins, sour cream, yogurt, bananas, avocados, chicken livers, and figs. These foods are high in tyramine, a precursor of norepinephrine. Normally, tyramine is deactivated in the gastrointestinal tract and liver, so large amounts do not reach the systemic circulation. When deactivation of tyramine is blocked by MAOIs, however, tyramine is absorbed systemically and transported to adrenergic nerve terminals, where it causes a sudden release of large amounts of norepinephrine. Hypertensive crisis can result. Several drugs can also interact with MAOIs to cause hypertensive crisis, for example, amphetamines, levodopa, and meperidine, and the antihistamines (including over-the-counter cough and cold remedies).

(1, 3, 4) These options are incorrect as seen in rationale (2).

66. ❹ As seen in question 65, rationale (2), levodopa, meperidine, and antihistamines can interact with MAOIs to cause hypertensive crisis.

(1, 2, 3) These options are incorrect as seen in answer 65, rationale (2).

67. ❶ Elavil, Tofranil, and Pamelor are tricyclic antidepressants.

2. Marplan, Nardil, and Parnate are MAOIs.

3. Lithium is an antimanic agent. Cogentin and Artane are cholinergic blockers used for treatment of symptoms of Parkinson's disease.

4. Haldol is a frequently used antipsychotic drug. Mellaril and Navane are antipsychotic/neuroleptic agents.

68. **④** A hyperactive manic patient can be dangerous to himself or herself and accidentally injure others. The nursing staff needs to meet and establish consistency of care and limit setting on the patient's behavior.

(1, 2, 3) Letting the patient know that the nursing staff will not tolerate his or her actions is a broad statement. The patient needs limits set on specific behavior, not on all of his or her behavior, and the staff must be consistent in setting these limits. It is not appropriate to threaten a patient with punishment. A hyperactive manic patient would not benefit from isolation. A hyperactive manic patient is constantly expressing feelings; therefore, he or she does not need any more time to express how he or she feels.

69. **③** The assault experienced by the client was sudden and arbitrary; she perceived it as life threatening; and her physical integrity was violated.

(1, 2) Memory of the event and the physical pain will cause her some psychological trauma because it is related to the violation of her physical integrity.

4. There are methods of preventing pregnancy if she is seen by the physician shortly after the rape occurred.

70. **②** The acute phase of the rape-trauma syndrome is confusion and disbelief, restless, and agitated motor activity.

(1, 3, 4) The long-term reorganization phase of rape-trauma syndrome include flashbacks, dreams, fears, and phobias.

71. **②** The patient's statement reflects use of the ego defense mechanism denial. This mechanism can be used unconsciously to protect the person from the emotionally overwhelming reality of the rape.

1. Attention-deficit disorder is a behavior disorder usually manifested before age 7 years that includes overactivity, chronic inattention, and difficulty dealing with multiple stimuli. It is not considered a temporary disorder.

3. Somatization can be defined as the expression of psychological stress through physical symptoms. Somatoform disorders have in common the presence of one or more physical complaints for which adequate physical explanation cannot be found.

4. Reaction formation (overcompensation) is the process of keeping unacceptable feelings or behaviors out of awareness by developing the opposite emotion or behavior.

72. **④** An appropriate intervention is to allow the patient time to talk at a comfortable pace. Assure her she is in a safe place and ask her questions in a nonjudgmental way.

◆ The nursing history includes the level of anxiety the victim is experiencing.

◆ Signs and symptoms of emotional trauma.

◆ Signs and symptoms of physical trauma.

1. The rape victim usually prefers to be with professionally trained personnel during her acute phase of rape-trauma syndrome.

2. During the acute phase of the rape-trauma syndrome, the patient is not comfortable with anyone touching her; she feels dirty and ashamed.

3. A patient in the acute phase of rape-trauma syndrome is confused, in shock, and afraid to be alone. A nurse should be with her at all times, but privacy should be provided.

73. **③** When taking a history from a patient in the acute phase of the rape-trauma syndrome, the nurse should determine what support system is available for her.

1. This is not the time to ask the patient if she will press charges against the man who raped her. The patient is in a state of shock and does not need any more problems to deal with at this time. It is the nurse's responsibility to save all evidence for the police.

2. All methods to prevent pregnancy should be provided for the rape victim. Contraceptive medication does not provide 100 percent protection.

4. The police will want to know if the patient knows the man who raped her, but this is not part of the nursing history.

74. **④** Allow the patient to verbalize negative expressions or feelings of self-blame. It will be through expressing her feelings that she will be able to deal with her psychological trauma.

1. It is important to allow the rape victim to make her own decisions so that she feels she has some control over her life. A rape victim feels that the man who raped her still controls her because he has made her feel so helpless.

2. Asking the patient many questions would only add to her trauma.

3. Reassuring the patient that her short dress and the way she acted had nothing to do with her being raped will make the patient feel even more guilty.

75. **④** Using a reflective communication technique is more helpful than discounting the victim's role. Self-blame serves to explain events that the victim otherwise finds incomprehensible.

(1, 2, 3) These options do not allow the patient to discuss her feelings.

76. **④** Agreeing to keep a follow-up appointment is a realistic short-term goal.

(1, 2, 3) These are not realistic short-term goals. Remember, the patient is still in the acute phase of the rape-trauma syndrome.

77. **①** The behavior that will indicate that the process of reorganization has occurred is feeling generally positive about self, sleeping and eating well, getting support from significant others, and being free of somatic reactions.

(2, 3, 4) These options reflect a continuation of the acute phase of rape-trauma syndrome.

78. **③** A family that is not supportive of a member of the family who has been raped may hold to the *myth* that nice girls do not get raped. Believing this myth allows the family to attribute blame to the victim.

(1, 2, 4) These statements are *facts* about rape and, if understood by the family, would prompt support.

79. **②** Explain that washing would destroy evidence. As uncomfortable as the client may be, she should not bathe until the physician's examination is completed. The collection of evidence is critical for the police investigation and may be used in court.

1. A patient may be given a basin of water to wash her hands and face. If given a basin of water with no instructions, she will take a total bath because she feels dirty all over.

3. Explaining to the client that every rape victim feels dirty is very degrading.

4. Taking a shower would destroy evidence, and although the raped victim does not want to be examined before she showers, it is for her benefit.

80. **③** The patient with a somatoform disorder will exaggerate or misinterpret physical symptoms.

(1, 2, 4) These options are incorrect as seen in rationale (4).

81. **①** The patient tells the nurse that she wishes her family and friends outside the hospital would pay more attention to her. The inference is that she is uninteresting and unpopular. The nurse's assessment is self-esteem disturbance.

(2, 3, 4) The scenario leads to a diagnosis of self-esteem disturbance as seen in rationale (1), whereas the other options do not.

82. **④** Hypochondriasis is the excessive preoccupation with one's physical health without the presence of any organic pathology.

1. Somatization is the expression of psychological stress through physical symptoms.

2. Psychosis is an extreme response to psychological or physical stressors that affect a person's affective psychomotor and physical behavior. Evidence of impairment in reality testing is manifested as hallucinations or delusions.

3. Projection is the unconscious attributing of one's own intolerable wishes, emotional feelings, or motivation to another person.

83. **①** Patients with somatoform conversion disorders go from physician to physician trying to establish a physical cause for their symptoms. When a psychological basis is suggested and a referral for counseling is offered, these patients reject both.

(2, 3, 4) These options are incorrect as seen in rationale (1).

84. **④** Focusing on the patient as a person rather than on his or her symptoms directs attention away from the symptoms. This approach eventually reduces the patient's need to gain attention by physical symptoms.

1. It is impossible for anyone to avoid all negative interactions, and psychiatric help is not necessary. However, psychological counseling would help.

2. Short-term goals would have to be implemented before long-term goals. The patient needs some psychological help before any goals can be established. The stem of the question did not say the patient was obese.

3. Verbalizing negative feelings about herself would increase her somatoform disorder. Verbalizing positive feelings about herself may increase her self-esteem.

85. **②** At the unconscious level, the somatoform disorder provides the patient with anxiety relief.

1. Somatoform disorder cannot be voluntarily controlled by the patient; however, with psychological therapy the patient can control the disorder and may be able to overcome it completely.

3. Somatoform disorder has no physiologic basis but does have a psychological basis.

4. There are no antipsychotic drugs that can control somatoform disorder; it is not a psychotic disorder.

86. **①** A nursing diagnosis for a somatoform disorder is impaired social interaction related to the unconscious need to focus on physical symptoms to feel more comfortable.

(2, 3, 4) These options are incorrect as seen in rationale (1).

87. **③** This option focuses on concern rather than the feelings the patient is expressing. This strategy prevents arguing about the reality of delusional beliefs and encourages the patient to express his feelings.

(1, 2, 4) These options are arguments that will increase the patient's anxiety and tenacity and encourage the patient to hold onto his delusion.

88. **②** Ideas of reference are misinterpretations of the verbalizations or actions of others that have special personal meanings (e.g., seeing a group of people talking, the individual assumes they are talking about him or her).

Schizophrenia is a severe disturbance of thought or association, characterized by impaired reality testing, hallucinations, delusions, and limited socialization.

(1, 3, 4) These options are incorrect as seen in rationale (2).

89. **②** Developmental theorist Harry Stack Sullivan suggests that a child raised with hostile inconsistent care, ridicule, or rejection will see the world as dangerous and frightening and act accordingly; this is one theory of the etiology of schizophrenia.

1. All children from a divorced family will always perceive the world as dangerous. Most children from divorced homes are happy and do not perceive the world as dangerous. When you see the word *all*, and always you should know that option probably is wrong.

3. Personal identity disturbance related to a traumatic event would be an appropriate diagnosis for a patient unable to recall his or her identify.

4. A child raised in a foster home may be very well adjusted; however, it would depend on the type of foster home. Some foster parents are very caring individuals, others are not.

90. **④** Common side effects of Thorazine are dry mouth, orthostatic hypotension, and shuffling gait.

(1, 2, 3) These options are incorrect as seen in rationale (4).

91. **②** If the patient knows what side effects to expect and that he or she can seek help from the physician if the side effects are severe, he or she usually will demonstrate more compliance. This gives the patient some feeling of control and will encourage him or her to take the medication.

1. A nurse should never advise a patient to reduce medication; this is the physician's responsibility.

3. A nurse should never tell a patient he or she will die if he or she does not take the medication; it is not a true statement.

4. Giving Thorazine IM does not decrease side effects of the medication.

92. ❸   Prolixin decanoate is a long-acting drug and can be given by injection every 1 to 4 weeks, thus reducing the daily opportunities for noncompliance. Prolixin decanoate and Thorazine are both antipsychotic-phenothiazine. Prolixin decanoate is a long-acting drug, and Thorazine is a short-acting drug.

1. Amitriptyline (Elavil) cannot be used to replace Thorazine because it is an antidepressant, not an antipsychotic agent.

2. Diazepam (Valium) is an anticonvulsant, sedative/hypnotic, and skeletal muscle relaxant.

4. Xanax is an antianxiety/sedative/hypnotic-benzodiazepine, and therefore, cannot be used to replace Thorazine.

93. ❷   Side effects of fluoxetine (Prozac) are insomnia, drowsiness, nervousness, convulsions, and sexual dysfunction.

(1, 3, 4) None of these are side effects of fluoxetine (Prozac).

94. ❶   Clues to hallucinations include rambling or talking aloud as though responding conversationally to someone, eyes looking around the room as though to find the speaker, and head tilting to one side as though listening intently.

(2, 3, 4) These options are incorrect as seen in rationale (1).

95. ❹   When giving a bath to a paranoid patient in the withdrawn phase of catatonic schizophrenia, the nurse should explain all physical care activities in simple, explicit terms, working with the patient as if he will respond.

(1, 2, 3) These options are incorrect as seen in rationale (4).

96. ❸   Solitary noncompetitive activities that require concentration are best for a patient having hallucinations. Solitary activity provides reality for the patient; it will help to decrease hallucinations.

(1, 2, 4) These options are incorrect as seen in rationale (3).

97. ❶   The most appropriate nursing diagnosis for a patient in the withdrawn phase of catatonic schizophrenia is self-care deficit. When patients are withdrawn, they will not properly care for themselves.

(2, 3, 4) These diagnoses are not as important as the self-care deficit diagnosis. It has a high priority because, if not acted on, the patient's life would be in danger.

98. ❹   Serve the client food in sealed containers and allow him access to lobby food machines. Patients perceive that foods that are in sealed containers and packages are safer.

1. Attempts to tube feed are seen as aggression and usually promote violence.

2. The patient needs psychological help; allowing the patient to leave the hospital can endanger his life.

3. It is against hospital policy to allow patients into the kitchen. A paranoid patient would still believe that the food was poisoned even if he was allowed in the kitchen.

99. ❸   To establish a relationship with a severely withdrawn schizophrenic patient, the nurse should sit facing the client for short periods, several times per day, accept silence, and state when the nurse will return. Short contacts are helpful to minimize the patient's and the nurse's anxiety. Accepting periods of silence helps establish a relationship.

1. Five minutes is not long enough to spend with a severely withdrawn patient. Giving directions and expecting a response will only upset the patient and the nurse.

2. One hour is too long to sit with a severely withdrawn patient, and he will not discuss how he feels.

4. A nurse should not place her or his hands on the patient's arm. The nurse should not expect a severely withdrawn patient to tell him or her when he or she should leave his room.

100. ❸   The nurse should indicate that he or she does not hear the voices the patient hears. Reality can be further emphasized by casting doubt on the patient's misinterpretation of reality by discrediting the voices, referring to them as "so-called voices."

(1, 2, 4) These options are incorrect as seen in rationale (3).

Chapter

22

Gerontology and Home Health Nursing

1. The age of 65 years has been chosen to signify the geriatric age group because of the number of psychosocial and physiologic changes that occur after this age.

2. Renal function: During the aging process, the ureters and bladder tend to lose muscle tone. The bladder may lose enough muscle tone to result in incomplete emptying, which increases the risk of urine retention and cystitis. The ability of the kidney to concentrate urine decreases, causing frequent urination and nocturia.

3. Fluid intake: Elderly people may choose to decrease fluid intake to alleviate urinary frequency and incontinence. The nurse should explain the hazards of dehydration and should encourage the elderly person to have at least 2000 mL of fluid intake per 24-h period, unless they have congestive heart failure (CHF) and must restrict fluids.

4. Sleep: The elderly generally tend to require less sleep than younger adults. The nurse should assist the elderly to relax and prepare for sleep and discourage naps during the day to assure more restful sleep patterns at night.

5. The nurse must treat the elderly as intelligent adults capable of comprehending events and making decisions about their own care. The elderly with pathologic conditions should be allowed to participate in their care to the degree that their mental and physical conditions will allow.

B. Physiologic Changes in Women

1. Decreased estrogen production during menopause can cause many physiologic changes in the female body. Changes in breast tissue result in less glandular tissue, reduced elasticity, and an increase in connective tissue and fat.

2. Relaxation of pelvic muscles in elderly women results in urinary incontinence. Teach patient Kegel exercises to strengthen the perineal muscle.

C. Physiologic Changes in Men

1. A decline in testosterone production occurs in the aging male but does not affect spermatogenesis.

2. Benign prostatic hypertrophy is common in elderly males, and symptoms of inability to initiate a stream of urine and frequent urination occur.

3. The prostate gland enlarges and compresses the urethra, causing urinary problems. Signs and symptoms depend on the extent of prostatic enlargement, the decrease in bladder capacity, and the decreased ability to concentrate urine. Because of all these conditions, the elderly male experiences frequency of urination.

4. Determination of prostate-specific antigen (PSA) level is the diagnostic test for prostate cancer.

II. ELDERLY PERSONS AND SAFETY CONSIDERATIONS

A. Vision Deficits

1. Vision loss in the elderly is common, and prevalence increases with age.

2. Cataracts, glaucoma, muscular degeneration, and diabetic retinopathy often cause visual problems in the elderly.

3. Loss of vision can result in injuries from falls or automobile crashes and can result in the patient taking the wrong dosage or the wrong medication. This significantly affects quality of life for elderly people.

4. To determine the amount of visual impairment, the nurse should question the patient regarding limitations to normal activities of daily living associated with poor vision. ("Does your vision make it difficult for you to feed yourself, read medication labels, handle money, or find your way around your home or outside your home?")

5. Determine whether the patient is using visual assistance devices, such as glasses, contact lenses, or magnifying lenses.

6. After complete assessment, the nurse should refer the patient with significant evidence of decreased visual acuity to an eye care specialist.

B. Degenerative Joint Disease

1. During the aging process, alterations in status and posture occur, especially among women.

2. The older adult faces many changes; loss of agility, flexibility, and mobility are common changes.

3. Degenerative joint diseases are particularly debilitating for the older adult.

4. Painful or immobile joints interfere with self-care activities and the ability to maintain locomotion, thus causing the elderly to lose an independent lifestyle.

5. Pain management of the many musculoskeletal disorders is a primary problem in the elderly.

6. Nursing interventions for the older adult with musculoskeletal disorders are focused on maintenance of mobility, safety, and independence.

7. Continuous activity promotes greater functioning in the geriatric client.

8. Exercise programs (e.g., swimming, walking) are beneficial to maintain or increase flexibility and strength.

9. Safety becomes a major problem for the elderly with musculoskeletal disorders because of the loss of agility, flexibility, and mobility.

10. Many elderly hospitalized patients receive treatment for injuries caused by their inability to properly maneuver an ambulatory aid (e.g., walker, crutches), resulting in a fall causing injuries.

11. Instruct the family and patient to provide a safe environment to reduce injury from falls by

    a. Removing small rugs

    b. Using night lights

    c. Using hand rails

    d. Using a cane or walker

    e. Properly using crutches

    f. Wearing sturdy shoes (without slippery soles)

    g. Wearing properly fitting shoes

    h. Clearing all pathways

    i. Wearing glasses if needed

    j. Instructing the patient on techniques to improve gait/ambulation, balance, and endurance

    k. Instructing the patient to avoid prolonged activities of walking, standing, and sitting, as well as sudden movements

    l. Avoiding slippery tub or shower; use nonskid mats

    m. Providing grab rails for tub, shower, and toilet

    n. Avoiding wet and slippery floors

    o. Removing furniture that is too low or too soft, that tips easily, or is on wheels

    p. Avoiding clutter in living area

    q. Selecting furniture that provides stability and support, such as chairs with arms

    r. Instructing the elderly to watch for pets underfoot and scattered pet food

12. Falls are the leading cause of death from injury for people age 65 years and older and are particularly common among those over age 85 years.

    a. Falls and fall-related injuries are of special concern in older adults because of the severity of injuries combined with long recovery periods and the threat of long-term health problems.

    b. In addition to the immediate pain and disability caused by the injury, falls are associated with loss of confidence in ability to function independently, restriction of physical and social activities, increased dependence, and increased need for long-term care.

C. Medications

1. Another threat to the safety of older adults is the use and misuse of medications. At least 10 to 40 percent of geriatric hospital admissions are associated with inappropriate drug administration.

2. Factors that contribute to medication noncompliance, misuse, and overuse are the following:

    a. Impaired vision and/or impaired hearing

    b. Complex drug regimen called *polypharmacy* (polypharmacy refers to physicians prescribing multiple drugs for a client), which is a fairly common practice that affects the elderly

    c. Physiologic changes associated with aging (e.g., decreased absorption, metabolism, and excretion of drugs)

    d. Problems with self-administration, such as failure to take the medications prescribed due to the inability to open drug containers, forgetfulness, and vision problems

    e. Failure to discard outdated or discontinued medication

    f. Lack of financial resources to purchase necessary medication (medication not covered by Medicare)

    g. Desire to avoid unpleasant side effects

    h. Sharing of prescription medication with spouse or others

i. Fear of drug dependency

j. Lack of knowledge or information about the reason for taking the medication and the prescribed regimen

k. Stopping medications when symptoms subside

l. Multiple prescriptions or related medications for the same condition from different providers

m. Complexity of drug regimens and number of drugs prescribed

n. Failure to report or to stop using self-medication with over-the-counter drugs

o. Interactions between different medications

p. Difficulty swallowing

q. Mistrust of health professionals

3. To help avoid problems associated with the elderly patient's self-administration of medication

a. Use a medication box that can be filled weekly and distribute the medication based on the day (e.g., Monday through Sunday) and time of day (morning, noon, evening before bed time).

b. Evaluate potential medication interactions whenever a new medication is prescribed and keep the physician informed.

c. Instruct the patient about possible side effects and symptoms of toxicity and explain what to do if they occur.

d. Encourage the patient to bring all medications when seeing a physician.

e. Help the patient make and maintain a list of all prescription and over-the-counter medications, including dosage, frequencies, purpose, and side effects.

f. Simplify the medication regimen as much as possible by working with the physician and pharmacist.

g. Ask the pharmacist to use large type print on labels.

h. Involve a caregiver with all details of the patient's medication regimen.

i. Allow the patient input into scheduling and other details of the medication regimen.

j. Assess the patient for memory loss, difficulty swallowing, noncompliance behavior, financial resources, and caregiver's ability to assist the patient with the medication regimen.

D. Geriatric Patient's Response to Medications

1. Because of more body fat, the effects and side effects of medications persist longer in the elderly patient, even after the medication is discontinued.

2. Because of less plasma albumin, less medication is protein bound and more medication is free to circulate in the elderly body.

3. Less medication is needed to achieve a given blood level because the elderly patient has less total body water.

4. The elderly patient has a slower liver metabolism and slower renal clearance; therefore, medications remain in the body longer.

5. The elderly patient generally has fewer brain cells, so less medication is needed to produce the desired effect when treating pathologic disorders of the brain.

E. Intravenous Administration of Medications

1. In addition to observing the effects of IV medication on the elderly, the nurse needs to be alert to the amount of fluid in which the drug is administered.

2. Information about intake and output, body weight, and specific gravity is useful for monitoring signs of fluid overload.

3. Declining cardiac and renal function make the elderly more susceptible to dehydration and to overhydration.

4. Signs of circulatory overload must be closely monitored, including elevated blood pressure, increased heart rate, coughing, shortness of breath, and other symptoms of pulmonary edema.

5. Close monitoring for IV infiltration and thrombophlebitis is necessary because of decreased sensation and fragile vessels and skin.

F. Administration of Oral Medications

1. The elderly sometimes have difficulty swallowing, so it is very important that they be given ample fluids, placed in a high-Fowler's position (if not contraindicated), and allowed ample time to swallow medications.

2. After each pill is administered and the patient has swallowed, the oral cavity should be examined to be sure that the patient was able to swallow the medication (some elderly patients may be unaware that the tablet is stuck to the roof of their dentures or under their tongue).

3. Enteric-coated and sustained-release tablets should not be crushed; therefore, the nurse should consult with the physician for an alternative form of the drug, if necessary.

4. Generally, capsules are not to be broken open or mixed with food or liquids. Medications are manufactured in capsule form so that the unpleasant taste is covered by the capsule.

5. If the effect of the medication is not changed, however, some medications can be combined with food and drink (e.g., juice or applesauce), which can make medications more palatable and prevent gastric irritation. Because this can be a problem if the full amount of food is not ingested, the patient should be informed when they are ingesting food or drink containing medication.

6. The nurse should provide proper oral hygiene after the administration of oral drugs. It is very important to prevent unpleasant aftertaste and reduce stomatitis and tooth decay.

III. MEDICATIONS FREQUENTLY ADMINISTERED TO THE ELDERLY

A. Antipsychotic Agents

1. Antipsychotic drugs are used to treat schizophrenia, bipolar disorder (manic episodes), major depressive episodes with psychotic features, delirium, and other organic mental disorders that cause delusions, hallucinations, or severe agitation.

2. Patients with dementia are prescribed antipsychotics to control aggression, distressing repetitive behavior, delusions, hallucinations, and other forms of agitation.

3. An acute illness can intensify preexisting psychotic symptoms (hallucination, delusions, bizarre behavior). Therefore, it is imperative that when antipsychotic drug therapy is being considered in an elderly person, the patient should first have a physical examination including laboratory studies to screen for possible physical illness.

4. Medications used for the treatment of psychiatric disorders can offer significant improvement to the client, but these medications also can have profound adverse effects in the older adult. Some of the adverse effects of these medications can lead to anorexia, constipation, incontinence, anemia, lethargy, sleep disturbance, confusion, and falling.

5. The lowest possible dosage should be used in the elderly patient and reactions observed closely.

B. Diuretics

1. The elderly are at greater risk for developing fluid and electrolyte imbalances, and the use of diuretics increases this risk considerably.

2. The nurse should be alert to dryness of the oral cavity, thirst, confusion, hypotension, and oliguria.

C. Sedative-Hypnotics and Barbiturates

1. Sedative-hypnotics are often prescribed to the elderly for the treatment of insomnia, nocturnal restlessness, acute confusion, and anxiety.

    a. It is not unusual for restlessness, insomnia, and nightmares to occur after sedatives are discontinued.

2. Side effects of these drugs are hypotension, drowsiness, and impaired coordination, which can lead to injury.

3. Barbiturates (e.g., Nembutal and Seconal) are *not recommended* for use in the elderly because these drugs are stored in adipose tissue, and the increased proportion of adipose tissue in the older adult's body can cause these drugs to accumulate and reach toxic levels.

4. The following nonbarbiturates are used for short-term treatment of insomnia: zaleplon (Sonata), quazepam (Doral), chloral hydrate (Chloral Hydrate (CAN)), and zolpidem (Ambien).

D. Laxatives

1. Reduced peristaltic activity, reduced fiber and fluid in the diet, and less activity are causes of constipation in the elderly.

2. Many elderly patients believe that they must have a daily bowel movement, which causes them to abuse laxatives. Laxatives are habit forming and compound the problem.

3. If elderly patients have difficulty with constipation, the nurse should encourage an increase in fiber and fluid in their diet and an increase in exercise.

4. If the patient feels the need to use a laxative, the nurse should recommend a bulk form of laxative, such as Metamucil, which absorbs fluid in the intestine and creates extra bulk, distending the intestine and increasing peristaltic activity.

IV. CHARACTERISTICS OF HOME HEALTH CARE FOR THE GERIATRIC PATIENT

A. Health Promotion and Illness Prevention

1. The movement from an illness-oriented "cure" perspective in acute care, hospital-based health settings to a focus on health promotion and primary health care in community-based settings, combined with changes in medical technology, cost consciousness, and an aging population, all have dramatically changed health care today.

2. Many nurses prefer the emphasis on health promotion and illness prevention that is a major focus of primary health care.

3. The registered nurse (RN) in a home health care setting gets to know patients and their families by seeing them in their own homes.

4. The RN's role involves the direct delivery of care: performing skills for which they were trained and that typically are associated with nursing practice (e.g., client assessment, taking vital signs, changing dressings, administering IV fluids, administering medications, inserting catheters), and using the same skills used in acute care settings, where patients typically are hospitalized for surgery or for treatment of serious medical conditions.

5. A major difference exists in the time spent in direct care of the patient.

    a. An ICU nurse spends 70 to 80 percent of his or her time in direct care provision.

    b. A nurse working on a general medical surgical unit spends approximately 50 to 60 percent of his or her time in direct care provision.

    c. A postpartum nurse spends approximately 40 to 50 percent of his or her time in direct care provision.

    d. A nurse in a psychiatric unit spends approximately 20 to 30 percent of his or her time in direct care provision.

    e. A nurse in home health can spend 30 to 40 percent of his or her time in direct care provision.

6. Although direct care provision is an important part of home health care nursing practice, this task tends to occupy less time than in acute care settings. As a result, many nursing students and some RNs who have very little knowledge about community-based practice often discount the nurse's importance in these health care settings. Another contributing factor is that the home health care nurse is not seen as the glamorous or heroic nurse working in the hospital as portrayed on television.

B. Collaborative Management

1. Home health nursing practice standard IX requires the RN to initiate and maintain an ongoing relationship with all health care providers working with the patient.

2. In health care, collaboration implies joint decision making regarding the plan of care with all professionals involved with the patient's care.

3. As the case manager, the RN must share the plan of care with all involved in the care and make recommendations and modifications based on their input.

4. Case conferences should be held regularly, particularly for patients with complicated or prolonged care, to share information among the providers and discuss the patient's response to the treatment plan.

5. The nurse must work with the physician to receive and outline the plan of care. Also, as the case manager, the RN coordinates the professionals who are involved in home health care. They include the following:

   a. *Nurses* have been the traditional providers of health care in the home. RNs provide skilled nursing services, coordinate care and use referral agents, and act as patient advocates.

   b. *Physical therapists* are used in most home care agencies. They assess the patient's needs for assistive devices that will support rehabilitation and safety and administer therapy procedures to meet patient's needs. They work on gross motor skills and rehabilitation.

   c. *Occupational therapists* assist the patient in restoring fine motor coordination, improving physical task-related to activities of daily living, and reaching the highest level of functioning possible.

   d. *Speech therapists* work with patients who have communication problems related to speech, language, hearing, as well as swallowing difficulties, to treat, manage, or alleviate these problems. Speech therapists also work with patients who have undergone a laryngectomy. They help them develop laryngeal, esophageal, or pharyngeal speech without the use of an artificial larynx. They teach the patient to swallow air and then gradually push the air back out to form words. If the patient is not successful with developing speech, an electronic larynx can be used.

   e. *Social workers* assist patients with social, emotional, and financial needs and refer clients to available community resources.

   f. *Registered dietitians* provide direct counseling and teaching for patients with special dietary needs and problems.

   g. *Home health aides* and *licensed practical nurses* (LPN) are paraprofessionals who assist in the home with a patient's personal care and basic nursing (e.g., bathing patient, taking vital signs, making the bed, assisting with self-administered medication, and light housekeeping). For Medicare reimbursement, home health aides must be supervised by an RN. The LPN can administer and perform other duties (e.g., wound care).

   h. *Other providers* may include laboratory technicians, eye specialists, chaplains, enterostomal therapists, pharmacists, and respiratory therapists.

6. Collaboration is an interdisciplinary approach wherein several health care professionals are responsible for various facets of care.

   a. Individuals from various professions work with the patient and the family or the caregivers to jointly determine the course of care.

   b. Through interaction, discussion, and coordination, goals are set and a plan of care is formed to meet the needs of the patient.

C. Skills the RN Needs for Home Health Practice

1. Skills needed for home health practice include:

   a. Managerial skills.

   b. Self-direction skills and the ability to work autonomously in a nonstructured atmosphere.

   c. Strong clinical skills, ability to function independently, and flexibility.

   d. A personality that is open and sincerely accepting of people's unique lifestyle and the associated effects that these lifestyles have on health.

   e. Ability to pay attention to incredible detail.

   f. Understanding that change can be very difficult and sometimes impossible.

   g. Excellent communication skills.

   h. Enjoys working with peers (a team player).

D. Advance Directive for Treatment

1. Laws have been passed by various legislative bodies to ensure patients' rights to direct their treatment.

2. The federal Patient Self-Determination Act requires that health care provider agencies receiving Medicare payments must inform all patients 18 years or older of their right to plan in advance for their care.

3. Failure to comply with the law can result in loss of Medicare payments.

4. Patients can indicate the life-sustaining treatments they do and do not want or designate an individual to make decisions on their behalf if they become unable to make their wishes known.

5. There two types of advance medical directives: a *living will* and a *durable power of attorney*.

   a. The *living will* records a patient's decision to decline life-prolonging treatment if he or she becomes terminally ill.

   b. The *durable power of attorney* names someone who will make health care decisions if the patient becomes unable to make them.

   c. Instructions in the advance directive should be very specific to ensure compliance with the patient's wishes (e.g., "If I become terminally ill, with no hope of recovery, I do not want to receive chemotherapy, nutrition, hydration, artificial respiration, or cardiopulmonary resuscitation.")

6. In addition to the federal Patient Self-Determination Act, many states have enacted laws regulating do-not-resuscitate (DNR) orders.

7. A *DNR order* means that no attempt will be made to revive heart or lung function if these activities stop.

8. Although the specifics of the laws vary from state to state, in general, a DNR request must be made by the patient or the family.

9. A DNR decision can be revoked at any time by the requesting party.

10. Home health nurses must be aware of requirements for informed decision making in health care and be able to assess the patient's desires with regard to advanced medical directives in compliance with the Home Care Bill of Rights.

EXAMINATION

1. The vital sign that the nurse should expect to be normal in a geriatric patient is
 1. An increase in breathing capacity.
 2. A lower body temperature.
 3. A decrease in peripheral resistance, causing a lower blood pressure.
 4. An increase in pulse rate causing an increase in stroke volume.

2. A female geriatric patient asks the nurse why she is bothered more with constipation now that she is older. The nurse's most helpful response is
 1. The stomach takes a longer time to empty, and your feeling of hunger is reduced, causing a reduction in appetite.
 2. Peristalsis is slower in your intestinal tract, and this causes constipation.
 3. Constipation can be the result of your poor appetite and all the medications you are taking.
 4. Inactivity, less fiber and fluid in your diet, and laxative abuse can contribute to your problem.

3. A patient age 82 years tells the nurse that he finds that he tires easily, but when he goes to bed, he only sleeps 5 to 6 h. Which response by the nurse would be most helpful in planning for rest and sleep?
 1. Evaluate your activity schedule, maybe your activities are too strenuous.
 2. More rest is required as you get older; therefore, your sleeping time should be increased.
 3. You may sleep less soundly because of muscle tension, tremors, environmental noises, or bladder distention.
 4. Satisfying, regular activities promote relaxation. You may need more rest during the day, but as you grow older you need less sleep.

4. A 65-year-old female patient, weighing 190 lb, tells the nurse that she frequently has joint pain and asks the nurse if she should increase her aspirin intake. The best response by the nurse is
 1. Complete bed rest and moist heat will relieve the joint pain.
 2. Heat will give relief, so take a warm tub bath and use a heating blanket when you sleep.
 3. A balanced diet that is rich in protein and minerals, weight reduction, and activity will promote optimal function with less pain.
 4. Aspirin is effective against pain; the more you take, the less pain you will have in your joints.

5. A patient has a slight hearing deficit, presbycusis, which results from changes in the ear due to the aging process. The nursing approach that would be the most appropriate when speaking with this patient is
 1. Talking slowly and distinctly in a low tone of voice.
 2. Writing out all important comments.
 3. Raising the voice and accentuating each word.
 4. Using sign language and gestures.

6. A female retired teacher tells the nurse that her skin is very dry, and she asks if taking a daily bath is too much. The best response by the nurse is
 1. Continue taking a daily bath, but avoid drying agents such as harsh soap. Follow the bath with an application of oil.
 2. Wash hands, face, under arms, and perineum area daily, and a bath every third or fourth day will provide cleanliness without drying the skin.
 3. Good skin condition depends on the hydration activity, oils, and good nutrition.
 4. Daily oil baths, use soft sheets, and give special attention to any skin breakdown.

7. The first time a home health nurse visits a 72-year-old woman, she complains of sudden loss of energy and appetite, is extremely nervous, and suffers from insomnia. The data that would seen to be the most significant cause of these symptoms is that the woman
 1. Has just sold her home.
 2. Has very little medical insurance.
 3. Is overweight and smokes a pack of cigarettes per day.
 4. Has been a widow for 5 years and lives alone.

8. An 81-year-old woman tells a home health nurse that she is unable to concentrate and states, "I am afraid I will lose all control." The best response by the nurse that will help her to define her fears is
 1. Do you think you will hurt yourself when you lose control?
 2. Are you afraid that you will become dependent on others?
 3. What is it that you fear you will lose control of?
 4. This must be difficult for you, but I am here to protect you.

9. The nurse is working with an 80-year-old woman in her home. The patient demonstrates a very high level of anxiety and asks the nurse for some medication to help her. The plan that will best help the patient is to
   1. Ask the physician to order the client 20 mg of Valium tid PO to reduce her anxiety.
   2. Communicate with her based on her level of anxiety.
   3. Give her instructions on techniques to reduce anxiety.
   4. Ask the physician to order the patient a medication to reduce her anxiety.

10. The nurse visits an immobile 82-year-old woman in her home. While doing a physical assessment, she discovers many bruises on the patient's body. The daughter tells the nurse that although her mother is a lot of work, she never feels any anger toward her mother. The nurse recognizes that this statement is a defensive mechanism of denial, which is
    1. Keeping unacceptable experiences in her conscious mind.
    2. Developing the opposite attitude to the way she feels.
    3. Giving a logical reason for something she did not want to happen.
    4. Rejecting something that is very disturbing to her.

11. An elderly, immobile female client has a quarter-sized reddened area on the coccyx. It is nonblanchable and was not present the day before. The most appropriate treatment is
    1. Place an egg crate mattress on the bed.
    2. Use OpSite to cover the area.
    3. Position the patient off her back until the area is no longer red and turn her every 2 h.
    4. Massage the area every 2 h.

12. The physician has ordered an occlusive dressing over a stage II decubitus ulcer. The most appropriate choice is
    1. Fine-meshed gauze covered with Telfa.
    2. DuoDERM, a hydrocolloid dressing.
    3. Antiseptic plastic spray.
    4. Karaya powder.

13. An elderly patient is sent home from the hospital following surgery to put a flap of skin over a decubitus. The home health nurse knows that the Jackson-Pratt drain in the wound is for the purpose of
    1. Observing the wound for bleeding or infected drainage.
    2. Providing an exit for infected drainage.
    3. Preventing fluid from forming a pocket and preventing grafting of the skin graft.
    4. Allowing the wound to heal from the outside in.

14. You visit an 83-year-old female client in her home to change an ischemic ulcer dressing on her ankle. The most appropriate treatment is

1. Wash wound with hydrogen peroxide and apply a cotton-filled pad.
2. Apply enzymatic debriding agent such as self-adhesive film (OpSite).
3. Irrigate wound with normal saline using a bulb syringe and leave wound uncovered.
4. Irrigate wound with normal saline and apply fine-meshed gauze covered with Telfa.

15. You are changing a dressing on an abdominal surgical wound of a 75-year-old obese male client. You notice that the edges are separating in a third of the wound and it is draining. Your best action will be to
    1. Observe for hemorrhage by pressing on the edges of the wound wearing sterile gloves. Force out as much drainage as possible and redress wound.
    2. Use sterile gloves and clean the wound with normal saline and hydrogen peroxide, dry the skin, and apply Band-Aid sutures to hold the wound together.
    3. Observe the wound for hemorrhage by pressing on edges of the wound wearing sterile gloves.
    4. Redress the wound, have patient remain in bed, and notify the physician to come to inspect the wound.

16. You are getting a 70-year-old patient out of bed when her abdominal dressing falls off because of wound dehiscence and evisceration has occurred. Your best action will be
    1. Redress the wound and notify the physician immediately.
    2. Add extra dressings to the wound to absorb the drainage and have the patient rest in bed until the physician arrives.
    3. Cover the wound with a sterile saline-soaked dressing, put the client in a low semi-Fowler's position, and notify the surgeon immediately.
    4. Using a sterile glove, gently push viscera back into the abdomen and notify the surgeon immediately.

17. A 75-year-old female is being cared for in her home after recovering from a fractured hip. The most helpful teaching the home health nurse can give this patient is that
    1. Postmenopausal women who take estrogen need to take more calcium than women not taking estrogen.
    2. Everyone over the age of 70 years who is taking calcium needs to have their blood tested for a calcium level once per month.
    3. The recommended amount of calcium intake for postmenopausal women not taking estrogen is 800 mg/day.
    4. To have her physician order calcium supplement, reduce her alcohol intake, avoid smoking, and eat foods high in calcium.

18. An 82-year-old man is being cared for in his home after a radical neck resection to remove a malignant tumor. The

physician has ordered blood from the patient be sent to the laboratory. The nurse knows that the mineral the physician is concerned about is

1. Calcium.
2. Iron.
3. Sodium.
4. Magnesium.

19. An 88-year-old man is diagnosed with an elevated serum calcium level due to prolonged immobilization. The home health nurse knows that the medications the physician will order to lower the serum calcium level are

1. Doxycycline calcium (Vibramycin Calcium syrup), polycarbophil (Mitrolan), and tolmetin sodium (Tolectin).
2. Prednisone, furosemide (Lasix), and salmon calcitonin (Calcimar).
3. Aztreonam (Azactam) and amcinonide (Cyclocort).
4. Methimazole (Tapazole), Levothyroxine (Synthroid), and strong iodine solution (Lugol's solution).

20. When receiving feedback from an elderly female patient about her understanding of her calcium supplement regimen, the statement that would lead you to believe that she understands the teaching you have done is

1. I will take the medication with meals.
2. I will limit the intake of foods high in calcium.
3. I will take the calcium with milk of magnesia to prevent constipation.
4. I will contact my physician if I feel tingling in my fingers or begin to urinate excessively.

21. The most common reason why the elderly sustain hip fractures is

1. Decreased calcium intake.
2. Decreased muscle strength.
3. Osteoporosis.
4. Decreased production of bone marrow.

22. Buck's traction is applied to an elderly woman's fractured leg. The nurse knows that an *inappropriate* reason for using Buck's traction is to

1. Immobilize the leg until the leg is healed.
2. Prevent further soft-tissue damage.
3. Reduce the fracture.
4. Reduce muscle spasm and pain.

23. Buck's traction is contraindicated if an elderly patient experienced the following

1. Bilateral lower leg ulcers.
2. Osteoarthritis.
3. Deformity of the affected leg.
4. Pelvic pain.

24. Following physician's orders for intermittent Buck's traction for an elderly patient, the correct nursing plan of care is to

1. Turn the patient on her unaffected side to give back rub and skin care.
2. Remove the traction every shift to observe for pressure areas and provide skin care.
3. Elevate the head of the bed to apply countertraction, observe for pressure areas, and provide skin care.
4. Raise the knee hatch to prevent the patient from sliding down in bed, observe for pressure areas, and provide skin care.

25. You are caring for an 83-year-old woman in her home. The daughter tells you that her mother fell on the bathroom floor and was returned to bed because she complained of severe pain in her right hip. To assess the fracture, you would

1. Observe for bruising over the right hip.
2. Move the right leg gently to see if the movement causes pain.
3. Observe for shortening of the affected leg.
4. Call the physician immediately.

26. A 92-year-old man is recuperating after a serious car accident that caused multiple bone fractures. The home health nurse's assessment that would require immediate nursing intervention would be

1. A rectal temperature of 100°F.
2. Feeling of fatigue and weakness.
3. An inability to cough productively 5 days after the accident.
4. Dyspnea and complaints of sharp chest pains.

27. The daughter of a 78-year-old woman tells the home health nurse who has cared for her mother for several months, "I am worried about my mother. She complains about her health more and more. I think she may be developing a serious disease." The *most* correct response by the nurse is

1. I have worked with your mother for 3 months, and she is just a complainer.
2. I will spend more time assessing your mother today. I may have overlooked some major problem.
3. The elderly sometimes will use physical complaints as an attention-getting mechanism. Try not to respond to her physical complaints and give her more attention when she is not complaining.
4. The elderly have many physical problems, so it is not unusual for them to complain a lot. I will leave you medication to give her when she complains to reduce her pain and anxiety.

28. A 70-year-old patient asks the home health nurse, "Will I become senile if I live to be 90 years old or older?" The *most* correct response by the nurse is

1. Some degree of cognitive impairment is common among the elderly and often increases with age. Some elderly people have little or no cognitive impairment,

and you may be one of the lucky ones. Genetics seem to be a contributing factor.

2. Many elderly patients develop Alzheimer's disease and dementia. The only thing you can do is to be prepared for that time in your life so that you will not be alone with no one to care for you. Try not to become engaged in a lot of social activities because this leads to alcohol abuse.

3. You are 70 years old and you are not senile, so you have nothing to worry about. If you were going to develop senility, you would have developed it by now. Stay active and that will help to prevent senility.

4. Alzheimer's disease develops at a relatively young age, so you have escaped that disease and senility does not develop until 70 years of age or older.

29. A 75-year-old man diagnosed with colon cancer asks the home health nurse if Medicare insurance will cover expenses if he has to go into a nursing home. The correct response by the nurse is

1. Medicare insurance will cover your medical expenses for as long as you live at home or in a nursing home.

2. Neither Medicare nor your private health insurance will cover long-term care at home or in the nursing home.

3. If you had bought a medical care supplement insurance or specific insurance that covers long-term care, you would have nothing to worry about because all of your bills would be paid for you.

4. Your private insurance company will cover the expenses that Medicare insurance will not cover.

30. The home health nurse is assessing an 83-year-old man. He complains of coughing up copious yellow sputum every morning and of having a fever for the past 2 days. The nurse should instruct the patient how to

1. Collect a sterile sputum before breakfast the next day so the nurse can send it to the laboratory.

2. Take a rectal temperature three times during the day and give that information to the nurse the next day.

3. Measure his intake and output and to keep a record for the visiting nurse.

4. Call and give the physician detailed information about his complaints.

31. A public health nurse presenting a program on breast self-examination realizes that certain aspects of the teaching would have to be reviewed when the nurse observed that several clients are

1. Observing their breast for symmetry while holding their arms above their heads.

2. Checking their nipples for alterations in size and shape.

3. Palpating their breast while in a sitting position.

4. Palpating their breast with the palmar surface of their extended fingers.

32. A 69-year-old woman recovering from a modified radical mastectomy asks the home health nurse how she can protect her daughter from breast cancer. The nurse tells the patient to have her daughter perform a breast examination

1. Several days before an expected menstrual period.

2. Two to three days after the completion of each menstrual period.

3. The same date every month, regardless of when menstruation occurs.

4. Halfway between menstrual periods, preferably after taking a shower.

33. An 82-year-old man is receiving phenytoin (Dilantin) therapy to control seizures and iron for anemia. The daughter told the home health nurse that her father had a seizure while sitting in a chair and fell on the floor an hour before the nurse arrived. The urine in the client's Foley bag is a pink color. The nurse should

1. Notify the physician immediately about the seizure and blood in urine.

2. Take the patient's vital signs and tell the daughter to encourage fluid intake to remove the blood from the kidneys and call the physician.

3. Take the patient's vital signs, and ask the client if he hurt himself when he fell and if he took his Dilantin as ordered.

4. If the client complains of lower back pain and blood pressure is elevated, call the physician.

34. A 90-year-old woman in end-stage renal failure has a red blood cell (RBC) count of 3.5 mL. The home health nurse anticipated that the physician will order

1. Enterogastrone.

2. Epogen.

3. Several blood transfusions.

4. Prolactin.

35. A 90-year-old male patient developed diabetes insipidus after a serious head injury. The patient says to the nurse, "My physician tells me that my body is not producing enough antidiuretic hormone. What medication is she giving me for that?" The correct response by the nurse is, "She is giving you

1. Pitressin, a synthetic antidiuretic hormone (ADH) that helps control blood volume by promoting water reabsorption in the renal tubules."

2. Insulin. It carries sugar into the cells to produce energy. If the cells cannot get sugar, the body will burn fat and you will develop ketoacidosis."

3. Synthroid to increase your metabolism. This will help to replace the antidiuretic you are missing."

4. Lasix. It will replace the antidiuretic hormone that you are missing."

36. You are a home health nurse caring for a 76-year-old woman diagnosed with chronic obstructive pulmonary disease (COPD). You know that the oxygen mask of choice for a COPD patient is a

1. Tracheostomy collar.

2. Simple mask.

3. Nonrebreathing mask.

4. Venturi mask.

37. A 62-year-old male client diagnosed with COPD is receiving intravenous aminophylline. One of the most common side effects for which the nurse should observe is

1. Bradycardia.

2. Hypotension.

3. Hypoventilation.

4. Oliguria.

38. In helping an elderly female client deal with the vicious cycle of her fear caused by dyspnea, the nurse should place primary emphasis in the teaching program on

1. Teaching about priorities in carrying out daily activities.

2. Education about the disease and breathing exercises.

3. Judicious use of aerosol therapy, especially nebulizers.

4. Learning how to prevent respiratory infections.

39. A 60-year-old male client diagnosed with cancer of the neck is scheduled for radical neck resection. During the preoperative period, the most important aspect of his care is

1. Maintain a cheerful and optimistic environment.

2. Keeping visitors to a minimum so that he can have time to think about his future living without cancer.

3. Assure the patient that his cancer is under control.

4. Assess patient's understanding of the procedure and expectation of bodily appearance after surgery.

40. An 80-year-old patient diagnosed with cancer is scheduled for chemotherapy at 2:00 PM. The nurse knows antiemetics will be administered

1. When chemotherapy is half-way through, at 3:00 PM, and again at 6:00 PM.

2. When chemotherapy is finished at 4:00 PM.

3. Before chemotherapy is started, at 1:30 PM, and during and after administration if needed.

4. After chemotherapy is started at 2:30 PM and again the next day if needed.

41. A 60-year-old man is diagnosed with pernicious anemia. The physician orders 0.2 mg of vitamin B_{12} IM. The home health nurse prepares to give

1. Folic acid.

2. Ascorbic acid.

3. Cholecalciferol.

4. Cyanocobalamin.

42. A 75-year-old male client is recovering after surgery for colon cancer. The home health nurse asks the patient if he would like to start changing the dressing on his colostomy. He says to the nurse, "You want me to change it because you can't stand to look at it." The nurse recognizes that the client is using the defense mechanism known as

1. Projection.

2. Reaction formation.

3. Displacement.

4. Intellectualization.

43. A 66-year-old man with a long history of alcohol abuse is receiving home health care for various medical and psychological problems. To give the patient greater responsibility for self-control, the nurse should initially plan to

1. Confront him with his alcohol abuse.

2. Discuss with him the different detoxification programs.

3. Assist him to identify and adopt more healthful coping patterns.

4. Administer antianxiety medication as needed.

44. A 62-year-old woman with a long history of alcohol abuse has diabetes mellitus. She has been in a detoxification program for 3 months. She tells the nurse that she feels better and that she now really realizes how much her alcohol abuse has affected her diabetes. The patient believes no further treatment for alcohol abuse is necessary. The nurse recognizes that

1. The patient has accepted her illness and now just needs to resist the alcohol.

2. The patient realizes how much alcohol is affecting her diabetes so she probably will not use alcohol again.

3. Her physician should be notified of her statement so that an aversion therapy can be started before she starts drinking alcohol again.

4. The patient lacks insight about the emotional aspect of her illness and she needs continued therapy.

QUESTIONS 45 TO 49

45. The home health nurse is caring for Mary Scott, an 85-year-old woman diagnosed as being in the early stage of dementia due to organic brain disease. This morning, Mary is very anxious because she is going to join a group of geriatric patients in recreational therapy. It would be most helpful for the nurse to

1. Remind Mary to dress quickly to avoid delaying the others.

2. Help Mary dress and tell her the time when recreational therapy begins.

3. Help Mary select appropriate attire and offer her assistance in getting dressed.

4. Allow Mary as much time as she needs but explain that she may be too late to go with the other patients, so she will miss her therapy.

46. Mary hoards leftovers from her meal tray, along with other seemingly valueless articles, and stuffs them in her dress

pockets "so the others won't steal them." You should plan to

1. Explain to Mary why putting food and other articles in her dress pocket can cause bacteria to grow in her pockets and cause a disease.
2. Give Mary a small bag in which to place selected personal articles and food of her own choosing.
3. Remove unsafe and soiled articles from Mary's belongings during the night.
4. Tell Mary it is your responsibility to keep her clean and safe, and ask her to give you everything in her pockets.

47. In planning activities for Mary, the nurse should

1. Plan a variety of activities that will keep Mary occupied.
2. Offer challenging activities to maintain Mary's contact with reality.
3. Provide familiar activities that Mary can successfully complete.
4. Make sure that Mary participates in many daily activities.

48. Mary likes to talk about her youth and, at times, has a tendency to confabulate (fill in gaps in memory). As her nurse, you should recognize that this behavior serves to

1. Promote self-esteem.
2. Remember herself when she was healthy and happy.
3. Attract attention to herself.
4. Prevent regression.

49. Mary frequently talks about "the good old days on the farm" where she was born. On the basis of an understanding of Mary's diagnosis, the nurse's most appropriate action is

1. Involving Mary in interesting diversional activities in a small group.
2. Allowing Mary to reminisce about her past and engage her in conversation about her past.
3. Gently remind Mary that those "good old days" are past and that she needs to think about the present and the future.
4. Introduce Mary to other neighbors her age so they can mutually share their past and present experiences.

End of Case

50. The home health nurse is caring for an 80-year-old widower with a history of hypertension. At the nurse's first home visit, the patient's blood pressure is 180/102. When the nurse asks him if he has been taking his medication, he replies, "I took the pill my doctor prescribed for me a few times last week, but it didn't help me feel any better, so I quit taking it." The best initial response by the nurse is

1. You must not be very concerned about your high blood pressure.
2. You really should try to take your medication the doctor ordered.

3. Taking pills are no fun, but your blood pressure is sky high, and if you don't take it, you will have a stroke.
4. Do you know why your doctor ordered the medication that you are no longer taking?

ANSWERS AND RATIONALES

1. ❷ A lower body temperature is normal for the geriatric patient.

1. Geriatric breathing capacity is decreased because of loss of elasticity.

3. There is an increase in peripheral resistance, which causes an increase in blood pressure.

4. The geriatric patient has a decrease in pulse and stroke volume.

2. ❹ The most helpful response by the nurse is "inactivity, less fiber and fluid in your diet, and laxative abuse can contribute to your problem."

(1, 2, 3) These responses are true about the aging process but *cannot* be controlled.

3. ❹ The most helpful response by the nurse is "satisfying, regular activities promote relaxation. You may need *more rest* during the day, but as you grow older you need *less sleep.*"

1. The nurse is presuming that the patient's activity schedule is too strenuous and may have assumed that this activity took place before going to bed.

2. *More rest* is required for the elderly, but *less sleep* is required, *not more.*

3. The nurse is presuming that the patient cannot sleep because of tremors and so forth; the client cannot control these problems.

4. ❸ A balanced diet that is rich in protein and minerals, weight reduction, and activity will promote optimal function with less pain. A good diet is important in preventing and managing musculoskeletal problems. Weight reduction will reduce the strain on joints, and activity promotes optimal function and reduces the complications of immobility.

1. Complete bed rest would increase joint pain, and moist heat is helpful for relieving pain but does not produce optimal function.

2. An electric blanket should not be used by the elderly because of the danger of burns; the sensitivity to pain is reduced in the elderly.

4. Aspirin will relieve pain but can cause serious gastrointestinal bleeding.

5. ❶ Talking slowly, distinctly, and in a low tone of voice is the most appropriate approach. The patient has a beginning hearing deficit, which involves difficulty with high-frequency sounds.

(2, 3, 4) These options are incorrect as seen in rationale (1).

6. ❷ The best response by the nurse is to "wash hands, face, under arms, and perineum area daily, and a bath every third or fourth day will provide cleanliness without drying the skin."

1. A bath every day is very drying for the skin, and using bath oil will not replace the natural oil of the skin.

3. This is a true statement but fails to answer the patient's concern about bathing every day.

4. Daily oil baths will not replace the natural oil in the skin. Soft sheets will feel good but will not hydrate the skin. Special attention to skin breakdown is important but will not hydrate the skin.

7. ❶ Based on Maslow's hierarchy of needs, safety is the next most important need of humans after physical needs. The home provides security, stability, and order.

(2, 3, 4) These options are incorrect as seen in rationale (1). These options would have occurred over time, not suddenly.

8. ❸ The best response by the nurse that will help the patient define her fears is "what is it that you fear you will lose control of?" This encourages the patient to discover what it is she fears, and discussing her fears will help relieve her anxiety and fear.

(1, 2) These options make a statement about what the nurse thinks the patient's fear is; they do not help the patient to discuss her fear.

4. The statement "This must be difficult for you, but I am here to protect you" does not encourage the patient to explore her fear.

9. ❹ Ask the physician to order a medication to relieve her anxiety is the most appropriate plan of care.

1. It is inappropriate for the nurse to tell the physician which medication to order. Valium 20 mg is a high dosage for a younger adult and is an extremely dangerous dosage for an elderly client.

(2, 3) When a patient is in a very high state of anxiety, trying to communicate with him or her is an impossible task. At a very high level of anxiety, the patient has difficulty communicating effectively. Therefore, he or she could not follow instructions on how to reduce anxiety. When a patient is in a very high state of anxiety, the nurse must ask questions and give directions that are simple and to the point.

10. ❹ The nurse recognizes that the daughter is using the defense mechanism of *denial* by rejecting something that is very disturbing to her. Many elderly people are abused in their own homes by family members.

1. Keeping unacceptable experiences in her mind is another defense mechanism (*repression*).

2. Developing the opposite attitude to the way one is feeling constitutes the defense mechanism of *reaction formation.*

3. Giving a logical reason for something constitutes the defense mechanism of *rationalization.*

11. ❸ Position the patient off her back until the area is no longer red. This area will need close watching so that no skin breakdown occurs. Turning the patient every 2 h is the best way to prevent decubitus ulcers from forming.

1. The egg crate mattress is helpful in preventing decubitus ulcers, but the patient still needs to be turned every 2 to 3 h.

2. OpSite is used if a decubitus ulcer develops.

4. Massaging the area every 2 h can increase damage to the skin. Massaging with lotion every 4 h would be helpful.

12. ❷ DuoDERM is the only occlusive dressing listed. It can be used to protect the wound mechanically and can débride small amounts of necrotic tissue.

(1, 3, 4) These options are incorrect as seen in rationale (2).

13. ❸ The purpose of a Jackson-Pratt drain is to prevent fluid from collecting in the wound. If fluid collects in the wound, a dead space is created and tissue cannot grow; the skin graft would not attach, and the decubitus would not heal.

(1, 2) A drain is used to remove fluid; if there was an infection, it would be treated with antibiotics.

4. A wound will heal from the inside out, not from the outside in. See rationale (3).

14. ❷ The most appropriate treatment is applying enzymatic debriding agents such as self-adhesive film (OpSite). Debriding of the wound removes the dead tissue and encourages the growth of new tissue.

(1, 3, 4) These options are incorrect as seen in rationale (2).

15. ❹ Redress the wound, have patient remain in bed, and notify the physician. Obese and diabetic patients have a higher risk for wound dehiscence and evisceration than the general population. Evisceration occurs when the viscera protrude through the disrupted wound. Dehiscence is the partial or complete separation of the wound edges.

(1, 2, 3) These options are incorrect as seen in rationale (4).

16. ❸ Cover the wound with a sterile saline-soaked dressing, put the patient in a low semi-Fowler's position, and notify the surgeon immediately.

(1, 2) A moist dressing must be used to prevent damage to the viscera.

4. Viscera should not be pushed back in to the abdomen because injury to the viscera can occur.

17. ❹ A physician's order of a calcium supplement is important for the elderly because of the danger of hypocalcemia. Many elderly use alcohol to reduce their depression. Alcohol interferes with bone calcium absorption. Some elderly are addicted to tobacco, which also interferes with calcium absorption. Therefore, hypercalcemia develops because the calcium is coming out of the bones and into the blood serum. The patient will develop all of the side effects of hypercalcemia (e.g., kidney stones).

1. Postmenopausal women who take estrogen need to take less calcium than women not taking estrogen. Estrogen increases bone the absorption of calcium.

2. It is not necessary for a patient at any age to have his or her blood calcium level evaluated every month. The only exception is a patient with hypercalcemia.

3. The recommended amount of calcium intake for postmenopausal women not taking estrogen is 1500 mg/day.

18. ❶ Malignant neoplasm causes hypercalcemia because cancer stimulates bone reabsorption, which increases serum calcium levels; calcium is pulled out of the bone and back into the blood. Other common causes of hypercalcemia are prolonged immobilization; ingestion of thiazide, diuretics, and lithium; and overzealous intake of calcium supplement, vitamin D, antacids containing calcium or phosphate, and estrogen.

(2, 3, 4) These options are incorrect as seen in rationale (1).

19. ❷ Prednisone, Lasix, and Calcimar are drugs used to reduce serum calcium levels. Prednisone antagonizes the effects of vitamin D and, therefore, decreases gastrointestinal absorption of calcium and inhibits bone reabsorption. In other words, less calcium from the bone will be pulled back into the blood serum. Lasix pulls calcium out by increasing urinary output. Calcimar reduces bone turnover by decreasing bone reabsorption.

(1, 3, 4) These options are incorrect as seen in rationale (2).

20. ❹ Urinating frequently will decrease the patient's serum calcium level because calcium is excreted. Tingling in fingers is a sign of hypocalcemia.

(1, 2, 3) These options are incorrect as seen in rationale (4).

21. ❸ Osteoporosis is the most common cause of hip fractures in the elderly. Osteoporosis appears to be a hereditary condition, but it is also caused by lifestyle (e.g., immobilization, diet). It is marked by excessive calcification and bone with a marbleized appearance.

1. Decreased calcium intake is not a specific enough answer; decreased a little or a lot? A patient can have the recommended calcium intake and still develop osteoporosis.

2. Decreased muscle strength is not related to hip fractures. The word *decrease* is vague and usually makes the option wrong.

4. Decreased bone marrow does not cause hip fractures. Bone marrow depression will cause anemia (RBCs), leukemia [white blood cells (WBCs)], and thrombocytopenia (platelets).

22. ❶ An inappropriate use of Buck's traction is for immobilizing the leg until it heals. This means that the patient would be immobile for several weeks, which this would cause all of the problems related to immobility.

(2, 3, 4) These options are correct reasons for using Buck's traction. If you got this question wrong, you may have difficulty answering negative questions. You can change this by reading each option and saying "yes, that is true" and then when reading an incorrect option, marking it because that is the right answer.

23. ❶ Buck's traction is contraindicated in the elderly patient who has a bilateral lower leg ulcer because the traction is applied directly to the skin, so it would irritate an existing ulcer. Many ulcers have serious drainage, which would create even more problems. Skin traction is also contraindicated in the presence of skin abrasions or wounds, dermatitis, varicose ulcers, peripheral neuropathies, and impaired circulation.

2. Buck's traction can be used on elderly patients with osteoarthritis. Osteoarthritis is a degenerative joint disease and is the most common type of arthritis.

3. Buck's traction can be used on a deformed leg.

4. One of the primary uses for Buck's traction is to relieve pelvic pain after a leg fracture.

24. ❷ The correct plan of care for an elderly patient with *intermittent* Buck's traction is to remove traction once every shift to observe pressure areas and to provide good skin care.

1. The patient cannot be turned on the affected side because a client cannot be turned while in Buck's traction and, if out of traction, would be turned on the unaffected side.

(3, 4) These options will cause the loss of countertraction and the effectiveness of the traction.

25. ❸ Shortening of the affected leg occurs because of the overriding of bone fragments.

1. The elderly bruise very easily; it is not an indication of a hip fracture.

2. Moving the affected leg would hurt after a fall and would not indicate right hip fracture.

4. You never call the physician until you have assessed the patient.

26. ❹ Dyspnea and complaints of sharp chest pain after a car accident that caused multiple bone fractures may be symptoms of a pulmonary embolus. The home health nurse needs to notify the physician immediately.

1. A slight rise in temperature could result from the inflammatory process; the temperature-regulating mechanism in the elderly may be slightly compromised, which can cause a slight elevation in body temperature for a longer period after an injury.

2. Feelings of weakness and fatigue are normal symptoms for a 92-year-old patient after a serious car accident.

3. An inability to cough *productively* 5 days after a car accident is a good indication of no respiratory infection. A productive cough means coughing up purulent sputum.

27. ❹ Hypochondriasis is used by some elderly patients as an attention-getting mechanism.

◆ Often, health professionals reinforce this behavior by reacting to physical complaints promptly but not reinforcing periods of good health and normal functioning.

◆ Health professionals may not respond to a request from the patient to sit and talk with him or her, but these professionals give undivided attention when the same person expresses physical complaints.

◆ The elderly may use hypochondriacal behavior as an effective means of controlling a spouse or children or as a means of socialization.

◆ Family members need to understand the dynamics of hypochondriacs so that they can learn to reinforce positive behavior and not manipulative behavior by the elderly patient. Also, family members need to understand that telling elderly people that "nothing is wrong" is of little help and only perpetuates the hypochondriacal behavior.

(1, 2, 3) These options are incorrect as seen in rationale (4).

28. **①** Some degree of cognitive impairment is relatively common among the elderly and often increases with age.

Senility, dementia, and Alzheimer's disease are not the same disease. *Senility* refers to growing old and the mental weakness that is sometimes associated with it. *Dementia* is an irrecoverable deteriorative mental state, with absence or reduction of intellectual faculties due to organic brain disease. *Alzheimer's disease* is a form of presenile dementia due to atrophy of frontal and occipital lobes.

◆ Alzheimer's disease usually occurs between ages 40 to 60 years, more often in women than men.

◆ Involves progressive irreversible loss of memory, deterioration of intellectual functions, apathy, speech and gait disturbance, and disorientation.

◆ May take from a few months to 4 or 5 years to progress to complete loss of intellectual function.

◆ Alzheimer's disease, dementia, stroke, pharmaceutical agents, and alcohol are frequently implicated as inducing cognitive changes.

◆ Approximately four million Americans have Alzheimer's disease, and 14 million Americans will have the disease by the year 2050 unless a cure or prevention is found.

◆ More than 70 percent of people with Alzheimer's disease live at home with care provided by family or friends; some have home health nurse assistance.

(2, 3, 4) These options are incorrect as seen in rationale (1).

29. **②** Neither Medicare nor private health insurance will pay for long-term health care in the home or in the nursing home. Families are beginning to invest in specific insurance that covers long-term care for the elderly.

1. This option is incorrect as seen in rationale (2).

3. It is true that families are beginning to invest in specific insurance that covers long-term care for the elderly. It is inappropriate to tell a 75-year-old man diagnosed with cancer that if he had just bought the long-term health insurance before he got cancer he would not have to worry about it now.

4. Private insurance companies will not pay for long-term health care unless the insurance is specific for long-term health care.

30. **①** The nurse should instruct the patient about how to collect a sterile sputum the next day before breakfast. Before breakfast is the best time to collect sputum because a large quantity of secretions collects in the lungs during the night if the patient has an infection. The physician will need the sputum to identify the organism so that an appropriate antibiotic can be ordered.

(2, 3, 4) These options are incorrect as seen in rationale (1).

31. **③** Palpating the breast while in a sitting position is an incorrect procedure for breast examination.

(1, 2, 4) These options are incorrect as seen in rationale (3).

32. **②** The correct response by the nurse is that the best time to do a breast examination is 2 to 3 days after the completion of each menstrual period.

(1, 3, 4) These options are incorrect as seen in rationale (2).

33. **③** The nurse should take the client's vital signs, and ask the client if he hurt himself when he fell and if he took his Dilantin. Dilantin turns urine pink. The patient may have forgotten to take his Dilantin, and the daughter may have given it to him after the seizure, turning the urine pink.

(1, 2, 4) These options are incorrect as seen in rationale (3).

34. **②** The physician ordered a hormone that normally is produced by the kidney to stimulate the bone marrow to produce RBCs. The synthetic hormone epoetin alfa (Epogen, Procrit), which mimics erythropoietin, has been developed for use in persons in end-stage renal failure.

(1, 3, 4) These options are incorrect as seen in rationale (2).

35. **①** Pitressin is a synthetic ADH that helps control blood volume by promoting water reabsorption in the renal tubules. If the pituitary gland cannot produce this medication, the patient would be urinating excessive amounts of urine.

(2, 3, 4) These options are incorrect as seen in rationale (1).

36. **④** A Venturi mask is used for COPD patients because it gives the most accurate amount of oxygen. Oxygen therapy for COPD patients must be administered in low accurate amounts.

1. A tracheostomy collar delivers oxygen and humidification via a tracheostomy; it must be connected to a nebulizer. Condensation must be drained often, and it is associated with risk for nosocomial respiratory infection, especially in the elderly. There was no indication in the question that this client had a tracheostomy.

2. Simple mask delivers low to medium concentration and must use liter flow greater than 5 L/min. It would not be used with a COPD patient.

3. Nonrebreathing mask delivers the highest concentration, 80 to 90 percent; the reservoir bag it must be kept inflated at all times. Risk of necrosis from snug fit; not for long-term use.

37. **②** Aminophyllin causes bronchial vasodilation and will cause hypotension when blood vessels are dilated.

(1, 3, 4) These options are incorrect as seen in rationale (2).

38. **②** Patients need to understand the disease is a physiologic event that is not always a life-threatening crisis. Learning breathing exercises will help the patient deal with his fears by helping him to have some control over his dyspnea.

(1, 3, 4) These options are incorrect as seen in rationale (2).

39. **④** Assess the patient's understanding of the procedure and expectation of bodily appearance after surgery.

(1, 2, 3) These options are incorrect as seen in rationale (4).

40. **③** Antiemetics are administered before chemotherapy is started, and during and after administration if needed. This is to try to prevent the severity of nausea and vomiting associated with chemotherapy.

(1, 2, 4) These options are incorrect as seen in rationale (3).

41. ❹ The nurse would prepare to give cyanocobalamin (vitamin B$_{12}$).

1. Folic acid (vitamin B$_9$) is needed for erythropoiesis; it increases RBC, WBC, and platelet formation.

2. Ascorbic acid (vitamin C) is needed for wound healing, collagen synthesis, antioxidant and carbohydrate metabolism, protein and lipid synthesis, and prevention of infections.

3. Cholecalciferol (vitamin D) is needed for regulation of calcium and phosphate levels, normal bone development, parathyroid activity, and neuromuscular functioning.

42. ❶ *Projection* is the attributing of unacceptable feelings and emotions to others. The patient does not want to look at the stoma, so he accuses the nurse; projecting his feeling to the nurse.

2. A *reaction formation* is the unconscious reversal of feelings or behavior. A person acts in a way that is opposite to how he or she feels. A nursing student dislikes a clinical instructor yet asks repeatedly to be assigned to that instructor.

3. In *displacement,* a person transfers an emotion from its original object to a substitute object. A child is angry at his mother, so he breaks his favorite toy or kicks the dog.

4. *Intellectualization* is the use of a mental reasoning process to deny facing emotions and feelings involved in a situation.

43. ❸ Assist the patient to identify and adopt more healthful coping patterns. The patient must learn to develop and use more helpful healthful mechanisms if drinking alcohol is to be stopped; the responsibility is with the patient because he must do the changing.

1. Confronting the patient will increase guilt and place her on the defense, and it will not foster the development of a trusting relationship.

(2, 4) These options are incorrect as seen in rationale (1).

44. ❹ The patient lacks insight about the emotional aspect of her illness, and she needs continued therapy by going to Alcoholics Anonymous (AA) meetings every day. It takes at least 1 year for an alcoholic person to break away from the use of alcohol, and many continue to attend AA meetings all of their life.

(1, 2, 3) These options are incorrect as seen in rationale (4).

45. ❸ Help the patient select appropriate attire and offer her assistance in getting dressed. This assists the client in decision making; a new situation may be very stressful for an elderly client with dementia.

(1, 2, 4) These options do not allow for shared decision making; hurrying the patient will lead to frustration, resentment, and guilt, and she may perceive these actions as punishment.

46. ❷ This allows the patient to exercise the right to decide which articles to keep and provides cleanliness. Working with the patient allows the nurse the opportunity to encourage her to keep solid foods and safe articles in her pockets. This allows her to make some decisions and have some feeling of control over her life.

(1, 3, 4) These options deceive the patient, limit judgment, and create mistrust. Explanations alone will not provide safety for this patient because of decreased attention span and memory.

47. ❸ Routines and familiarity with activities or environment provide for a sense of security. The feeling of security is very important to a client experiencing disorientation.

1. Change is poorly tolerated; frustration and inability to accomplish tasks lead to anxiety and lowered self-esteem.

2. Challenging activities can be frustrating and can lead to hostility or withdrawal.

4. Decreased physical capacity and attention span limits activity participation; anxiety and frustration can result.

48. ❶ Confabulation is used as a defense mechanism against embarrassment caused by a lapse of short-term memory; it increases her self-esteem.

2. This can be accomplished but usually is not the purpose of reminiscence and is not the purpose of confabulation.

3. Although many elderly fear being forgotten or losing others' affection, this is not the main reason for confabulation.

4. Regression is a defense mechanism in which the individual moves back to earlier developmental behavior.

49. ❷ Allowing Mary to reminisce about her past and engaging her in conversation about her past encourages verbalization. This gives Mary a feeling of security and decreases her sense of isolation.

1. Mary will have difficulty functioning in a small group of strangers because of her anxiety and short-term memory loss.

3. Gently reminding Mary that those "good old days" are past and that she needs to think about the present and the future will discourage verbalization of her feelings and will increase anxiety.

4. Introducing Mary to other neighbors her age may be impossible. There may not be anyone her age in the neighborhood. If someone is 85 years old, they may not want to visit with Mary.

50. ❹ The best response by the nurse is, "Do you know why your doctor ordered the medication that you are no longer taking?" Baseline data must be known before the nurse can begin to educate the patient about the importance of taking his medication.

(1, 2, 3) These options are judgmental. They do not help the nurse to develop a working relationship with the patient and do not help the patient to understand why he needs to take his blood pressure medication.

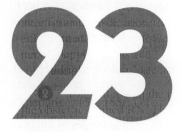

Chapter

23

Registered Professional Nurses as Managers and as Delegators of Tasks to Unlicensed Assistive Personnel (ULP)

◆ Community-based nursing differs from hospital nursing in that the community-based setting requires that the nurse understand aspects of the patient's life that will impact nursing practice.

◆ It is helpful to know how nursing in the hospital and in the community differ from public health nursing. The nurse as a manager will function differently in each setting, but some basic principles of management remain the same.

A. Nursing in the Hospital Setting

1. In the hospital setting, the health care provider is in control and the patient may feels powerless.

2. Admission to the hospital, especially when it is the patient's first time, is a cold, frightening experience.

3. A hospital gown usually replaces the patient's clothing, and personal items, such as watches, glasses, wallet, dentures and jewelry, may temporarily be removed from the patient.

4. Different types of procedures and treatments are scheduled and performed on a routine basis with little or no input from the patient.

5. Physical examinations may be conducted by numerous health professionals with little or no input from the patient.

6. Behaviors considered normal at home are considered unacceptable in the hospital. For example, if a husband gets in bed with his wife and holds her close to him.

7. Many questions, some of them very personal, are asked numerous times; the rationale on the significance of the questions asked is rarely provided.

8. The strict hospital routines are done for specific and valid reasons. This process controls the environment, provides an efficient and safe workplace for the nurse, and meets the needs of the critically ill patient in an efficient manner.

9. Many different services, for example, pharmacy and dietary, are on site and can be accessed by telephone.

10. Equipment and supplies needed for patient care are readily available.

11. Replacement and maintenance of equipment are carried out on an orderly and systematic basis.

12. Although the nurse may be exposed to more organisms in the hospital than in other settings, universal/standard precautions are strictly enforced. Isolation equipment and supplies are readily available in the hospital setting.

13. Health professionals expect the patient to be compliant; the patient can be labeled noncompliant by the staff and treated accordingly.

14. Documentation usually can be completed manually or by computer in a relatively short time.

15. The nurse is in one location so that no more travel is involved once the nurse is at work.

16. Coworkers in the immediate area are available for consultation.

B. Nursing in the Community Setting: Home

1. Community health nursing has a new name: community-based nursing.

2. When a patient is at home, not in the hospital, the situation is completely reversed.

3. The patient, not the nurse, is in control.

4. Nurse collaboration is limited; usually practice is alone.

5. Nurse works in an unknown environment, and safety is a concern.

6. The patient knows the environment, so support is in place (family/friends/pets).

7. The patient is in control of personal items, schedules, and routine.

8. Nurse must adapt to patient's situation and lifestyle.

9. The patient maintains self-determination and lifestyle.

10. The patient can be himself or herself.

11. The quality of home life can range from happy and well adjusted to unhappy and maladjusted.

12. When the patient knows that he or she can make choices and that these decisions determine their lives, he or she feels in control.

13. Pets can play a very significant role in the life of a patient, especially one who lives alone.

14. The family may not have a means of transportation for health-related activities. The nurse should know that a passenger in his or her car makes the nurse liable. Many home health agencies have a policy that does not permit transporting anyone.

15. The nurse working in a community setting has advantages and disadvantages.

    a. Flexibility in planning their day; traveling and working alone.

    b. Limited nurse collaboration is especially difficult when the need for verification of assessment occurs (e.g., lung sounds, heart rhythm, etc.).

    c. Using universal/standard precautions protects the nurse in most situations in the community settings.

    d. Documentation is lengthy and very time consuming.

    e. The nurse may encounter many different family members, each with his or her own idea of what kind of care the patient should receive.

C. Nursing in the Public Health Setting

1. Public health departments have the responsibility of maintaining the health of the community as a whole.

2. This includes diverse duties such as inspecting restaurants for sanitation, providing for immunization programs, and treating venereal disease and tuberculosis.

3. The exact responsibilities are specific to the laws and funding of each community. Some public health departments also provide nurses, who make home visits to offer a variety of supportive services.

4. These services are directed at health maintenance (e.g., teaching clients how to manage their own care or following-up on communicable disease treatment).

5. Care through public health departments usually is free or provided at cost.

D. Nurses as Case Managers in the Health Care Setting

1. Case management is a collaborative process that assesses, plans, implements, coordinates, monitors, and evaluates the options and services to meet an individual's needs using communication and available resources to promote a high-quality, cost-effective outcome.

2. Basically, case management makes the health care system work by ensuring that the patient is at the right level of care at the right time in his or her illness or injury and by encouraging a high quality of care at the correct price.

3. Professional case managers exist in every organization that pays for health care services.

4. The case manager working with patients who have highly expensive illnesses can control cost while maintaining quality care.

5. These benefits occur because the case manager ensures that the necessary resources are available and coordinated, implemented, and monitored as needed.

6. A case manager is like a tour guide, leading patients through the complex health care system.

7. Case management offers services that not only encourage early discharge but also help prevent hospitalization or rehospitalization. This is accomplished by facilitating communication among persons at all levels within the hospital and external post-discharge health care teams, and then implementing or coordinating care needs using existing community resources.

8. Most important, the case manager is expected to encourage and empower the patient to understand and gain control over his or her own medical care; to become an educated consumer; to be more aware of health care cost and seek alternatives when services are limited or excluded from the patient's insurance package; and to know how to find and use community resources.

9. This empowerment is very important because many patients in the case management system eventually may require long-term or chronic care.

10. Clients should be referred to case management as early in the case as possible so that referrals can be made as soon as risks or needs are identified.

11. In most cases, case management is a win–win situation for everyone; the patient, health care provider, insurance company, and the organization offering case management services.

12. There are no guidelines for case management services; each case is individual and the success of case management is directly related to the skills of the case manager and his or her ability to be a team player; his or her knowledge of treatment modalities and community resources; and his or her willingness to be available to the patient in times of crisis or as the patient's condition changes.

13. Case managers are no different than any other registered nurse (RN) when delegating responsibility and authority to subordinates such as licensed practical nurses (LPNs) and other nonprofessionals (e.g., nursing aides, nursing assistants). They need to ensure that goals and objectives are met in a safe and timely manner.

14. The National Case Management Task Force developed criteria for certified case managers.

   a. The applicant must pass a examination for certification as a Certified Insurance Rehabilitation Specialist.

   b. The applicant must have an employment history that validates his or her employment experience.

   c. A job description must include responsibility for patient advocacy and empowerment.

   d. Along with the application, the employer must validate the fact that the individual has direct contact with patients in need of case management services.

E. Nurses as Delegators and Supervisors of Unlicensed Personnel

1. In conversation in the workplace, delegation and supervision are often used interchangeably, even though they have significantly different legal and practice applications.

   a. Supervision

   (1) RNs provide supervision in a number of settings and situations (e.g., community-based nursing, hospitals).

   (2) Supervision is the active process of directing, guiding, and influencing the outcome of licensed and unlicensed assistive personnel (UAP) or unlicensed personnel (ULP) in the performance of an activity or task. These are just broad titles used to cover LPN nurses' aides, technicians, and other assistive personnel.

   (3) In the hospital setting, the RN provides clinical supervision by being physically present or immediately available while activity is being performed.

   b. Delegation

   (1) Delegation is the transfer of responsibility for performance of a task from one individual to another.

   (2) The delegation of an activity passes on the responsibility for task performance but *not* the accountability for the process or the outcome of the task.

   (3) The RN delegator has greater knowledge and a higher degree of judgment than the UAP.

   (4) Direct delegation is the verbal direction by the RN to the UAP regarding an activity or task in a specific nursing care situation.

   (5) Indirect delegation usually is an approved list of activities or tasks that have been established in the policies and procedures of a health care facility.

   (6) Indirect delegation offers convenience and consistency in establishing parameters for the utilization of an UAP in a health care facility. It cannot be used as a substitute for the professional, independent judgment of the RN. It is the RN who must delegate specific tasks based on his or her assessment of the patient, the patient's condition, and the UAP's training and ability to carry out the delegated task safely.

   (7) In delegating, the RN must use professional judgment to decide which patient care activities can be delegated to whom, and under what circumstances.

   (8) Some tasks that require specific nursing knowledge and/or skill are more appropriate for the RN to delegate to a licensed practical nurse (LPN) or licensed vocational nurse (LVN) rather than to a ULP.

   (9) Unlike ULPs, LPNs/LVNs are trained in a state-approved program and must successfully complete a standardized examination. They are able to perform some tasks or functions that UAPs cannot.

   (10) LPNs/LVNs are licensed and, therefore, are held accountable for their own actions. The RN, however, is still responsible for overall client assessment, planning, and evaluations.

   (11) An example of the RN's responsibility for delegating tasks to the ULP can be seen in the performance of an admission assessment and the development of a plan of care for the newly admitted patient.

      (a) The RN cannot delegate to a ULP patient care activities that include the care of the nursing process and require specialized nursing knowledge, judgment, and/or skill. These activities include the following:

         (i) The initial nursing assessment and any subsequent assessment

         (ii) Interventions that require professional nursing knowledge, judgment, and skills (e.g., counseling, teaching)

         (iii) Determination of the nursing diagnosis

         (iv) Development of the nursing plan of care

         (v) Evaluation of the client's progress in relation to the plan of care

      (b) The RN can delegate to a ULP the following direct client care activities used to meet basic human needs: feeding the patient, ambulating, taking vital signs, grooming, toileting, dressing, socialization, assisting the patient with self-care deficit, transportation, bathing, bed making, moving the patient in bed, collecting, reporting, and documentation of related data, which are reported to the RN who uses the information in making clinical judgments about patient care.

F. Nurses as Managers in All Areas and Levels of Nursing Practice

1. RNs are involved with leadership and management tasks at every level and area of practice. The understanding of management tasks is becoming more important because of

a. Increase in number of community-based nursing settings

b. Tightening of budgets at all levels

c. Sweeping changes in the rules and regulations of state and Federal government policies

2. These changes necessitate the need for greater efficiency in the delivery of health care.

3. Leadership and management share some similarities. Both suggest that someone is in charge and assisting workers.

a. The difference is how this is done.

4. *Leadership* can be described as having the capacity to guide and the ability to influence, lead, enable, and inspire.

a. Leadership is accomplished by participating in or guiding the activity.

5. *Management* is the act of controlling, directing, arranging, handling, or supervising an activity.

a. This is accomplished by being *responsible* for the activity and controlling its movement.

b. Management once reserved entirely for the director of nursing service is now included in job descriptions of RNs, LPNs, and LVNs in long-term care facilities.

6. Nursing management in long-term care is identified as follows:

a. LVNs/LPNs are in the lowest level of management called *first-line managers.*

b. RNs are identified at the next higher level of management and identified as *second-line managers.*

c. Directors of nursing service (RN or BSN) are identified as *third-line managers.*

Note: ULP (e.g., nursing assistants) are not licensed caregivers and are not included in management.

7. In long-term care, ULPs are educated according to a federal government training program and are placed on a registry in the state where they work.

8. First-line managers in long-term care are responsible for the residents' care and the delegation of tasks to ULPs on the unit to which they are assigned.

9. They are also responsible for residents' assessment, documentation, communication, and networking with family, visitors, staff, and other disciplines.

a. Other first-line managers' responsibilities include assessing areas of safety and evaluating the implementation of policies and procedures.

10. A second-line manager (RN) is involved in

a. Staff development, coordinating personnel

b. Teaching facility policies and nursing procedure to the staff

c. Assuring continuity and safe delivery of care to residents

d. Problem solving and disciplining

e. Hiring and firing

11. A nursing assistant cannot

a. Administer medication

b. Perform treatments

c. Assess or evaluate residents

d. Manage the unit

12. Guidelines for an RN demonstrating a new task to ULP or an LVN/LPN: The RN can demonstrate new tasks to the ULP, which include

a. Explaining why the procedure is done

b. Assembling appropriate equipment

c. Demonstrating safety measures

d. Demonstrating steps slowly, in correct order

e. Asking questions

f. Requesting return demonstration

g. Identifying specific outcomes of the task that should be reported to the nurse in charge of the patient

13. The second-line manager RN follows these steps in problem solving:

a. Obtain the facts.

(1) Interview each person involved in the issue independently.

(2) Inspect equipment or check sources to verify facts; gather information from policy and procedure manuals.

b. Identify the issue.

(1) Focus on problem.

(2) Look at individual's beliefs and cultural issues.

c. Make decisions.

(1) Base decision on facts, issues, and resources.

(2) Weigh the outcome of decision.

d. Take action.

(1) Verbalize and document decision.

(2) Remember "no action" is still a decision.

e. The prior description of nurses as managers in long-term care facilities is fundamentally the same for nurses as for managers in the hospital or any other health care facility.

(1) Nurses as managers in the hospital work under different titles (e.g., coordinator, quality assurance nurse, infection control, or unit supervisor/charge nurse).

EXAMINATION

Note: On this examination, you must assign an LPN, RN, or ULP to each option. The nursing titles can be used more than once, and every title does not have to be used. (Use answer sheet in back of book.)

Note: Information or diseases covered in the disease section of this book are added here for a more complete understanding of diseases.

Note: The term *general care* used in these questions means taking vital signs, measuring and recording intake and output (I&O), feeding the patient, ambulating and bathing the patient, and so forth.

1. The following patients have been assigned to you, the RN. delegate the following patients' general care to a registered nurse (RN), licensed practical nurse (LPN), and unlicensed personnel (ULP).

   1. A 60-year-old patient with congestive heart failure (CHF) on the second day after admission to the hospital.
   2. A 40-year-old patient with myocardial infarction (MI), new admission to the hospital.
   3. A 70-year-old patient with chronic renal failure, new admission.
   4. A 30-year-old patient with secondary polycythemia, on the second day after admission.

2. A 50-year-old patient has been admitted to the hospital with severe renal failure. Delegate the following tasks to an RN, LPN, and ULP.

   1. Assessment of the patient at the time of admission.
   2. Administration of medications.
   3. Urinary Foley care and measuring output.
   4. Working with a patient to develop short-term goals.

3. A 52-year-old male patient has been admitted to the hospital diagnosed with CHF. Delegate the following tasks to an RN, LPN, and ULP.

   1. Irrigate central line.
   2. Change abdominal dressing.
   3. IV push 20 mg of Lasix.
   4. Report slow decubitus ulcer healing to RN.

4. The following patients have been assigned to you. Delegate their general care to an RN, LPN, and ULP. A patient with

   1. Asthma on the day of admission to the hospital.
   2. Viral hepatitis on the second day after admission.
   3. Liver abscess on the second day of admission.
   4. Chronic glomerulonephritis on the third day after admission.

5. You are caring for a 90-year-old female on the second day in the hospital after a colon resection surgery. Delegate the following interventions to an RN, LPN, and ULP.

   1. Administer IV push medication.
   2. Aspirin PO.
   3. Use restraints as prescribed.
   4. Insert a nasogastric tube.

6. A 28-year-old woman has been admitted to the hospital with a diagnosis of appendicitis. Which of the following skills would you delegate to an RN, LPN, and ULP?

   1. Vital signs and I&O on the day of admission.
   2. Evaluate the patient's vital signs.

   3. Assess abdominal pain.
   4. Administer intravenous fluids.

7. You are caring for a 90-year-old woman on her second day in the hospital after hip replacement. Which of the following tasks would you delegate to an RN, LPN, and ULP?

   1. Bathe and turn the client.
   2. Listen and answer the family's and patient's basic concerns.
   3. Remove Buck's traction per physician's orders.
   4. Administer blood.

8. A 52-year-old man is admitted to the hospital with severe herpes zoster and you have on your team a female RN, 28 years of age; a female LPN, 52 years of age; and a male ULP, 30 years old. Delegate the following skills to them.

   1. Bathe the client.
   2. Administer medications.
   3. Apply calamine lotion as prescribed.
   4. Observe the patient for hearing loss.

9. Patients with the following diagnosis have been assigned to you. Delegate their general care to an RN, LPN, and ULP. A client with

   1. Scarlet fever.
   2. Meningitis.
   3. Encephalitis.
   4. Diverticulitis.

10. The following patients have been assigned to your care. Delegate their general care to an RN, LPN, and ULP. A client with

    1. Intussusception 2 days after admission to the hospital.
    2. Diabetes mellitus and a blood sugar level of 52 mg/dL.
    3. Diabetes insipidus and specific gravity of 1.010.
    4. Down syndrome, age 20 years, with white blood cell (WBC) count of 10,000 mL.

11. A 20-year-old man is admitted to the hospital with a diagnosis of a brain tumor, and he has a cast on his left leg. Delegate the following assessments or interventions to an RN, LPN, and ULP.

    1. Teach the patient relaxation methods.
    2. Provide diversional activities for the patient to decrease discomfort and help to relieve the fear of surgery.
    3. Assess the patient's neurovascular status.
    4. Look for swelling on right leg, which may indicate vascular constriction of the extremity.

12. A 50-year-old man is in the hospital recovering from an old MI and a cardiac bypass graft (CABG) times three. He states that he is afraid he will have another MI. Delegate the following nursing assessment or interventions to an RN, LPN, and ULP.

    1. Check color, pulse, and temperature of the patient's legs.

2. Teach the patient about the need for daily exercise and the importance of following the cardiac diet.

3. Assess the patient's respiration status, cardiac rhythm, and electrocardiogram (ECG).

4. Help the patient to verbalize his fear of having another MI.

13. A 40-year-old woman is admitted to the hospital diagnosed with intestinal obstruction. Delegate the following nursing assessment or interventions to an RN, LPN, and ULP.

   1. Assess patient for relief of pain after administration of analgesic.

   2. Change the patient's position frequently for comfort.

   3. Maintain a calm, restful environment for the patient.

   4. Assess pain and abdominal distention per physician's orders.

14. Delegate the following patients' general care to an RN, LPN, and ULP. A client hospitalized with

   1. Hypertension and blood pressure of 180/104.

   2. Emphysema and experiencing severe dyspnea on the first day in the hospital.

   3. Ulcerative colitis on the first day in the hospital.

   4. Prostate cancer on the second day in the hospital.

15. Delegate an RN, LPN, and ULP in a community-based setting (home) to an appropriate assessment or intervention.

   1. Coordinate nursing activity in the home.

   2. Direct care of client (e.g., redressing an open wound).

   3. Check for the amount of urine excreted in 24 h, taking vital signs, and weighing the patient daily.

   4. Assess the patient's and family's emotional status, coping mechanisms, and support systems.

16. Delegate an RN, LPN, and ULP in a community-based nursing setting (long-term care facility) to an appropriate task.

   1. Teach facility policies and nursing procedures to the staff or to family members.

   2. Observe for dyspnea and weakness during exertion.

   3. Administer treatments (e.g., cleaning, draining wound).

   4. Suction a tracheostomy tube.

17. Assign an RN, LPN, and ULP in a community-based nursing setting (long-term care facility) to an appropriate task.

   1. Communication between levels of nursing.

   2. Work on quality assurance.

   3. Report nausea and vomiting (time frequency and amount).

   4. Inspect mouth for moisture, color, and ulceration.

18. Assign an appropriate task to an RN, LPN, and ULP in a community-based nursing setting (case management) caring for a patient with Parkinson's disease.

   1. Administer drug treatment and offer emotional support.

   2. Encourage and empower the patient to understand and gain control over his or her medical care.

   3. Ensure that the needs of the patient are met.

   4. Help the patient develop long- and short-term goals.

19. Delegate an RN, LPN, and ULP in a community-based nursing setting (home) to an appropriate task. The patient is diagnosed with chronic glomerulonephritis.

   1. Instruct the patient on a low-sodium diet.

   2. Assess the patient's laboratory data.

   3. Encourage small frequent feedings and provide good oral hygiene.

   4. Assist and evaluate the patient's ability to cope with any fluid.

20. Delegate an RN, LPN, and ULP in a community-based nursing setting (long-term care facility) to the following management levels.

   1. First-line manager.

   2. Second-line manager.

   3. Area supervisor.

   4. Assistant.

ANSWERS AND RATIONALES

1.

LPN 1. CHF patient on the second day after admission is not considered as critical as a new MI patient or the patient with polycythemia.

RN 2. MI patient on the first day of admission to the hospital would be assigned to an RN because of the patient's critical condition.

ULP 3. Chronic renal failure client on the first day of admission to the hospital can be delegated to the ULP. Renal failure is chronic, and that situation will not change because the patient is 70 years old and will not be a candidate for a kidney transplant.

RN 4. A patient with secondary polycythemia should be delegated to an RN because the patient must be monitored for hypoxemia and blood clots due to hyperviscosity of the blood. He or she also has an increased risk for paradoxical hemorrhage; this can be due to defective platelet function.

2.

RN 1. Assessment of a patient at the time of admission is the responsibility of the RN.

LPN 2. Administration of medication can be delegated to an LPN. He or she can give all medication except IV pushes.

ULP 3. Urinary Foley care and measuring output can be delegated to the ULP. These skills are within the domain of the ULP and do not require specialized nursing knowledge, judgment, and/or skill.

RN 4. An RN should work with a patient to develop short-term goals. Nursing activities that include the nursing process (assessment, diagnosis, planning, and evaluation, which require specialized knowledge, judgment, and/or skill) should be delegated to an RN.

3.

RN 1. Irrigating a central line should be delegated to an RN because it requires special knowledge, judgment, and skill.

LPN 2. Changing an abdominal dressing can be delegated to an LPN because he or she has the required skill and knowledge to perform this task as a result of to training and education on how to change dressings.

RN 3. An IV push is a very dangerous procedure and should be done by someone trained and educated on how to safely administer an IV push.

ULP 4. A ULP can report slow decubitus ulcer healing to an RN. Reporting information to an RN about the patient's condition and care is an important part of ULP responsibility.

4.

RN 1. An RN should be delegated to care for an asthma patient on the day of admission to the hospital. Having a patent airway is a very high priority for a patient. The RN has the education and training to work with the critically ill.

LPN 2. An LPN can be delegated to work with a patient diagnosed with viral hepatitis. Viral hepatitis type A is highly contagious and usually is transmitted by the fecal or oral route. The LPN has been educated to know and understand how to prevent transmission of this disease.

ULP 3. A ULP can be delegated to work with a patient diagnosed with a liver abscess on the second day of admission to the hospital. A liver abscess is not considered life threatening if treated in a timely manner. The organism causing the abscess is treated with long-term antibiotic therapy. This is not a contagious disease.

LPN 4. An LPN can be delegated to care for a patient diagnosed with chronic glomerulonephritis on the third day of admission. If this was acute glomerulonephritis, an RN would be delegated to care for this patient. The patient with acute glomerulonephritis will have mild to severe hypertension as a result of renin release. This is a relatively common disease that follows a streptococcal infection of the respiratory tract. Glomerulonephritis that is mild will resolve within 2 weeks. Patient care for acute or mild glomerulonephritis is primarily supportive. It is most common in boys ages 3 to 7 years but can occur at any age. Remember, this disease is not treated with antibiotics because it is an antigen–antibody reaction (immunologic response to *Streptococcus*). Protein must be given in small amounts using (high biologic value). Protein makes the kidney work harder. Monitoring vital signs and laboratory val-

ues is important, and the LPN can report problems to the RN.

5.

RN 1. An IV push can be administered only by an RN.

LPN 2. An LPN can give by mouth (PO) medication; a ULP cannot give aspirin or any other medication in the hospital.

ULP 3. The use of restraints on a patient when prescribed by a physician can be delegated to the ULP because he or she must remove and apply restraints when bathing patients. This skill is within the ULP domain.

LPN 4. An LPN can be delegated to the task of inserting a nasogastric tube. If the LPN has a problem inserting the tube, he or she can consult with an RN.

6.

ULP 1. A ULP can be delegated the task of vital signs and I&O; these skills are within the ULP domain.

RN 2. Evaluation is part of the core of the nursing process and, therefore, must be delegated to an RN.

RN 3. Assessing is part of the core of the nursing process and, therefore, must be delegated to the RN.

LPN 4. Administering IV fluids is within the LPN domain; however, he or she cannot give IV pushes.

7.

LPN 1. An LPN can be delegated to bathe and turn a 90-year-old patient. Hip dislocation is a major concern this early after hip surgery; therefore, a ULP should not be delegated these tasks.

ULP 2. Listening and answering family and patient's concerns can be delegated to a ULP. When a ULP takes water into a patient's room or removes urine from the Foley, the family and patient may ask the ULP questions. This is within the ULP domain. The ULP cannot teach the patient, but it saves the RN and LPN time by having the ULP answer basic questions.

LPN 3. Removing Buck's traction can be delegated to an LPN. This is skin traction and very simple to remove. LPNs are trained to perform this procedure.

RN 4. Administration of blood should be delegated to an RN. Some hospitals will not allow an LPN to administer blood. When possible, an RN should be delegated for this task because of the complications associated with the administration of blood.

8.

ULP 1. Bathing this patient can be delegated to a 30-year-old male ULP.

LPN 2. (1, 3, 4) Administering medication to this patient, applying calamine lotion, and checking for hearing loss can be delegated to a 52-year-old female LPN. The 28-year-old RN cannot be assigned to a client with herpes zoster (shingles) because she might be pregnant. Herpesvirus varicella-zoster is the same virus that causes chickenpox and, in its latent stage, causes herpes zoster (shingles). Congenital varicella can affect infants whose mothers had an acute varicella infection in their first or early second trimester.

9.

ULP 1. The general care of a patient diagnosed with scarlet fever can be delegated to a ULP. Scarlet fever usually follows streptococcal pharyngitis or wound infection. It is most common in children 2 to 10 years old. Penicillin or erythromycin is used to treat the disease. Complications from the disease are rare.

RN 2. The general care of a patient diagnosed with meningitis should be delegated to an RN. Meningitis almost always is a complication of another bacterial infection. Manifestations of meningitis are fever, increased intracranial pressure, nuchal (back of neck) rigidity, positive Brudzinski's and Kerning's sign, sinus arrhythmias, and many other central nervous system symptoms. If you do not know what Brudzinski's and Kerning's signs are, look them up, write them down, and learn them. You may be asked about these signs on the RN board examination. From these signs and symptoms, you now know why an RN should care for this patient.

RN 3. The general care of a patient diagnosed with encephalitis should be delegated to an RN. Encephalitis is a severe inflammation of the brain, usually caused by a mosquito-borne or, in some areas, a tick-borne virus. The acute illness begins with a sudden onset of fever, headache, and vomiting and progresses to signs and symptoms of meningeal irritation (stiff neck and back) and neuronal damage (drowsiness, coma, paralysis, convulsions). After the acute phase of illness, coma can persist for days or weeks. During the acute phase, the RN must assess neurologic functions often.

LPN 4. The general care of a patient diagnosed with diverticulitis can be delegated to an LPN. Diverticulitis can be mild or severe. In diverticulitis, undigested food mixed with bacteria accumulates in the diverticular sac, forming a hard mass. This substance interferes with the blood supply to the thin walls of the sac, making them more susceptible to attack by colonic bacteria. Inflammation follows and, if severe, can lead to intestinal perforation, abscess and peritonitis, obstruction, or hemorrhage. Management of mild diverticulitis involves teaching the patient about bowel and dietary habits and explaining why and how diverticular sacs form. Make sure that the patient understands the importance of dietary roughage and the harmful effects of constipation. Advise the patient to start this diet after the colon inflammation is eliminated. Meningitis and encephalitis are more acute diseases; therefore, they should be delegated to the RN. Answering delegation questions correctly is easy if you have a good knowledge about the most commonly occurring diseases; you then know to delegate the most acutely ill to an RN, the next most seriously ill to the LPN, and the less seriously ill to the ULP.

10.

LPN 1. A patient diagnosed with intussusception 2 days after admission can be delegated to an LPN for general care. Intussusception is a telescoping of a portion of the bowel into an adjacent distal portion. Intussusception is most common in infants and occurs three times more often in males than in females. The cause is unknown. Treatment for children is a barium enema; if this is not successful in forcing the bowel back into place, surgery is performed but manual reduction is attempted first. In adults, surgery is always the treatment of choice.

RN 2. A patient diagnosed with diabetes mellitus and a blood sugar of 52 mg/dL should be assigned to an RN. Normal blood glucose is 60 to 120 mg/dL. A blood sugar of 52 mg/dL is low, and the patient is in a state of hypoglycemia. If not treated, the patient can lose consciousness, go into a coma, and die.

LPN 3. A patient diagnosed with diabetes insipidus can be delegated to an LPN. Diabetes insipidus results from a deficiency of circulating vasopressin, also called antidiuretic hormone (ADH). Secondary diabetes insipidus results from removal of the pituitary gland (hypophysectomy) or other neurosurgery or head trauma that damages the neurohypophyseal structure. It also can be caused by infection and vascular lesions. Primary diabetes insipidus accounts for 50 percent of patients and is familial or idiopathic. Signs and symptoms are extreme polyuria (usually 4–16 liters [L] of dilute urine but sometimes as much as 30 L/day). As a result, the patient is thirsty and drinks great quantities of water to compensate for the body's water loss. Other signs and symptoms are constipation, muscle weakness, hypotension, and a very low specific gravity of less than 1.005. Treatment is various forms of vasopressin. Because this patient may have severe hypotension and muscle weakness, an LPN rather than a ULP should care for the patient.

ULP 4. A patient admitted to the hospital with Down syndrome and a WBC count of 10,800 mL can be delegated to a ULP because normal WBCs are 5000 to 10,000 mL for an adult. Down syndrome is caused by an aberration in which chromosome 21 has three copies instead of the normal one. If the mother of the child is a carrier, she has a 10 percent chance of having a baby with Down syndrome; a carrier father has a less than 5 percent chance. Down syndrome patients have an IQ between 30 and 50; however, social performance usually is beyond that expected for mental age. Commonly, they have congenital heart disease (septal deficit of pulmonary or aortic stenosis), megacolon, and pelvic bone abnormalities. Their genitals are poorly developed, and puberty is delayed. Females may menstruate and be fertile. Males usually are infertile with low serum testosterone levels.

11.

LPN 1. An LPN can be delegated responsibility for the general care of a patient with a brain tumor and a leg in a cast. The cause of the brain tumor is unknown. A patient with a brain tumor requires supportive care, documentation of seizure activity (occurrence, nature, and duration), monitoring of client's safety, and administration of anticonvulsive drugs, as ordered. The LPN can perform all of these tasks.

ULP 2. A ULP can be delegated the intervention of providing diversional activities for the patient to decrease discomfort and help to relieve the fear of surgery.

RN 3. The RN should be delegated the task of assessing the patient's neurovascular status. The RN needs to continuously assess for changes in neurologic status and for increased intracranial pressure (ICP). Assess pupillary dilation and, if any dilation occurs, immediately report to physician. These assessments are within the RN's domain.

ULP 4. A ULP can be delegated the intervention to look for swelling on the right leg; there is no indication that the right leg is injured. If swelling occurs, he or she will report this to the RN in charge.

12.

LPN 1. An LPN can be delegated the intervention to check color and temperature of the patient's legs. A vein or artery is required for CABG surgery. Usually, the mammary artery or the saphenous vein in the leg is used. When the saphenous vein is used, the leg must be checked frequently to determine if there is adequate circulation.

RN 2. The RN should be delegated the task of teaching this patient the need for daily exercise and the importance of following the cardiac diet because these two activities are so vital to his recovery and further health. This teaching requires specialized knowledge and skills.

RN 3. An RN should be delegated the task of assessing this patient's respiration status, cardiac rhythm, and ECG because this requires specialized knowledge, judgment, and skills.

LPN 4. The LPN can be assigned the intervention of helping this patient verbalize his fear of having another MI.

13.

LPN 1. The LPN can be delegated the task of assessing this patient's relief of pain after the administration of an analgesic. The LPN could be the nurse administering the pain medication to the patient, so it would be an appropriate task. This assessment is basic and does not require special knowledge or skill.

ULP 2. Delegating the task of changing this patient's position frequently to the ULP is appropriate. This intervention is within the ULP domain.

ULP 3. The delegating of an intervention of maintaining a calm, restful environment to a ULP is appropriate and is within her or his domain. This patient could be cared for by a ULP because the patient's acuity level does not require an RN or LPN for general care. Therefore, the ULP could perform interventions (2) and (3) at the same time.

RN 4. Measuring and assessing the patient's abdominal distention should be delegated to the RN. This assessment requires special knowledge. If the RN assesses that the abdominal distention and pain have increased so much that the intestines may perforate from the pressure, the RN must notify the physician immediately; failure to do so can cause serious injury or death to the client.

14.

RN 1. The general care of a patient with severe hypertension of 180/104 should be delegated to the RN. This patient may have a cerebrovascular accident (CVA). Controlling the blood pressure and knowing the early signs and symptoms of a CVA or other complications require special knowledge.

RN 2. A patient with emphysema experiencing severe dyspnea on the day of admission should be delegated to an RN because managing airway patency demands special knowledge and skills. If this task is not accomplished, the patient will die. Remember that when delegating, you do not want to harm the patient; this thought is helpful when delegating tasks and personnel.

LPN 3. A patient with an ulcerative colitis the first day in the hospital can be delegated to an LPN. Ulcerative colitis is an inflammatory, often chronic, disease that affects the mucosa and submucosa of the colon. It is diagnosed by sigmoidoscopy, and biopsy can help confirm the diagnosis. A colonoscopy is required to determine the extent of disease. Bowel preparation is needed prior to the colonoscopy. Bowel preparation includes 2 days of clear liquid along with a strong cathartic, and on the day of admission an enema is given. Many physicians are now ordering 1 day of clear liquid and a gallon of Colyte or GoLYTELY; an enema is not usually needed. Accurately recording I&O and monitoring fluid and electrolytes are important interventions for this patient before and after diagnostic or surgical procedures. Also, administering antidiarrhea medication (e.g., Lomotil), steroids, and hyperalimentation (TPN) requires an LPN. If complications occur, the LPN knows to consult with an RN.

ULP 4. The general care of a patient diagnosed with prostate cancer the second day in the hospital can be delegated to a ULP. Prostate cancer is the second most common neoplasm found in men older than 50 years and the third leading cause of male cancer death. Prostate carcinoma seldom produces symptoms until well advanced. This patient will not die suddenly or have any major complications from the cancer before surgery; therefore, the general care of this patient can be assigned to a ULP.

15.

RN 1. An RN would be delegated the task of coordinating nursing activity in a home health care situation. The role of the RN in a community setting involves management of the nurse's time, limited resources, other personnel, and program management of the patient's care. The management role includes planning, organizing, coordinating, marketing, controlling and evaluating care, and care delivery.

LPN 2. The LPN is involved in direct care of the patient in a community-based setting. Wound care is one of the most common services an LPN provides in a home health care setting.

ULP 3. Interventions of checking urinary output every 24 h, taking vital signs, and weighing the patient can all be delegated to a ULP because these skills are within his or her domain.

RN 4. Assessing the patient's and family's emotional status, coping mechanisms, and support systems requires special knowledge and judgment skills; therefore, such assessments must be delegated to the RN.

16.

RN 1. An RN should be delegated the task of teaching facility policies and nursing procedures to the staff or to family members. There are some basic simple tasks that family members can and want to do for their loved one. Teaching and delegating tasks requires special knowledge.

ULP 2. Observing for dyspnea and weakness during exertion can be delegated to a ULP. The ULP often ambulates a patient, and this is a good time to observe for dyspnea and weakness and to report any occurrence to the RN.

LPN 3. The LPN can be delegated to administer treatments such as cleaning a wound that has a drain. He or she has been trained in sterile technique.

LPN 4. Suctioning a tracheostomy tube can be delegated to an LPN. He or she has been trained to do this procedure.

17.

LPN 1. Because an LPN working in a long-care facility is given so much responsibility (e.g., charge nurse, medication nurse, managing supplies), he or she is responsible for communication between levels of nursing.

RN 2. The RN should be delegated to work on quality assurance. Quality assurance programs in health care agencies are required for reimbursement of services and for accreditation by the Joint Commission on Ac-

creditation of Healthcare Organizations (JCAHO). The concept of *quality assurance* refers to the accountability of the health profession to society for the quality, quantity, appropriateness, and cost of health services provided. The RN has the special skills and knowledge needed to perform this task.

ULP 3. The ULP can be delegated the responsibility of reporting the time, frequency, and amount of vomiting. This is within his or her domain.

ULP 4. The ULP can be delegated the task of inspecting the client's mouth for moisture, color, and ulceration and reporting this to the RN.

18.

LPN 1. Administering drug treatment (e.g., dopamine) and emotional support can be delegated to the LPN.

RN 2. (2, 3) The RN is the case manager and is responsible for encouraging and empowering the patient to understand and gain control over his or her own medical care and to ensure that the needs of the patient are met.

RN 4. Helping the patient establish long- and short-term goals should be delegated to an RN. This is the core of the nursing process.

19.

LPN 1. The LPN can be delegated to instruct the patient on a low-sodium diet. This requires very basic instructions.

RN 2. The RN should be delegated to assess the patient's laboratory data, especially blood urea nitrogen (BUN), creatinine, and proteinuria.

ULP 3. The ULP can be delegated to encourage small frequent feedings and provide good oral hygiene.

RN 4. Assisting and evaluating the patient's ability to cope with any fluid and dietary restrictions that are ordered would be delegated to the RN. Evaluation is in the core of the nursing, process and assisting a patient to cope takes special knowledge and skills.

20.

LPN 1. First-line manager in a long-term facility would be an LPN.

RN 2. Second-line manager would be an RN.

RN 3. Area supervisor would be an RN.

ULP 4. Assistant would be a ULP.

Chapter 24

New Category of Application Questions on the RN State Board Exam

QUESTIONS 1 TO 20: PRIORITIZING PATIENT CARE

1. Four adult patients with the following medical diagnosis have been assigned to you. Using nursing priority skills, which of the patients will you assess first? The patient with a medical diagnosis of
   1. Bacterial meningitis, second day in the hospital.
   2. Ménière's disease, first day in the hospital.
   3. Diabetes mellitus, third day in the hospital.
   4. Graves' disease, second day in the hospital.

2. An airplane crash occurs near the hospital. You are asked to discharge an adult patient. Using nursing priority skills, which of the patients will you discharge? The patient with a medical diagnosis of
   1. Acquired immunodeficiency syndrome (AIDS), first day in the hospital.
   2. Hemophilia, first day in the hospital.
   3. Sickle cell anemia, second day in the hospital.
   4. Aplastic anemia, second day in the hospital.

3. You are an RN on a medical/surgical unit and assigned to four adult patients. Using nursing priority skills, which of the following patients will you see first? The patient with a medical diagnosis of
   1. Chronic obstructive pulmonary disease (COPD), 40 years of age, second day in the hospital.
   2. Myocardial infarction (MI), 60 years of age, second day in the hospital.
   3. Systemic lupus erythematosus (SLE), 30 years of age, third day in the hospital.
   4. Rocky mountain fever, 25 years of age, second day in the hospital.

4. An obstetric-trained RN is transferred to your medical/surgical unit from an obstetrics unit to work in place of the RN who went home ill. Using nursing priority skills, which two adult patients will you assign to the obstetric RN? The patients with medical diagnosis of
   1. Cystic fibrosis, and a breast cancer patient (postoperatively), their third day in the hospital.
   2. Total hip replacement and a renal failure, their first day in the hospital.
   3. Multiple sclerosis (MS) and gangrene of the left large toe, their first day in the hospital.
   4. Congestive heart failure and a Guillain-Barré syndrome, their first day in the hospital.

5. As the charge nurse on the medical/surgical unit, which adult patient will you assign to your most experienced RN? The patient with a medical diagnosis of
   1. Hypothyroidism, first day in the hospital, scheduled for diagnostic testing.
   2. Leukoplakia vulvae, first day in the hospital, scheduled for biopsy.
   3. Severe prolapsed mitral valve scheduled for a valve replacement, second day in the hospital.
   4. Deep thermal burns (deep-thickness burns) over the lower half of the body caused by a scalding water accident, first day in the hospital.

6. An RN from a pediatric unit is assigned to the medical/surgical critical care unit to replace an RN who is home with a sick child. Which patient will you assign to this RN?
   1. A 5-year-old child with hydrocephalus, second day in the hospital for surgical/medical management of shunt.
   2. A 3-year-old child with nephrotic syndrome, first day in the hospital.
   3. A 5-month-old child with spina bifida, first day in the hospital.
   4. An 8-year-old with cystic fibrosis, fourth day in the hospital.

7. An RN from an obstetric unit is assigned to the pediatric intensive care unit to replace an RN who is home sick with the flu. Which patient will you assign to this RN?
   1. A 1-month-old baby with pyloric stenosis, second day in the hospital.
   2. A 2-year-old child with bacterial meningitis, second day in the hospital.
   3. A newborn baby with esophageal atresia, first day in the hospital.
   4. A 5-month-old baby with intracranial pressure (ICP), first day in the hospital.

8. You have just finished hearing report on the patients you will be caring for today. Using the following information given to you, which of the patients will you assess first?
   1. A 75-year-old woman, second day in the hospital, with a diagnosis of severe hypertension and congestive heart failure.
   2. A 64-year-old woman, diagnosed with coronary insufficiency, first day in the hospital.
   3. A 48-year-old woman, first day in the hospital, complaining of chest pain and headache.
   4. A 28-year-old woman, first day in the hospital, with signs and symptoms of cardiogenic shock.

9. You are the head nurse on a medical/surgical unit, and you have been instructed by the nurse supervisor to send home one of the patients on your unit to make room for a patient injured in a car accident. You will send home the
   1. A 38-year-old male, third day in the hospital, diagnosis hydronephrosis.
   2. A 48-year-old male, fourth day in the hospital, diagnosis pheochromocytoma.
   3. A 58-year-old male, second day in the hospital, diagnosis Buerger's disease.
   4. A 26-year-old female, second day in the hospital, diagnosis polycythemia vera.

10. You are the charge nurse on a pediatric unit. Which of the following patients will you assign to your most experienced RN? The child with a diagnosis of
    1. Nephrotic syndrome, 3-year-old, third day in the hospital.

    2. Failure to thrive syndrome, 1-year-old, first day in the hospital.
    3. Bacillary dysentery, 4-year-old, second day in the hospital.
    4. Botulism, 2-year-old, first day in the hospital.

11. A medical surgical nurse has been assigned to your pediatric unit. Which of the following patients will you assign this nurse? The child's first day in the hospital with a diagnosis of
    1. Hirschsprung's disease, 2-week old.
    2. Celiac disease, 5-month-old.
    3. Intussusception, 4-month-old.
    4. Malignant optic nerve tumor, 3-year-old.

12. You are assigned four babies on an obstetric unit. Which new baby will you assess first? The baby with a diagnosis of
    1. Myelocele, a spinal defect.
    2. Phenylketonuria (PKU).
    3. Pyloric stenosis.
    4. Esophageal atresia.

13. You have listened to report on the patients you will care for on a pediatric unit. Which one of the four patients assigned to you will you assess immediately after report? The child with a diagnosis of
    1. Hydrocephalus, 3-year-old, first day in the hospital.
    2. Gastroenteritis, 4-year-old, second day in the hospital.
    3. Bacillary dysentery, 3-year-old, first day in the hospital.
    4. Cystic fibrosis, 4-year-old, third day in the hospital.

14. You are the charge nurse on a pediatric unit. Which of the following patients will you assign to an obstetrical RN transferred to your unit? The child diagnosed with
    1. ABO hemolytic disease, 1-week-old, third day in the hospital.
    2. Cystic fibrosis disease, 2-week-old, first day in the hospital.
    3. Cerebral palsy, 1-month-old, first day in the hospital.
    4. Bacterial meningitis, 6-year-old, second day in the hospital.

15. You were assigned four patients admitted to the psychiatric unit yesterday. Which patient will you assess first? A patient diagnosed with
    1. Panic disorder, second day in the hospital.
    2. Anorexia nervosa, first day in the hospital.
    3. Bipolar disorder, 2 weeks in the hospital.
    4. Major depression, first week in the hospital.

16. You are the charge nurse on a psychiatric unit. Which of the following patients will you assign to your most experienced RN? The patients were admitted 3 days ago to the unit with a diagnosis of

1. Bipolar disorder.
2. Alzheimer's disease.
3. Paranoid personality.
4. Borderline personality.

17. You are the head nurse on a psychiatric unit, and you have been instructed by the nurse supervisor to send home one of the patients on your unit to make room for an emergency admission. Which of the following patients will you send home? The patient diagnosed with
    1. Schizoid avoidance personality, first day on the unit.
    2. Passive-aggressive personality, second day on the unit.
    3. Major depression, second day on the unit.
    4. Borderline personality disorder, fourth day on the unit.

18. You are the charge nurse on a psychiatric unit. Which of the following patients will you assign to your most inexperienced RN? The patients were admitted to the unit yesterday. The patient diagnosed with
    1. Schizophrenic disorder
    2. Borderline personality disorder
    3. Obsessive-compulsive disorder
    4. Major depression.

19. You have just finished receiving reports on the patients you will be caring for today. Using the following information, you will assess which patient first?
    1. A 50-year-old man with a diagnosis of borderline personality disorder, third day in the hospital. He tells the nurse that "All nurses are bad and I hate every one of you. I am angry and I want all of you to know it."
    2. A 20-year-old male patient is admitted with a cocaine addiction. This is his first day on the unit. His vital signs have shown some improvement. He tells the nurse, "I have finally accepted God's help and I know I can now stop using cocaine. Therefore, I really don't need to be in this place any longer."
    3. A 30-year-old patient with a diagnosis of passive-aggressive personality. This is his first day on the unit. He tells the nurse, "I know you don't appreciate or care about me, but that is OK, you have to do what you have to do."
    4. A 20-year-old female with a diagnosis of obsessive-compulsive disorder. This is her second day on the unit. She tells the nurse, "This place is driving me crazy. No one understands that I have to do what I have to do, or I will die."

20. You are assigned to a musculoskeletal unit in the AM. The following four patients have been admitted to the unit during the night. Using the following information, you will assess which patient first?
    1. Male patient with a cast on his left ankle with signs of severe edema. The patient has complained to the nurse during the night that the pain in his ankle is getting worse.
    2. A female patient in Buck's traction, with a hip fracture.
    3. Female patient with a left shoulder rotator cuff injury scheduled for surgery at 3 PM. She tells the nurse, "I am having stabbing sharp pain in my back every time I move and the pain medication is not helping me."
    4. A male patient scheduled for open reduction on his left tibia at 1:00 PM. He has a large amount of ecchymoses covering the injured area.

QUESTIONS 21 TO 30: CASE HISTORY

Patient's diagnosis was made the day of admission to the hospital. The patient you will assign to a psychiatric-trained RN transferred to a medical/surgical unit is the patient diagnosed with

21. 1. Cerebral palsy, second day in the hospital.
    2. Trigeminal neuralgia, second day in the hospital.
    3. Rape-trauma syndrome, first day in the hospital.
    4. Hyperactive active manic patient, third day in the hospital.

22. 1. Pancreatic cancer, third day in the hospital.
    2. Pernicious anemia, second day in the hospital.
    3. Bulimia, second day in the hospital.
    4. Major depression, second day in the hospital.

23. 1. Alcohol and cocaine, approximately 16 years of age, fourth day in the hospital.
    2. Muscular dystrophy, 30 years of age, second day in the hospital.
    3. Alzheimer's disease, 80 years of age, third day in the hospital.
    4. Bell's palsy, 98 years of age, second day in the hospital.

24. 1. Esophageal varices, 68 years of age, second day in the hospital.
    2. Anorexia nervosa, 19 years of age, second day in the hospital.
    3. Gastritis, 53 years of age, third day in the hospital.
    4. Ulcerative colitis, 43 years of age, second day in the hospital.

25. 1. Bipolar disorder, with a new diagnosis of cancer, 28 years of age, second day in the hospital.
    2. Toxic shock syndrome, 17 years of age, first day in the hospital.
    3. Parkinson's disease demonstrating signs of depression, 30 years of age, second day in the hospital.
    4. Spinal hyperreflexia/quadriplegic, 18 years of age, first day in the hospital.

26. 1. Dilated cardiomyopathy, third day in the hospital.
    2. Alcohol abuse, first day in the hospital.
    3. Rheumatoid arthritis, first day in the hospital.
    4. Infectious mononucleosis, second day in the hospital.

27. 1. Simple goiter, first day in the hospital.
    2. Hyperparathyroidism, second day in the hospital.
    3. Noncompliant diabetic mellitus, third day in the hospital.
    4. Epilepsy, third day in the hospital.

28. 1. Reye's syndrome, 15 years of age, second day in the hospital.
    2. Parkinson's disease, 23 years of age, second day in the hospital.
    3. Spinal cord injury caused by lifting the front of a car, 18 years of age, third day in the hospital.
    4. Sexually abused 16-year-old, third day in the hospital.

29. 1. Pneumothorax, first day in the hospital.
    2. Adenomyosis, second day in the hospital.
    3. Amenorrhea, second day in the hospital.
    4. Agoraphobia, first day in the hospital.

30. 1. Advanced Alzheimer's disease and pneumonia, first day in the hospital.
    2. Schizoid avoidance personality and sickle cell anemia, second day in the hospital.
    3. Senile dementia and bronchiectasis, first day in the hospital.
    4. Coma with dehydration, first day in the hospital.

End of Case

QUESTIONS 31 TO 40: CASE HISTORY

Patient's diagnosis was made the day of admission to the hospital. The patient you will assign to a medical/surgical trained RN transferred to an obstetric unit is the patient diagnosed with

31. 1. Respiratory distress, 1 day old.
    2. Hypoglycemia, 4 days old.
    3. Subnormal temperature, age 2 hours after birth.
    4. PKU, age 5 hours after birth.

32. 1. Respiratory syncytial virus (RSV), 1 day old.
    2. PKU, 2 days old.
    3. Galactosemia, 1 day old.
    4. Cerebral palsy, 3 days old.

33. 1. A 30-year-old mother's fetus is given a nonstress test and the result is considered a nonreactive nonstress test, mother's first day in hospital.
    2. A 40-year-old with degenerative changes in her uterus, late in her pregnancy, first day in the hospital.
    3. A 20-year-old with Braxton Hicks contractions and a positive Homan's sign in calf of leg, second day in the hospital.
    4. A 32-year-old with placenta previa, scheduled for a cesarean section, first day in the hospital.

34. 1. Breech presentation, 16 years of age, first day in the hospital.
    2. Postdelivery/active syphilis, 30 years of age, second day in the hospital.
    3. Active labor, active gonorrhea, 25 years of age, first day in the hospital.
    4. Threatening abortion with moderate vaginal bleeding, 38 years of age, 5 months pregnant, first day in the hospital.

35. 1. Pregnant 8 months with swollen cervix and dysuria, second day in the hospital.
    2. Uterine rupture during labor, 41 years of age, first day in the hospital.
    3. Ectopic pregnancy, 30 years of age, 3 months pregnant, first day in the hospital.
    4. Abruptio placenta with vaginal bleeding, 28 years of age, first day in the hospital.

36. 1. Hyperbilirubinemia, 4-day-old infant.
    2. Cocaine-addicted neonate.
    3. Lethargic neonate.
    4. Erythema toxicum neonatorum, 1-day-old infant.

37. 1. Respiratory distress, 3-day-old infant.
    2. Telangiectatic nevi, 1-day-old infant.
    3. Postmaturity, 43-week-old infant, weight 12 lb, hypoglycemic, 1-day-old infant.
    4. Elevated temperature of 104°F, 1-day-old infant.

38. 1. Endometritis related to membranes rupture 24 h before delivery of fetus.
    2. Active herpes simplex virus type 2 (HSV-2) in active labor.
    3. Threatening abortion, 9 weeks of gestation.
    4. Narcotic-addicted mother in active labor.

39. 1. Human immunodeficiency virus, 3-day-old infant.
    2. Congenital heart defect neonate.
    3. Kernicterus, neonate.
    4. Elevated temperature of 105°F, 3-day-old infant.

40. 1. Episiotomy infection, temperature of 105°F, second day in the hospital.
    2. Postpartum depression (blues), third day postdelivery.
    3. Soft fundus, with vaginal bleeding, first day in the hospital.
    4. Ectopic pregnancy, scheduled for laparotomy, first day in the hospital.

End of Case

QUESTIONS 41 TO 45: CASE HISTORY

Patient's diagnosis was made the day of admission to the hospital. The patient you will assign to a pediatric-trained RN transferred to a psychiatric unit is the patient diagnosed with

41. 1. Alzheimer's disease, second day in the hospital.
    2. Paranoid schizophrenia, third day in the hospital.

3. Borderline personality, fourth day in the hospital.

4. Obsessive-compulsive disorder, first day in the hospital.

42. 1. Schizoid avoidance personality disorder, second day in the hospital.

2. Borderline personality disorder, third day in the hospital.

3. Obsessive-compulsive disorder, fourth day in the hospital.

4. Paranoid, first day in the hospital.

43. 1. Delusional disorder, first day in the hospital.

2. Cocaine withdrawal, fourth day in the hospital.

3. Passive-aggressive personality, third day in the hospital.

4. Panic disorder, third day in the hospital.

44. 1. Phobic disorder, first day in the hospital.

2. Anorexia nervosa, first day in the hospital.

3. Bipolar disorder, first day in the hospital.

4. Major depression, third day in the hospital.

45. 1. Schizophrenia, first day in the hospital.

2. Angry outbursts, episodes of hitting coworkers, first day in the hospital.

3. Passive-aggressive personality, first day in the hospital.

4. Alcohol abuse, first day in the hospital.

End of Case

QUESTIONS 46 TO 52: CASE HISTORY

Patient's diagnosis was made the day of admission to the hospital. The patient you would assign to an orthopedic-trained RN transferred to a neurologic unit is the patient diagnosed with

46. 1. Myasthenia gravis, first day in the hospital.

2. Guillain-Barré syndrome, first day in the hospital.

3. Malignant brain tumor, third day in the hospital.

4. Spinal cord injury and paresthesia, second day in the hospital.

47. 1. Tetanus, second day in the hospital.

2. Parkinson's disease, third day in the hospital.

3. Lou Gehrig's disease, first day in the hospital.

4. Huntington's disease, fourth day in the hospital.

48. 1. Trigeminal neuralgia, second day in the hospital.

2. Epilepsy, first day in the hospital.

3. Brain attack, second day in the hospital.

4. Cerebral aneurysm, fourth day in the hospital.

49. 1. Guillain-Barré syndrome, first day in the hospital.

2. Comatose, first day in the hospital.

3. Brain abscess, third day in the hospital.

4. Bell's palsy, second day in the hospital.

50. 1. Lou Gehrig's disease, third day in the hospital.

2. Spinal hyperreflexia, third day in the hospital.

3. Trigeminal neuralgia, second day in the hospital.

4. Paraplegia, first day in the hospital.

51. 1. Malignant brain tumor, third day in the hospital.

2. Herpes zoster, first day in the hospital.

3. Peripheral neuritis, first day in the hospital.

4. Huntington's disease, third day in the hospital.

52. 1. Parkinson's disease, second day in the hospital.

2. Brain attack, first day in the hospital.

3. Epilepsy, second day in the hospital.

4. Multiple sclerosis, first day in the hospital.

End of Case

QUESTIONS 53 TO 57: CASE HISTORY

Patient's diagnosis was made the day of admission to the hospital. The patient you will assign to obstetric-trained RN transferred to a medical/surgical unit is the patient diagnosed with

53. 1. Cardiogenic shock, second day in the hospital.

2. Congestive heart failure, fourth day in the hospital.

3. MI, fourth day in the hospital.

4. Spontaneous angina, second day in the hospital.

54. 1. Stenosis of the mitral valve, third day in the hospital.

2. Rheumatic fever, fourth day in the hospital.

3. Ventricular tachycardia, second day in the hospital.

4. Dilated cardiomyopathy, third day in the hospital.

55. 1. Ulcerative colitis, second day in the hospital.

2. Severe Cohn's disease, third day in the hospital.

3. Diverticulosis disease, second day in the hospital.

4. Bleeding peptic ulcer, third day in the hospital.

56. 1. Breast cancer, first day in the hospital.

2. Lung cancer, second day in the hospital.

3. Progressive disseminated histoplasmosis, second day in the hospital.

4. Acute tuberculosis, third day in the hospital.

57. 1. Pulmonary embolism, third day in the hospital.

2. Pulmonary edema, second day in the hospital.

3. Spontaneous pneumothorax, first day in the hospital.

4. Lung abscess, second day in the hospital.

End of Case

QUESTIONS 58 TO 64: CASE HISTORY

Patient's diagnosis was made the day of admission to the hospital. The patient you will assign to gynecology-trained RN transferred to a medical/surgical unit is the patient diagnosed with

58. 1. Pancreatitis, third day in the hospital.

2. Pancreatic cancer, fourth day in the hospital.

    3. Pernicious anemia, second day in the hospital.

    4. Dysmenorrhea, first day in the hospital.

59. 1. Laryngeal cancer, third day in the hospital.

    2. Endometriosis, first day in the hospital.

    3. Acute cystitis, second day in the hospital.

    4. Paralytic ileus, fourth day in the hospital.

60. 1. Amenorrhea, first day in the hospital.

    2. Glomerulonephritis, second day in the hospital.

    3. Appendicitis, first day in the hospital.

    4. Hepatitis, fourth day in the hospital.

61. 1. Adenomyosis, second day in the hospital.

    2. Benign prostate hypertrophy, third day in the hospital.

    3. Urinary retention, first day in the hospital.

    4. Urethritis, fourth day in the hospital.

62. 1. Nephrotic syndrome, third day in the hospital.

    2. Hyperkalemia, first day in the hospital.

    3. Hydronephrosis, second day in the hospital.

    4. Breast cancer, first day in the hospital.

63. 1. Acute cystitis, first day in the hospital.

    2. Bladder cancer, third day in the hospital.

    3. Female infertility related to chlamydia infection, first day in the hospital.

    4. Total cystectomy, third day in the hospital.

64. 1. Nephrotic syndrome, second day in the hospital.

    2. Urinary retention, first day in the hospital.

    3. Peritonitis, fourth day in the hospital.

    4. Infertility related to dysfunctional uterine bleeding, first day in the hospital.

QUESTIONS 65 TO 70: CASE HISTORY

Patient's diagnosis was made the day of admission to the hospital. The patient you will assign to orthopedic-trained RN transferred to a medical/surgical unit is the patient diagnosed with

65. 1. Paget's disease, third day in the hospital.

    2. Spontaneous pneumothorax, first day in the hospital.

    3. Colitis, second day in the hospital.

    4. Marfan's syndrome, second day in the hospital.

66. 1. Peripheral neuropathy, third day in the hospital.

    2. Addison's disease, second day in the hospital.

    3. Kaposi's sarcoma, third day in the hospital.

    4. Amputation left leg, third day in the hospital.

67. 1. Squamous cell carcinomas, second day in the hospital.

    2. Multiple myeloma, third day in the hospital.

    3. Rheumatoid arthritis, second day in the hospital.

    4. Hodgkin's disease, third day in the hospital.

68. 1. Cushing's disease, fourth day in the hospital.

    2. Gout, second day in the hospital.

    3. Malignant melanoma, third day in the hospital.

    4. Toxoplasmosis, third day in the hospital.

69. 1. Hip fracture, first day in the hospital.

    2. Hypertension, first day in the hospital.

    3. Hypothyroidism, second day in the hospital.

    4. Trigeminal neuralgia, second day in the hospital.

70. 1. Parkinson's disease, third day in the hospital.

    2. Compound fracture of the femur, first day in the hospital.

    3. Leg ulcers, first day in the hospital.

    4. Renal calculi, third day in the hospital.

End of Case

QUESTIONS 71 TO 85: PRIORITIZING ADMINISTRATION OF MEDICATIONS

Physicians ordered the following medications for four different patients to be administered at 12 noon. These four patients have been in the hospital for 1 day and have the following diagnosis. Which of these patients should receive his or her medications first? The patient diagnosed with

71. 1. Hypertension, drug ordered is Inderal PO.

    2. Congestive heart failure, drug ordered is Digoxin IV.

    3. Chronic open-angle glaucoma, drug ordered is Diamox.

    4. Epilepsy generalized seizure, drug ordered is Dilantin IV.

72. 1. Pulmonary edema, drug ordered is Lasix PO.

    2. Intrinsic asthma, drug ordered is Aminophylline IV.

    3. Hypertension, drug ordered is Vasotec PO.

    4. Congestive heart failure, drug ordered is Accupril IV.

73. 1. Congestive heart failure, drug ordered is Lanoxin IV.

    2. Severe hypertension, drug ordered is Nipride IV.

    3. Cardiac dysrhythmias, drug ordered is Pronestyl PO.

    4. Old MI, drug ordered is Zocor IV.

74. 1. Ventricular dysrhythmia, drug ordered is Lidocaine IV, first day in the hospital.

    2. Brain attack, drug ordered is Heparin IV, third day in the hospital.

    3. Total knee replacement, drug ordered is Fragmin SC, fourth day in the hospital.

    4. Anemia caused by chemotherapy, drug ordered is Epogen SC, first day in the hospital.

75. 1. Endometriosis, drug ordered is Depo-Provera IV.

    2. Addison's disease, drug ordered is Cortone IV.

    3. Atherosclerosis in coronary arteries, drug ordered is Lopid IV.

    4. Raynaud's disease, drug ordered is Inderal PO.

76. 1. Cryptosporidium, drug ordered is Amphotericin B IV.

    2. Hepatitis B, drug ordered is Cortef IV.

3. Acute open-angle glaucoma, drugs ordered are Betoptic and Pilocar, two drops in eyes at 12 noon.

4. Systemic mycoses, drug ordered is Amphotericin B IV.

77. 1. Hepatic encephalopathy, drugs ordered are Lactulose PO and Neomycin PO.

2. Human immunodeficiency virus, drug ordered is Pyridoxine PO.

3. Pernicious anemia, drug ordered is Cyanocobalamin PO.

4. Bipolar disorder, drug ordered is Lithium PO.

78. 1. Nephrotic syndrome, drug ordered is Solu-Medrol IV.

2. Cerebral palsy, drug ordered is Diazepam PO.

3. Multiple sclerosis, drug ordered is Lioresal PO.

4. Cystic fibrosis, drug ordered is Viokase PO.

79. 1. Meningitis (bacterial), with signs of increased intracranial pressure, drugs ordered are Dilantin IV and Mannitol IV.

2. Asthma, drugs ordered are Aminophylline PO and cortisone PO.

3. Ménière's disease, drugs ordered are Dramamine and Hydro-Diuril PO.

4. Nephrotic syndrome, drugs ordered are Lasix and Solu-Medrol IV.

80. 1. Ulcerative colitis, drugs ordered are Lomotil and Donnatal PO.

2. Cirrhosis of the liver, drugs ordered are Aqua Mephyton PO and Spironolactone PO.

3. Pernicious anemia, drug ordered is Cyanocobalamin IM.

4. Brain abscess, drugs ordered are Mannitol IV, Dexamethasone IV, and Penicillin G (aqueous) IV.

81. 1. Myasthenia gravis, drugs ordered are Neostigmine and Mestinon.

2. Parkinson's disease, drug ordered is Sinemet PO.

3. Hypoparathyroidism, drug ordered is Calcium gluconate IV.

4. Hyperparathyroidism, drug ordered is Didronel IV.

82. 1. Hyperosmolar coma, drug ordered is 100 units of humulin R insulin in 500 mL of normal saline (NS).

2. Diabetic ketoacidosis, drug ordered is 40 units of Humulin R insulin in 300 mL of NS.

3. Diabetes insipidus, drug ordered is Pitressin SC.

4. Hypothyroidism (myxedema), drug ordered is Synthroid IV.

83. 1. Cushing's disease, drug ordered is mitotane (Lysodren) PO.

2. Pheochromocytoma, drugs ordered are Inderal IV and Capoten IV.

3. Deep thermal burns on lower fourth of body, drug ordered is Silvadene cream.

4. Congestive heart failure, drugs ordered are Lasix PO and Digoxin PO.

84. 1. Bipolar 1 disorder, manic type, drug ordered is Lithium Carbonate PO.

2. Severe panic disorder, drug ordered is Tofranil.

3. Obsessive-compulsive disorder, drugs ordered are Xanax and Prozac PO.

4. Major depression, drugs ordered are Tofranil and Zoloft PO.

85. 1. Preeclampsia, drugs ordered are Magnesium Sulfate and Hydralazine.

2. Postpartum bleeding, drug ordered is continuous IV infusion of Oxytocin.

3. Premature rupture of membranes at 38 weeks of gestation, drug ordered is Pitocin IV.

4. Precipitated labor drug ordered at 39 weeks of gestation, drug ordered is Pitocin.

86. Using the numbers 1 to 13, establish the correct procedure for insertion of an intravenous catheter.

____ Distend veins by applying tourniquet 8 to 10 inches above site, tap vessel or have patient open and close fist, or hang arm over side of the bed.

____ Hold skin taut to stabilize vein.

____ Clean site with alcohol swab, start at center and work outward.

____ Explain procedure, check ID.

____ Put on sterile gloves.

____ Insert catheter bevel up (direct method: thrust catheter through skin and vein in one smooth motion; indirect method: first pierce skin, then vessel).

____ When you see blood return, advance catheter one-fourth inch and then remove tourniquet.

____ Lessen the angle and advance catheter, watch for flashback of blood.

____ Secure catheter.

____ Attach IV tubing.

____ Begin IV infusing.

____ Check for infiltration or hematoma.

____ Withdraw needle from catheter, advance up to hub.

87. Check the boxes A to F that are related to iron deficiency anemia.

A. ____ Bleeding
B. ____ Iron PO extended-release
C. ____ Vitamin B_{12}
D. ____ Milk
E. ____ Decreased hemoglobin
F. ____ Premature infants

88. Using the numbers 1 to 6, put the cardinal movements of labor in their correct order.

____ Expulsion
____ Restitution
____ Extension
____ External rotation (shoulder rotation)
____ Internal rotation
____ Engagement, descent, and flexion

89. Check the boxes 1 to 5 that are related to placenta previa.
1. ____ Placenta separation prior to delivery of fetus
2. ____ Painless vaginal bleeding
3. ____ Suspected vaginal bleeding occurring after 24 weeks of gestation
4. ____ Bleeding is associated with stretching and thinning of the lower uterine segment
5. ____ Bleeding may be concealed

QUESTIONS 90 TO 96: FILL IN THE BLANK

90. You would anticipate the physician administering the medication ____ to a patient diagnosed with bradycardia.

91. You would anticipate the physician administering the medication ____ to a patient diagnosed with ventricular dysrhythmias.

92. You are caring for a patient diagnosed with thyroid cancer the first day after a thyroidectomy. The patient shows signs of muscle excitability. Your first and correct interventions will be ____ and ____.

93. When surgery for hyperparathyroidism is contraindicated, you will anticipate that the medical management of this patient's high calcium level by the physician will include ____ and ____.

94. The test used to assess for prostate cancer is ____.

95. The leading cause of death of people 65 years and older is ____.

96. The recommended milliliters of fluid that the elderly should intake in 24 h is ____.

QUESTIONS 97 TO 99: SELECT THE BEST ANSWER FROM WITHIN THE PARENTHESES

97. The effect of medications last (longer or shorter) in the elderly?

98. Is (more or less) medication needed to achieve a given blood level in the elderly?

99. When teaching a patient with a broken left tibia how to climb the stairs, you will tell him or her to put up the (right foot or left foot) first?

QUESTION 100: PROVIDE THE ANSWER

100. Name two of the most common medications used to treat congestive heart failure.

ANSWERS AND RATIONALES

1. **❶** Bacterial meningitis is a serious central nervous system (CNS) disease caused by an invasion of the meninges by bacteria. Can cause increased intracranial pressure (ICP) and death of the brain. This patient is still in very serious condition because he or she has been in the hospital for only 2 days and it takes several days for the antibiotics to control the bacteria. This will be the first patient you will assess in this scenario.

2. Ménière's disease is an inner ear disorder that causes vertigo, nausea, and vomiting. This is not a life-threatening disorder. The patient is put on bed rest and treated with Dramamine and antiemetics. Long-term management includes a diuretic and restricted sodium intake. This patient will be the fourth patient you will assess in this scenario.

3. Diabetic mellitus is a chronic disease resulting from a deficiency or resistance to insulin. Episodes of hyperglycemia and hypoglycemia can be serious but usually can be treated successfully. Remember you are not caring for the patient when he or she was first admitted. This will be the third patient you will assess.

4. Graves' disease (hyperthyroidism) is excess of the thyroid hormones T_3 and T_4. The most dangerous signs are hypertension and tachycardia; both of these conditions usually are treated successfully but they can be very dangerous. This will be the second patient you will assess in this scenario. Although this is the patient's second day and the patient's symptoms of hypertension and tachycardia are being treated, you will assess this patient second.

2. **❸** You will discharge from the hospital the patient with a diagnosis of sickle cell anemia. The main treatment of sickle cell anemia is hydration, and this process would be completed by the second day. Bone marrow transplant may also be considered but would occur at a later date.

1. A patient with AIDS is characterized by progressive decline of the immune system. The patient becomes very susceptible to opportunistic infections. A patient with AIDS on his or her first day in the hospital probably will be in crisis.

2. A patient with hemophilia has a bleeding disorder, and this condition must be under control before he or she can be sent home. This is the patient's first day in the hospital.

4. Aplastic anemia can be a life-threatening disease. Platelets, white blood cells (WBCs), and red blood cells (RBCs) will be decreased. This is only the second day in the hospital for this patient.

3. **❷** You will assess the patient with the diagnosis of an MI first because this patient had an MI yesterday, so he or she could have another MI or develop ventricular arrhythmias. Once a patient has developed a blood clot, the probability of developing another is greater. Death from an MI can be swift, so assessing symptoms early and continuously is very important. This patient's age is 60 years; therefore, the patient is more at risk for a medical crisis than the other patients who are younger.

1. COPD is a chronic disease. This is the patient's second day in the hospital, so treatment would be established. You would assess this patient because you may have to perform tracheobronchial suctioning in order to maintain a clear airway.

3. SLE is a chronic disease in which tissue and cells are damaged by pathogenic autoantibodies. The body produces antibodies against its own cells. Thrombosis in vessels of any size can be a major problem. Renal effects include hematuria, proteinuria, and renal failure. This is the third day in the hospital, and the patient's treatment would be established. Death will not occur rapidly as it can with an MI.

4. Rocky Mountain spotted fever is transmitted by a tick bite. This disease can be fatal but usually can be treated with antibiotics. You will assess this patient last. The patient will have received antibiotics for 3 days.

4. ❸ You will assign the patients diagnosed with multiple sclerosis and with gangrene of the left toe to the obstetric-trained RN. Remember when an obstetric-trained RN is assigned to a medical/surgical unit, you will always assign that RN to the patient who has the least life-threatening situation because there usually are no obstetric patients on a medical/surgical unit. The patient diagnosed with gangrene, first day in the hospital, will be under medical assessment to determine if the left large toe will have to be amputated. The patient can care for himself or herself with only minimum assistance. The patient will be on antibiotics, which the obstetric RN can administer. The other patient that you will assign to the obstetric-trained RN is the patient with a diagnosis of multiple sclerosis. MS is the gradual demyelination of the myelin sheath in the brain and spinal cord. Signs are muscle weakness, paralysis, ataxia (defective muscle coordination), urinary incontinence, blurred vision, and mood swings. Seventy percent of these patients can lead active and productive lives, so this patient will also be assigned to the obstetric-trained RN. Remember MS is a major cause of chronic disability in young adults.

1. Cystic fibrosis is the most common fatal genetic disease of white children. The average life expectancy is 24 years, with maximum survival of 30 to 40 years. Cystic fibrosis is generalized dysfunction of the exocrine glands, affecting multiple organ system in varying degrees of severity. The enzymes secreted from the pancreas becomes so tenacious that they plug the pancreatic ducts, causing cells to atrophy and destroy their ability to produced enzymes. Therefore, amylase, lipase, and trypsin cannot reach the duodenum. Lipase breaks down fat, trypsin breaks down protein, and amylase breaks down starches. Cystic fibrosis causes the lung to fill with mucus, leading to a serious threat to life. The child must be suctioned frequently. The child may expectorate as much as 200 to 300 mL of blood in 24 h. This patient will be assigned to a medical/surgical RN. The patient diagnosed with breast cancer, third day in the hospital, will also need the care of a medical/surgical–trained RN. This patient is in her early postoperative state and needs the care of a medical/surgical–trained RN.

2. A patient with total hip replacement must be moved in or out of bed very carefully. An obstetric-trained RN nurse would not have these skills. The patient in renal failure, first day in the hospital, may be in a life-threatening situation and needs the care of a trained medical/surgical RN.

4. A patient with congestive heart failure (CHF) has serious heart and lung problems and should not be in the care of an obstetric-trained RN. CHF is a chronic disease, and patients with chronic disorders usually are not in immediate danger of death. However, this is the patient's first day in the hospital, so this patient would require more care than if it was his or her third or fourth day in the hospital. A patient with Guillain-Barré syndrome has demyelination of the nerves, which causes muscle weakness that usually ascends from the legs to chest and facial nerves in approximately 24 to 72 h. Supportive tracheal intubation may be needed. Recovery usually is spontaneous and complete in 95 percent of patients.

5. ❸ A patient with severe prolapsed mitral valve scheduled for a valve replacement will be in serious condition, and you must assign this patient to the most competent registered nurse. Prolapsed mitral valve can lead to severe arrhythmias and CHF.

1. A patient diagnosed with hypothyroidism, first day in the hospital, will be the second patient you will assign to an experienced RN. This patient will have bradycardia and hypotension and will be receiving Synthroid to control these symptoms.

2. Leukoplakia vulvae is an atrophic disease that affects the female external genitalia. It is seen most often in older women and is characterized by severe itching of the skin. Without medical intervention, the skin may undergo malignant degeneration. This patient could be assigned to a less experienced RN or LPN.

4. A patient with deep thermal burns over the lower half of the body you will assign to an RN who has worked with other patients with burn injuries. The burns are on the lower half of the body, so the patient's airway is not a problem. This will be the second patient you will assess. The nurse will assess urinary function because of the location of the burns. If these burns were on the upper half of the body, this patient would be in critical condition and you will have assessed this patient first. Remember the upper half of the body includes the neck and head.

6. ❹ You will assign the pediatric RN to the most critical pediatric patient you have, the 8-year-old with cystic fibrosis. See answer 4, rationale (1) for more information.

1. The 5-year-old child with hydrocephalus, second day in the hospital, is in for the surgical/medical management of a head shunt. Special care is needed, but the child usually is not in critical condition. Hydrocephalus is an excessive accumulation of cerebrospinal fluid (CSF) within the ventricular spaces of the brain. It occurs most often in newborns, but it also can occur in adults as a result of injury or disease. In infants, hydrocephalus enlarges the head. In both infants and adults, the resulting compression can damage brain tissue. With early detection and surgical intervention, prognosis improves but remains guarded. Without surgery, prognosis is poor. Mortality may result from increased ICP in persons of all ages; infants also may die prematurely of infection and malnutrition.

2. The 3-year-old with nephrotic syndrome, first day in the hospital, has large amounts of protein excreted through the urine.

This reduces the serum albumin level, which causes the fluid to shift from the intervascular system to body cavities, causing some degree of hypotension. Treatment consists of bed rest and a high-protein diet. This child needs special care but is not in as critical condition as is the patient with cystic fibrosis.

3. Spina bifida is the incomplete closure of one or more vertebrae without protrusion of the spinal cord or meninges. It is often accompanied by a depression with a tuft of hair. This baby needs special care because of the baby's age and the possibility, although rare, of neurologic defect.

7. ❸ You will assign the obstetric RN to the baby who is most critically ill, the newborn with esophageal atresia. Remember, you assign to an obstetric nurse an obstetric patient if there is one on the unit. Remember, the 1-month-old, 2-year-old, and 5-month-old children are pediatric patients, not obstetric patients. A newborn with esophageal atresia, first day in the hospital, will require emergency surgery because of the danger of aspiration.

1. Pyloric stenosis is hypertrophy of the circular muscle of the pylorus. At approximately 3 weeks of age, the infant begins to regurgitate small amounts of milk immediately after feeding. The vomit is propelled the distance of several feet. This baby must be monitored for aspiration but is not as serious as the newborn with esophageal atresia, and the 3-week-old is not an obstetric patient.

2. The 2-year-old child diagnosed with bacterial meningitis, second day in the hospital, needs to be assigned to the most experienced RN who has worked with pediatric patients diagnosed with bacterial meningitis because injury to the brain is irreversible; therefore, very close monitoring is important to prevent increased ICP.

4. A 5-month-old baby diagnosed with ICP, first day in the hospital, will be assigned to the most competent RN who has worked with patients diagnosed with ICP because damage to the brain is irreversible.

8. ❹ The patient you will assess first is the 28-year-old woman, first day in the hospital, with signs and symptoms of cardiogenic shock. Cardiogenic shock is any condition that causes severe dysfunction of the left ventricle, such as MI or severe CHF. This is a crisis situation; the patient may die.

1. The 75-year-old patient diagnosed with severe hypertension and CHF will be the second patient you will assess. This patient must be assessed carefully to be sure medications are controlling the woman's hypertension and CHF.

2. The 64-year-old woman diagnosed with coronary insufficiency, first day in the hospital, will be the third patient you will assess. This patient's coronary arteries are partially occluded, and the patient will undergo angioplasty or atherectomy and possibly stent insertion.

3. The 48-year-old woman, first day in the hospital, complaining of chest pain and headache will be the fourth patient you will see. The chest pain is not a cardiac condition because that would be diagnosed by the second day.

9. ❹ You will send home the 26-year-old female, second day in the hospital, diagnosis polycythemia Vera. *Vera* means

chronic and *polycythemia* means excessive RBCs. By the second day, this patient's RBC volume will be reduced by phlebotomy and hydration, and the patient needs to be ambulatory to prevent thrombosis. Therefore, this patient can be discharged from the hospital with instructions to make an appointment with her physician.

1. Hydronephrosis is distention of the renal pelvis caused by obstruction. The most common causes are benign prostatic hypertrophy, urethral strictures, and calculi. Signs and symptoms usually are severe renal pain and gross urinary abnormalities, such as hematuria, pyuria, and dysuria, alternating oliguria and polyuria, or complete anuria. Treatment is surgical removal of the obstruction by prostatectomy or dilation of urethra.

2. Pheochromocytoma is a tumor that results in hyperactivity of the adrenal gland. It is a catecholamine-secreting tumor usually found in the adrenal medulla. The excessive amounts of catecholamines (epinephrine, norepinephrine, and dopamine) secreted by the adrenal medulla produce severe signs and symptoms of hypertension, tachycardia, and hyperglycemia.

3. Buerger's disease is inflammation and subsequent thrombus formation in small and medium arteries and sometimes veins resulting in decreased blood flow to the feet and legs. This disorder may produce ulceration and eventually gangrene. Buerger's disease produces intermittent claudication in the calf of the legs.

10. ❹ You will assign your most competent RN to care for the 2-year-old, diagnosis botulism, first day in the hospital. Botulism is a life-threatening paralytic illness that results from an exotoxin produced by gram-positive bacterium *Clostridium botulinum*. Botulism usually results from ingestion of inadequately cooked contaminated foods. Treatment consists of IV fluids and IM administration of botulinum antitoxin.

1. Nephrotic syndrome is a condition characterized by marked proteinuria, hypoalbuminemia, hyperlipemia, and edema. Prognosis is highly variable, depending on the underlying cause. The dominant clinical feature of nephrotic syndrome is mild to severe dependent edema of the ankles, sacrum, or periorbital region, especially in children. Accompanying symptoms may include orthostatic hypotension, lethargy, anorexia, and depression. Major complications are malnutrition, infection, coagulation disorders, and thromboembolic vascular occlusion. Effective treatment of nephrotic syndrome is correction of vascular volume deficit, a high-protein diet, sodium restriction, diuretics for edema, and antibiotics for infection. This 3-year-old needs to be assigned to an RN that has cared for children having renal disorders. This child is 3 years old, third day in the hospital, and is not as critical as the 2-year-old, first day in the hospital.

2. Failure to thrive syndrome is also known as maternal deprivation. Failure to thrive is a common disorder of infancy. The child tends to be unlivable, stiff, and rigid, is uncomforted and unyielding to cuddling or holding, and is very slow to smile or socially respond to others. Treatment includes nutritional intake and loving care, and meeting the emotional needs of the infant. The younger the child, the better the prognosis because the child will not have had as long a history of maternal deprivation. This

baby needs to be assigned to an RN who loves to work with very young children.

3. Bacillary dysentery is an acute intestinal infection caused by the bacterium *Shigella*. Prognosis is good. Mild infections usually subside within 10 days; severe infection may persist for 2 to 6 weeks. Signs and symptoms include high fever, diarrhea, nausea, vomiting, irritability, and abdominal pain. Treatment of bacillary dysentery includes low-residue diet and replacement of fluids and electrolytes with IV infusion of normal saline, with electrolytes in sufficient quantities to maintain a urine output of 40 to 50 mL/h. Antibiotics may be useful. Antidiarrheals (e.g., Lomotil) that slow intestinal motility are contraindicated in the treatment of bacillary dysentery because it delays the excretion of *Shigella* and prolongs the fever and diarrhea. This patient may be assigned to an RN who has cared for children with dysentery.

11. **❹**   You will assign the medical surgical RN to the 3-year-old child diagnosed with a malignant optic nerve tumor. The child will have to be assessed for increased intracranial and intraocular pressures, and the medical/surgical nurse has the experience of working with increased intracranial and intraocular pressures in adult patients. This is also the oldest of the children, but none of them are obstetric patients and all of the other diseases occur only in children. This is a slow-growing tumor; signs and symptoms include visual deficits (decreased acuity), which can cause blindness. Surgical excision is sometimes possible when only one optic nerve is involved. Chemotherapy may be beneficial for children younger than 5 years and is preferable because radiation is very destructive to the tissue of very young children.

1. Hirschsprung's disease is a congenital disease of the large intestine characterized by the absence or marked reduction of parasympathetic ganglion cells in the intestinal wall. This disorder impairs intestinal mobility and causes severe constipation. Without prompt treatment, an infant with colon obstruction may die of shock within 24 h. The newborn fails to pass meconium within 24 to 48 h, shows signs of obstruction, bile-stained or fecal vomiting, abdominal distention, and overflow diarrhea caused by enterocolitis.

2. Celiac disease is characterized by poor food absorption and intolerance of gluten, a protein in wheat and wheat products. With treatment (eliminating gluten from the patient's diet) prognosis is good, but residual bowel changes persist in adults. Advise elimination of wheat, barley, rye, and oats and foods made from these grains, such as bread. Suggest substitution of corn and rice. Advise the parents to consult a dietitian for a gluten-free diet, which is high in protein and low in carbohydrates and fats. Instruct patient to read all labels before buying food products to be sure they are gluten-free.

3. Intussusception is telescoping of the bowel into an adjacent distal portion. Intussusception is most common between the ages of 4 and 11 months. The cause is unknown. If intussusception is severe, it may be fatal if treatment is delayed more than 24 h. Signs and symptoms include "current jelly" stools, which contain a mixture of blood and mucus, and a tender, distended abdomen with a palpable, sausage-shaped abdominal mass. For

treatment of hydrostatic reduction, the radiologist drips a barium solution into the rectum from a height of approximately 3 inches, then fluoroscopy traces the progress of the barium. If this procedure is successful, the bowel is pushed back into place. If the hydrostatic reduction (barium enema) fails, surgery is performed.

12. **❹**   You would assess the baby with esophageal atresia first. This is caused by the failure of the embryonic esophagus and trachea to develop and separate correctly. In the most common abnormality, the upper section of the esophagus terminates in a blind pouch. Esophageal atresia usually is a surgical emergency. Preoperative and postoperative suctioning is required to prevent aspiration.

1. Myelocele is like spina bifida; it rarely causes neurologic deficits. In myelocele, there is incomplete closure of one or more vertebrae, causing protrusion of the spinal content in an external sac. This sac contains meninges, CSF, and a portion of the spinal cord.

2. PKU is an inborn error in phenylalanine metabolism, resulting in high serum levels of phenylalanine, causing mental retardation. Early detection and treatment can minimize this cerebral damage. Almost all states now require screening for PKU at birth. The infant should be reevaluated after he has received dietary protein for 24 to 48 h. Treatment consists of restricting intake of the amino acid phenylalanine to keep phenylalanine blood levels between 3 and 9 mg/dL. Lofenalac powder or Pregestimil powder is substituted for milk in the diets of affected infants. Dietary restriction usually is continued throughout life.

3. Pyloric stenosis: see answer 7, rationale (1).

13. **❹**   You would assess the child diagnosed with cystic fibrosis first because of the danger of respiratory arrest. See answer 4, rationale (1).

1. Hydrocephalus: see answer 6, rationale (1).

2. Gastroenteritis is characterized by diarrhea, nausea, vomiting, and abdominal cramping. Gastroenteritis has many causes, such as bacteria (responsible for acute food poisoning), viruses, or ingestion of toxin, plants, toadstools, or food allergens.

3. Bacillary dysentery is an acute intestinal infection caused by the bacterium *Shigella*. Prognosis is good with prompt treatment.

14. **❶**   You would assign the baby diagnosed with ABO hemolytic disease to the obstetric nurse. The obstetric RN would have worked with babies diagnosed with ABO hemolytic disease. ABO incompatibility occurs between mother and fetus in approximately 25 percent of pregnancies. Although ABO incompatibility is more common than Rh isoimmunization, it is less severe. Signs and symptoms of ABO incompatibility include jaundice, which usually appears in newborns in 24 to 48 h. Diagnosis is made by a weak to moderately positive Coombs' test and elevated serum bilirubin levels. Treatment is blood transfusion with blood of the same group and Rh type as that of the mother. Because infants with ABO incompatibility respond so well to phototherapy, exchange transfusion is seldom necessary. Unlike Rh isoimmunization, which always follows sensitization during a previous pregnancy, ABO incompatibility is likely to develop in a firstborn infant.

A fetus with Rh-positive cells will experience hemolysis and anemia. To compensate, the fetus increases the production of RBCs and erythroblast (immature RBCs). Extensive hemolysis results in the release of large amounts of unconjugated bilirubin, which the liver is unable to conjugate and excrete, causing hyperbilirubinemia and hemolytic anemia. Administration of RhoGAM immune human globulin to an unsensitized Rh-negative mother as soon as possible after birth of an Rh-positive infant prevents complications in subsequent pregnancies.

2. Cystic fibrosis disease is a generalized dysfunction of the exocrine glands, affecting multiple organs in varying degrees of severity. The clinical effects may become apparent soon after birth or may take years to develop. The sodium and chloride concentrations of sweat normally increase with age. The respiratory system accumulates thick, tenacious secretions in the bronchioles and alveoli, eventually leading to severe atelectasis and emphysema. Pneumonia, emphysema, or atelectasis usually causes death. Obstruction of the pancreatic duct results in deficiency of trypsin, amylase, and lipase, preventing the conversion and absorption of protein, starch, and fat, respectively, in the intestinal tract. The undigested food is excreted in bulky, foul-smelling, pale stools. The inability to absorb fat produces deficiency of fat-soluble vitamins (A, D, E, and K), leading to clotting problems, retarded bone growth, and delayed sexual development.

The child's diet should be low in fat, high in protein, high in calories, salt tablets, and soluble vitamins (A, D, E, and K).

3. Cerebral palsy is the most common cause of crippling in children. The spastic form of cerebral palsy is the most common, affecting 70 percent of patients. This form is characterized by hyperactive, deep tendon reflexes; rapid alternating muscle contractions and relaxation; muscle weakness; underdevelopment of affected limbs; muscle contraction in response to manipulation; and a tendency toward contractures. Typically, a child with spastic cerebral palsy walks on his toes with a scissor gait, crossing one foot in front of the other. In early diagnosis, the infant has difficulty sucking or keeping nipple or food in his or her mouth; seldom moves voluntarily; and crosses his or her legs when lifted from behind rather than pulling the legs up like a normal infant. Infants at high risk for cerebral palsy include those with low birth weight and babies with low Apgar scores at 5 min.

Treatment includes braces or splints; range-of-motion-exercises to minimize contractures; orthopedic surgery; phenytoin (Dilantin); and muscle relaxants.

4. Bacterial meningitis is a serious CNS infection caused by an infection of the meninges by bacteria. For more information see answer 7, rationale (2).

15. ❹ You would assess the patient diagnosed with major depression first because he or she may be suicidal. Signs and symptoms, which include weight loss of 1 lb/week without dieting; insomnia; energy loss; fatigue; loss of interest or pleasure in activities; decreased sex drive; and difficulty with concentration. Recurrent suicide thoughts or death wishes may cause the patient to commit suicide.

1. Panic disorder is a brief period of intense apprehension or fear; it may last minutes or hours. The patient will have a history of three or more panic attacks within 3 weeks that are unrelated to life-threatening situations and not related to phobias, thus confirming panic disorder.

During a panic attack, the patient will have symptoms of chest pain, palpitations, dyspnea, choking or smothering feeling, shaking and trembling, and fear of going crazy. When caring for this patient, your role is primarily supportive. Your goal is to help the patient develop effective coping mechanisms to manage the anxiety.

2. Anorexia nervosa probably is a mental disorder characterized by self-imposed starvation and consequent emaciation. Anorexia nervosa usually develops in a patient whose weight is normal or who may be 4 or 5 lb overweight. Treatment aims to promote weight gain. Patient is offered frequent, small portions of food and drink. Discuss with patient the need for food in a matter-of-fact manner. Encourage patient to recognize and assert her feelings freely. If she understands that she can be assertive, she may gradually learn that expressing her true feelings will not result in her losing control of herself. Remember that the patient may use manipulation and lying as mechanisms to preserve the only control she feels she has in her life. The patient's family may need therapy to uncover and correct faulty family interactions.

3. Bipolar disorder is marked by severe pathologic mood swings ranging from euphoria to sadness. The patient has separate episodes of mania (elation) and depression that can begin anytime after adolescence. This illness is associated with significant mortality; 20 percent of patients die as a result of suicide, many just as the depression lifts. Drug therapy consists of monoamine oxidase inhibitors (MAOIs) such as phenelzine (Nardil) and the tricyclic antidepressant imipramine (Tofranil). This patient has been in the hospital 2 weeks, so medication would begin to be effective.

16. ❹ The patient diagnosed with borderline personality you would assign to your most experienced RN. These patients have impulsive and unpredictable behavior in self-damaging areas: spending, gambling, substance abuse, shoplifting, and overeating; they are very manipulative, pitting others (including staff) against each other. You need a very experienced RN to care for this patient.

1. Bipolar disorder, see answer 15, rationale (3).

2. Alzheimer's disease is primary degenerative dementia accounting for more than half of all dementias. The cause is unknown. Signs and symptoms are insidious initially. The patient experiences forgetfulness, recent memory loss, deterioration in personal hygiene, progressive difficulty in communication, severe deterioration in memory, and loss of motor function that results in loss of communication and inability to write or speak. The patient becomes very susceptible to infection and accidents. The RN needs to offer emotional support to the patient and

family. Protect the patient from injury by providing a safe, structural environment. Teach family about the disease.

3. The patient diagnosed with paranoid personality is very suspicious, concerned with hidden motives, social isolation, poor self-image, coldness, detachment, and absence of tender feelings. The patient needs to feel in control, is argumentative, is conflict with authority, and is jealous. This patient would be the second in line to be assigned to an experienced RN. The reason this patient is not the first in line to be assigned to an experienced RN is because he or she is not manipulative.

17. ❶ You will send home the patient diagnosed with schizoid avoidance personality. A patient with schizoid personality is suspicious, hypersensitive to criticism, is subject to social withdrawal, and has poor self-image. Schizoid patients are not schizophrenic. Schizoid patients maintain a firm grip on reality. Their major problem is their inability to relate warmly to other people. Schizoid patients rarely, if ever, appear to experience anger or joy. This patient can be sent home because he or she is not a danger to self or others. He or she is reclusive and lives with parents or in isolation.

2. Patients with passive-aggressive personality tend to perceive the world, and themselves, as negative. For example, these patients search for mistakes, faults, and injustices in almost all situations. They have low self-confidence and resentment toward authority figures. The passive-aggressive person avoids seeking adaptive solutions through learning and problem solving; therefore, it is not surprising that he or she often develops anxiety and depressive episodes as well as suicidal crisis; therefore, this will not be the patient you discharge from the hospital.

3. Major depression, see answer 15, rationale (4).

4. Borderline personality disorders, see answer 16, rationale (4).

18. ❸ You will assign the patient with a diagnosis of obsessive-compulsive disorder to your most <u>inexperienced</u> RN. This behavior is manifested by physically repetitive touching, doing and undoing (opening and closing doors and rearranging things), washing hands repeatedly. This patient is not a danger to self or others. Allow the patient time to carry out the ritualistic behavior until he or she can be distracted into some other activity. Blocking these behaviors raises anxiety to an intolerable level. Encourage the patient to express his or her feelings about anxiety that causes the compulsive behavior.

1. Schizophrenic disorder is marked mainly by withdrawal into self and failure to distinguish reality from fantasy. The *Diagnostic and Statistical Manual of Mental Disorders, Fourth Edition* (DSM IV) recognizes five types of schizophrenia: catatonic, paranoid, disorganized, undifferentiated, and residual. An estimated two million Americans may suffer from the disease. No single symptom or characteristic is present in all schizophrenic disorders. The five subtypes differ markedly. This group of disorders is marked mainly by withdrawal into self and failure to distinguish reality from fantasy. *Paranoid schizophrenia* is characterized by persecutory or grandiose delusional thought content and delusional jealousy. These conditions may be associated with patient's anger, argumentativeness, and violence. This type of schizophrenia tends to develop in later life.

2. Borderline personality disorders, see answer 16, rationale (4).

4. Major depression, see 15, rationale (4).

19. ❷ You will assess the 20-year-old male patient with a diagnosis of cocaine addiction first. This is the patient's first day in the hospital. He is still in critical condition. The patient must be monitored very closely for seizures, ventricle fibrillation, and cardiac standstill. This patient is in a life-threatening situation.

1. Borderline personality disorders, see 16, rationale (4).

3. Passive-aggressive personality, see answer 17, rationale (2).

4. Obsessive-compulsive disorders, see answer 18, rationale (3).

20. ❶ You would assess first the patient with a cast on his left ankle with signs of severe edema, who is complaining of pain in that area. This is a sign of compartment syndrome, which is an increase of pressure within the closed space of the tissue compartment. This can create sufficient pressure to obstruct circulation and cause venous and arterial occlusion. As ischemia continues, muscle and nerve cells are destroyed. Delayed treatment can result in irreversible muscle and nerve damage. This can produce a useless or severely impaired extremity.

2. Buck's traction is generally used for temporary immobilization and stabilization of a fractured hip or fracture of the femoral bone.

3. A rotator cuff injury is very painful. The patient is not scheduled for surgery until 3:00 PM, so there is no need to assess this patient first.

4. The patient scheduled for open reduction of his left tibia at 1:00 PM and has ecchymoses covering the injured area is not in need of immediate assessment. Ecchymosis is the discoloration of skin as a result of the broken bone injury surrounding tissue. The nurse should reassure the patient that this process is normal.

21. ❸ You would assign the psychiatric-trained RN to the patient experiencing rape-trauma syndrome. This patient needs psychological support. The rape victim experiences powerlessness, loss of control, fear, shame, guilt, humiliation, rage, and feelings of being contaminated or "dirty," all of which may be overwhelming. The psychiatric nurse is trained to work with patients having psychological problems, not medical problems.

1. Cerebral palsy, see answer 14, rationale (3).

2. Trigeminal neuralgia (tic douloureux) is a painful disorder caused by one or more branches of the fifth cranial (trigeminal) nerve that produces paroxysmal attacks of excruciating facial pain. It occurs mostly in people older than 40 years, in women more often than in men, and on the right side more often than on the left side. Trigeminal neuralgia can subside spontaneously, with remissions lasting for several months to 1 year. Treatment consists of oral administration of Tegretol or Dilantin. If medical measures fail or attacks become increasingly frequent or severe, neurosurgical procedures may provide permanent relief.

4. Hyperactive active manic individuals experiencing a manic episode have an inflated view of their importance. ("I'm so important that the president of the USA needs my advice on

international affairs.") The episode presents as an elevated or irritable mood. Symptoms include a decreased need for sleep, talkativeness, flights of ideas, and distractibility. They may speculate on a risky business venture because they believe they understand the big picture of business. People have lost everything in such periods of manic thinking. They will go on expensive spending sprees. This patient can be treated with medication, which will help control his or her moods. This is the patients third day in the hospital.

22. **4** You would assign the psychiatric-trained RN to the patient diagnosed with major depression. This is the only patient in this scenario who has a psychological problem; therefore, the patient would be assigned to the psychiatric-trained RN.

1. Pancreatic cancer is second only to cancer of the colon as the deadliest gastrointestinal (GI) cancer. Prognosis is poor, and most patients die within 1 year after diagnosis.

2. Pernicious anemia is characterized by decreased gastric production of hydrochloric acid and deficiency of intrinsic factors, a substance normally secreted by parietal cells of the gastric mucosa that is essential for vitamin B_{12} absorption. Familial incidence of pernicious anemia suggests a genetic predisposition. Gastrectomy, either partial or complete, will result in a decrease in intrinsic factor and hydrochloric acid causing pernicious anemia. The patient will have to take vitamin B_{12} by IM injection for the rest of his or her life.

3. There are three core criteria for bulimia nervosa. (1) Recurrent episodes of uncontrolled binge eating (eating an unusually large amount of food in a short period of time). (2) Various behaviors designed to control shape and weight, such as extreme dieting, excessive exercising, self-induced vomiting, taking laxatives or diuretics, use of diet pills, or abuse of enemas/suppositories. (3) Persistent overconcern with body shape and weight. This patient needs psychological support, but not as much as the patient diagnosed with major depression.

23. **1** The patient diagnosed with the abuse of alcohol and cocaine you will assign to the psychiatric-trained RN. This 16-year-old is a chemically dependent patient who will need psychological support. This patient needs to recover from the dependency and addiction; however, the potential for relapse also must be addressed. The patient will have postacute withdrawal; these symptoms include difficulty in thinking clearly; managing feelings, emotions, and stress; remembering things; and sleeping. The nurse should confirm that arrangements for aftercare, outpatient counseling, and self-help support group meetings are made before discharge.

2. Muscular dystrophy is a group of congenital disorders characterized by progressive symmetric wasting of skeletal muscles without neural or sensory defects. Paradoxically, these wasted muscles tend to enlarge because of connective tissue and fat deposits, giving an erroneous impression of muscle strength. Four main dystrophies occur, with Duchenne's muscular dystrophy accounting for 50 percent of all cases.

Duchenne's muscular dystrophy generally strikes during early childhood and results in death within 10 to 15 years of onset. This is an X-linked recessive disorder, affecting males most often. Duchenne's muscular dystrophy begins insidiously between the ages of 3 and 5 years. Initially it affects legs and pelvic muscles, but eventually it spreads to the involuntary muscles. Muscle weakness produces a waddling gain, toe walking, and lordosis (abnormal anterior convexity of the spine). Later in the disease, progressive weakening of cardiac muscle causes tachycardia, ECG abnormalities, and pulmonary complications. Death commonly results from sudden heart failure or severe respiratory infection.

3. Alzheimer's disease or dementia of the Alzheimer's type is the form of dementia commonly seen in the elderly. It is the most prevalent of all nonreversible dementias, accounting for 50 to 75 percent of all diagnosed cases of dementia.

The criteria for dementia of the Alzheimer's type are as follows:

a. *Amnesia:* inability to learn new information or to recall previously learned information

b. *Agnosia:* failure to recognize or identify objects despite intact sensory function

c. *Aphasia:* language disturbance that can manifest in both understanding and expressing the spoken word

d. *Apraxia:* inability to perform motor activities despite intact motor function (e.g., ability to grab a doorknob but not knowing what to do with it.)

Language disability progresses from expressive aphasia to receptive aphasia to mindless repetition of words. *Behavior* progresses from indifference to agitation. *Memory dysfunction* progresses from recent memory loss to recent/remote memory loss and can reach the point where the patient does not know his or her own name. *Motor function* is spared except in the advanced stage. *In this advanced stage,* the patient eventually becomes emaciated, helpless, and bedridden. The most frequent cause of death is pneumonia and other infections, with malnutrition and dehydration as contributing factors.

4. Bell's palsy is a disease of the seventh cranial nerve (facial) that produces unilateral facial weakness or paralysis. Onset is rapid. It occurs most often in persons younger than 60 years. In 80 to 90 percent of patients, it subsides spontaneously, with complete recovery in 1 to 8 weeks. If recovery is partial, contractures may develop on the paralyzed side of the face. Bell's palsy usually produces unilateral facial weakness, occasionally with aching pain around the angle of the jaw or behind the ear. On the weak side, the mouth droops (causing the patient to drool saliva from the corner of the mouth), and taste perception is lost over the anterior portion of the tongue. The patient's ability to move the eye on the weak side is impaired. Advise patient to protect the eye by covering it with an eye patch, especially when outdoors.

24. **2** Anorexia nervosa is a more dangerous disorder than bulimia nervosa. You would assign the patient diagnosed with anorexia nervosa to the psychiatric-trained RN because this patient has serious psychological problems.

◆ *Anorexia nervosa:* disorder characterized by restrictive eating resulting in emaciation, amenorrhea, disturbance in body image, and an intense fear of becoming obese.

◆ *Amenorrhea:* absence of menstruation.

(a) *Binge:* eating an unusually large amount of food in a relatively short period of time

(b) *Restricting type:* during an episode of anorexia nervosa, the person *does not* engage in recurrent episodes of binge eating or purging.

(c) *Binge eating/purging type:* during an episode of anorexia nervosa, the person engages in recurrent episodes of binge eating and purging.

◆ *Bulimia nervosa:* disorder characterized by binge eating, purging, and overconcern with body shape and weight.

There are four criteria for anorexia nervosa:

1. Refusal to maintain body weight at or above a minimum normal weight for age and height

2. Intense fear of gaining weight or becoming fat, even though the person is underweight

3. Disturbance in the way in which one's body weight or shape is experienced, overvaluing of shape or weight, or denial of seriousness of low weight

4. In females, the absence of at least three consecutive menstrual cycles

1. Esophageal varices is caused by portal hypertension (elevated pressure in the portal vein), which occurs when blood flow meets increased resistance. The disorder is the result of cirrhosis of the liver. Bleeding of dilated tortuous veins often causes massive hematemesis, requiring emergency treatment to control hemorrhage and prevent hypovolemic shock. Placement of a Minnesota or Sengstaken-Blakemore tube may help control hemorrhage by applying pressure on bleeding site.

3. Gastritis, an inflammation of the gastric mucosa, may be acute or chronic. Acute gastritis, the most common stomach disorder, produces mucosal reddening, edema, hemorrhage, and erosion. Gastritis is common in persons with pernicious anemia (as chronic atrophic gastritis). Although gastritis can occur at any age, it is more prevalent in the elderly. Acute gastritis usually results from the gram-negative bacterium *Helicobacter pylori;* ingestion of alcoholic beverages; irritating drugs, such as nonsteroidal antiinflammatory agents; aspirin; spicy foods; caffeine; and tobacco. Treatment usually consists of eliminating gastric irritants and taking antacids, mucosal protectants, and antisecretory agents. If the cause is *H. pylori,* then an antibiotic (e.g., Flagyl) will be used to eradicate the bacteria.

4. Ulcerative colitis is an inflammatory, often chronic, disease that affects the mucosa of the colon. It usually begins in the rectum and sigmoid colon and often extends upward into the entire colon; it rarely affects the small intestine. Severity ranges from a mild, localized disorder to a fulminant disease that may cause a perforated colon, progressing to potentially fatal peritonitis and toxemia. Ulcerative colitis occurs primarily in young adults, especially women. The cause of is unknown. The goals of treatment are to control inflammation, replace nutritional losses and blood volume, and prevent complications. Supportive treatment includes bed rest, IV fluid replacement, and clear liquid diet. Drug therapy includes adrenal corticosteroids, such as prednisone and hydrocortisone, antispasmodics such as tincture of belladonna, and antidiarrheals such as Lomotil.

25. ❶ You would assign the patient diagnosed with bipolar disorder to the psychiatric-trained RN. All of the other diagnoses are medical. Bipolar disorders are those in which individuals experience the extremes of mood polarity. Persons may feel very euphoric or very depressed. Although the term *bipolar* is the accepted diagnostic terminology, many professionals, and much of the professional literature, still use the term *manic-depressive.* Often mood swings are not severe enough to warrant hospitalization; however, problems with everyday life still occur. *Hypomania* is the term for an elevated state that is less intense than full mania.

a. Bipolar episodes are divided into bipolar I and bipolar II. There are six categories of bipolar I. In bipolar I, the patient must have a history of a manic episode.

b. Bipolar II: Patient has experienced major depression and a hypomanic episode (but not a manic episode).

c. Cyclothymic disorder: For a period of 2 years, the patient has had numerous periods of *hypomanic symptoms* and numerous periods of a depressed mood. The patient is never symptom-free for more than 2 months at a time. The patient has *never* experienced major depression.

See answer 15, rationale (3) for more information on bipolar disorder.

2. Toxic shock syndrome (TSS) is an acute bacterial infection caused by penicillin-resistant *Staphylococcus aureus,* generally in association with continuous use of tampons during the menstrual period. It usually affects menstruating women younger than 30 years. A strong correlation exists between TSS and use of superabsorbent tampons. Incidence is rising, and the recurrence rate is approximately 30%. Signs and symptoms of TSS include fever over 104°F, vomiting, diarrhea, headache, decreased level of consciousness, rigors, conjunctival hyperemia, and vaginal hyperemia and discharge. Severe hypotension occurs with hypovolemic shock. Within a few hours of onset, a deep red rash develops, especially on the palms and soles, and later desquamates. Treatment consists of IV antistaphylococcal antibiotics that are beta-lactamase–resistant, such as oxacillin, nafcillin, and methicillin. To reverse shock, expect to replace fluids with saline solution and colloids, as ordered.

3. Parkinson's disease, see answer 28, rationale (2).

4. Spinal hyperreflexia occurs most often in quadriplegics and is an emergency, requiring immediate attention. Autonomic dysreflexia is an exaggerated autonomic response that may occur with spinal cord injury. Most common with cervical and high thoracic injuries. Signs and symptoms include severe hypertension and bradycardia. Treatment and prevention include emptying the bowel or bladder on a regular basis and immediately

if hyperreflexia occurs. Atropine is given to raise the heart rate in bradycardia. Emotional support is given and antihypertensive drugs are administered.

26. ❷ You would assign the patient diagnosed with alcohol abuse to the psychiatric-trained RN. Alcohol is considered to be both a psychological and a biologic disorder. Psychological treatment emphasizes behavioral management techniques. Biologic studies have shown genetic predisposition as the single most significant factor identifying alcoholism. The patient with a diagnosis of alcohol abuse, first day in the hospital, needs psychological support so that he or she will stay in treatment.

1. Dilated cardiomyopathy results from extensively damaged myocardial muscle fibers. This disorder interferes with myocardial metabolism and grossly dilates the ventricles without proportional compensatory hypertrophy, causing the heart to become very large and to contract poorly during systole. Dilated cardiomyopathy leads to intractable CHF, arrhythmias, and emboli. Because this disease usually is not diagnosed until it is in the advanced stages, prognosis is generally poor. The cause is unknown.

3. Rheumatoid arthritis is a chronic inflammatory disease that primarily attacks peripheral joints and surrounding muscles, tendons, ligaments, and blood vessels. Spontaneous remissions and unpredictable exacerbations mark the course of the potentially crippling disease. Rheumatoid arthritis usually requires lifelong treatment and sometimes surgery. Rheumatoid arthritis occurs three times more often in females than males.

4. Infectious mononucleosis is an acute infectious disease caused by the Epstein-Barr virus (EBV). It primarily affects young adults. Symptoms of mononucleosis mimic those of other infectious diseases and include fever, sore throat, and cervical lymphadenopathy (the hallmarks of the disease), as well as hepatic dysfunction, increased lymphocytes and monocytes, and development and persistence of heterophil antibodies. Prognosis is excellent and major complications are uncommon. EBV is spread by the oropharyngeal route and via blood transfusions.

27. ❸ A patient diagnosed with diabetes mellitus and is not following his or her doctor's orders is called *noncompliant*. The person's blood sugar level will be higher than normal. This patient will need psychological support to help him or her realize the importance of following the diabetic regimen. The patient needs to understand the long-term complications of diabetes, which include retinopathy, nephropathy, atherosclerosis, and peripheral and autonomic neuropathy. Peripheral neuropathy usually affects the hands and feet and may cause numbness or pain. The other three patients do not require the same level of physiologic support as this patient needs.

1. Simple goiter, thyroid gland enlargement that is not caused by inflammation or a neoplasm, is commonly classified as endemic or sporadic. *Endemic goiter* is usually due to inadequate dietary intake of iodine, which leads to inadequate secretion of thyroid hormone. Iodized salt prevents this deficiency. *Sporadic goiter* commonly results from ingestion of large amounts of goitrogenic foods or use of goitrogenic drugs. Goitrogenic foods contain agents that decrease thyroxine production and

include rutabagas, cabbage, soybeans, peanuts, peaches, peas, strawberries, and spinach. Thyroid enlargement may range from a single, small nodule to massive, multinodular goiter. Because simple goiter does not alter the patient's metabolic state, clinical features arise solely from thyroid enlargement and include respiratory distress and dysphagia from compression of the trachea and esophagus and swelling and distention of the neck.

2. Hyperthyroidism is a metabolic imbalance that results from thyroid hormone overproduction. The most common form of hyperthyroidism is Graves' disease, which increases thyroxine production, enlarges the thyroid gland (goiter), and causes multiple system changes. Incidence of Graves' disease is highest between the ages of 30 and 40 years. Graves' disease may result from genetic or immunologic factors. The classic symptoms of Graves' disease are an enlarged thyroid (goiter), nervousness, heat intolerance, weight loss despite increased appetite, sweating, diarrhea, tremor, and palpitations. Treatment includes antithyroid drugs that inhibit thyroid hormone synthesis, such as Tapazole and propylthiouracil (PTU). Initial effects of potassium iodide solution (SSKI) or Lugol's begin to occur within the first 24 h; peak effects develop within 10 to 15 days. One of these iodine solutions together with PTU or Tapazole is administered for the last 10 days prior to subtotal thyroid thyroidectomy.

4. Epilepsy is a condition of the brain marked by susceptibility to recurrent seizures associated with abnormal electrical discharge of neurons in the brain. In about half of all cases of epilepsy, the cause is unknown. However, some possible causes include (1) birth trauma (e.g., inadequate oxygen supply to the brain, blood incompatibility, or hemorrhage); (2) infectious diseases (e.g., meningitis or encephalitis); (3) brain abscess, tumor of the brain, head injury or trauma; (4) metabolic disorders (e.g., hypoglycemia or hypoparathyroidism); and (5) cerebrovascular accident (e.g., hemorrhage, thrombosis, or embolism).

28. ❹ You would assign the sexually abused patient to the psychiatric-trained RN because this patient will have the most psychological problems. See answer (21), rationale 3 for more information.

1. Reye's syndrome is a noninflammatory encephalopathy associated with fatty infiltration of the viscera for which no other chemical or clinical explanation can be found. Typically, symptoms are seen following a viral illness, but a definitive cause has not been identified. Viral infections most strongly associated with the onset of Reye's syndrome are influenza types A and B and varicella. Use of aspirin has also been strongly linked to the onset of the syndrome but is not involved in every case. Even though the American Academy of Pediatrics and the Centers for Disease Control and Prevention have issued warnings against the use of salicylates in children with possible varicella or influenza infection, the link between salicylates and Reye's syndrome remains a topic of intense discussion.

2. Parkinson's disease characteristically produces progressive muscle rigidity, akinesia, and involuntary tremor. Deterioration progresses for an average of 10 years, at which time death usually results from aspiration pneumonia or some other

infection. Parkinson's disease, one of the most common crippling diseases in the United States, affects men more often than women. Although the cause of Parkinson's disease is unknown, study of the extrapyramidal brain nuclei has established that a dopamine deficiency prevents affected brain cells from performing their normal inhibitory function within the CNS. The cardinal symptoms of Parkinson's disease are muscle rigidity and akinesia, and an insidious tremor that begins in the fingers (unilateral pill-roll tremor). It also produces a high-pitched monotone voice; drooling; masklike facial expression; loss of posture control (patient walks with body bent forward); and dysarthria, dysphagia, or both.

3. Most serious spinal injuries result form motor vehicle accidents, falls, diving into shallow water, and gunshot wounds. Less serious injuries result from lifting heavy objects and minor falls.

29. **❹** You would assign the psychiatric RN to the patient diagnosed with agoraphobia. A patient with agoraphobia has a great fear of being alone or of being in public places from which escape might be difficult. Normal activities that involve being in crowds, on a busy street, or in a crowded store are avoided. Exposure to these conditions may cause the individual to panic. The psychiatric nurse will know how to help this patient overcome his or her fear.

1. A pneumothorax is a collection of air or gas in the pleural cavity. The gas enters as the result of a perforation through the chest wall or the pleura covering the lung (visceral pleura).

2. Adenomyosis is a benign invasive growth of the endometrium into the muscular layer of the uterus.

3. Amenorrhea is the absence or suppression of menstruation; normal before puberty, after menopause, and during pregnancy and lactation. The most common causes of abnormal amenorrhea are *congenital abnormalities of the reproductive tract; metabolic disorders* (e.g., obesity, malnutrition, diabetes); *systemic diseases* (e.g., syphilis, tuberculosis, nephritis); *emotional disorders* (e.g., anorexia nervosa); *endocrine disorders* (e.g., especially those involving the ovaries, pituitary, thyroid, and adrenal glands); and *hormonal imbalance* of estrogen, progesterone, or follicle-stimulating hormone.

30. **❷** You will assign the psychiatric-trained RN to the patients diagnosed with schizoid avoidance personality and sickle cell anemia. The schizoid patients are not schizophrenic; the distinguishing characteristics of a schizoid patient are the following:

a. Schizoid patients maintain a firm grip on reality.

b. Their major problem in their inability to relate warmly to other people.

c. They often are reclusive and live with parents or in isolation.

d. They seem to have little need for human contact or comfort. This deficiency is compensated for by an active fantasy life.

e. The diagnostic criteria for schizoid personality disorder are designed to separate this disorder from the more disturbed schizophrenia.

f. No conclusive studies implicate genetic or biologic features.

g. Schizoid patients rarely, if ever, appear to experience anger and joy.

h. Schizoid patients indicate little, if any, desire to have sexual experiences with another person.

Remember, a psychiatric nurse transferred to a medical/surgical floor you will always assign to a patient with a psychological disorder or to the patient with the least serious medical diagnosis.

Sickle cell anemia is a congenital hemolytic anemia that occurs primarily but not exclusively in blacks. It results from a defective hemoglobin molecule (hemoglobin S) that causes RBCs to roughen and become sickle shaped, causing chronic ill health (fatigue, dyspnea on exertion, swollen joints), periodic crises, long-term complications, and premature death. Penicillin prophylaxis can decrease morbidity and mortality from bacterial infections. Half of such patients die by their early twenties; few live to middle age. Characteristically, sickle cell anemia produces tachycardia, cardiomegaly, systolic and diastolic murmurs, pulmonary infarctions (which may result in cor pulmonale), chronic fatigue, unexplained dyspnea or dyspnea on exertion, hepatomegaly, jaundice, pallor, joint swelling, aching bones, chest pains, ischemic leg ulcers (especially around the ankles), and increased susceptibility to infection. Such symptoms usually do not develop until after age 6 months because large amounts of fetal hemoglobin protect infants for the first few months after birth. Treatment includes prophylaxis penicillin, hydration, packed red cell transfusion, and analgesics.

1. Alzheimer's disease, see answer 16, rationale (2).

Pneumonia occurs in people with immune deficiencies, especially the elderly and children younger than 2 years. Pneumonia is an acute infection of the lung parenchyma that often impairs gas exchange. Prognosis is generally good for people who have normal lungs and adequate host defenses before the onset of pneumonia; however, bacterial pneumonia is the fifth leading cause of death in debilitated patients. Symptoms of early bacterial pneumonia are coughing, sputum production, pleuritic chest pain, shaking chills, and fever. Physical signs vary widely, ranging from diffuse, fine rales to signs of localized or extensive consolidation and pleural effusion.

3. Senile dementia occurs in the aged and is characterized by progressive mental deterioration with loss of memory, especially for recent events, and occasional intercurrent attacks of excitement.

Bronchiectasis is a condition marked by chronic abnormal dilation of bronchi and destruction of bronchial walls. Because of the availability of antibiotics for treatment of acute respiratory tract infections, the incidence of bronchiectasis has dramatically decreased in the past 20 years. This disease results from conditions associated with repeated damage to bronchial walls, abnormal mucobronchial walls, and abnormal mucociliary clearance, which causes breakdown of supporting tissue adjacent to airways. Conditions include cystic fibrosis; immunologic disorders; recurrent, inadequately treated bacterial respiratory tract infections, such as tuberculosis; as a complication of measles, pneumonia, pertussis, or influenza; and inhalation of corrosive gas or repeated aspiration of gastric juices into the lungs.

4. Coma is deep sleep, an abnormal deep stupor occurring in illness, as a result of the illness or due to an injury. The patient cannot be aroused by external stimuli. More than 50 percent of cases are a result of trauma to the head or circulatory accidents in the brain caused by hypertension, arteriosclerosis, thrombosis, tumor, abscess formation, or insufficient flow of blood to the brain. Other frequent causes of coma are acute infections of the brain (meninges), effect of drugs (alcohol, barbiturates), trauma caused by severe accidents, and exposure to gases or fumes. The level of consciousness is measured using the Glasgow Coma Scale. Comas are diagnosed by the absence of motor and verbal response and eye opening.

31. **❷** You would assign the medical/surgical-trained RN transferred to an obstetric unit to the 4-day-old infant diagnosed with hypoglycemia. The medical/surgical nurse has had experience working with hypoglycemic patients, and this is the oldest baby in the unit.

1, 3, 4. All three of these babies require the care of an obstetric-trained RN.

32. **❹** You would assign the medical/surgical trained–RN to the 3-day-old baby diagnosed with cerebral palsy because this is the oldest baby in the unit and the disease is not life threatening. See answer 14, rationale (3) for more information.

1. RSV is a highly contagious pathogen. Its primary effect is on the lower respiratory tract. RSV is the only viral disease that has it maximum impact during the first few months of life (incidence peaks at age 2 months). The organism is transmitted from person to person by respiratory secretions and has an incubation period of 4 to 5 days.

2. PKU, see answer 12, rationale (2).

3. A 1-day-old baby diagnosed with galactosemia needs the care of a trained obstetric RN because of the morbidity and mortality resulting from classic galactosemia; prompt recognition of clinical signs and immediate treatment are imperative. Shortly after birth, drops of blood are drawn from the heel and tested for lactose enzyme. If enzyme is not present, the infant will be given soy-based formula. In severe cases, the symptoms begin within the first day of life. Untreated children who survive the neonatal period usually have neurologic deficits and mental retardation. Warn parents to read medication and food product labels carefully to avoid foods containing lactose. Lactose and galactose restriction are lifelong in children with classic galactosemia. Babies with severe respiratory distress require endotracheal intubation and mechanical ventilation.

33. **❸** You will assign the medical/surgical-trained RN to the patient with Braxton Hicks contractions, which are intermittent, painless uterine contractions that may occur every 10 to 20 min. They occur after the third month of pregnancy. These contractions do not represent true labor pains but are often so interpreted. The sign is not present in every pregnancy.

Homan's sign is pain in the calf of the leg when the toes are passively dorsiflexed. This is a sign indicating a possible blood clot in the deep veins but is not positive proof. A positive diagnosis is made by ultrasound or MRI. This patient will stay in bed until a positive diagnosis is made.

1. Nonstress test (NST) is the most widely used technique for antepartum evaluation of the fetus. The basis for NST is that the normal fetus will produce characteristic heart rate patterns in response to fetal movement. In the healthy fetus with an intact CNS, 90 percent of gross fetal body movement is associated with acceleration of fetal heart rate. *This response can be blunted by hypoxia, acidosis, drugs (analgesics, barbiturates, and beta blockers), fetal sleep, and some congenital anomalies.* Generally accepted criteria for a reactive tracing are as follows:

a. Two or more accelerations of 15 bpm lasting for 15 seconds over a 20-min period

b. Normal baseline rate

c. Long-term variability amplitude of 10 or more bpm

If the test does not meet these criteria after 40 min, it is considered nonreactive. In this case, future assessments are needed with a contraction stress test or biophysical profile. A noninvasive dynamic assessment of fetus by ultrasonography is external fetal monitoring.

2. Degenerative changes in the patient's uterus occur most often in patients with a diagnosis of diabetes mellitus type I, and assessment of the fetus is imperative.

4. A 32-year-old with placenta previa scheduled for a cesarean section would be assigned to an obstetric nurse because close fetal assessment is imperative.

34. **❷** The medical/surgical–trained RN will be assigned to the 30-year-old woman with a diagnosis of active syphilis postdelivery because she has cared for other women with active syphilis on the medical/surgical unit. The rest of the options deal directly with obstetric problems.

1. Breech presentation is a common abnormality of delivery where the baby's buttock presents rather than the head. This is a very difficult, delivery especially for a 16-year-old.

3. A patient in active labor diagnosed with gonorrhea will be assigned to an obstetric-trained RN. Gonorrhea can be transmitted to the newborn in the form of ophthalmia neonatorum during vaginal birth by direct contact with gonococcal organism in the cervix.

4. A 38-year-old, 5-month pregnant woman threatening abortion with moderate vaginal bleeding needs medical and psychological support from a trained obstetric RN.

35. **❶** You will assign the 8-month-pregnant woman with a swollen cervix and dysuria to the medical/surgical–trained RN because the woman is not in active labor. A swollen cervix is not a dilated cervix, and the swelling may be from an infection.

2. Uterine rupture during labor could cause death of mother and fetus.

3. Ectopic pregnancy is one in which the fertilized ovum is implanted outside the uterine cavity. Approximately 90 percent of ectopic pregnancies occur in the uterine (fallopian) tube. Ectopic pregnancy is responsible for 10 percent of all maternal deaths.

4. Abruptio placenta is separation of the placenta prior to delivery of the fetus. Varying degrees of placental separation can occur. Most women who present with vaginal bleeding will have increased uterine tone, boardlike abdomen, and abdominal back pain. Bleeding may be concealed within the uterus. Fetal stress is present in more than 50 percent of cases.

36. **④** You will assign the medical/surgical trained–RN to the 1-day-old baby diagnosed with erythema toxicum neonatorum. Erythema toxicum neonatorium is a benign, self-limited occurrence of firm, yellow-white papules or pustules 1 to 2 mm in size that are present in approximately 50 percent of full-term infants. The cause is unknown, and the lesions disappear without need for treatment. Remember you will assign a medical/surgical-trained RN transferred to an obstetric unit to the patient with the least life-threatening diagnosis or to the patient with a medical/surgical problem.

1. Neonatal hyperbilirubinemia occurs in 50 percent of term and 80 percent of preterm newborns. Bilirubin levels must be assessed, and a level greater than 12 mg/dL may indicate either an exaggeration of the physiologic handicap or presence of disease. Kernicterus, the most serious complication of neonatal hyperbilirubinemia, is caused by the precipitation of bilirubin in neuronal cells, resulting in their destruction. Cerebral palsy, epilepsy, and mental retardation may occur if the infant survives kernicterus.

2. Cocaine-dependent neonates do not experience a process of withdrawal seen with narcotics (e.g., opium, morphine, codeine, and heroin). Cocaine-exposed infants suffer from neurotoxic effect of the drug. Signs of exposure include defects such as hydronephrosis, congenital heart disease, skull defects, limb reductions, and neurologic abnormalities.

3. A heroin-dependent neonate will show signs of lethargy, but other causes must be evaluated. The neonate must be continually assessed by an obstetric-trained RN.

37. **②** You will assign the medical/surgical trained RN to the 1-day-old infant with a diagnosis telangiectatic nevi. Telangiectatic nevi is birthmark that may occur anywhere on the skin but is seen most frequently on the face and thighs.

1, 3, 4. The 1-day-old infant in respiratory distress, the infant born weighing 12 lb, and the 1-day-old infant with a 104°F temperature must be in the care of an obstetric-trained RN. These three infants need to be assessed continually. All of these infants are only 1 day old, and the infant assigned to the medical/surgical trained RN is 3 days old. The premature baby weighing 12 lb may have a low blood sugar level. Neonates born to diabetic women usually weigh more than neonates born to nondiabetic women and are usually premature. This information was intentionally not given to you so you can learn to deduct from the information given you. You will need good deduction skills for your RN State Board Examination.

38. **①** You will assign the patient diagnosed with endometritis to the medical/surgical–trained RN. This is the least difficult patient to care for. Endometritis is produced by bacterial invasion of the endometrium.

2, 4. These three patients are in active labor and therefore need an obstetric-trained RN.

3. A patient threatening to abort a 9-week-old fetis needs to be cared for an obstetric-trained RN.

39. **①** You will assign the medical/surgical–trained RN to the 3-day-old patient with a diagnosis of human immunodeficiency virus (HIV). It is estimated that globally more than one million children born to HIV-infected women acquire the virus each year. Typically, the HIV-infected neonate is asymptomatic at birth. These infants tend to be of lower birth weight than those born to noninfected mothers.

2. Congenital heart defects (CHDs) are anatomic abnormalities in the heart that are present at birth, although they may not be diagnosed immediately. Ventricular septal defects, constituting more than 20 percent of all CHDs, is the most common type of acyanotic lesion. Tetralogy of Fallot, constituting 10 percent of all CHDs, is the most common type resulting in cyanosis. After prematurity, CHDs are the next major cause of death in the first year of life. The causes of CHDs are unknown in more than 90 percent of cases. Maternal factors associated with a higher incidence of CHD include maternal rubella, alcoholism, diabetes, poor nutrition, and age greater than 40 years.

3. Kernicterus, the most serious complication of neonatal hyperbilirubinemia, is caused by the precipitation of bilirubin in neuronal cells, resulting in their destruction. Cerebral palsy, epilepsy, and mental retardation may occur if the infant survives kernicterus.

4. A 3-day-old baby with an elevated temperature of 105°F must be cared for by an obstetric-trained RN. The cause must be determined quickly so that the condition can be treated and brain damage from the very high temperature prevented. Measures must be taken immediately to reduce the temperature.

40. **①** You will assign the medical/surgical–trained RN to the patient with a diagnosis of episiotomy infection with a temperature of 105°F. The medical/surgical RN will have worked with patients with infection and high fevers, and this is the least difficult patient. The other three patients have very serious diagnoses.

2. Postpartum depression can cause the patient to want to kill herself or her baby, and the patient may not be capable of caring for her baby.

3. The patient with a diagnosis of a soft fundus and vaginal bleeding must be monitored closely to prevent further bleeding. The fundus must be massaged often to regain firmness.

4. Ectopic pregnancy, see answer 35, rationale (3).

41. **①** In this situation there is no pediatric patient, so you will assign the pediatric-trained RN to the patient with the least difficult psychiatric diagnosis. Patients diagnosed with Alzheimer's disease often are transferred to psychiatric unit for drug treatment of agitation or aggressive behavior and for psychological counseling. Overall care is focused on supporting the patients' abilities and compensating the abilities they have lost. Establish an effective communication system with the patient and the family to help them adjust to the patient's altered cognitive abilities. The patient usually admitted to a psychiatric unit is in the early stages of the disease and usually are not in the unit for very long.

2. Paranoid personality, see answer 16, rationale (3).

3. Borderline personality, see answer 16, rationale (4).

4. Obsessive-compulsive disorder, see answer 18, rationale (3).

42. ❸ You will assign the pediatric-trained RN to the patient with a diagnosis of obsessive-compulsive disorder, fourth day in the hospital. This patient will have received some psychological help in the 4 days, and this patient will be the least difficult to care for compared to the other three patients. For more information see answer 18, rationale (3).

1, 2, 4. These options are incorrect as seen in rationale (3).

43. ❹ You will assign the pediatric-trained RN to the patient with a diagnosis of panic disorder. This is the easiest patient to care for because the patient does not have as serious a psychiatric disorder as the other patients. This patient is not a danger to self or others. For more information see answer 15, rationale (1).

1, 2, 3 Are incorrect as seen in rationale (4).

44. ❶ You will assign the pediatric-trained RN to the patient with a diagnosis of phobic disorder. Phobic disorders are intense, irrational fear responses to an external object, activity, or situation. Anxiety is experienced if the person comes into contact with the dreaded object or situation. Phobias persist even though phobic persons recognize that they are irrational. Persons can control the intensity of anxiety simply by avoiding the object or situation they fear. This is the easiest patient to care for compared to the other three patients, and this patient is not a danger to self or others.

2, 3, 4. These options are incorrect as seen in rationale (1).

45. ❹ You will assign the pediatric-trained RN to the patient with a diagnosis of alcohol abuse, first day in the hospital. The patient usually will not show signs of withdrawal from alcohol the first day in the hospital. Withdrawal symptoms occur approximately 3 to 4 days after the person stops the intake of alcohol. Withdrawal from alcohol can be painful, scary, and even lethal. As the person abstains from alcohol, he or she begins to reap the consequences of the CNS irritation caused by alcohol: tremulousness, nervousness, anxiety, anorexia, nausea and vomiting, insomnia and other sleep disturbances, rapid pulse, high blood pressure, profuse perspiration, diarrhea, fever, unsteady gait, difficulty concentrating, exaggerated startle reflex, and a craving for alcohol or other drugs. As the withdrawal symptoms become more pronounced, hallucinations can occur. The body is in a state of alcohol toxicity and needs detoxification. It is important for the patient undergoing the detoxification process to have a secure environment. Sedation, nutritional supplements, multivitamins, B complex, and magnesium are also recommended during and up to 5 months after detoxification. A calm, secure environment is important because the physical experience of withdrawal can be dramatically influenced by emotional and psychological distress. Sedation can be used to slow and thus ameliorate (moderation of a condition) the withdrawal

process and to calm the anxious, hallucinating, or delirious patient.

1, 2, 3. These options are incorrect as seen in rationale (4).

46. ❹ You will assign the orthopedic-trained RN to the patient with a diagnosis of spinal cord injury and paresthesia. Paresthesia is the sensation of numbness, prickling, or tingling and heightened sensitivity. Paresthesia is not an indication of a serious spinal cord injury. An example of serious spinal cord injuries would be a newly diagnosed quadriplegic. The patient with paresthesia may be able to move himself or herself in bed but would may need help getting out of bed and walking. Paresthesia usually is an indication of a pinched spinal cord nerve. Remember the orthopedic-trained RN has worked with patients with bone disorders. The spinal cord consists of bones and nerves. All bones in the body are very closely related to nerves.

1, 2, 3. These three patients have very serious neurologic problems, and they need a neurology-trained RN to work with them.

47. ❷ You will assign the orthopedic-trained RN to the patient with a diagnosis of Parkinson's disease, third day in the hospital. This patient is not in any immediate danger. This is a chronic, progressive disease caused by dopamine deficiency that prevents affected brain cells from functioning. The cardinal symptoms of Parkinson's disease are muscle rigidity and akinesia, and an insidious tremor that begins in the fingers (unilateral pill-roll tremor), increases during stress or anxiety, and decreases with purposeful movement and sleep. Muscle rigidity results in resistance to passive muscle stretching, which may be uniform (lead-pipe rigidity) or jerky (cogwheel rigidity). Akinesia causes the patient to walk with difficulty. It also produces a high-pitched monotone voice; drooling; masklike facial expression; loss of posture control (patient walks with body bent forward); and dysarthria, dysphagia, or both. Because there is no cure for Parkinson's disease, the primary aim of treatment is to relieve symptoms and keep the patient functional as long as possible. Treatment consists of physical therapy and drugs that usually include levodopa, a dopamine replacement that is most effective during early stages. Because the side effects of dopamine can be serious, levodopa is now frequently given in combination with carbidopa to halt peripheral dopamine synthesis (carbidopa plus levodopa [Sinemet]).

1. Tetanus is caused by the anaerobic spare-forming, gram-positive bacillus *Clostridium*. Transmission is through a puncture wound that is contaminated with soil, dust, or animal excretions containing *Clostridium tetani*. If tetanus develops, the patient will require airway maintenance and a muscle relaxant such as diazepam (Valium) to decrease muscle rigidity and spasm. The patient diagnosed with tetanus has a life-threatening disease and must be cared for by a neurology-trained RN. Remember that within 72 h after puncture wound, a patient who has *not* had tetanus immunization within 10 years needs a booster injection of tetanus toxoid.

3. Amyotrophic lateral sclerosis (ALS; Lou Gehrig's disease) is a chronic, progressively debilitating disease. It is fatal within 2 to 5 years after diagnosis. Reportedly, more than 30,000

Americans have ALS; approximately 5000 are newly diagnosed each year. ALS and other motor neuron diseases may result from several causes. Patients with ALS develop atrophy and weakness, especially in the muscles of the feet and hands. Other signs include impaired speech; difficulty chewing, swallowing, and breathing, particularly if the brainstem is affected; and, occasionally, choking and excessive drooling. Mental deterioration usually does not occur, but patients may become depressed as a reaction to the disease. No effective treatment exists for ALS. Management aims to control symptoms and provide emotional, psychological, and physical support. This patient may have difficulty swallowing and breathing; therefore, the patient must be under the care of a neurology-trained RN, not an orthopedic-trained RN.

4. Huntington's disease is a hereditary disease in which degeneration in the cerebral cortex and basal ganglia causes chronic progressive chorea and mental deterioration, ending in dementia. Huntington's disease usually strikes persons between the ages of 25 and 55 years. Death usually results 10 to 15 years after onset, from suicide, CHF, or pneumonia. The cause is unknown. Because this disease is transmitted as an autosomal dominant trait, either sex can transmit and inherit the disease. Each child of a parent with the disease has a 50 percent chance of inheriting it; however, the child who does not inherit it cannot pass it on to his own children. Because of hereditary transmission, Huntington's disease is prevalent in areas where affected famili ave lived for several generations. Onset is insidious. The pa t eventually becomes totally dependent (emotionally and physically) through loss of musculoskeletal control and develops progressively severe choreic movements. Chorea is a nervous condition marked by involuntary muscular twitching of the limbs or facial muscles. Ultimately, the patient with Huntington's disease develops progressive dementia, although the dementia does not always progress at the same rate as the chorea. Dementia can be mild at first but eventually severely disrupts the personality. Because Huntington's disease has no known cure, treatment is supportive, protective, and symptomatic. Because patients know that they have only 10 to 15 years to live and mental deterioration cannot be stopped, they can become very depressed and attempt suicide. This patient has been cared for by neurology-trained RN for 3 days, and a patient with Huntington's disease needs continuity of care.

48. ❶ You will assign the orthopedic-trained RN to the patient with a diagnosis of trigeminal neuralgia. None of the options have a patient with an orthopedic diagnosis, so you will assign the orthopedic-trained RN to the easiest patient. For more information see answer 21, rationale (2).

2. Epilepsy is a very dangerous disorder. For more information see answer 27, rationale (4).

3. Brain attack (stroke) is a very dangerous disease because increased ICP can cause irreversible brain damage. Brain attack results from one of four events: (1) Blood clot (2) Other material, etc. (3) Decreased blood flow to an area of the brain, etc. (4) Ruptures of cerebral blood vessels, etc.

4. Cerebral aneurysm is localized dilation of a cerebral artery that results from a weakness in the arterial wall. Its most common form is the berry aneurysm, a saclike outpouching in a cerebral artery. Cerebral aneurysms usually arise at an arterial junction in the circle of Willis, the circular anastomosis forming the major cerebral arteries at the base of the brain. Cerebral aneurysms often rupture and cause subarachnoid hemorrhage. Prognosis is guarded. Probably half of patients suffering subarachnoid hemorrhages die immediately; of those who survive untreated, 40 percent die of the effects of hemorrhage; another 20 percent die later from recurring hemorrhage. With new and better treatment, prognosis is improving.

49. ❹ You will assign the orthopedic-trained RN to the patient with a diagnosis of Bell's palsy because this patient's diagnosis is not life threatening. Bell's palsy is a disease of the seventh cranial nerve (facial) that produces unilateral facial weakness or paralysis. Onset is rapid. It occurs most often in those younger than 60 years. In 80 to 90 percent of patients, it subsides spontaneously, with complete recovery in 1 to 8 weeks. If recovery is partial, contractures may develop on the paralyzed side of the face.

1. Guillain-Barré syndrome is an acute, rapidly progressive, potentially fatal form of polyneuritis that causes muscle weakness. Recovery is spontaneous and complete in approximately 95 percent of patients, although mild motor or reflex deficits in the feet and legs may persist. The precise cause is unknown, but it may be caused by a cell-mediated immunologic attack on peripheral nerves in response to a virus or to an influenza vaccination. Significant complications of Guillain-Barré syndrome include mechanical ventilatory failure, aspiration, pneumonia, sepsis, joint contractures, and deep venous thrombosis. Unexplained autonomic nervous system involvement may cause sinus tachycardia or bradycardia, hypertension, postural hypotension, or loss of bladder and bowel sphincter control.

2. A coma is an abnormal deep stupor occurring in illness, as a result of illness, or due to an injury. The patient cannot be aroused by external stimuli. More than 50 percent of cases are a result of trauma to the head or circulatory accidents in the brain caused by hypertension, arteriosclerosis, thrombosis, tumor, abscess formation, or insufficient flow of blood to the brain. Other frequent causes of coma are acute infections of the brain or meninges.

Nursing care for patients in comas, regardless of the cause, includes maintaining a patent airway, monitoring vital signs, performing a neurologic assessment every 4 h, assessing the patient's level of consciousness, and maintaining fluid and electrolyte balance. Also maintain the patient's skin integrity, provide passive range-of-motion exercises, protect the patient's eyes from corneal irritation, and prevent the complications of immobilization. It is important to keep in mind that the level of coma may permit the patient to be aware of the surroundings and to hear all that is said.

3. A brain abscess is a collection of pus within the substance of the brain itself. It may occur by direct invasion of the brain

from intracranial trauma or surgery; by spread of infection from nearby sites such as the sinuses, ears, and teeth (paranasal sinus infections, otitis media, dental sepsis); or by spread of infection from other organs (lung abscess, infective endocarditis). Brain abscess is a complication encountered increasingly in patients whose immune systems have been suppressed through either therapy or disease. To prevent brain abscesses, promptly treat otitis media, mastoiditis, sinusitis, dental infections, and systemic infections. The clinical manifestations of a brain abscess result from alterations in intracranial dynamics (edema, brain shift), infection, or the location of the abscess. Headache usually is worse in the morning. Vomiting is common. Focal neurologic signs (weakness of an extremity, decreasing vision, seizures) may occur, depending on the site of the abscess. There may be a change in the patient's mental alertness as reflected in lethargic, confused, irritable, or disoriented behavior. Fever may or may not be present. Repeated neurologic examinations and continuing assessment of the patient are necessary to determine accurately the location of the abscess. Computed tomography is invaluable in showing the site of the abscess, following the evolution and resolution of suppurative lesions, and determining the optimum time for surgical intervention. The goal of management is to eliminate the abscess. Brain abscess is treated with antimicrobial therapy and surgery. Antimicrobial treatment is given to eliminate the causative organism or reduce its virulence. Large intravenous doses usually are prescribed preoperatively to penetrate brain tissue and brain abscess. The therapy is continued postoperatively. Corticosteroids may be given if the patient shows evidence of an increasing neurologic deficit to help reduce the inflammatory cerebral edema. Anticonvulsant medications (phenytoin, phenobarbital) may be given as prophylaxis against seizures.

50. ❸ You would assign the orthopedic-trained RN to the patient with the diagnosis of trigeminal neuralgia because this is not a life-threatening disease. For more information see answer 21, rationale (2).

1. Lou Gehrig's disease, see answer 47, rationale (3).

2. Spinal hyperreflexia (autonomic dysreflexia) occurs most often in quadriplegics and is an emergency requiring immediate attention. Autonomic dysreflexia is an exaggerated autonomic response that may occur with spinal cord injury. Symptoms are severe hypertension, bradycardia, and a pounding headache usually triggered by bladder distention. Treatment and prevention include emptying the bladder on a regular basis and immediately if hyperreflexia occurs. Atropine is given to treat bradycardia and antihypertensive drugs to treat hypertension.

4. Paraplegia refers to loss of motion and sensation in the lower extremities and all or part of the trunk as a result of damage to the thoracic or lumbar spinal cord or to the sacral root. It most frequently follows trauma due to accidents and gunshot wounds but may be the result of spinal cord lesions (intervertebral disc, tumor, and vascular lesions), multiple sclerosis, infections and abscesses of the spinal cord, and congenital defects. The patient faces a lifetime of great disability, requiring ongoing follow-up and the care of a number of health professionals, including the physician, rehabilitation nurse, occupational therapist, physical therapist, psychologist, social worker, rehabilitation engineer, and vocational counselor at different times as the need arises. Paraplegic patients may have autonomic dysreflexia, but quadriplegics have a much greater change because of greater nerve damage. Long-term complications or paraplegia include bladder and kidney infections, pressure sores with complications of sepsis, osteomyelitis, fistulas, and depression. Flexor muscle spasms may be particularly disabling. The patient requires extensive rehabilitation, which will be less difficult if appropriate nursing management has been carried out during the acute phase of the injury or illness. Nursing care is one of the determining factors in the success of the rehabilitation program. The main objective is for the patient to live as independently as possible in the home community.

51. ❷ You will assign the orthopedic-trained RN to the patient with a diagnosis of herpes zoster, which is not a life-threatening diagnosis. The other three patients have diseases that could be life threatening. Herpes zoster is acute, unilateral, segmental inflammation of the dorsal root ganglia caused by infection with the herpesvirus varicella-zoster, which also causes chickenpox. Prognosis is good unless the infection spreads to the brain. Eventually, most patients recover completely except for corneal damage and visual impairment. Occasionally, neuralgia persists for months or years. Symptoms including severe deep pain, pruritus, and paresthesia or hyperesthesia (increased sensitivity to sensory stimuli such as pain or touch) develop, usually on the trunk and occasionally on the arms and legs. Such pain may be continuous or intermittent and usually lasts from 1 to 4 weeks. The primary goal of treatment is to relieve itching and neuralgic pain with calamine lotion or another antipruritic and aspirin, codeine, or another analgesic if neuralgic pain is severe.

1. Among the malignant brain tumors (neoplasms), the most common type in adults are gliomas and meningiomas (slow-growing tumors). Brain tumors cause CNS changes by invading and destroying tissues and by secondary effects, mainly compression of the brain, cranial nerves, and cerebral vessels; causing cerebral edema; and increased ICP. Generally, clinical features result from increased ICP; these features vary with the tumor type, location, and degree of invasion. The onset of symptoms usually is insidious, and symptoms depend on the location of the tumor in the brain. For example, a tumor on the optic nerve would cause visual problems. Treatment includes removing a resectable tumor, reducing a nonresectable tumor, relieving cerebral edema or ICP, relieving symptoms, and preventing further neurologic damage.

3. Peripheral neuritis is inflammation of peripheral nerves, usually associated with a degenerative process. Causes include Guillain-Barré syndrome, tetanus, malaria, tuberculosis, and diabetes. Peripheral neuritis is also associated with peripheral vascular disease.

4. Huntington's disease, see answer 47, rationale (4).

52. ❶ You will assign the patient with a diagnosis of Parkinson's disease to the orthopedic-trained RN. This is a chronic disease, and this patient is not in a life-threatening situation. For more information see answer 28, rationale (2).

2. Brain attacks, see answer 48, rationale (3).

3. Epilepsy, see answer 27, rationale (4).

4. Multiple sclerosis, see answer 4, rationale (3).

53. ➋ You will assign the patient with a diagnosis of CHF to the obstetric-trained RN. This is a chronic condition, and the option did not indicate that this patient was in severe CHF. The patient has been in the hospital for 4 days, you would expect the patient's medical condition would have improved, therefore, the patient is not in a crisis situation; the other three patients have life-threatening diseases.

1. Cardiogenic shock, sometimes called pump failure, is a condition of diminished cardiac output that severely impairs tissue perfusion. It reflects severe left ventricular failure and occurs as a serious complication in nearly 15 percent of all patients hospitalized with acute myocardial infarction (MI). Cardiogenic shock typically affects patients whose area of infarction exceeds 40 percent of muscle mass; in such patients, the fatality rate may exceed 85 percent. Most patients with cardiogenic shock die within 24 h of onset. Prognosis for those who survive is extremely poor.

3. In MI, reduced blood flow through one of the coronary arteries results in myocardial ischemia and necrosis. In cardiovascular disease, which is the leading cause of death in the United States and western Europe, death usually results from cardiac damage or complications of MI. Mortality is high when treatment is delayed, and almost half of sudden deaths due to an MI occur before hospitalization, within 1 h of the onset of symptoms. Prognosis improves if vigorous treatment begins immediately. The goals of treatment are to relieve chest pain, stabilize heart rhythm, reduce cardiac workload, revascularize the coronary artery, and preserve myocardial tissue. Arrhythmias are the predominant problem during the first 48 h after the infarction. The most dangerous arrhythmia is ventricular fibrillation.

4. Spontaneous angina occurs suddenly with no known cause, and it can cause MI, which may lead to CHF.

54. ➋ You will assign the obstetric-trained RN to the patient with a diagnosis of rheumatic fever, fourth day in the hospital. This patient will have received effective management to eradicate the streptococcal infection, relieving symptoms, preventing recurrence, and reducing the chance of permanent cardiac damage. During the acute phase, treatment includes penicillin or erythromycin for patients with penicillin hypersensitivity. Salicylates, such as aspirin, relieve fever and minimize joint swelling and pain. If carditis is present or salicylates fail to relieve pain and inflammation, corticosteroids may be used. Rheumatic fever appears to be a hypersensitivity reaction to a group A beta-hemolytic streptococcal infection, in which antibodies manufactured to combat streptococci react and produce characteristic lesions at specific tissue sites, especially in the heart and joints. In 95 percent of patients, rheumatic fever characteristically follows a streptococcal infection that appeared a few days to 6 weeks earlier. A temperature of at least 100.4°F (38°C) occurs, and most patients complain of migratory joint pain or polyarthritis. The most destructive effect of rheumatic fever is carditis, which develops in up to 50 percent of patients and may affect the endocardium, myocardium, pericardium, or heart valves. This patient is not in a life-threatening situation; the other three patients have very serious diseases and cannot be assigned to an obstetric-trained RN.

1. Mitral stenosis is the narrowing of the valve by valvular abnormalities, fibrosis, or calcification that obstructs blood flow from the left atrium to the left ventricle. Consequently, left atrial volume and pressure rise, and the chamber dilates. Greater resistance to blood flow causes pulmonary hypertension, right ventricular hypertrophy, and, eventually, right ventricular failure. Also, inadequate filling of the left ventricle produces low cardiac output.

3. In ventricular tachycardia, the rate is greater than 100 bpm and usually is 140 to 250 bpm. The danger of ventricular tachycardia is that it can progress to ventricular fibrillation, which is a life-threatening situation. Conditions that lead to arrhythmias include hypoxemia, electrolyte imbalance, fever, emotional and physical stress, hyperthyroidism, caffeine, epinephrine, and atropine.

4. The cause of dilated cardiomyopathy is unknown. Predisposing factors include alcohol abuse, high blood pressure, infections, and pregnancy. If associated with pregnancy, it may disappear. Dilated cardiomyopathy probably is the most common cardiomyopathy, and it leads to CHF. It is characterized by gross dilation of the heart with interference in systolic function. Unlike hypertropic cardiomyopathy, in which ventricular filling is impaired, dilated cardiomyopathy is characterized by impaired systolic ejection function.

55. ➌ You will assign the obstetric-trained RN to the patient with the diagnosis of diverticulosis disease. Remember, when an obstetric RN is transferred from the obstetric unit, you will assign the RN to the easiest patient because there usually is no obstetric patient on a medical/surgical unit. Diverticular disease consists of outpouchings of the intestine. When diverticula are *not* inflamed, the condition is called *diverticulosis,* and the patient may be asymptomatic. When inflammation is present, the condition is referred to as *diverticulitis.*

Diet may be a contributing factor because lack of roughage reduces fecal residue, narrows the bowel lumen, and leads to higher intraabdominal pressure during defecation. *Diverticulitis* is inflammation of the outpouching of the intestine. This condition is very dangerous because the inflamed pouches may break open and gastric content would enter the peritoneum, causing peritonitis. *Peritonitis* is inflammation of the peritoneum, the membrane coat lining the abdominal cavity.

1. Ulcerative colitis, see answer 24, rationale (4).

2. In severe Crohn's disease, the inflammation severely involves segments of bowel and the inflamed areas are separated from each other by "skip areas" of apparently normal bowel. In 50 percent of patients with Crohn's disease of the colon, the rectum is spared. In contrast to ulcerative colitis, Crohn's disease is characterized by chronic inflammation extending through all layers of the intestinal wall. Whether or not the small bowel

or colon is involved, the basic pathologic process is the same. The patient with severe Crohn's disease may have frequent liquid stools (10–20 stools per day) containing blood and pus. The patient with severe Crohn's disease may have fever, abdominal pain, and diarrhea, often without blood and weight loss. Rectal bleedings are distinctly less common than with ulcerative colitis. Electrolyte abnormalities, especially hypokalemia, reflect the degree of diarrhea, often without blood and weight loss.

4. Hemorrhage occurs when ulcers perforate blood vessels. Hemorrhage varies from minimal bleeding, manifested by occult blood in the stool (melena), to massive bleeding, in which the patient vomits bright red blood (hematemesis). Monitor vital signs every 15 to 30 min. Early recognition of changes in vital signs and an increase in the amount and redness (blood) of nasogastric drainage often signal massive upper GI bleeding. The danger is that the ulcer perforates the stomach, and gastroduodenal contents enter the peritoneal cavity, causing chemical peritonitis, bacterial septicemia, and hypovolemic shock. Symptoms include sudden, sharp, severe pain beginning in the midepigastrium. Diminished peristalsis or ileus may develop.

56. ❶ You will assign the obstetric-trained RN to the patient with a diagnosis of breast cancer, first day in the hospital. This patient is not in an immediate life-threatening situation. The other three patients are diagnosed with lung disease that may obstruct their airway.

2. Most experts agree that lung cancer is attributable to inhalation of carcinogenic pollutants by a susceptible host. Who is most susceptible? Any smoker over age 40 years, especially if he began to smoke before age 15 years, has smoked a whole pack or more per day for 20 years, or works with or near asbestos. Although prognosis generally is poor, it varies with the extent of spread at the time of diagnosis and cell type growth rate. Because early-stage lung cancer usually produces no symptoms, this disease is often in an *advanced stage* at diagnosis.

3. Histoplasmosis is a fungal infection caused by *Histoplasma capsulatum.* It is found in the faces of birds and in soil contaminated by their feces (e.g., chicken coop farms). The primary acute disease is benign; the progressive disseminated disease is fatal in approximately 90 percent of patients. Without proper chemotherapy, chronic pulmonary histoplasmosis is fatal in 50 percent of patients within 5 years. Progressive disseminated histoplasmosis causes hepatosplenomegaly, general lymphadenopathy, anorexia, weight loss, fever, and possibly ulceration of the tongue, palate, epiglottis, and larynx, with resulting pain, hoarseness, and dysphagia. It also may cause endocarditis, meningitis, pericarditis, and adrenal insufficiency.

4. With acute or chronic infection caused by *Mycobacterium tuberculosis,* the primary focus of infection is in the lungs. However, mycobacteria commonly exist in other parts of the body, such as the kidney and the lymph nodes. Isolate the infectious patient in a quiet, well-ventilated room until he is no longer contagious. Teach the patient to cough and sneeze into tissues and to dispose of all secretions properly. Place a covered trash can nearby or tape a waxed bag to the side of the bed for disposal of used tissues. Instruct the patient to wear a mask when outside

of his room. Visitors and hospital personnel should wear masks when they are in the patient's room.

57. ❹ You will assign the obstetric-trained RN to the patient with a diagnosis of lung abscess. All four of these patients are diagnosed with a lung disease. This patient has the least chance of developing airway obstruction. Lung abscess is often the result of aspiration of oropharyngeal contents. Poor oral hygiene with dental or gingival (gum) disease is strongly associated with putrid lung abscess. Lung abscess is a lung infection accompanied by pus accumulation and tissue destruction. The clinical effects of lung abscess include a cough that may produce bloody, purulent, or foul-smelling sputum, pleuritic chest pain, dyspnea, excessive sweating, chills, fever, headache, malaise, diaphoresis, and weight loss. Treatment consists of prolonged antibiotic therapy, often lasting for months, until radiographic resolution or definite stability occurs. Symptoms usually disappear in a few weeks. Postural drainage may facilitate discharge of necrotic material into upper airways where expectoration is possible; oxygen therapy may relieve hypoxemia. Poor response to therapy required resection of the lesion.

1. Pulmonary embolism generally results from dislodged thrombi originating in the leg veins. More than half of such thrombi arise in the deep veins of the legs and usually are multiple. Predisposing factors to pulmonary embolism include long-term immobility, chronic pulmonary disease, CHF or atrial fibrillation, thrombophlebitis, polycythemia vera, thrombocytosis, cardiac arrest, defibrillation, cardioversion, autoimmune hemolytic anemia, sickle cell disease, varicose veins, recent surgery, advanced age, pregnancy, lower extremity fractures or surgery, burns, obesity, vascular injury, malignancy, or oral contraceptives. Total occlusion of the main pulmonary artery is rapidly fatal; smaller or fragmented emboli produce symptoms that vary with the size, number, and location of the emboli. Usually the first symptom of pulmonary embolism is dyspnea, which may be accompanied by anginal or pleuritic chest pain. Other clinical features include tachycardia, productive cough (possibly blood-tinged), low-grade fever, and pleural effusion. Treatment is designed to maintain adequate cardiovascular and pulmonary functions during resolution of the obstruction and to prevent recurrence of embolic episodes. Because most emboli largely resolve within 10 to 14 days, treatment consists of oxygen therapy, as needed, and anticoagulation with heparin to inhibit new thrombus formation.

2. Pulmonary edema usually results from left ventricular failure due to arteriosclerotic, hypertensive, cardiomyopathic, or valvular cardiac disease. In such disorders, the compromised left ventricle requires increased filling pressures to maintain adequate output; these pressures are transmitted to the left ventricle, causing hypertrophy and ultimately left ventricular failure. Symptoms include dyspnea on exertion, paroxysmal nocturnal dyspnea, tachycardia, tachypnea, increased blood pressure, and diastolic (S_3) gallop. With severe pulmonary edema, respiration becomes labored and rapid, with more diffuse crackles and coughing productive of frothy, blood sputum. Tachycardia increases and dysrhythmias may occur. Skin

becomes cold, clammy, diaphoretic, and cyanotic. Blood pressure falls, and pulse becomes thready as cardiac output falls.

3. Spontaneous pneumothorax usually occurs in otherwise healthy adults aged 20 to 40 years. Air leakage from ruptured congenital blebs adjacent to the visceral pleural surface, near the apex of the lung, causes this form of pneumothorax. The cardial features of pneumothorax are sudden sharp, pleuritic pain (exacerbated by movement of the chest, breathing, and coughing); asymmetric chest wall movement; shortness of breath; and cyanosis. In moderate to severe pneumothorax, profound respiratory distress may develop, with signs of tension pneumothorax; weak and rapid pulse; pallor; neck vein distention; and anxiety. Treatment is conservative for spontaneous pneumothorax, in which there are no signs of increased pleural pressure (indicating tension pneumothorax), lung collapse is less than 30 percent, and the patient shows no signs of dyspnea or other indications of physiologic compromise. Such treatment consists of bed rest; careful monitoring of blood pressure, pulse rate, and respirations; oxygen administration; and, possibly, needle aspiration of air with a large-bore needle attached to a syringe. If more than 30 percent of the lung is collapsed, treatment to reexpand the lung includes placing a thoracostomy tube in the second or third intercostal space in the midclavicular line, connected to an underwater seal.

58. ❹ You will assign the gynecology-trained RN to the patient with the diagnosis dysmenorrhea. This is the only diagnosis that is related to a female reproductive organ. Whenever possible, you will always assign an RN to a patient with a diagnosis that is related to the RN's training; in this case, the RN's expertise was in gynecology. Dysmenorrhea is painful menstruation.

1, 2, 3. These options are incorrect as seen in rationale (4).

59. ❷ You will assign the gynecology-trained RN to the patient with a diagnosis of endometriosis. This is the only diagnosis that is related to a female reproductive organ. Endometriosis is the presence of endometrial tissue outside the lining of the uterine cavity. Active endometriosis usually occurs between the ages of 30 and 40 years, especially in women who postpone child-bearing. It is uncommon before age 20 years. Severe symptoms of endometriosis may have an abrupt onset or may develop over many years. Generally, this disorder becomes progressively severe during the menstrual years and tends to subside after menopause.

1, 3, 4. These options are incorrect as seen in rationale (2).

60. ❶ You will assign the gynecology-trained RN to the patient with a diagnosis of amenorrhea. This is the only diagnosis that is related to a female reproductive organ. Amenorrhea is the abnormal absence or suppression of menstruation.

2, 3, 4. These options are incorrect as seen in rationale (1).

61. ❶ You will assign the gynecology-trained RN to the patient with a diagnosis of adenomyosis. This is the only diagnosis that is related to a female reproductive organ. Adenomyosis is a benign invasive growth of the endometrium into the muscular layer of the uterus.

2, 3, 4. These options are incorrect as seen in rationale (1).

62. ❹ You will assign the gynecology-trained RN to the patient with a diagnosis of breast cancer. This is the only diagnosis that is related to a female organ. The definition of gynecology is the study of disease of the female reproductive organs, including the breast.

1, 2, 3. These options are incorrect as seen in rationale (4).

63. ❸ You will assign the gynecology-trained RN to the patient with a diagnosis of infertility related to chlamydia infection. This is the only diagnosis that is related to a female reproductive organ. Chlamydia infection negatively influences tubal function and impedes fertility.

1, 2, 4. These options are incorrect as seen in rationale (3).

64. ❹ You will assign the gynecology-trained RN to the patient with a diagnosis of infertility related to dysfunctional uterine bleeding. This is the only diagnosis that is related to a female reproductive organ. Dysfunctional uterine bleeding refers to abnormal endometrial bleeding without recognizable organic lesions. Prognosis varies with the cause. Dysfunctional uterine bleeding usually results from an imbalance in the hormonal–endometrial relationship, where persistent and unopposed stimulation of the endometrium by estrogen occurs. Disorders that cause sustained high estrogen levels are polycystic ovary syndrome, obesity, and immaturity of the hypothalamic-pituitary-ovarian mechanism (in postpubertal teenagers). Diagnostic studies must rule out other causes of excessive vaginal bleeding, such as organic, systemic, psychogenic, and endocrine causes, including malignancy, polyps, incomplete abortion, pregnancy, and infection. Primary treatment is designed to control endometrial growth and reestablish a normal cyclic pattern of menstruation. If drug therapy is ineffective, dilation and curettage (D&C) serves as a supplementary treatment by removing a large portion of the bleeding endometrium. Also, a D&C can help determine the original cause of hormonal imbalance and can aid in planning further therapy. Regardless of the primary treatment, the patient may need iron replacement or transfusions of packed cells or whole blood, as indicated, because of anemia caused by recurrent bleeding.

1, 2, 3. These options are incorrect as seen in rationale (4).

65. ❶ You will assign the orthopedic-trained RN to the patient with a diagnosis of Paget's disease. This is the only diagnosis that is related to orthopedics. Paget's disease is a slowly progressive metabolic bone disease characterized by an initial phase of excessive bone resorption (osteoclastic phase), followed by a reactive phase of excessive abnormal bone formation (osteoblastic phase). The new bone structure, which is chaotic, fragile, and weak, causes painful deformities of both external contour and internal structure. Paget's disease usually localizes in one or several areas of the skeleton (most frequently the lower torso), but occasionally skeletal deformity is widely distributed. It can be fatal, particularly when it is associated with CHF (widespread disease creates a continuous need for high cardiac output). Primary treatment consists of drug therapy and includes calcitonin (a hormone, given subcutaneously or IM) or etidronate (Didronel IV); both are calcium regulators used to retard bone resorption. Although calcitonin requires long-tern maintenance therapy, there is noticeable improvement after the first few weeks.

2, 3, 4. These options are incorrect as seen in rationale (1).

66. ❹ You will assign the orthopedic-trained RN to the patient with diagnosed left leg amputation. Amputation of an extremity often is necessary as a result of progressive peripheral vascular disease, trauma (crushing injuries, burns, frostbite, electrical burns), congenital deformities, or malignant tumor. Of all these causes, peripheral vascular disease accounts for the majority of amputations of lower extremities.

Amputation is really reconstructive surgery designed to improve the patient's quality of life. It is used to relieve symptoms and to facilitate improved function. If the health care team is able to communicate a positive attitude, the patient will adjust to the amputation and actively participate in the rehabilitative plan.

Loss of an extremity requires major adjustments. The patient's perception of the amputation must be understood by the health care team. The patient must adjust to a permanent change in body image, which must be incorporated in such a way that self-esteem is not lost. Physical mobility and/or ability to perform activities of daily living are altered, and the patient needs to learn how to modify activities and environment to accommodate the use of mobility aids and assistive devices. The rehabilitation team is multidisciplinary (patient, nurse, physician, social worker, psychologist, prosthetist, vocational rehabilitation worker) and will help the patient achieve the highest possible level of function and participation in life activities.

1, 2, 3. These options are incorrect as seen in rationale (4).

67. ❸ You will assign the orthopedic-trained RN to the patient with a diagnosis of rheumatoid arthritis. In rheumatoid arthritis, abnormal or altered IgG antibodies develop after a genetically susceptible individual is exposed to an antigen. The altered IgG antibodies are not recognized as "self," and the individual forms an antibody against them, an antibody known as *RF*. By aggregating into complexes, RF generates inflammation. Eventually, cartilage damage by inflammation triggers additional immune responses, including activation of complement. This in turn attracts polymorphonuclear leukocytes and stimulates release of inflammatory mediators, which enhance joint destruction. Rheumatoid arthritis is a chronic, systemic, inflammatory disease that primarily attacks peripheral joints and surrounding muscles, tendons, ligaments, and blood vessels. Spontaneous remissions and unpredictable exacerbations mark the course of this potentially crippling disease. Rheumatoid arthritis usually requires lifelong treatment and, sometimes, surgery. The orthopedic-trained RN has worked with bone and joint disease/problems. The other three diagnoses are not bone or joint related.

1, 2, 4. These options are incorrect as seen in rationale (3).

68. ❷ You will assign the orthopedic-trained RN to the patient with a diagnosis of gout. Gout is a metabolic disease marked by urate deposits, which cause painfully arthritic joints. It can

strike any joint but favors those in the feet. especially the toes. Although the exact cause of primary gout is unknown, it seems to be linked to a genetic defect in purine metabolism, which causes overproduction of uric acid (hyperuricemia), retention of uric acid, or both. Treatment for chronic gout aims to decrease serum uric acid level. Continuing maintenance dosage of allopurinol is often given to suppress uric acid formation or control uric acid levels, preventing further attacks. However, this powerful drug should be used cautiously in patients with renal failure.

3. Cushing's disease, see answer 83, rationale (1).

3, 4. These options are incorrect as seen in rationale (2).

69. ❶ You will assign the orthopedic-trained RN to the patient with a diagnosis of hip fracture. There is a high incidence of hip fractures among elderly people because their bones are brittle from osteoporosis and they fall readily from weakness of the quadriceps muscles as well as from general frailty due to age and a sedentary lifestyle. Falls in the elderly also occur because of conditions that produce decreased cerebral arterial perfusion (transient ischemic attacks, anemia, emboli, cardiovascular disease, and drug effects). Because of the fracture, the leg is shortened, adducted, and externally rotated. The patient may complain of slight pain in the groin or on the medial side of the knee. With most fractures of the femoral neck, the patient is in pain, is unable to move the leg without significantly increased pain, and is able to achieve some comfort with the leg slightly flexed in external rotation. Temporary skin traction in the form of Buck's extension may be applied to reduce muscle spasm, to immobilize the extremity, and to relieve pain. Sand bags or a trochanter roll may be used to control the external rotation. The goal of surgical treatment of hip fractures is to obtain a satisfactory fixation so that the patient can be mobilized quickly and thereby avoid secondary medical complications. Operative treatment consists of (1) reduction of the fracture and internal fixation or (2) replacement of the femoral head with prosthesis (hemiarthroplasty).

2, 3, 4. These options are incorrect as seen in rationale (1). These three diagnoses are not related to orthopedics. If there are no orthopedic diagnoses, then you will assign the orthopedic-trained RN to patient with the least life-threatening diagnosis.

70. ❷ You will assign the orthopedic-trained RN to the patient with a diagnosis of compound fracture of the femur, first day in the hospital. In a compound femur fracture, when the bone is broken, an external wound leads down to the site of the fracture or fragments of bone protrude through the skin. Considerable force is required to break the shaft of the femur in adults. Most of these fractures are seen in the young male who has been involved in a vehicular accident or has fallen from a height. Frequently, these patients have associated multiple trauma problems.

The patient presents with an enlarged, deformed, painful thigh. The patient cannot move the hip or the knee. The fracture may be transverse, oblique, spiral, or comminuted. Frequently, the patient with this fracture is in impending shock because loss of 2 to 3 units of blood into the tissues is common. An expanding thigh may indicate continued bleeding.

Assessment includes checking neurovascular status of the extremity, especially circulatory perfusion of the foot. (Check popliteal and pedal pulses and toe capillary refill.) A Doppler ultrasound monitoring device may be needed to assess blood flow.

1, 3, 4. These options are incorrect as seen in rationale (2).

71. ❹ The first medication you will administer is Dilantin (phenytoin) IV to the patient diagnosed with epilepsy. Epilepsy is a condition of the brain marked by a susceptibility to recurrent seizures (paroxysmal events associated with abnormal electrical discharges of neurons in the brain). If seizure medication is not administered in a timely manner, the patient may develop status epilepticus. Status epilepticus (acute prolonged seizure activity) is a series of generalized convulsions that occur without full recovery of consciousness between attacks. It is considered a major medical emergency. Status epilepticus produces cumulative effects. Vigorous muscular contraction imposes a heavy metabolic demand and can interfere with respirations. Some respiratory arrest occurs at the height of each seizure, producing venous congestion and hypoxia of the brain. Repeated episodes of cerebral anoxia and swelling may lead to irreversible and fatal brain damage. Duration of Dilantin is 6 to 12 h. The maintenance dose is 300 mg/day. Remember, a medication ordered for the IV route usually is an indication of the severity of the disease. Given the shortage of RNs, the number of patients to whom the RN gives medications has greatly increased. As a result, medications are not always given in a timely manner, and the RN needs to know which medication must be given first and which patient must be assessed first. The patient with epilepsy must be assessed first and frequently because prolonged seizure activity can cause brain damage. Also, other factors can cause seizures, such as fever, meninigitis, brain abscess, hypoglycemia or hypoparathyroidism, and many cerebrovascular disorders. Therefore, giving seizure medication first will help to prevent seizures. Also, this patient will be assessed first.

1, 2, 3. These options are incorrect as seen in rationale (4).

72. ❷ The first medication you will administer is the aminophylline IV to the patient diagnosed with asthma. Aminophylline IV is a bronchodilator used to reduce bronchospasm and increase lung vital capacity. Asthma is a chronic reactive airway disorder that produces episodic, reversible airway obstruction via bronchospasms, increased mucous secretion, and mucosal edema. Its symptoms range from mild wheezing and dyspnea to life-threatening respiratory failure. Intrinsic asthma is not related to specific allergens. Factors such as a common cold, respiratory tract infections, exercise, emotions, and environmental pollutants may trigger an attack. Aspirin or other nonsteroidal antiinflammatory drugs also may be a factor. The attacks of intrinsic asthma may become more severe and frequent with time and can progress to chronic bronchitis and emphysema. Some patients will develop mixed asthma. Mixed asthma is the most common form of asthma. An asthma attack may begin dramatically, with simultaneous onset of severe multiple symptoms, or insidiously, with gradually increasing respiratory distress. Mixed asthma has characteristics of both the extrinsic and the intrinsic forms. Typically an acute asthmatic attack causes sudden dyspnea, wheezing, tightness in the chest, and cough with thick, clear or yellow sputum. The patient may feel as if he is suffocating. During a severe attack, the patient may be unable to speak more than a few words without pausing for breath. A patient's airway is a priority, so you will administer the aminophylline PO first, but if seizure medication were an option, then it would be given first and asthma medication second. Remember, the asthma patient will develop breathing problems but usually will respond quickly to bronchial dilators. If the diagnosis is *acute* asthmatic attack, then asthma medication will be given first and the doctor's order will be aminophylline IV, not PO.

1. Lasix PO is not considered a crisis drug. If the patient's pulmonary edema is severe, then the physician would order Lasix IV.

3. When a patient's blood pressure is extremely high, the physician will order nitride IV, not Vasotec PO. The fact that the antihypertensive medication ordered was PO tells you that the patient's blood pressure was not severely elevated.

4. CHF is a chronic disease. Accupril drug classification is an antihypertensive drug. Accupril is an angiotensin-converting enzyme (ACE) inhibitor. With CHF, the patient's blood pressure will be elevated due to fluid retention. Severe CHF can be life threatening, but this option did not use the word severe.

73. ❷ The first medication you will give is nitride to the patient with a diagnosis of severe hypertension. Severe hypertension can become a hypertensive crisis. Hypertensive crisis is an acute, life-threatening rise in blood pressure (diastolic may be over 120 mm Hg). It may develop in hypertensive patients after abrupt discontinuation of antihypertensive medication; increased salt consumption; increased production of renin, epinephrine, and norepinephrine; and increased stress. This emergency requires immediate and vigorous treatment to lower blood pressure and thereby prevent cerebrovascular accident, left heart failure, and pulmonary edema.

1, 3, 4. These options are incorrect as seen in rationale (2).

74. ❶ The first medication you will give is lidocaine IV to the patient with a diagnosis of ventricular dysrhythmia. The danger of ventricular dysrhythmia is that it can easily go into ventricular fibrillation. In ventricular fibrillation, there is no cardiac output; this is a life-threatening situation.

2, 3, 4. These options are incorrect as seen in rationale (1).

75. ❷ You will administer Cortone IV to the patient with a diagnosis of Addison's disease (adrenal insufficiency). Addison's disease, caused by a deficiency of cortical hormones, results when the adrenal cortex is surgically removed with bilateral adrenalectomy or is destroyed, often as a result of idiopathic atrophy or infections such as tuberculosis or histoplasmosis. Inadequate secretion of adrenocorticotropic hormone (ACTH) from the pituitary gland results in adrenal insufficiency because of decreased stimulation of the adrenal cortex. The symptoms of adrenocortical insufficiency may also result from sudden cessation of exogenous adrenocortical hormonal therapy, which suppresses the body's normal response to stress and interferes with normal feedback mechanisms. Addison's disease has a characteristic clinical picture. The chief clinical manifestations include muscular weakness, anorexia, GI symptoms, fatigue, and emaciation, generalized dark pigmentation of the skin, hypotension, low blood sugar, low serum sodium level, and high serum potassium level. In severe cases, the disturbances of sodium and potassium metabolism may be marked with depletion of sodium and water and severe chronic dehydration. As the disease progresses, with acute hypotension developing due to hypocorticism, the patient moves into addisonian crisis, which is a medical emergency marked by cyanosis, fever, and the classic signs of shock: pallor, apprehension, rapid and weak pulse, rapid respirations, and low blood pressure. In addition, the patient may complain of headache, nausea, abdominal pain, and diarrhea and show signs of confusion and restlessness.

1, 3, 4. These options are incorrect as seen in rationale (2).

76. ❸ The first medications you will administer are Betoptic and Pilocar to the patient with a diagnosis of acute open-angle glaucoma. Pilocar increases aqueous humor outflow, and its use is especially important for treatment of acute open-angle glaucoma and after surgical iridectomy; also for treatment of acute *angle-closed* glaucoma. Betoptic is used to decrease the production of aqueous humor in acute open-angle glaucoma. If glaucoma is not treated in a timely manner, blindness may occur.

1, 2, 4. These options are incorrect as seen in rationale (3). These three diseases will not cause immediate injury to the patient if these medications are not given in a timely manner.

77. ❶ The first medication you will administer is lactulose and neomycin to the patient with a diagnosis of hepatic encephalopathy. Hepatic encephalopathy develops when liver is no longer able to break down ammonia into urea (byproduct of protein metabolism). The ammonia will go to the brain and cause encephalopathy.

In patients with severe cirrhosis of the liver, hepatic encephalopathy (coma) can occur from intake of excessive amounts of protein but most often is caused by bleeding from esophageal varices resulting from portal hypertension. The blood from the esophagus enters the stomach and is used as protein.

Ammonia absorption can be decreased by administration of lactulose. Lactulose is an osmotic laxative agent that prevents the absorption of ammonia from the colon into the blood and thereby reduces blood ammonia levels. Absorbed lactulose is excreted in urine. Neomycin sulfate is used to reduce ammonia-forming bacteria in the GI tract.

Signs and symptoms include decreased level of consciousness. Patient demonstrates personality changes and fluctuating neurologic signs, such as flapping tremors of the hands, confusion, and impaired speech.

2, 3, 4. These options are incorrect as seen in rationale (1). These diseases are not immediately life threatening, so these medications do not have to be given first.

78. ❹ The first medication you will administer is Viokase to the patient with the diagnosis of cystic fibrosis. Viokase replaces pancreatis enzymes that help to digest and absorb fat, protein, and carbohydrates. With cystic fibrosis, these enzyme secretions become so tenacious that they plug the ducts, creating back pressure on the acinar cells, which causes cells to atrophy and destroys their ability to produce enzymes. Therefore, amylase, lipase, and trypsin cannot reach the duodenum. Lipase breaks down fat, trypsin breaks down protein, and amylase breaks down starches.

Pulmonary congestion exists in almost all children with cystic fibrosis because the large amount of mucus in the lungs is a serious threat to life. This person must receive Viokase on time or the lung will fill with mucus.

Without pancreatic enzymes, children are unable to digest fat and protein. Thus, quantities of fat and protein pass undigested through the intestinal tract, causing large, bulky, greasy stools (steatorrhea).

Cystic fibrosis (CF) is a common inherited recessive disorder and is the most common fatal genetic disease in white children. When both parents are carriers, there is a one in four chance with each pregnancy that the child will have CF. Reaching adulthood is now a realistic expectation for infants with CF.

1, 2, 3. These options are incorrect as seen in rationale (4). These three diseases are not an immediate life-threatening disease; therefore, none of these medications will have to be given first.

79. ❶ The first medications you will administer are Dilantin IV and mannitol IV. See answer 71, rationale (4) for information on why giving seizure medications first is a priority. Acute prolonged seizure activity can cause brain damage. The fact that Dilantin and mannitol will be administered IV gives you information that this patient is in immediate danger of increased ICP.

2, 3, 4. These options are incorrect as seen in rationale (1). The patient diagnosed with asthma has an order for aminophylline PO and cortisone PO; that tells you that the patient is not in a life-threatening situation. If the patient were in a life-threatening situation, the doctor would have ordered aminophylline IV and cortisone IM.

80. ❹ The first medications you will administer are mannitol IV, dexamethasone sodium phosphate IV, and penicillin G (aqueous) IV to the patient diagnosed with a brain abscess. Brain abscess is a free or encapsulated collection of pus usually found in the temporal lobe, cerebellum, or frontal lobes. It can vary in size and may occur singly or multilocularly (many cells or compartments). Brain abscess has a relatively low incidence. Although it can occur at any age, it is most common in persons between the ages of 10 and 35 years and is rare in the elderly. Untreated brain abscess usually is fatal. With treatment, prognosis is only fair, and approximately 30 percent of patients develop seizures. Brain abscess usually is secondary to another infection, especially otitis media, sinusitis, dental abscess, and mastoiditis. Treatment for a brain abscess includes mannitol, an osmotic diuretic used to reduce ICP; dexamethasone, a corticosteroid used to reduce inflammation, which will help to decrease cerebral edema; and penicillin G (aqueous) is an antibiotic used to treat severe infections. Penicillin G must be administered by IV, and no other medication should be given through that IV line. It is important to administer these drugs first to decrease ICP, prevent seizures, and prevent brain cell destruction.

1. Ulcerative colitis is an inflammatory, often chronic disease that affects the mucosa of the colon. It usually begins in the rectum and sigmoid colon and often extends upward into the entire colon. The hallmark of ulcerative colitis is recurrent bloody diarrhea, often containing pus and mucus, interspersed with asymptomatic remissions. Lomotil is an antidiarrheal medication used to reduce stool volume. Donnatal is used to provide an anticholinergic/antispasmodic effect on the bowel. This is not a life-threatening diagnosis.

2. Aqua Mephyton (vitamin K) is administered to a patient with cirrhosis of the liver to prevent esophageal bleeding. Vitamin K is necessary for production of prothrombin. Vitamin K is stored in the liver, so this patient would be low on vitamin K. Spironolactone is a potassium-sparing diuretic used to reduce ascites. Spironolactone can be administered only by the oral route.

3. Pernicious anemia is caused by a deficiency in cyanocobalamin (vitamin B_{12}).

81. ❸ The first medication you will administer is calcium gluconate IV to the patient diagnosed with hypoparathyroidism. Hypoparathyroidism is a deficiency of parathyroid hormone (PTH) caused by disease, injury, congenital malfunction of the parathyroid glands, or after a thyroidectomy. The thyroidectomy procedure can cause temporary damage to the parathyroid gland. Because the parathyroid gland primarily regulates calcium balance, hypoparathyroidism causes hypocalcemia, producing neuromuscular symptoms ranging from paresthesia to tetany. Tetany may cause seizures. The doctor's order for calcium gluconate IV should have indicated to you that the patient's calcium level was very low.

1. Myasthenia gravis is an autoimmune disease that causes a failure in transmission of nerve impulses because of ineffective acetylcholine release. Treatment is symptomatic. Anticholinesterase drugs, such as neostigmine and Mestinon, counteract fatigue and muscle weakness and allow approximately 80 percent of normal muscle function. However, these drugs become less effective as the disease worsens. If this option was myasthenia *crises,* then these medications may not be effective and the patient is put on respiratory support until respiratory function begins to improve.

2. Parkinson's disease, see answer 28, rationale (2).

4. Hyperparathyroidism is characterized by overactivity of one or more of the four parathyroid glands, resulting in excessive secretion of PTH. Such hypersecretion of PTH promotes bone resorption and leads to hypercalcemia and hypophosphatemia. In turn, increased renal and GI absorption of calcium occurs. Increased calcium can cause renal stones, muscle weakness, and bone degeneration. Treatment may include surgery, IV hydration, and medications (Didronel or calcitonin, which are calcium

regulators that slow abnormal bone reabsorption, thus reducing bone formation).

82. ❶ The first medication you will administer is 100 units of Humulin R insulin in 500 mL of NS. Hyperosmolar coma usually occurs in patients with type II non–insulin-dependent diabetes mellitus (NIDDM). Treatment can be very difficult because of resistance to insulin action in target tissue. Both type I insulin-dependent diabetes mellitus (IDDM) and type II NIDDM can be insulin resistant. Hyperosmolar coma patients usually are insulin resistant. They are in a state of profound dehydration resulting from sustained hyperglycemia diuresis, and patients are unable to drink sufficient water to keep up with urinary fluid losses. Seizure activity may be present. The 100 units of insulin in 500 mL of NS allows for hydration. The rate of administration depends on the rate needed to correct hyperglycemia and dehydration.

2. The patient in diabetic ketoacidosis is given 40 units of Humulin R in 300 mL of NS. The amount of insulin ordered is significantly less than the 100 units of insulin ordered for the patient in hyperosmolar coma. The reason is that it is not as difficult to treat a patient in diabetic ketoacidosis. The patient in a hyperosmolar coma state is in a more life-threatening situation and must be assessed first. The rate at which the insulin in NS is administered depends on the rate needed to correct hyperglycemia and dehydration.

3. Diabetes insipidus results from a deficiency of circulating vasopressin (also called antidiuretic hormone [ADH]). Primary diabetes insipidus (50 percent of patients) is familial or idiopathic in origin. Secondary diabetes insipidus results from intracranial neoplastic or metastatic lesions, hypophysectomy, or head trauma, which damages the neurohypophyseal structures. The hypothalamus synthesizes vasopressin. The posterior pituitary gland stores vasopressin and releases it into general circulation, where it causes the kidneys to reabsorb water by making the distal and collecting tubule cells permeable to water. The absence of vasopressin in diabetes insipidus allows the filtered water to be excreted in the urine instead of being reabsorbed. Diabetes insipidus typically produces extreme polyuria (usually 4–16 L/day of dilute urine, but sometimes as much as 30 L/day). As a result, the patient is extremely thirsty and drinks great quantities of water to compensate for the body's water loss. *Note:* Pituitary diabetes insipidus should not be confused with nephrogenic diabetes insipidus, a rare congenital disturbance of water metabolism that results from renal tubular resistance to vasopressin.

Pitressin is a synthetic ADH. If this medication is not given in a timely manner, the patient will not be in a life-threatening situation, but may show signs of dehydration.

4. Synthroid is a synthetic thyroid hormone given to patients with hypothyroidism (myxedema) to control their symptoms. For more information see answer 5, rationale (1).

83. ❷ The first medications you will administer are Inderal (beta blocker) IV and Capoten (ACE inhibitor) IV. A patient with pheochromocytomas will have excessive amounts of catecholamines causing severe hypertension and tachycardia, leading to a life-threatening situation for brain attack or MI. For more information see answer 9, rationale (2).

1. Cushing's syndrome is a cluster of clinical abnormalities due to excessive levels of adrenocortical hormones (particularly cortisol) or related corticosteroids and, to a lesser extent, androgens and aldosterone. Drug therapy is mitotane (Lysodren) PO, which inhibits corticosteroid synthesis. Its unmistakable signs include rapidly developing adiposity of the face (moon face), neck, and trunk, and purple striae on the skin. Cushing's syndrome is most common in females. Prognosis depends on the underlying cause. Prognosis is poor in untreated persons and in those with untreatable ectopic ACTH-producing carcinoma or metastatic adrenal carcinoma. In approximately 70 percent of patients, Cushing's syndrome results from excess production of ACTH or excessive administration of steroids over a long period of time. Signs and symptoms include diabetes mellitus, hypokalemia, and pathologic fracture due to decreased bone mineralization. Fat pads over upper back (buffalo hump) and on the face (moon face); slender legs and arms; peptic ulcers; emotional lability; hypertension; increased susceptibility to infection; decreased lymphocyte production; suppression of antibody formation; sodium and secondary fluid retention; and amenorrhea occur. Treatment includes restoration of hormone balance; radiation or drug therapy may be required. Surgery may be required; bilateral adrenalectomy or hypophysectomy or pituitary irradiation may be necessary. If the pituitary or adrenal gland is removed, cortisol therapy is essential during and after surgery to help the patient tolerate the physiologic stress imposed by surgery.

3. Deep thermal burns, see answer 5, rationale (4).

4. In CHF, the heart fails as a pump. It cannot perfuse the kidney. When the kidney is not perfused, it releases renin and aldosterone. Aldosterone retains sodium (Na), which retains water, and this increases the amount of fluid saved. Osmotic pressure is increased by the rising sodium concentration leading to release of ADH. ADH increases renal tubular reabsorption of water. Renin is a powerful vasoconstrictor that causes hypertension and increases the workload of the heart. The three mechanisms of compensation that enable the weakened heart to continue to meet the metabolic demands of the body are tachycardia, ventricular dilation, and hypertrophy of the myocardium. The fact that Lasix and digoxin are ordered PO tells you that the patient's CHF is not severe.

84. ❹ The first medications you will administer are Tofranil and Zoloft PO (these drugs cannot be given IV, IM, or SC) to the patient diagnosed with major depression. This patient has the serious diagnosis, and the condition is a danger to her. This patient may commit suicide. For more information see answer 15, rationale (4).

1. Bipolar disorder, see answer 15, rationale (3).

2. Panic disorder, see answer 15, rationale (1).

3. Obsessive-compulsive disorder, see answer 18, rationale (3).

85. ❷ The first medication you will administer is continuous IV infusion of oxytocin to the patient with a diagnosis of postpartum bleeding. Early recognition and acknowledgment of the diagnosis of postpartum bleeding is critical to care management. The first step is to evaluate the contractility of the uterus. If the uterus is hypotonic, management is directed toward increasing contractility and minimizing blood loss.

The initial management of excessive postpartum bleeding is firm massage of the uterine fundus, expression of any clots in the uterus, elimination if any bladder distention, and continuous IV infusion of 10 to 40 units of oxytocin added to 1000 mL of Ringer's lactate or NS solution. If the uterus fails to respond to oxytocin, a 0.2-mg dose of ergonovine (Ergotrate) or methylergonovine (Methergine) may be given intramuscularly to produce sustained uterine contractions.

Postpartum bleeding is a life-threatening situation and must be treated immediately.

1, 3, 4. These diagnoses may become life-threatening situations, but the postpartum bleeding is an immediate life-threatening situation.

86. 1. Explain procedure, check ID.

2. Distend vein by applying tourniquet 8 to 10 inches above site, tap on vessel or have patient open and close fist, or hang over side of bed.

3. Clean site with alcohol swab, start at center and work outward.

4. Put on sterile gloves.

5. Hold skin taut to stabilize vein.

6. Insert catheter bevel up (direct method: thrust catheter through skin and vein in one smooth motion; indirect method: first pierce skin, then vessel).

7. Lessen the angle and advance catheter, watch for flashback of blood

8. When you see blood return, advance catheter one-fourth inch and then remove tourniquet.

9. Withdraw needle from catheter, advance catheter up to hub.

10. Secure catheter.

11. Attach IV tubing.

12. Begin IV infusing.

13. Check for infiltration or hematoma.

87. Related to iron deficiency anemia: ❸ Iron PO extended release; ❺ Decreased hemoglobin; ❻ Premature infants.

Not related to iron deficiency anemia: A. Bleeding; C. Vitamin B₁₂, D. Milk.

88. The correct order for the cardinal movements: 1. Engagement, descent, and flexion; 2. Internal rotation; 3. Extension; 4. Restitution; 5. External rotation (shoulder rotation); 6. Expulsion.

89. Related to placenta previa: ❷ Painless vaginal bleeding; ❸ Suspected vaginal bleeding occurring after 24 weeks of gestation; ❹ Bleeding is associated with stretching and thinning of the lower uterine segment.

Not related to placenta previa: 1. Placenta separation prior to delivery of the fetus; 5. Bleeding may be concealed.

90. Atropine

91. Lidocaine

92. Trousseau's and Chvostek's sign

93. Hydration and Didronel

94. Prostate-specific antigen level

95. Falls

96. 2000 mL

97. Longer

98. Less

99. Right foot

100. Lasix and Lanoxin (digoxin)

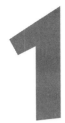
Simple Math Methods

INTERNATIONAL SYSTEM OF UNITS AND CONVENTIONAL UNITS

Most Commonly Used Weights

1,000,000 micrograms (μg) = 1 gram (g)
1000 micrograms (μg) = 1 milligram (mg)
60 milligrams (mg) = 1 grain (gr)
15 grains (gr) = 1 gram (g)
1 grain (gr) = .064779 gram (g)
1000 grams (g) = 1 kilogram (kg)
1000 milligrams (mg) = 1 gram (g)
500 mg = 0.5 g
50 mg = 0.05 g
5 mg = 0.005 g
1 mg = 0.001 g

Students, memorize this. It will really help you with your medication problems.

1/100 grain = 0.6 mg
1/150 grain = 0.4 mg
1/200 grain = 0.3 mg

Always set up math problems in the following way: divide what is ordered by what is available (on hand) multiplied by the form the medication is packaged in (e.g., mg, mL, g, etc.). For example:

Ordered: 2 grams. On hand: 500 mg/1 tablet
On hand: 500-mg tablets
2 g/500 mg × 1 tablet

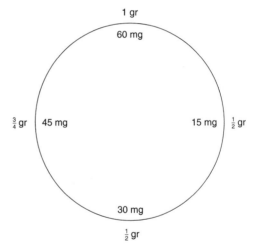

A. $\dfrac{2\text{g (ordered)} \times 1 \text{ tablet}}{500 \text{ mg (have)}}$

B. $\dfrac{2000 \text{ mg (ordered)}}{500 \text{ mg (have)}} = 4\,(500 \text{ mg tablets})$

(2 g converted to mg by moving the decimal point three places to the right)

C. $\dfrac{20 \text{ mg}}{5 \text{ mg}} \times \text{ tablet} = 4 \text{ tablets}$

SIMPLE MATH METHOD 1

Changing Grams (g) to Grains (gr)

(Grams to grains is larger to smaller; therefore, multiply.)
To change g ordered to gr on hand, take the number of gr in 1 g (15 gr) and multiply 15 gr by the number of g ordered.

(15 gr = 1 g)

Convert

A. 15 gr (15 gr in a g)
  × (g ordered)
  _____
  gr ordered

B. 15 gr (15 gr in a g)
  × 2 g (ordered)
  _____
  30 gr (g converted to gr)

Example 1 (g to gr)

Ordered: 4 g
On hand: 120-gr tablets

A. *Set it up*

$$\frac{4 \text{ g (ordered)}}{120 \text{ gr (on hand)}} \times 1 \text{ tablet}$$

B. *Convert*

15 gr

$$\times \frac{4 \text{ g (ordered)}}{60 \text{ gr}}$$

C. *Replace g with gr*

$$\frac{60 \text{ gr}}{120 \text{ gr}} \times 1 \text{ tablet}$$

Answer: 0.5 or ½ tablet = 60 gr ordered

Math Practice Exercise 1 (g to gr)

1. The physician orders 3 g Bactrim PO q6h. The nurse has on hand 15-gr Bactrim tablets. How many tablets would the nurse administer?
2. The physician orders 2 g Gantrisin PO q4h. The nurse has on hand 15-gr Gantrisin tablets. How many tablets would the nurse administer?

Answers for Math Practice 1 (g to gr)

1. A. *Set it up*

$$\frac{3 \text{ g}}{15 \text{ gr}} \times 1 \text{ tablet}$$

B. *Convert*

15 gr
$$\times 3 \text{ g (grams ordered)}$$
_____
45 grains (grams changed to gr)
(15 gr = 1 g)

C. *Replace g with gr*

$$\frac{45 \text{ g}}{15 \text{ g}} \times 1 \text{ tablet}$$

D. 3 × 1 tablet = 3

Answer: Administer *three* 15-gr tablets

2. A. *Set it up*

$$\frac{2 \text{ g}}{15 \text{ gr}} \times 1 \text{ tablet}$$

B. *Convert*

15 gr
$$\times 2 \text{ g (grams ordered)}$$
_____
30 grains (grams changed to gr)
(15 gr = 1 g)

C. *Replace g with gr*

$$\frac{30 \text{ g}}{15 \text{ g}} \times 1 \text{ tablet}$$

D. 2 × 1 tablet = 2

Answer: Administer *two* 15 gr tablets

SIMPLE MATH METHOD 2

Changing Grains (gr) Ordered to Grams (g) on Hand

(Grains to grams is smaller to larger; therefore, divide.)
Divide the number of grains (gr) in 1 gram (15 gr) into grains ordered.

(15 gr = 1 g) $\dfrac{\text{gr}}{15 \text{ gr}} = \text{g}$

Example 2 (gr to g)

Ordered: 3 gr of Deferoxamine PO q4h
On hand: 0.4-g tablets (15 gr = 1 g)

2. A. *Set it up*

$$\frac{3 \text{ gr (ordered)}}{0.4 \text{ g (on hand)}} \times 1 \text{ tablet}$$

B. *Convert*

3 gr ÷ 15 gr/g = 0.2 g

C. *Replace g with gr*

$$\frac{0.2 \text{ g (ordered)}}{0.4 \text{ g (on hand)}} \times 1 \text{ tablet}$$

D. ½ × 1 tablet = ½ tablet

Answer: ½ tablet

Math Practice Exercise 2 (gr to g)

1. The physician orders 60 gr. The nurse has on hand 4-g tablets. How many tablets would the nurse administer?
2. The physician orders 45 gr PO q3. The nurse has on hand 3-g tablets. How many g would the nurse administer?

Answers for Math Practice 2 (gr to g)

1.   (15 gr = 1 g)

A. *Set it up*

$$\frac{60 \text{ gr (ordered)}}{4 \text{ g (on hand)}} \times 1 \text{ tablet}$$

B. *Convert*

60 gr ÷ 15 gr/g = 4 g

C. *Replace g with gr*

$$\frac{4 \text{ g (ordered)}}{4 \text{ g (on hand)}} \times 1 \text{ tablet} = 1 \text{ tablet}$$

Answer: 1 tablet

2.   (15 gr = 1g)

A. *Set it up*

$$\frac{45 \text{ gr (ordered)}}{3 \text{ g (on hand)}} \times 1 \text{ tablet}$$

B. *Convert*

45 gr ÷ 15 gr/g = 3 g

C. *Replace g with gr*

$$\frac{3 \text{ g (ordered)}}{3 \text{ g (on hand)}} \times 1 \text{ tablet} = \text{tablet}$$

Answer: 1 tablet

SIMPLE MATH METHOD 3

Changing Milligrams (mg) Ordered to Grains (gr) on Hand

(Milligrams to grains is smaller to larger; therefore, divide.) Divide the number of milligrams (mg) in 1 grain (gr) (60 mg) into milligrams ordered.

(60 mg = 1 gr) mg (ordered) ÷ 60 mg/1 g = _____ gr

Example 3 (mg to gr)

The physician orders 180 mg Bactrim PO q6h. The nurse has on hand 3-gr tablets. How many tablets would the nurse administer?

(60 mg= 1 gr)

Set it up   *Convert*

A. $\dfrac{180 \text{ mg (ordered)}}{3 \text{ gr (on hand)}} \times 1 \text{ tablet}$ B. $\dfrac{180 \text{ mg}}{60 \text{ mg}} = 3 \text{ gr}$

Replace mg with gr

C. $\dfrac{3 \text{ gr (ordered)}}{3 \text{ gr (on hand)}} \times 1 \text{ tablet} = 1 \text{ tablet}$

The nurse has a 3-gr tablet available, which is the same as a 180-mg tablet.

Answer: 1 tablet

Math Practice Exercise 3 (mg to gr)

1. The physician orders 60 mg aspirin q3 PRN for pain. The nurse has on hand 1-gr tablets. How many tablets would the nurse administer?

2. The physician orders 120 mg aspirin. The nurse has on hand 2 gr tablets. How many tablets would the nurse administer?

Answers for Math Practice 3 (mg to gr)

1. (60 mg = 1 gr)

   Set it up   *Convert*

   A. $\dfrac{60 \text{ mg (ordered)}}{1 \text{ gr (on hand)}}$ B. 60 mg (ordered) ÷ 60 mg/1 gr = 1 gr

   Replace gr with g

   C. $\dfrac{1 \text{ gr (ordered)}}{1 \text{gr (on hand)}} \times 1 \text{ tablet} = 1 \text{ tablet}$

   Answer: 1 tablet

2. (60 mg = 1 gr)

   Set it up   *Convert*

   A. $\dfrac{120 \text{ mg (ordered)}}{2 \text{ gr (on hand)}}$ B. 120 mg (ordered) ÷ 60 mg/1 gr = 1 gr

   Replace mg with gr

   C. $\dfrac{2 \text{ gr (ordered)}}{2 \text{ gr (on hand)}} \times 1 \text{ tablet} = 1 \text{ tablet}$

   Answer: 1 tablet

SIMPLE MATH METHOD 4

Changing Grains (gr) Ordered to Milligrams (mg) on Hand

(Grains to milligrams is larger to smaller; therefore, multiply.) Multiply the number of milligrams (mg) in 1 grain (gr) (60 mg) times the number of grains ordered.

(60 mg = 1 gr)

Set it up   *Convert*

A. gr (ordered) × 60 mg/gr   B. 10 gr (ordered) × 60 mg/gr = 600 mg

Answer: 600 mg

Example 4 (gr to mg)

The physician orders 2 gr of Talwin q4h PRN for pain. The nurse has on hand 60-mg tablets. How many tablets would the nurse administer q4h?

(60 mg = 1 gr)

Set it up   *Convert*

A. $\dfrac{2 \text{ gr (ordered)}}{60 \text{ mg}} \times 1 \text{ tablet}$ B. 2 gr (ordered) × 60 mg/gr = 120 mg

Replace mg with gr

C. $\dfrac{120 \text{ mg}}{60 \text{ mg}} \times 2 \text{ tablets}$ D. 2 × 1 = 2 tablets

Answer: 2 tablets

Math Practice Exercise 4 (gr to mg)

1. The physician orders 5 gr ASA PO q4-6h PRN for fever. The nurse has on hand 300-mg tablets. How many tablets would the nurse administer?

2. The physician orders 2 gr PO. The nurse has on hand 120-mg tablets. How many tablets would the nurse administer?

Answers for Math Practice 4 (gr to mg)

1. (60 mg = 1gr)

   Set it up   *Convert*

   A. $\dfrac{5 \text{ gr (ordered)}}{300 \text{ mg}} \times 1 \text{ tablet}$ B. 5 gr (ordered) × 60 mg/gr = 300 mg

   Replace gr with mg

   C. $\dfrac{300 \text{ mg}}{300 \text{ mg}} \times 1 \text{ tablet} = 1 \text{ tablet}$

   Answer: 1 tablet

2. (60 mg = 1 gr)

   Set it up   *Convert*

   A. 2 gr (ordered)   B. 2 gr (ordered) × 60 mg/gr = 120 mg

C. $\dfrac{120 \text{ mg}}{120 \text{ mg}} \times \text{tablet} = 1 \text{ tablet}$

Answer: 1 tablet

SIMPLE MATH METHOD 5

Change Grams (g) Ordered to Milligrams (mg) on Hand

(Grams to milligrams is larger to smaller: therefore, multiply.) To change grams (g) to milligrams (mg), move the decimal point three places to the right, or multiply the number of grams times 1000.

A. 1 g = 1000 mg   B. 0.02 g = 20 mg

or

A. $1000 \text{ mg} \times \dfrac{1 \text{ g}}{1000 \text{ mg}}$ B. $1000 \text{ mg} \times \dfrac{0.002 \text{ g}}{20 \text{ mg}}$

A. 0.2 g = 200 mg   B. 0.0020 g = mg
$\Longrightarrow$ 2 places

Example 5 (g to mg)

The physician orders 0.1 g of Pepcid. The nurse has on hand 100 mg/mL. To change 0.1 g ordered to mg on hand, move the decimal point two places to the right.

Set it up

A. $\dfrac{0.1 \text{ g (ordered)}}{100 \text{ mg (on hand)}} \times 1 \text{ mL}$

Convert

B. 0.1 g = 100 mg, move decimal point two places to the right ($\Longrightarrow$ 2 places) 0.1 g = 100 mg
0.1 g = 100 mg

or

0.1 g × 1000 mg/g = 100 mg

Replace g with mg

C. $\dfrac{100 \text{ mg (ordered)}}{100 \text{ mg (on hand)}} \times 1 \text{ mL}$

D. 1 × 1 mL = 1 mL

Answer: 1 mL

Math Practice Exercise 5 (g to mg)

1. The physician orders ascorbic acid 0.25 g IM qd. The nurse has on hand ascorbic acid 500 mg/mL. How many mL would the nurse administer?

2. The physician orders 0.05 g of Demerol. The nurse has on hand 50 mg/mL. How many mL would the nurse administer?

Answers for Math Practice 5 (g to mg)

1. Change 0.25 g ordered to mg on hand (500 mg/mL on hand).

Set it up

A. $\dfrac{0.25 \text{ g (ordered)}}{500 \text{ mg (on hand)}} \times 1 \text{ mL}$

Convert

B. 0.25 g to mg, move decimal point two places to the right ($\Longrightarrow$ 2 places) 0.25 g = 250 mg

or

0.25 g × 1000 mg = 250 mg

Replace g with mg

C. $\dfrac{250 \text{ mg (ordered)}}{500 \text{ mg (on hand)}} \times 1 \text{ mL}$

D. $\frac{1}{2} \times 1 \text{ mL} = \frac{1}{2} \text{ mL or } 0.5 \text{ mL}$

Answer: 0.5 mL

2. *Set it up*

A. $\dfrac{0.05 \text{ g (ordered)}}{50 \text{ mg (on hand)}} \times 1 \text{ mL}$

Convert

B. 0.05 g to mg, move decimal point two places to the right ($\Longrightarrow$ 2 places) 0.05 g = 50 mg

or

0.05 g × 1000 mg = 50 mg

Replace g with mg

C. $\dfrac{50 \text{ mg (ordered)}}{50 \text{ mg (on hand)}} \times 1 \text{ mL}$

D. 1 × 1 mL = 1 mL

Answer: 1 mL

SIMPLE MATH METHOD 6

Changing milligrams (mg) ordered to grams (g) on hand

(Multiply by 0.001, move decimal point 3 places to the left, or 1 mg = 0.001 g.)
Multiply the number of grams (g) in 1 milligram (mg) (0.001 g) times the number of milligrams (mg) ordered.

1 mg = 0.001 g × mg ordered
0.001 g × 600 mg ordered = 0.6 g
or
600 mg; move three decimal points to the left
($\Leftarrow$ 3 places)

Answer: 0.6 g

Example 6 (mg to g)

The physician orders 350 mg. The nurse has on hand 0.035-g tablets. How many tablets would the nurse administer?

Set it up

A. $\dfrac{350 \text{ mg (ordered)}}{.035 \text{ g (on hand)}} \times 1 \text{ tablet}$

Convert

B. 350 mg to g; move decimal point three places to the left
($\Leftarrow$ 3 places)
350 mg = 0.035 g

Replace mg with g

C. $\dfrac{.035 \text{ g (ordered)}}{.035 \text{ g (on hand)}} \times 1 \text{ tablet} = 1 \text{ tablet}$

Answer: 1 tablet

Math Practice Exercise 6 (mg to g)

1. The physician orders 56 mg. The nurse has on hand 0.056-g tablets. How many tablets would the nurse administer?

2. The physician orders 6000 mg. The nurse has on hand 2-g tablets. How many tablets would the nurse administer?

Answers for Math Practice 6 (mg to g)

1. Change 56 mg ordered to g on hand (0.056-g tablets on hand).

Set it up

A. $\dfrac{56 \text{ mg (ordered)}}{0.056 \text{ g (on hand)}} \times 1 \text{ tablet}$

Convert

B. 56 mg to g, move decimal point three places to the left
($\Leftarrow$ 3 places)
0.056 mg = 56 g

Replace mg with g

C. $\dfrac{0.056 \text{ g (ordered)}}{0.056 \text{ g (on hand)}} \times 1 \text{ tablet} = 1 \text{ tablet}$

Answer: 1 tablet

2. Change 6000 mg ordered to g on hand (2-g tablets on hand).

Set it up

A. $\dfrac{6000 \text{ mg (ordered)}}{2 \text{ g (on hand)}} \times 1 \text{ tablet}$

Convert

B. 6000 mg to g, move decimal point three places to the left
($\Leftarrow$ 3 places)
6000 mg = 6 g

Replace mg with g

C. $\dfrac{6 \text{ g}}{2 \text{ g}} \times 1 \text{ tablet} = 3 \text{ tablet}$

D. $3 \times 1 \text{ tablet} = 3 \text{ tablets}$

Answer: Three 2-g tablets

SIMPLE MATH METHOD 7

Changing a Fraction of a Grain (gr) to Milligrams (mg)

(Grains to milligrams is larger to smaller; therefore, multiply.) When a prescription has a *fraction of a weight* ordered, the nurse must determine what *fraction* that is of the whole unit weight on hand (mg, g, or gr).
The physician orders Atropine 1/150 gr IM. The nurse has on hand 0.4 mg/1 mL (60 mg = 1 gr).

Set it up

A. $\dfrac{1/150 \text{ gr (ordered)}}{0.4 \text{ mg (on hand)}} \times 1 \text{ mL}$

Convert

B. $1/150 \text{ gr} \times 60 \text{ mg} = \dfrac{60 \text{ mg}}{150 \text{ gr}} = 0.4 \text{ mg}$

Replace gr with mg

C. $\dfrac{0.4 \text{ mg}}{0.4 \text{ mg}} \times \text{mL} = 1 \text{ mL}$

Answer: 1 mL

Example 7 Fractions (gr to mg)

The physician orders atropine injection of 1/200 gr. The nurse has on hand 0.3 mg/mL. How many mL will the nurse administer?

Set it up

A. $\dfrac{1/200 \text{ gr (ordered)}}{0.3 \text{ mg (on hand)}} \times 1 \text{ mL}$

Convert

B. $1/200 \text{ gr} \times 60 \text{ mg} = \dfrac{60 \text{ mg}}{200 \text{ gr}} = 0.3 \text{ mg}$

Replace gr with mg

C. $\dfrac{0.3 \text{ mg}}{0.3 \text{ mg}} \times 1 \text{ mL} = 1 \text{ mL}$

Answer: 1 mL

Math Practice Exercise 7 Fractions (gr to mg)

1. The physician orders Decaject 1/120 gr IM. The nurse has on hand 0.2 mg/mL. How many mL would the nurse administer?

2. The physician orders colchicine 1/60 gr IM. The nurse has on hand 1 mg/mL. How many mL would the nurse administer?

Answers for Math Practice 7 Fraction (gr to mg)

1.   (60 mg = 1 gr)

Set it up

A. $\dfrac{1/120 \text{ gr (ordered)}}{0.2 \text{ mg (on hand)}} \times 1 \text{ mL}$

Convert

B. $1/120 \text{ gr} \times 60 \text{ mg} = \dfrac{60 \text{ mg}}{120 \text{ gr}} = 0.5 \text{ mg}$

Replace gr with mg

C. $\dfrac{0.5 \text{ (ordered)}}{0.2 \text{ (on hand)}} \times 1 \text{ mL}$

D. $2.5 \text{ mL} \times 1 \text{ mL} = 2.5 \text{ mL}$

Answer: 2.5 mL

2. (60 mg = 1 gr)

Set it up

A. $\dfrac{1/60 \text{ gr (ordered)}}{1 \text{ mg/mL (on hand)}}$

Convert

B. $1/60 \text{ gr} \times 60 \text{ mg} = \dfrac{60 \text{ mg}}{60 \text{ gr}} = 1 \text{ mg}$

Replace gr with mg

C. $\dfrac{1 \text{ mg (ordered)}}{1 \text{ mg (on hand)}} \times 1 \text{ mL}$

D. $1 \times 1 \text{ mL} = 1 \text{ mL}$

Answer: 1 mL

SIMPLE MATH METHOD 8

Changing a Fraction of a Gram (g) to Milligrams (mg)

(Grams to milligrams is larger to smaller; therefore, multiply.) The physician orders Amcill 0.5 g. The nurse has on hand 500-mg tablets.

(1 g = 1000 mg)
Set it up

A. $\dfrac{1/2 \text{ g (ordered)}}{500 \text{ mg (on hand)}} \times 1 \text{ tablet}$

Convert

B. $1/2 \text{ g} \times 1000 \text{ mg} = \dfrac{1000 \text{ mg}}{2} = 500 \text{ mg}$

Replace g with mg

C. $\dfrac{500 \text{ mg}}{500 \text{ mg}} \times 1 \text{ tablet}$

D. $1 \times 1 \text{ tablet} = 1 \text{ tablet}$

Answer: One 500-mg tablet

Example 8 Fractions (g to mg)

The physician orders Stilbestrol 1/5 g. The nurse has on hand 400-mg tablets. How many tablets would the nurse administer?

(1 g = 1000 mg)
Set it up

A. $\dfrac{1/5 \text{ g (ordered)}}{400 \text{ mg (on hand)}} \times 1 \text{ tablet}$

Convert

B. $1/5 \text{ g} \times 1000 \text{ mg} = \dfrac{1000 \text{ mg}}{5 \text{ g (ordered)}} = 200 \text{ mg}$

Replace g with mg

C. $\dfrac{200 \text{ mg (on hand)}}{400 \text{ mg (ordered)}} \times 1 \text{ tablet}$

D. $1/2 \times 1 \text{ tablet} = \frac{1}{2} \text{ tablet}$

Answer: ½ tablet or 200 mg

Math Practice Exercise 8 Fractions (g to mg)

1. The physician orders 1/5 g. The nurse has on hand 200 mg/mL. How many mL would the nurse administer?

2. The physician orders 1/10 g. The nurse has on hand 100-mg tablets. How many tablets would the nurse administer?

Answers for Math Practice 8 Fraction (g to mg)

1. Change 1/5 g ordered to mg on hand, which is 200 mg/mL.

(1 g = 1000 mg)
Set it up

A. $\dfrac{1/5 \text{ g (ordered)}}{200 \text{ mg (on hand)}}$

Convert

B. $1/5 \text{ g} \times 1000 \text{ mg} = \dfrac{1000 \text{ mg}}{5 \text{ g (ordered)}}$
$= 200 \text{ mg / mL}$

Replace g with mg

C. $\dfrac{200 \text{ mg (on hand)}}{200 \text{ mg (ordered)}} \times 1 \text{ mL}$

D. $1 \times 1 \text{ mL} = 1 \text{ mL}$

Answer: 1 mL

2. Change 1/10 g ordered to mg on hand, which is 100-mg tablets.

(1 g = 1000 mg)
Set it up

A. $\dfrac{1/10 \text{ g (ordered)}}{100 \text{ mg (on hand)}} \times 1 \text{ tablet}$

Convert

B. $1/10 \text{ g} \times 1000 \text{ mg} = \dfrac{1000 \text{ mg (on hand)}}{10 \text{ g (ordered)}}$
$= 100 \text{ mg}$

Replace g with mg

C. $\dfrac{100 \text{ mg}}{100 \text{ mg}} \times 1 \text{ tablet}$

D. $1 \times 1 \text{ tablet} = 1 \text{ tablet}$

Answer: 1 tablet

SIMPLE MATH METHOD 9

Changing a Fraction of a Gram (g) to Grains (gr)

(Grams to grains is larger to smaller; therefore, multiply.)

(1 g = 15 gr)

Set it up

A. $\dfrac{1/5 \text{ g (ordered)}}{3 \text{ gr (on hand)}} \times 1$ tablet

Convert

B. $1/5 \text{ g} \times 15 \text{ gr} = \dfrac{15}{5}$
   $= 3 \text{ gr}$

Replace g with gr

C. $\dfrac{3 \text{ gr}}{3 \text{ gr}} \times 1$ tablet $= 1$ tablet

Answer: 1 tablet

Example 9 Fractions (g to gr)

The physician orders 1/3 g codeine. The nurse has on hand 10-gr tablets. How many tablets would the nurse administer?

(1 g = 15 gr)

Set it up

A. $\dfrac{1/3 \text{ g (ordered)}}{10 \text{ gr (on hand)}} \times 1$ tablet

Convert

B. $1/3 \text{ g} \times 15 \text{ gr} = \dfrac{15 \text{ gr}}{3 \text{ gr}}$
   $= 5 \text{ gr}$

Replace g with gr

C. $\dfrac{5}{10} = 0.5$ or $\frac{1}{2}$ tablet

Answer: ½ tablet

Math Practice Exercise 9

1. The physician orders 1/3 g. The nurse has on hand 5-gr tablets. How many tablets would the nurse administer?

2. The physician orders 1/5 g of aspirin. The nurse has on hand 3-gr tablets. How many tablets would the nurse administer?

Answers for Math Practice 9 Fraction (g to gr)

1. (1 g = 15 gr)

   Set it up

   A. $\dfrac{1/3 \text{ g (ordered)}}{5 \text{ gr (on hand)}} \times 1$ tablet

   Convert

   B. $1/3 \text{ g} \times 15 \text{ gr} = \dfrac{15 \text{ gr}}{3 \text{ g}} = 5 \text{ gr}$

Replace g with gr

C. $\dfrac{5 \text{ gr}}{5 \text{ gr}} = 1$ tablet $\times 1$ tablet
   $= 1$ tablet

Answer: 1 tablet

2. *Set it up*

   A. $\dfrac{1/5 \text{ g (ordered)}}{3 \text{ gr}} \times 1$ tablet

   Convert

   B. $1/5 \text{ g} \times 15 \text{ gr} = \dfrac{15 \text{ gr}}{5} = 3 \text{ gr}$

   Replace g with gr

   C. $\dfrac{3 \text{ gr}}{3 \text{ gr}} \times 1$ tablet   D. 1×1 tablet $= 1$ tablet

Answer: 1 tablet

SIMPLE MATH METHOD 10

Working Math Questions when the Weight Ordered and the Weight on Hand are the Same Equivalent

Divide the equivalent ordered by the equivalent on hand.

$$\frac{\text{ordered}}{\text{on hand}} = \frac{30 \text{ mg (ordered)}}{15 \text{ mg tablets (on hand)}}$$
$$= 2 \text{ tablets}$$

Answer: 2 tablets

Example 10 (Same Equivalents)

1. The physician orders 50 mg of Demerol PO PRN for pain. The nurse has on hand 100-mg tablets. How many tablets will the nurse administer? (Divide what you have on hand by what is ordered.)

Set it up

A. $\dfrac{50 \text{ mg (ordered)}}{100 \text{ mg (on hand)}} \times 1$ tablet

B. $\frac{1}{2} \times 1$ tablet $= \frac{1}{2}$ or 0.5 tablet

Answer: 0.5 tablet

2. The physician orders 30 gr of aspirin PO PRN for pain. The nurse has on hand 15-gr aspirin tablets. How many tablets will the nurse administer? (Divide what is on hand by what is ordered.)

Set it up

A. $\dfrac{30 \text{ gr (ordered)}}{15 \text{ gr (on hand)}} \times 1$ tablet

B. 2×1 tablet $= 2$ tablets

Answer: Two 15-gr tablets

Math Practice Exercise 10 (Same Equivalents)

1. The physician orders 100-mg Demerol tablets PRN for pain. The nurse has on hand 50-mg tablets. How many tablets would the nurse administer?

2. The physician orders 10 mg Valium IM HS. The nurse has on hand 5 mg/mL. How many mL would the nurse administer?

3. The physician orders phenobarbital 80 mg SC q8h PRN. The nurse has on hand phenobarbital 40 mg/mL. How many mL would the nurse administer?

4. The physician orders Seconal 50 mg IM HS PRN. The nurse has on hand 250 mg/5 mL of Seconal. How many mL would the nurse administer?

Answers for Math Practice 10 (Same Equivalents)

1. A. $\dfrac{100 \text{ mg (ordered)}}{50 \text{ mg (on hand)}} \times 1 \text{ tablet}$

   B. 2×1 tablet $= 2$ tablets

Answer: 2 tablets

2. A. $\dfrac{10 \text{ mg (ordered)}}{5 \text{ mg (on hand)}} \times 1 \text{ mL}$

   B. $2 \times 1 \text{ mL} = 2 \text{ mL}$

Answer: 2 mL

3. A. $\dfrac{80 \text{ mg (ordered)}}{40 \text{ mg (on hand)}} \times \text{ mL}$

   B. $2 \times 1 \text{ mL} = 2 \text{ mL}$

Answer: 2 mL

4. A. $\dfrac{50 \text{ mg (ordered)}}{250 \text{ mg (on hand)}} \times 5 \text{ mL}$

   B. $0.2 \times 5 \text{ mL}$ on hand $= 1 \text{ mL}$

Answer: 1 mL

SIMPLE MATH METHOD 11

Working Math Questions when the Weight Ordered and the Weight on Hand are the Same Equivalent and Both are Fractions

Divide the fraction equivalent *ordered* by the fraction equivalent *on hand*.

$$\frac{\text{(fraction) ordered}}{\text{(fraction) on hand}} = \text{answer}$$

Remember, when dividing by a fraction, invert the fraction and multiply.

Example 11 (Fractions Same Equivalents)

1. The physician orders atropine gr 1/100 IM. The nurse has on hand atropine gr 1/150/mL. How many mL with the nurse administer?

   Set it up

   A. $\dfrac{1/100 \text{ gr (ordered)}}{1/150 \text{ gr (on hand)}} \times 1 \text{ mL}$

   Convert

   B. $\dfrac{1}{100 \text{ gr}} \times \dfrac{150}{1} \times 1 \text{ mL}$

   C. $\dfrac{150}{100} \times 1 \text{ mL}$

   D. $1.5 \times 1 \text{ mL} = 1.5 \text{ mL}$

Answer: 1.5 mL

2. The physician orders morphine gr 1/16 SC q4h. The nurse has on hand morphine gr 1/4/mL. How many mL will the nurse administer? Remember, when dividing by a fraction, invert and multiply.

   Set it up

   A. $\dfrac{1/16 \text{ gr (ordered)}}{1/4 \text{ gr (on hand)}} \times 1 \text{ mL}$

   B. $\dfrac{1}{16 \text{ gr}} \times \dfrac{4 \text{ gr}}{1} \times 1 \text{ mL}$

   C. $\dfrac{4}{16} \times 1 \text{ mL} = 0.25 \times 1 \text{ mL}$
   $= 0.25 \text{ mL}$

Answer: 0.25 mL

Math Practice Exercise 11 (Same Equivalents)

1. The physician orders morphine gr 1/4 IM q3h PRN for pain. The nurse has on hand morphine gr 1/8/mL. How many mL would the nurse administer?

2. The physician orders morphine gr 1/5 SC q3h PRN for pain. The nurse has on hand morphine gr 1/8/mL. How many mL would the nurse administer?

3. The physician orders atropine gr 1/200 IM 8:00 AM. The nurse has on hand atropine gr 1/100/mL. How many mL would the nurse administer?

Answers for Math Exercise 11 (Fractions Same Equivalents)

   Set it up

1. A. $\dfrac{1/4 \text{ gr (ordered)}}{1/8 \text{ gr (on hand)}} = \times 1 \text{ mL}$

   or

   B. $\dfrac{1}{4} \times \dfrac{8}{1} \times 1 \text{ mL}$

   C. $\dfrac{8}{4} \times 1 \text{ mL} = 2 \times 1 \text{ mL}$

Answer: 2 mL

Set it up

2. A. $\dfrac{1/5 \text{ gr (ordered)}}{1/8 \text{ gr (on hand)}} \times 1 \text{ mL}$

   or

   B. $\dfrac{1}{5} \times \dfrac{8}{1} \times 1 \text{ mL}$

   C. $\dfrac{8}{5} \times 1 \text{ mL}$

   D. $1.6 \times 1 \text{ mL} = 1.6 \text{ mL}$

Answer: 1.6 mL

Set it up

A. $\dfrac{1/200 \text{ gr (ordered)}}{1/100 \text{ gr (on hand)}} \times 1 \text{ mL}$

B. $\dfrac{1}{200} \times \dfrac{100}{1} \times 1 \text{ mL}$

C. $\dfrac{100}{200} \times 1 \text{ mL} = \dfrac{1}{2} \times 1 \text{ mL}$

Answer:

D. 0.5 mL

SIMPLE MATH METHOD 12

Comprehensive Practice Exercise

1. Vibramycin 200 mg IV q6h. On hand Vibramycin 10 mg/mL.
   Administer_____mL.

2. Demerol 100 mg IM q3h PRN for pain. On hand Demerol 50 mg/mL.
   Administer_____mL.

3. Haldol 3 mg IM qid. On hand Haldol 5 mg/mL.
   Administer_____mL.

4. Digoxin 0.2 mg IM qd. On hand Digoxin 0.5 mg/2 mL.
   Administer_____mL.

5. Aminophylline 100 mg IV q6h. On hand Aminophylline 500 mg/mL.
   Administer_____mL.

6. Demerol 50 mg IM q3h PRN for pain. On hand Demerol 50 mg/0.5 mL.
   Administer_____mL.

7. Atropine gr 1/200. On hand atropine 0.4 mg/mL.
   Administer_____mL.

8. Solu-Cortef 100 mg IM q6. On hand Solu-Cortef 250 mg/ 2 mL.
   Administer_____mL.

9. Valium 15 mg IV stat. On hand 5 mg/mL.
   Administer_____mL.

10. Digoxin (Lanoxin) 0.25 mg IV qd. On hand digoxin 0.5 mg/2 mL.
    Administer_____mL.

11. Cleocin 50 mg IV q8h. On hand Cleocin 300 mg/2 mL.
    Administer_____mL.

12. Phenobarbital 33 mg IM PRN. On hand phenobarbital 66 mg/mL.
    Administer_____mL.

13. Dilaudid 2 mg IM q3h PRN. On hand Dilaudid 4 mg/ mL.
    Administer_____mL.

14. Gentamicin 60 mg IV q6h. On hand gentamicin 20 mg/ mL.
    Administer_____mL.

15. Penicillin G procaine 400,000 U IM q8h. On hand penicillin G procaine 200,000 U/5 mL.
    Administer_____mL.

16. Penicillin 200,000 U PO tid. On hand penicillin 400,000 U/2 mL.
    Administer_____mL.

17. Decadron 0.5 mg PO q6h. On hand Decadron 0.25-mg tablets.
    Administer_____tablets.

18. Lanoxin 0.25 mg PO qid. On hand Lanoxin 0.125-mg tablets.
    Administer _____tablets.

19. Keflex 250 mg PO qid. On hand Keflex 0.25-g capsules.
    Administer_____capsules.

20. Prednisone 7.5 mg PO tid. On hand prednisone 2.5-mg tablets.
    Administer_____tablets.

21. Flagyl 750 mg PO tid. On hand Flagyl 250-mg tablets.
    Administer_____tablets.

22. Aspirin 0.6 g PO q3h PRN for pain. On hand aspirin 5-gr tablets.
    Administer_____tablets.

23. KCl elixir 40 mEq PO bid with juice. On hand KCl 20 mEq/15 mL.
    Administer_____mL.

24. Solu-Cortef 0.05 g IM q4h. On hand Solu-Cortef 250 mg/2 mL.
    Administer_____mL.

25. Keflex Neutral 50 mg IV q6h. On hand Keflex Neutral 1 g/ 10 mL.
    Administer_____mL.

26. Atropine sulfate injection 1 gr/150 atropine sulfate. On hand atropine sulfate 0.4 mg/2 mL.
    Administer_____mL.

Answers for Comprehensive Exercise 12

1. 20 mL	14. 3 mL
2. 2 mL	15. 10 mL
3. 9 M	16. 1 mL
4. 0.8 mL	17. 2 tablets
5. 0.2 mL	18. 2 tablets
6. 0.5 mL	19. 1 capsule
7. 0.75 mL	20. 3 tablets
8. 0.8 mL	21. 3 tablets
9. 3 mL	22. 2 tablets
10. 1 mL	23. 30 mL
11. 0.3 mL	24. 0.4 mL
12. 0.5 mL	25. 0.5 mL
13. 0.5 mL	26. 2 mL

DIGOXIN

Digoxin is packaged 0.5 mg/2 mL. Therefore,

0.5 mg $= 2$ mL
0.25 mg $= 1$ mL——0.25 is $\frac{1}{2}$ of 0.5
0.125 mg $= 0.5$ mL——0.125 is $\frac{1}{2}$ of 0.25
0.0625 mg $= 0.25$ mL——0.0625 is $\frac{1}{2}$ of 0.125

1. $\dfrac{0.25 \text{ (ordered)}}{0.5 \text{ (on hand)}} = 0.05 \times 2 \text{ mL} = 1 \text{ mL}$

2. $\dfrac{125 \text{ (ordered)}}{0.5 \text{ (on hand)}} = 0.25 \times 2 \text{ mL} = 0.5 \text{ mL}$

3. $\dfrac{0.0625 \text{ (ordered)}}{0.5 \text{ (on hand)}} = 0.125 \times 2 \text{ mL} = 0.25 \text{ mL}$

SIMPLE MATH METHOD 13

Examples 13 IV (Intravenous)

1. The physician orders heparin 600 U/h. How many units of heparin will be added to 100 mL NS if the IV is infusing at 5 mL/h? Divide ordered by what is on hand times the form of the medication.

   A. $\dfrac{100 \text{ mL NS (ordered)}}{5 \text{ mL/h (on hand)}} = 20 \text{ mL/h} = 600 \text{ U/h}$

   B. $\dfrac{600 \text{ U/h} \times 20 \text{ mL/h}}{12,000 \text{ U}}$ to be added to IV

   Formula A

   $\dfrac{100 \text{ mL solution}}{\text{mL/h}} = \text{mL/h} \times \text{U/h}$
   $= \text{U of heparin to be added to mL of solution}$

Formula B

$\dfrac{\times \text{U}}{100 \text{ mL}} = \dfrac{600 \text{ U/h (ordered)}}{5 \text{ mL/h (ordered)}}$

$\dfrac{600}{5 \text{ mL}} = 120 \times 100$

$= 1200$ U to be added to IV

2. The physician orders 800 U/h; the pharmacy sends 12,000 U/250 mL NS. The nurse will infuse the IV at *what rate*?

   A. $\dfrac{12000 \text{ U heparin}}{250 \text{ mL NS}} = 48 \text{ units/mL}$

   Answer: 48 U/mL

   B. $\dfrac{800 \text{ U heparin IV}}{48 \text{ U mL}} = 17 \text{ mL/h}$

   Answer: 17 mL/h

   Formula A

   $\dfrac{\text{heparin (ordered)}}{\text{IV solution}} = \text{U/mL}$

   $\dfrac{\text{U/h}}{\text{U/mL}} = \text{mL/h}$

   Formula B

   $\dfrac{800 \text{ U}}{x \text{ mL}} = \dfrac{1200 \text{ U}}{250 \text{ mL}}$

   $12,000x = 800 \times 250$
   $12,000x = 200,000$
   $x = 16.6 \text{ or } 17 \text{ mL/h}$

3. The physician orders aminophylline 50 mg/h; the pharmacy sends 1 g aminophylline/500 mL NS. The nurse will infuse the IV at what rate?

   $\dfrac{50 \text{ mg/h}}{1000 \text{ mg (1 gm)}} x\ 500 \text{ mL} = \times \text{ mL/h}$

   $\dfrac{50}{1000} = \dfrac{x}{500}$

   $1000\, x = 25,000$
   $x = 25 \text{ mL/h}$

   Answer: 25 mL/h

4. The physician orders 3 mg morphine/h. How much morphine needs to be added to the 100 mL D$_5$ $\frac{1}{2}$ if the flow rate is 10 mL/h?

   $\dfrac{3 \text{ mg/h}}{x \text{ mg}} \times 100 \text{ mL} = 10 \text{ mL/h}$

   $\dfrac{3}{x} = \dfrac{10}{100}$

   $10\, x = 300$
   $x = 30 \text{ mg}$

   Answer: 30 mg

5. The physician orders heparin 750 U/h. On hand is 15,000 U in D_5W 250 mL. At what rate is the IVAC to be set?

$$\frac{750 \text{ U/h}}{15,000 \text{ U}} \times 250 \text{ mL} = x \text{ mL/h}$$

$$\frac{750}{15,000} = \frac{x}{250}$$

$$15,000\,x = 1875$$

$$x = 12.5 \text{ mL}$$

Answer: 12.5 mL

6. The physician orders D_5W 1000 mL q8h. The drip (gtt) factor is 15 (gtt/mL). How many gtt/min should the IV be set?

A. $$\frac{1000 \text{ mL}}{8 \text{ h}} = 125 \text{ mL/h}$$

B. This shortcut can be used because there are 60 seconds in 1 minute and 60 minutes in 1 hour; therefore, divide.

$$\frac{60}{15} = 4$$

Then divide 4 into 125 mL/h.

C. First determine how many mL/h, then see what the drop factor is. It will be one of the following:

Drop factor	Divide into	Allows you to divide by
10 gtt	60 min	6
12 gtt	60 min	5
15 gtt	60 min	4
20 gtt	60 min	3
60 gtt	60 min	1

$$\frac{60 \text{ m}}{10\,(\text{gtt factor})} = 6 \qquad \frac{60 \text{ m}}{12\,(\text{gtt factor})} = 5$$

$$\frac{60 \text{ m}}{15\,(\text{gtt factor})} = 4 \qquad \frac{60 \text{ m}}{60\,(\text{gtt factor})} = 1$$

D. Then divide *mL/h* by *the dividing factor* to determine *gtt/min*.

$$\frac{\text{mL/h}}{\text{the dividing factor}} = \text{gtt/min}$$

7. The physician orders 1000 mL $D_5\frac{1}{2}$, administered over a period of 10 h with a drop factor of 20 gtt/mL.

A. How many mL/h?

$$\frac{1000 \text{ mL}}{10 \text{ h}} = 100 \text{ mL}$$

B. How many gtt/min? Drop factor is 20; divide by 3.

$$\frac{100 \text{ mL/h}}{3 \text{ h}} = 33 \text{ gtt/min}$$

8. Cytoxan 475 mg in 250 mL $D_5\frac{1}{2}$ administered over 2 h, with a drop factor of 15 gtt/mL.
A. How many mL/h?

$$\frac{250 \text{ mL}}{2 \text{ h}} = 25 \text{ mL}$$

B. How many gtt/min?
Drop factor is 15; divide by 4.

$$\frac{125 \text{ mL/h}}{4 \text{ h}} = 31 \text{ gtt/min}$$

9. $D_5\frac{1}{4}$ 500 mL + 5.5 mEq KCl administered over 2 h. Drop factor is 60 (gtt/mL).

A. How many mL/h?

$$\frac{500 \text{ ml } D_5\frac{1}{4}}{2 \text{ h}} = 250 \text{ mL/h}$$

B. How many gtt/min?
gtt factor is 60; divide by 1.

$$\frac{250 \text{ mL/h}}{1 \text{ gtt factor}} = 250 \text{ gtt/min}$$

Simple Math Exercise 13

1. Packed RBCs IV 120 mL. Administer over 4 h; drop factor is 12 (gtt/mL).
   A. How many mL/h?
   B. How many gtt/min?

2. Blood plasma 500 mL. Administer over 4-h; drop factor is 15 gtt/mL.
   A. How many mL/h?
   B. How many gtt/min?

3. Ringer's lactate solution 1500 m:. Administer over 12-h period. Drop factor is 10 gtt/min.
   A. How many mL/h?
   B. How many gtt/min?

4. 0.9% NS 1000 mL plus 30,000 U heparin. Infuse at 1000 U of heparin/h; drop factor is 60 gtt/min.
   A. Amount of heparin/mL?
   B. How many mL/h?
   C. How many gtt/min?

Answers for Simple Math Exercise 13

1. A. 30 mL   B. 6

2. A. 125 mL/h   B. 31 gtt/min

3. A. 125 mL/h   B. 20 gtt/min

4. A. 30 U heparin/mL   B. 33.3 mL/h

   C. 34 gtt/min

Note:

A. $$\frac{30,000 \text{ U heparin/mL}}{1000 \text{ mL NS}} = 30 \text{ U heparin/mL}$$

B. $$\frac{1000 \text{ U/h}}{30 \text{ U heparin}} = 33.3 \text{ mL/h}$$

C. $\dfrac{33.3\ \text{mL/h}}{1} = 34\ \text{gtt/min}$

gtt factor is 60 gtt/mL; dividing factor is 1.

Note: 33.3 gtt is rounded up to 34 gtt/min.

Determining mg for kg Weight

To determine mg for kg weight of a child, take mg of medication ordered times the weight of the child in kg. This equals the mg desired.

    The physician orders neomycin sulfate 10.3 mg/kg q4h. The child weighs 5 kg. Which of the following dosages would the child receive within a *24-h period?*

A. 50 mg/day
B. 100 mg/day
C. 309 mg/day
D. 408 mg/day

    10.3 mg (ordered) × 5 kg = 51.5 mg
    Daily dosage: Take 51.5 mg × 6 = 308 mg in a 24-h period.

Converting from Pounds (lb) to Kilograms (kg)

To convert from pounds to kilograms, divide by 2.2. Round kilograms to the nearest tenth. If body weight is measured in pounds, convert pounds to kilograms when dosage recommendations are based on weight in pounds.

Example A

Find the number of kg in 98 lb.

$$(2.2\ \text{lb} = 1\ \text{kg})$$
$$\dfrac{98}{2.2} = 44.5\ \text{kg}$$

Answer: 98 lb = 44.5 kg

Exercise A

1. 220 lb	4. 80 lb
2. 66 lb	5. 60 lb
3. 44 lb	6. 28 lb

Answers to Exercise A

1. 220 lb = 100 kg	4. 80 lb = 37 kg
2. 66 lb = 30 kg	5. 60 lb = 28 kg
3. 44 lb = 20 kg	6. 28 lb = 13 kg

Appendix

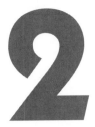

Normal Laboratory Values

The tables in this appendix list only the most common tests, their normal values, and possible etiologies for abnormal values. Laboratory values may vary with different techniques and/or different laboratories; therefore, hospitals will show a slight difference in normal values.

PART I: COMPLETE BLOOD COUNT

Hematology	Reference Values	Comments
1. Hemoglobin (Hgb): vehicle for oxygen carbon dioxide transport	Adult: Male: 13.5–18.0 g/dL Female: 12–16 g/dL Child: 11–16 g/dL	◆ Hemoglobin levels decrease after severe hemorrhage but change may not occur until 3 to 4 h later.
2. Hematocrit (Hct)	Male: 40–54% Female: 36–46%	◆ Hematocrit is an effective indicator of body fluid volume. A large fluid loss and dehydration increase hematocrit level (occurs because of hemoconcentration). ◆ It usually takes 4–8 h for the hematocrit to increase after fluid loss. ◆ Hct is a measure of the percentage of RBCs in the total blood volume.
3. WBC count	Adult: 5000–10,000 mL Child (2 years): 6000–17,000 μL	◆ If WBC levels are significantly increased, the change could be due to infection.
4. RBC count	Adult: Male: 4.5–6.0 μL Female: 4.0–5.0 μL Elderly: Male: 3.7–6.0 μL Female: 4.0–5.0 μL Child: 3.8–5.5 μL	◆ RBC level is decreased when patient hemorrhages, has anemia, and is overhydrated. ◆ RBC level increases in dehydration and polycythemia.

Hematology	Reference Values	Comments
5. Platelet count	Adult: 150,000–400,000 μL	◆ Platelet count is monitored during and after blood loss and acute trauma. ◆ A low platelet count (thrombocytopenia) will cause bleeding. If platelet count is markedly decreased, hemorrhage might occur.

6. Hematocrit (Hct)
Packed red cell volume (PVC)
	Adult:
	  Male: 40–54%
	  Female: 36–46%
	Elderly:
	  Male: 38–42%
	  Female: 38–41%
	Child:
	  1–3 years: 29–40%
	  4–10 years: 36–38%
		◆ HCT level decreases when the patient has one of the following anemias: aplastic, hemolytic, folic acid deficiency, pernicious, or sickle cell.
		◆ HCT level is increased in dehydration and polycythemia vera.

PART II: ELECTROLYTE LEVELS

Electrolyte (Serum)	Reference Values	Comments
1. Potassium (K)	3.5–5.0 mEq/L	◆ In kidney failure or during shock, potassium excess will occur (hyperkalemia).
2. Sodium (Na)	135–145 mEq/L	◆ If patient is receiving liter of IV saline solution and kidney failure occurs, an increase in serum sodium level will occur (hypernatremia).
3. Calcium (Ca)	4.5–5.5 mEq/L	◆ Thyroidectomy causes trauma to the parathyroids and may cause calcium deficit (hypocalcemia). ◆ Drugs that decrease calcium level include aspirin, corticosteroids, heparin, and oral contraceptives.

PART III: ARTERIAL BLOOD GASES

Adults and children have approximately the same arterial blood gas (ABG) values.

	Adult or Child	Newborn	Comments
1. pH	7.35–7.45	7.34–7.46	◆ pH <7.35 indicates acidosis—either respiratory or metabolic. ◆ pH >7.45 indicates alkalosis—either respiratory or metabolic.
2. PCO_2 PO_2	35–45 mEq/L 75–100 mEq/L	26–41 mEq/L 60–70 mEq/L	◆ PCO_2 reflects the adequacy of alveolar ventilation. When there is alveolar damage, carbon dioxide (CO_2) cannot escape. CO_2 combines with water to form carbonic acid, causing an acidotic state. ◆ When the patient is hypoventilating, CO_2 is blown off and respiratory alkalosis occurs. Chronic obstructive lung disease is a major cause of respiratory acidosis.
3. HCO_3	21–28 mEq/L	16–24 mEq/L	◆ Bicarbonate (HCO_3) is an alkaline substance that comprises over half of the total buffer base in the blood. When there is a significant reduction is HCO_3 and an increase in acids, metabolic acidosis occurs.
4. Oximeter	95–100%		

ACID–BASE BALANCE

	pH	PCO_2	HCO_3
Metabolic acidosis	↓	↑	↓
Metabolic alkalosis	↑	↓	↑
Respiratory acidosis	↓	↑	↓
Respiratory alkalosis	↑	↓	↑

Causes of Acid–Base Imbalance

1. Respiratory acidosis (pH ≤7.35; PCO_2 ≥45 mm Hg): Chronic obstructive lung disease (e.g., emphysema, chronic bronchitis, pneumonia).

2. Respiratory alkalosis (pH ≥7.45; PCO_2 ≤35 mm Hg): Salicylate toxicity in the early phase, hysteria (hyperventilation), and pulmonary embolism.

3. Metabolic acidosis (pH ≤7.35; HCO_3 ≤24 mEq/L): Diabetic ketoacidosis, severe diarrhea, starvation/ malnutrition, shock, burns, kidney failure, and acute myocardial infarction.

4. Metabolic alkalosis (pH ≥7.45; HCO_3 ≥28 mEq/L): Severe vomiting, suction, peptic ulcer, potassium loss, and excess administration of bicarbonate.

PART IV: BLOOD CHEMISTRY

Chemistry (Blood)	Reference Values	Comments
1. Glucose	Adult: 60–120 mg/dL Child: 60–120 mg/dL Neonate: 30–60 mg/dL	◆ Serum glucose level must be evaluated according to time of day blood is drawn. For example, a glucose level of 135 mg/dL may be normal if taken 1 h after eating, but it may be abnormal if the patient is fasting. ◆ Critical values: <50 mg/dL or >400 mg/dL
2. Prothrombin time (PT) (plasma)	11–12.5 s	◆ The major use of the PT test is to monitor oral anticoagulant [warfarin sodium (Coumadin)] therapy. Antidote for Coumadin overdose is vitamin K.
3. Partial thromboplastin time (PTT)	60–70 s and activated partial thromboplastin time (aPTT) 30–40	◆ The major use of the PTT test is to monitor anticoagulant therapy heparin. Antidote for heparin is protamine sulfate.
4. Creatinine (serum)	Adult: .05–1.2 mg/dL Child: 0.3–0.7 mg/dL	◆ Is excreted only by the kidney. The following renal disorders will cause increased creatinine level: glomerulonephritis, pyelonephritis, acute tubular necrosis, urinary obstruction, kidney failure, and hepatic failure.
5. Blood urea nitrogen (BUN)	Adult: 10–20 mg/dL Child: 5–18 mg/dL	◆ BUN is the amount of urea nitrogen in the blood. Urea is formed in the liver as an end-product of protein metabolism.
6. Prostatic Acid phosphatase (PAP) (serum)	Adult: 0–3.1 mg/mL	◆ Found in highest concentration in the prostate gland and is used to diagnose end-stage prostatic carcinoma and to monitor the efficiency of treatment. Elevated levels of PAP are seen in patients with prostatic cancer that has metastasized beyond the capsule to other parts of the body, especially to the bone. Treatment of prostatic cancer is surgery and estrogen therapy.
7. Prostate-specific antigen (PSA)	Men: 0–4.0 ng/mL	◆ PSA is functionally and immunologically distinct from PAP. PSA is localized in both normal prostatic epithelial cells and prostatic carcinoma cells. PSA has proved to be the most prognostically reliable marker for monitoring recurrence of prostatic carcinoma; however, this test does not have the sensitivity or specificity to be considered an ideal tumor marker. ◆ The most useful approach to date may be age-specific PSA reference ranges, which are based on the concept that blood PSA concentration is dependent on patient age. The increase in PSA with advancing age is attributed to four major factors: prostate enlargement, increasing inflammation, presence of microscopic but clinically insignificant cancer, and leakage of PSA into the serum.

PART IV: BLOOD CHEMISTRY (CONTINUED)

Chemistry (Blood)	Reference Values	Comments
8. Specific gravity	Adult: 1.016–1.022	◆ Specific gravity will be increased in dehydration and decreased in hydration.
9. Urine pH	Adult: 4.6–8.0	◆ Bacteria will grow faster in urine with a high pH (alkaline). Cranberry juice may be used to increase urine acidity.
10. Direct Coombs' test		◆ Used to detect autoantibodies against RBCs, which can cause cellular damage.
		◆ Erythroblastosis fetalis, lymphomas, lupus erythematosus, infectious mononucleosis, hemolytic anemia, and use of some drugs (e.g., quinidine) are all associated with the production of autoantibodies against RBCs.
11. Lithium	Adult: 0.6–1.2 mEq/L	◆ Used for treatment of manic-depressive illness and as maintenance therapy to prevent or diminish frequency and intensity of manic episodes.
12. Dilantin	Adults: 10–20 μg/mL	◆ Prevention/treatment of seizures and treatment of digitalis-induced arrhythmias.
13. Digoxin (Lanoxin)	Adult: 0.8–2.0 mg/mL (levels >2.4 mg/mL are toxic)	◆ Increases intracellular calcium and allows more calcium to enter the myocardial cell during depolarization via a sodium/potassium pump mechanism; this increases force of contraction (positive inotropic effect), increases renal perfusion (seen as diuretic effect in patients with CHF), decreases heart rate (negative chronotropic effect), and decreases AV node conduction.

LIQUID CONVERSION

30 mL (cc) = 1 ounce (oz)   500 mL (cc) = 1 pint (pt)

1000 mL (cc) = 1 quart (qt)   15 mL (cc) = 1 tablespoon (T)

= 1 liter (L)   5 mL (cc) = 1 teaspoon (tsp)

Teaching Dietary Guidelines for Patient

1. Tyramine-Rich Foods (important to avoid with MAOIs and some antihypertensives)

  a. Avocados, bananas, beer, bologna, cheeses, chocolate, liver, red wine, salami, smoked fish

2. Potassium-Rich Foods (important to eat with potassium-wasting diuretics)

  a. Avocados, bananas, broccoli, cantaloupe, dried fruits, grapefruit, instant coffee, nuts, oranges, peaches, potatoes, prunes, salt substitute, sunflower seeds, spinach, tomatoes

3. Calcium-Rich Foods (important for women after menopause and for patients in hypocalcemic states)

  a. Broccoli, canned salmon, canned sardines, clams, cream soups (made with milk), spinach, dairy products, milk, molasses, oysters, tofu

4. Urine Acidifiers (important in maintaining excretion of some drugs and in treating and preventing urinary tract infection)

  a. Cheese, cranberries, eggs, fish, grains, plums, poultry, prunes, red meats

5. Iron-Rich Foods (important in maintaining RBCs)

  a. Beets, dried beans/peas, dried fruit, enriched grains, leafy-green vegetables, organ meats (liver, heart, kidney)

6. Low-Sodium Foods (important in CHF, hypertension, fluid overload)

  a. Egg yolk, fresh vegetables, fresh fruit, grits, honey, jam/jellies, lean meats, lima beans, macaroons, potatoes, poultry, pumpkin, red kidney beans, sherbet, unsalted nuts

7. High-Sodium Foods (important to avoid eating in CHF, hypertension, fluid overload)

  a. Barbeque (BBQ), beer, buttermilk, butter, canned soups, canned seafood, cured meats, microwave dinners, cookies, mixes, tomato ketchup, TV dinners, pretzels, pickles, snack foods, sauerkraut, canned vegetables

Index

ANSWER SHEETS

Chapter 11 • Diseases, Medications, and Nutrition

Exam I

1.____	16.____	31.____	46.____	61.____	76.____	91.____
2.____	17.____	32.____	47.____	62.____	77.____	92.____
3.____	18.____	33.____	48.____	63.____	78.____	93.____
4.____	19.____	34.____	49.____	64.____	79.____	94.____
5.____	20.____	35.____	50.____	65.____	80.____	95.____
6.____	21.____	36.____	51.____	66.____	81.____	96.____
7.____	22.____	37.____	52.____	67.____	82.____	97.____
8.____	23.____	38.____	53.____	68.____	83.____	98.____
9.____	24.____	39.____	54.____	69.____	84.____	99.____
10.____	25.____	40.____	55.____	70.____	85.____	100.____
11.____	26.____	41.____	56.____	71.____	86.____	
12.____	27.____	42.____	57.____	72.____	87.____	FIRST
13.____	28.____	43.____	58.____	73.____	88.____	EXAM
14.____	29.____	44.____	59.____	74.____	89.____	GRADE
15.____	30.____	45.____	60.____	75.____	90.____	____

Exam II

1.____	16.____	31.____	46.____	61.____	76.____	91.____
2.____	17.____	32.____	47.____	62.____	77.____	92.____
3.____	18.____	33.____	48.____	63.____	78.____	93.____
4.____	19.____	34.____	49.____	64.____	79.____	94.____
5.____	20.____	35.____	50.____	65.____	80.____	95.____
6.____	21.____	36.____	51.____	66.____	81.____	96.____
7.____	22.____	37.____	52.____	67.____	82.____	97.____
8.____	23.____	38.____	53.____	68.____	83.____	98.____
9.____	24.____	39.____	54.____	69.____	84.____	99.____
10.____	25.____	40.____	55.____	70.____	85.____	100.____
11.____	26.____	41.____	56.____	71.____	86.____	
12.____	27.____	42.____	57.____	72.____	87.____	SECOND
13.____	28.____	43.____	58.____	73.____	88.____	EXAM
14.____	29.____	44.____	59.____	74.____	89.____	GRADE
15.____	30.____	45.____	60.____	75.____	90.____	____

Exam III

1._____	16._____	31._____	46._____	61._____	76._____	91._____
2._____	17._____	32._____	47._____	62._____	77._____	92._____
3._____	18._____	33._____	48._____	63._____	78._____	93._____
4._____	19._____	34._____	49._____	64._____	79._____	94._____
5._____	20._____	35._____	50._____	65._____	80._____	95._____
6._____	21._____	36._____	51._____	66._____	81._____	96._____
7._____	22._____	37._____	52._____	67._____	82._____	97._____
8._____	23._____	38._____	53._____	68._____	83._____	98._____
9._____	24._____	39._____	54._____	69._____	84._____	99._____
10._____	25._____	40._____	55._____	70._____	85._____	100._____
11._____	26._____	41._____	56._____	71._____	86._____	
12._____	27._____	42._____	57._____	72._____	87._____	THIRD
13._____	28._____	43._____	58._____	73._____	88._____	EXAM
14._____	29._____	44._____	59._____	74._____	89._____	GRADE
15._____	30._____	45._____	60._____	75._____	90._____	_____

ANSWER SHEETS

Chapters 12 and 13 • Fluid & Electrolyte and Renal & Urinary Disorders

Exam I

1._____	16._____	31._____	46._____	61._____	76._____	91._____
2._____	17._____	32._____	47._____	62._____	77._____	92._____
3._____	18._____	33._____	48._____	63._____	78._____	93._____
4._____	19._____	34._____	49._____	64._____	79._____	94._____
5._____	20._____	35._____	50._____	65._____	80._____	95._____
6._____	21._____	36._____	51._____	66._____	81._____	96._____
7._____	22._____	37._____	52._____	67._____	82._____	97._____
8._____	23._____	38._____	53._____	68._____	83._____	98._____
9._____	24._____	39._____	54._____	69._____	84._____	99._____
10._____	25._____	40._____	55._____	70._____	85._____	100._____
11._____	26._____	41._____	56._____	71._____	86._____	
12._____	27._____	42._____	57._____	72._____	87._____	FIRST
13._____	28._____	43._____	58._____	73._____	88._____	EXAM
14._____	29._____	44._____	59._____	74._____	89._____	GRADE
15._____	30._____	45._____	60._____	75._____	90._____	_____

Exam II

1._____	16._____	31._____	46._____	61._____	76._____	91._____
2._____	17._____	32._____	47._____	62._____	77._____	92._____
3._____	18._____	33._____	48._____	63._____	78._____	93._____
4._____	19._____	34._____	49._____	64._____	79._____	94._____
5._____	20._____	35._____	50._____	65._____	80._____	95._____
6._____	21._____	36._____	51._____	66._____	81._____	96._____
7._____	22._____	37._____	52._____	67._____	82._____	97._____
8._____	23._____	38._____	53._____	68._____	83._____	98._____
9._____	24._____	39._____	54._____	69._____	84._____	99._____
10._____	25._____	40._____	55._____	70._____	85._____	100._____
11._____	26._____	41._____	56._____	71._____	86._____	
12._____	27._____	42._____	57._____	72._____	87._____	SECOND
13._____	28._____	43._____	58._____	73._____	88._____	EXAM
14._____	29._____	44._____	59._____	74._____	89._____	GRADE
15._____	30._____	45._____	60._____	75._____	90._____	_____

Exam III

1._____	16._____	31._____	46._____	61._____	76._____	91._____
2._____	17._____	32._____	47._____	62._____	77._____	92._____
3._____	18._____	33._____	48._____	63._____	78._____	93._____
4._____	19._____	34._____	49._____	64._____	79._____	94._____
5._____	20._____	35._____	50._____	65._____	80._____	95._____
6._____	21._____	36._____	51._____	66._____	81._____	96._____
7._____	22._____	37._____	52._____	67._____	82._____	97._____
8._____	23._____	38._____	53._____	68._____	83._____	98._____
9._____	24._____	39._____	54._____	69._____	84._____	99._____
10._____	25._____	40._____	55._____	70._____	85._____	100._____
11._____	26._____	41._____	56._____	71._____	86._____	
12._____	27._____	42._____	57._____	72._____	87._____	THIRD
13._____	28._____	43._____	58._____	73._____	88._____	EXAM
14._____	29._____	44._____	59._____	74._____	89._____	GRADE
15._____	30._____	45._____	60._____	75._____	90._____	_____

ANSWER SHEETS

Chapter 14 • Gastrointestinal, Accessory Organ, and Nutritional Anemia Disorders

Exam I

1._____	16._____	31._____	46._____	61._____	76._____	91._____
2._____	17._____	32._____	47._____	62._____	77._____	92._____
3._____	18._____	33._____	48._____	63._____	78._____	93._____
4._____	19._____	34._____	49._____	64._____	79._____	94._____
5._____	20._____	35._____	50._____	65._____	80._____	95._____
6._____	21._____	36._____	51._____	66._____	81._____	96._____
7._____	22._____	37._____	52._____	67._____	82._____	97._____
8._____	23._____	38._____	53._____	68._____	83._____	98._____
9._____	24._____	39._____	54._____	69._____	84._____	99._____
10._____	25._____	40._____	55._____	70._____	85._____	100._____
11._____	26._____	41._____	56._____	71._____	86._____	
12._____	27._____	42._____	57._____	72._____	87._____	FIRST
13._____	28._____	43._____	58._____	73._____	88._____	EXAM
14._____	29._____	44._____	59._____	74._____	89._____	GRADE
15._____	30._____	45._____	60._____	75._____	90._____	_____

Exam II

1._____	16._____	31._____	46._____	61._____	76._____	91._____
2._____	17._____	32._____	47._____	62._____	77._____	92._____
3._____	18._____	33._____	48._____	63._____	78._____	93._____
4._____	19._____	34._____	49._____	64._____	79._____	94._____
5._____	20._____	35._____	50._____	65._____	80._____	95._____
6._____	21._____	36._____	51._____	66._____	81._____	96._____
7._____	22._____	37._____	52._____	67._____	82._____	97._____
8._____	23._____	38._____	53._____	68._____	83._____	98._____
9._____	24._____	39._____	54._____	69._____	84._____	99._____
10._____	25._____	40._____	55._____	70._____	85._____	100._____
11._____	26._____	41._____	56._____	71._____	86._____	
12._____	27._____	42._____	57._____	72._____	87._____	SECOND
13._____	28._____	43._____	58._____	73._____	88._____	EXAM
14._____	29._____	44._____	59._____	74._____	89._____	GRADE
15._____	30._____	45._____	60._____	75._____	90._____	_____

Exam III

1._____	16._____	31._____	46._____	61._____	76._____	91._____
2._____	17._____	32._____	47._____	62._____	77._____	92._____
3._____	18._____	33._____	48._____	63._____	78._____	93._____
4._____	19._____	34._____	49._____	64._____	79._____	94._____
5._____	20._____	35._____	50._____	65._____	80._____	95._____
6._____	21._____	36._____	51._____	66._____	81._____	96._____
7._____	22._____	37._____	52._____	67._____	82._____	97._____
8._____	23._____	38._____	53._____	68._____	83._____	98._____
9._____	24._____	39._____	54._____	69._____	84._____	99._____
10._____	25._____	40._____	55._____	70._____	85._____	100._____
11._____	26._____	41._____	56._____	71._____	86._____	
12._____	27._____	42._____	57._____	72._____	87._____	THIRD
13._____	28._____	43._____	58._____	73._____	88._____	EXAM
14._____	29._____	44._____	59._____	74._____	89._____	GRADE
15._____	30._____	45._____	60._____	75._____	90._____	_____

ANSWER SHEETS

Chapter 15 • Cardiovascular and Peripheral Vascular Disorders

Exam I

1._____	16._____	31._____	46._____	61._____	76._____	91._____
2._____	17._____	32._____	47._____	62._____	77._____	92._____
3._____	18._____	33._____	48._____	63._____	78._____	93._____
4._____	19._____	34._____	49._____	64._____	79._____	94._____
5._____	20._____	35._____	50._____	65._____	80._____	95._____
6._____	21._____	36._____	51._____	66._____	81._____	96._____
7._____	22._____	37._____	52._____	67._____	82._____	97._____
8._____	23._____	38._____	53._____	68._____	83._____	98._____
9._____	24._____	39._____	54._____	69._____	84._____	99._____
10._____	25._____	40._____	55._____	70._____	85._____	100._____
11._____	26._____	41._____	56._____	71._____	86._____	
12._____	27._____	42._____	57._____	72._____	87._____	FIRST
13._____	28._____	43._____	58._____	73._____	88._____	EXAM
14._____	29._____	44._____	59._____	74._____	89._____	GRADE
15._____	30._____	45._____	60._____	75._____	90._____	_____

Exam II

1._____	16._____	31._____	46._____	61._____	76._____	91._____
2._____	17._____	32._____	47._____	62._____	77._____	92._____
3._____	18._____	33._____	48._____	63._____	78._____	93._____
4._____	19._____	34._____	49._____	64._____	79._____	94._____
5._____	20._____	35._____	50._____	65._____	80._____	95._____
6._____	21._____	36._____	51._____	66._____	81._____	96._____
7._____	22._____	37._____	52._____	67._____	82._____	97._____
8._____	23._____	38._____	53._____	68._____	83._____	98._____
9._____	24._____	39._____	54._____	69._____	84._____	99._____
10._____	25._____	40._____	55._____	70._____	85._____	100._____
11._____	26._____	41._____	56._____	71._____	86._____	
12._____	27._____	42._____	57._____	72._____	87._____	SECOND
13._____	28._____	43._____	58._____	73._____	88._____	EXAM
14._____	29._____	44._____	59._____	74._____	89._____	GRADE
15._____	30._____	45._____	60._____	75._____	90._____	_____

Exam III

1._____	16._____	31._____	46._____	61._____	76._____	91._____
2._____	17._____	32._____	47._____	62._____	77._____	92._____
3._____	18._____	33._____	48._____	63._____	78._____	93._____
4._____	19._____	34._____	49._____	64._____	79._____	94._____
5._____	20._____	35._____	50._____	65._____	80._____	95._____
6._____	21._____	36._____	51._____	66._____	81._____	96._____
7._____	22._____	37._____	52._____	67._____	82._____	97._____
8._____	23._____	38._____	53._____	68._____	83._____	98._____
9._____	24._____	39._____	54._____	69._____	84._____	99._____
10._____	25._____	40._____	55._____	70._____	85._____	100._____
11._____	26._____	41._____	56._____	71._____	86._____	
12._____	27._____	42._____	57._____	72._____	87._____	THIRD
13._____	28._____	43._____	58._____	73._____	88._____	EXAM
14._____	29._____	44._____	59._____	74._____	89._____	GRADE
15._____	30._____	45._____	60._____	75._____	90._____	_____

ANSWER SHEETS

Chapter 16 • Respiratory Disorders

Exam I

1._____	9._____	17._____	25._____	33._____	41._____	49._____
2._____	10._____	18._____	26._____	34._____	42._____	50._____
3._____	11._____	19._____	27._____	35._____	43._____	
4._____	12._____	20._____	28._____	36._____	44._____	
5._____	13._____	21._____	29._____	37._____	45._____	FIRST
6._____	14._____	22._____	30._____	38._____	46._____	EXAM
7._____	15._____	23._____	31._____	39._____	47._____	GRADE
8._____	16._____	24._____	32._____	40._____	48._____	_____

Exam II

1._____	9._____	17._____	25._____	33._____	41._____	49._____
2._____	10._____	18._____	26._____	34._____	42._____	50._____
3._____	11._____	19._____	27._____	35._____	43._____	
4._____	12._____	20._____	28._____	36._____	44._____	
5._____	13._____	21._____	29._____	37._____	45._____	SECOND
6._____	14._____	22._____	30._____	38._____	46._____	EXAM
7._____	15._____	23._____	31._____	39._____	47._____	GRADE
8._____	16._____	24._____	32._____	40._____	48._____	_____

Exam III

1._____	9._____	17._____	25._____	33._____	41._____	49._____
2._____	10._____	18._____	26._____	34._____	42._____	50._____
3._____	11._____	19._____	27._____	35._____	43._____	
4._____	12._____	20._____	28._____	36._____	44._____	
5._____	13._____	21._____	29._____	37._____	45._____	THIRD
6._____	14._____	22._____	30._____	38._____	46._____	EXAM
7._____	15._____	23._____	31._____	39._____	47._____	GRADE
8._____	16._____	24._____	32._____	40._____	48._____	_____

ANSWER SHEETS

Chapter 17 • Orthopedic Disorders

Exam I

1.___	9.___	17.___	25.___	33.___	41.___	49.___
2.___	10.___	18.___	26.___	34.___	42.___	50.___
3.___	11.___	19.___	27.___	35.___	43.___	
4.___	12.___	20.___	28.___	36.___	44.___	
5.___	13.___	21.___	29.___	37.___	45.___	FIRST
6.___	14.___	22.___	30.___	38.___	46.___	EXAM
7.___	15.___	23.___	31.___	39.___	47.___	GRADE
8.___	16.___	24.___	32.___	40.___	48.___	___

Exam II

1.___	9.___	17.___	25.___	33.___	41.___	49.___
2.___	10.___	18.___	26.___	34.___	42.___	50.___
3.___	11.___	19.___	27.___	35.___	43.___	
4.___	12.___	20.___	28.___	36.___	44.___	
5.___	13.___	21.___	29.___	37.___	45.___	SECOND
6.___	14.___	22.___	30.___	38.___	46.___	EXAM
7.___	15.___	23.___	31.___	39.___	47.___	GRADE
8.___	16.___	24.___	32.___	40.___	48.___	___

Exam III

1.___	9.___	17.___	25.___	33.___	41.___	49.___
2.___	10.___	18.___	26.___	34.___	42.___	50.___
3.___	11.___	19.___	27.___	35.___	43.___	
4.___	12.___	20.___	28.___	36.___	44.___	
5.___	13.___	21.___	29.___	37.___	45.___	THIRD
6.___	14.___	22.___	30.___	38.___	46.___	EXAM
7.___	15.___	23.___	31.___	39.___	47.___	GRADE
8.___	16.___	24.___	32.___	40.___	48.___	___

ANSWER SHEETS

Chapter 18 • Neurologic Disorders

Exam I

1._____	9._____	17._____	25._____	33._____	41._____	49._____
2._____	10._____	18._____	26._____	34._____	42._____	50._____
3._____	11._____	19._____	27._____	35._____	43._____	
4._____	12._____	20._____	28._____	36._____	44._____	
5._____	13._____	21._____	29._____	37._____	45._____	FIRST
6._____	14._____	22._____	30._____	38._____	46._____	EXAM
7._____	15._____	23._____	31._____	39._____	47._____	GRADE
8._____	16._____	24._____	32._____	40._____	48._____	_____

Exam II

1._____	9._____	17._____	25._____	33._____	41._____	49._____
2._____	10._____	18._____	26._____	34._____	42._____	50._____
3._____	11._____	19._____	27._____	35._____	43._____	
4._____	12._____	20._____	28._____	36._____	44._____	
5._____	13._____	21._____	29._____	37._____	45._____	SECOND
6._____	14._____	22._____	30._____	38._____	46._____	EXAM
7._____	15._____	23._____	31._____	39._____	47._____	GRADE
8._____	16._____	24._____	32._____	40._____	48._____	_____

Exam III

1._____	9._____	17._____	25._____	33._____	41._____	49._____
2._____	10._____	18._____	26._____	34._____	42._____	50._____
3._____	11._____	19._____	27._____	35._____	43._____	
4._____	12._____	20._____	28._____	36._____	44._____	
5._____	13._____	21._____	29._____	37._____	45._____	THIRD
6._____	14._____	22._____	30._____	38._____	46._____	EXAM
7._____	15._____	23._____	31._____	39._____	47._____	GRADE
8._____	16._____	24._____	32._____	40._____	48._____	_____

ANSWER SHEETS

Chapter 19 • Obstetric, Neonatal, and Gynecologic Disorders

Exam I

1._____	16._____	31._____	46._____	61._____	76._____	91._____
2._____	17._____	32._____	47._____	62._____	77._____	92._____
3._____	18._____	33._____	48._____	63._____	78._____	93._____
4._____	19._____	34._____	49._____	64._____	79._____	94._____
5._____	20._____	35._____	50._____	65._____	80._____	95._____
6._____	21._____	36._____	51._____	66._____	81._____	96._____
7._____	22._____	37._____	52._____	67._____	82._____	97._____
8._____	23._____	38._____	53._____	68._____	83._____	98._____
9._____	24._____	39._____	54._____	69._____	84._____	99._____
10._____	25._____	40._____	55._____	70._____	85._____	100._____
11._____	26._____	41._____	56._____	71._____	86._____	
12._____	27._____	42._____	57._____	72._____	87._____	FIRST
13._____	28._____	43._____	58._____	73._____	88._____	EXAM
14._____	29._____	44._____	59._____	74._____	89._____	GRADE
15._____	30._____	45._____	60._____	75._____	90._____	_____

Exam II

1._____	16._____	31._____	46._____	61._____	76._____	91._____
2._____	17._____	32._____	47._____	62._____	77._____	92._____
3._____	18._____	33._____	48._____	63._____	78._____	93._____
4._____	19._____	34._____	49._____	64._____	79._____	94._____
5._____	20._____	35._____	50._____	65._____	80._____	95._____
6._____	21._____	36._____	51._____	66._____	81._____	96._____
7._____	22._____	37._____	52._____	67._____	82._____	97._____
8._____	23._____	38._____	53._____	68._____	83._____	98._____
9._____	24._____	39._____	54._____	69._____	84._____	99._____
10._____	25._____	40._____	55._____	70._____	85._____	100._____
11._____	26._____	41._____	56._____	71._____	86._____	
12._____	27._____	42._____	57._____	72._____	87._____	SECOND
13._____	28._____	43._____	58._____	73._____	88._____	EXAM
14._____	29._____	44._____	59._____	74._____	89._____	GRADE
15._____	30._____	45._____	60._____	75._____	90._____	_____

Exam III

1._____	16._____	31._____	46._____	61._____	76._____	91._____
2._____	17._____	32._____	47._____	62._____	77._____	92._____
3._____	18._____	33._____	48._____	63._____	78._____	93._____
4._____	19._____	34._____	49._____	64._____	79._____	94._____
5._____	20._____	35._____	50._____	65._____	80._____	95._____
6._____	21._____	36._____	51._____	66._____	81._____	96._____
7._____	22._____	37._____	52._____	67._____	82._____	97._____
8._____	23._____	38._____	53._____	68._____	83._____	98._____
9._____	24._____	39._____	54._____	69._____	84._____	99._____
10._____	25._____	40._____	55._____	70._____	85._____	100._____
11._____	26._____	41._____	56._____	71._____	86._____	
12._____	27._____	42._____	57._____	72._____	87._____	THIRD
13._____	28._____	43._____	58._____	73._____	88._____	EXAM
14._____	29._____	44._____	59._____	74._____	89._____	GRADE
15._____	30._____	45._____	60._____	75._____	90._____	_____

ANSWER SHEETS

Chapter 20 • Growth, Development, and Early Childhood Diseases

Exam I

1.___	16.___	31.___	46.___	61.___	76.___	91.___
2.___	17.___	32.___	47.___	62.___	77.___	92.___
3.___	18.___	33.___	48.___	63.___	78.___	93.___
4.___	19.___	34.___	49.___	64.___	79.___	94.___
5.___	20.___	35.___	50.___	65.___	80.___	95.___
6.___	21.___	36.___	51.___	66.___	81.___	96.___
7.___	22.___	37.___	52.___	67.___	82.___	97.___
8.___	23.___	38.___	53.___	68.___	83.___	98.___
9.___	24.___	39.___	54.___	69.___	84.___	99.___
10.___	25.___	40.___	55.___	70.___	85.___	100.___
11.___	26.___	41.___	56.___	71.___	86.___	
12.___	27.___	42.___	57.___	72.___	87.___	FIRST
13.___	28.___	43.___	58.___	73.___	88.___	EXAM
14.___	29.___	44.___	59.___	74.___	89.___	GRADE
15.___	30.___	45.___	60.___	75.___	90.___	___

Exam II

1.___	16.___	31.___	46.___	61.___	76.___	91.___
2.___	17.___	32.___	47.___	62.___	77.___	92.___
3.___	18.___	33.___	48.___	63.___	78.___	93.___
4.___	19.___	34.___	49.___	64.___	79.___	94.___
5.___	20.___	35.___	50.___	65.___	80.___	95.___
6.___	21.___	36.___	51.___	66.___	81.___	96.___
7.___	22.___	37.___	52.___	67.___	82.___	97.___
8.___	23.___	38.___	53.___	68.___	83.___	98.___
9.___	24.___	39.___	54.___	69.___	84.___	99.___
10.___	25.___	40.___	55.___	70.___	85.___	100.___
11.___	26.___	41.___	56.___	71.___	86.___	
12.___	27.___	42.___	57.___	72.___	87.___	SECOND
13.___	28.___	43.___	58.___	73.___	88.___	EXAM
14.___	29.___	44.___	59.___	74.___	89.___	GRADE
15.___	30.___	45.___	60.___	75.___	90.___	___

Exam III

1. _____	16. _____	31. _____	46. _____	61. _____	76. _____	91. _____
2. _____	17. _____	32. _____	47. _____	62. _____	77. _____	92. _____
3. _____	18. _____	33. _____	48. _____	63. _____	78. _____	93. _____
4. _____	19. _____	34. _____	49. _____	64. _____	79. _____	94. _____
5. _____	20. _____	35. _____	50. _____	65. _____	80. _____	95. _____
6. _____	21. _____	36. _____	51. _____	66. _____	81. _____	96. _____
7. _____	22. _____	37. _____	52. _____	67. _____	82. _____	97. _____
8. _____	23. _____	38. _____	53. _____	68. _____	83. _____	98. _____
9. _____	24. _____	39. _____	54. _____	69. _____	84. _____	99. _____
10. _____	25. _____	40. _____	55. _____	70. _____	85. _____	100. _____
11. _____	26. _____	41. _____	56. _____	71. _____	86. _____	
12. _____	27. _____	42. _____	57. _____	72. _____	87. _____	THIRD
13. _____	28. _____	43. _____	58. _____	73. _____	88. _____	EXAM
14. _____	29. _____	44. _____	59. _____	74. _____	89. _____	GRADE
15. _____	30. _____	45. _____	60. _____	75. _____	90. _____	_____

ANSWER SHEETS

Chapter 21 • Psychiatric Disorders

Exam I

1._____	16._____	31._____	46._____	61._____	76._____	91._____
2._____	17._____	32._____	47._____	62._____	77._____	92._____
3._____	18._____	33._____	48._____	63._____	78._____	93._____
4._____	19._____	34._____	49._____	64._____	79._____	94._____
5._____	20._____	35._____	50._____	65._____	80._____	95._____
6._____	21._____	36._____	51._____	66._____	81._____	96._____
7._____	22._____	37._____	52._____	67._____	82._____	97._____
8._____	23._____	38._____	53._____	68._____	83._____	98._____
9._____	24._____	39._____	54._____	69._____	84._____	99._____
10._____	25._____	40._____	55._____	70._____	85._____	100._____
11._____	26._____	41._____	56._____	71._____	86._____	
12._____	27._____	42._____	57._____	72._____	87._____	FIRST
13._____	28._____	43._____	58._____	73._____	88._____	EXAM
14._____	29._____	44._____	59._____	74._____	89._____	GRADE
15._____	30._____	45._____	60._____	75._____	90._____	_____

Exam II

1._____	16._____	31._____	46._____	61._____	76._____	91._____
2._____	17._____	32._____	47._____	62._____	77._____	92._____
3._____	18._____	33._____	48._____	63._____	78._____	93._____
4._____	19._____	34._____	49._____	64._____	79._____	94._____
5._____	20._____	35._____	50._____	65._____	80._____	95._____
6._____	21._____	36._____	51._____	66._____	81._____	96._____
7._____	22._____	37._____	52._____	67._____	82._____	97._____
8._____	23._____	38._____	53._____	68._____	83._____	98._____
9._____	24._____	39._____	54._____	69._____	84._____	99._____
10._____	25._____	40._____	55._____	70._____	85._____	100._____
11._____	26._____	41._____	56._____	71._____	86._____	
12._____	27._____	42._____	57._____	72._____	87._____	SECOND
13._____	28._____	43._____	58._____	73._____	88._____	EXAM
14._____	29._____	44._____	59._____	74._____	89._____	GRADE
15._____	30._____	45._____	60._____	75._____	90._____	_____

Exam III

1._____	16._____	31._____	46._____	61._____	76._____	91._____
2._____	17._____	32._____	47._____	62._____	77._____	92._____
3._____	18._____	33._____	48._____	63._____	78._____	93._____
4._____	19._____	34._____	49._____	64._____	79._____	94._____
5._____	20._____	35._____	50._____	65._____	80._____	95._____
6._____	21._____	36._____	51._____	66._____	81._____	96._____
7._____	22._____	37._____	52._____	67._____	82._____	97._____
8._____	23._____	38._____	53._____	68._____	83._____	98._____
9._____	24._____	39._____	54._____	69._____	84._____	99._____
10._____	25._____	40._____	55._____	70._____	85._____	100._____
11._____	26._____	41._____	56._____	71._____	86._____	
12._____	27._____	42._____	57._____	72._____	87._____	THIRD
13._____	28._____	43._____	58._____	73._____	88._____	EXAM
14._____	29._____	44._____	59._____	74._____	89._____	GRADE
15._____	30._____	45._____	60._____	75._____	90._____	_____

ANSWER SHEETS

Chapter 22 • Gerontology and Home Health Nursing

Exam I

1._____	9._____	17._____	25._____	33._____	41._____	49._____
2._____	10._____	18._____	26._____	34._____	42._____	50._____
3._____	11._____	19._____	27._____	35._____	43._____	
4._____	12._____	20._____	28._____	36._____	44._____	
5._____	13._____	21._____	29._____	37._____	45._____	FIRST
6._____	14._____	22._____	30._____	38._____	46._____	EXAM
7._____	15._____	23._____	31._____	39._____	47._____	GRADE
8._____	16._____	24._____	32._____	40._____	48._____	_____

Exam II

1._____	9._____	17._____	25._____	33._____	41._____	49._____
2._____	10._____	18._____	26._____	34._____	42._____	50._____
3._____	11._____	19._____	27._____	35._____	43._____	
4._____	12._____	20._____	28._____	36._____	44._____	
5._____	13._____	21._____	29._____	37._____	45._____	SECOND
6._____	14._____	22._____	30._____	38._____	46._____	EXAM
7._____	15._____	23._____	31._____	39._____	47._____	GRADE
8._____	16._____	24._____	32._____	40._____	48._____	_____

Exam III

1._____	9._____	17._____	25._____	33._____	41._____	49._____
2._____	10._____	18._____	26._____	34._____	42._____	50._____
3._____	11._____	19._____	27._____	35._____	43._____	
4._____	12._____	20._____	28._____	36._____	44._____	
5._____	13._____	21._____	29._____	37._____	45._____	THIRD
6._____	14._____	22._____	30._____	38._____	46._____	EXAM
7._____	15._____	23._____	31._____	39._____	47._____	GRADE
8._____	16._____	24._____	32._____	40._____	48._____	_____

ANSWER SHEETS

Chapter 23 • Registered Professional Nurses as Managers and as Delegators of Tasks to Unlicensed Assistive Personnel (ULP)

Exam I

1) 1._____ 2._____ 3._____ 4._____
2) 1._____ 2._____ 3._____ 4._____
3) 1._____ 2._____ 3._____ 4._____
4) 1._____ 2._____ 3._____ 4._____
5) 1._____ 2._____ 3._____ 4._____
6) 1._____ 2._____ 3._____ 4._____
7) 1._____ 2._____ 3._____ 4._____
8) 1._____ 2._____ 3._____ 4._____
9) 1._____ 2._____ 3._____ 4._____
10) 1._____ 2._____ 3._____ 4._____

11) 1._____ 2._____ 3._____ 4._____
12) 1._____ 2._____ 3._____ 4._____
13) 1._____ 2._____ 3._____ 4._____
14) 1._____ 2._____ 3._____ 4._____
15) 1._____ 2._____ 3._____ 4._____
16) 1._____ 2._____ 3._____ 4._____
17) 1._____ 2._____ 3._____ 4._____
18) 1._____ 2._____ 3._____ 4._____
19) 1._____ 2._____ 3._____ 4._____
20) 1._____ 2._____ 3._____ 4._____

FIRST EXAM GRADE _____

Exam II

1) 1._____ 2._____ 3._____ 4._____
2) 1._____ 2._____ 3._____ 4._____
3) 1._____ 2._____ 3._____ 4._____
4) 1._____ 2._____ 3._____ 4._____
5) 1._____ 2._____ 3._____ 4._____
6) 1._____ 2._____ 3._____ 4._____
7) 1._____ 2._____ 3._____ 4._____
8) 1._____ 2._____ 3._____ 4._____
9) 1._____ 2._____ 3._____ 4._____
10) 1._____ 2._____ 3._____ 4._____

11) 1._____ 2._____ 3._____ 4._____
12) 1._____ 2._____ 3._____ 4._____
13) 1._____ 2._____ 3._____ 4._____
14) 1._____ 2._____ 3._____ 4._____
15) 1._____ 2._____ 3._____ 4._____
16) 1._____ 2._____ 3._____ 4._____
17) 1._____ 2._____ 3._____ 4._____
18) 1._____ 2._____ 3._____ 4._____
19) 1._____ 2._____ 3._____ 4._____
20) 1._____ 2._____ 3._____ 4._____

SECOND EXAM GRADE _____

Exam III

1) 1._____ 2._____ 3._____ 4._____
2) 1._____ 2._____ 3._____ 4._____
3) 1._____ 2._____ 3._____ 4._____
4) 1._____ 2._____ 3._____ 4._____
5) 1._____ 2._____ 3._____ 4._____
6) 1._____ 2._____ 3._____ 4._____
7) 1._____ 2._____ 3._____ 4._____
8) 1._____ 2._____ 3._____ 4._____
9) 1._____ 2._____ 3._____ 4._____
10) 1._____ 2._____ 3._____ 4._____

11) 1._____ 2._____ 3._____ 4._____
12) 1._____ 2._____ 3._____ 4._____
13) 1._____ 2._____ 3._____ 4._____
14) 1._____ 2._____ 3._____ 4._____
15) 1._____ 2._____ 3._____ 4._____
16) 1._____ 2._____ 3._____ 4._____
17) 1._____ 2._____ 3._____ 4._____
18) 1._____ 2._____ 3._____ 4._____
19) 1._____ 2._____ 3._____ 4._____
20) 1._____ 2._____ 3._____ 4._____

THIRD EXAM GRADE _____

ANSWER SHEETS

Chapter 24 • New Category of Application Questions on the RN State Board Exam

Exam I

1.____	16.____	31.____	46.____	61.____	76.____	91.____
2.____	17.____	32.____	47.____	62.____	77.____	92.____
3.____	18.____	33.____	48.____	63.____	78.____	93.____
4.____	19.____	34.____	49.____	64.____	79.____	94.____
5.____	20.____	35.____	50.____	65.____	80.____	95.____
6.____	21.____	36.____	51.____	66.____	81.____	96.____
7.____	22.____	37.____	52.____	67.____	82.____	97.____
8.____	23.____	38.____	53.____	68.____	83.____	98.____
9.____	24.____	39.____	54.____	69.____	84.____	99.____
10.____	25.____	40.____	55.____	70.____	85.____	100.____
11.____	26.____	41.____	56.____	71.____	86.____	
12.____	27.____	42.____	57.____	72.____	87.____	FIRST
13.____	28.____	43.____	58.____	73.____	88.____	EXAM
14.____	29.____	44.____	59.____	74.____	89.____	GRADE
15.____	30.____	45.____	60.____	75.____	90.____	____

Exam II

1.____	16.____	31.____	46.____	61.____	76.____	91.____
2.____	17.____	32.____	47.____	62.____	77.____	92.____
3.____	18.____	33.____	48.____	63.____	78.____	93.____
4.____	19.____	34.____	49.____	64.____	79.____	94.____
5.____	20.____	35.____	50.____	65.____	80.____	95.____
6.____	21.____	36.____	51.____	66.____	81.____	96.____
7.____	22.____	37.____	52.____	67.____	82.____	97.____
8.____	23.____	38.____	53.____	68.____	83.____	98.____
9.____	24.____	39.____	54.____	69.____	84.____	99.____
10.____	25.____	40.____	55.____	70.____	85.____	100.____
11.____	26.____	41.____	56.____	71.____	86.____	
12.____	27.____	42.____	57.____	72.____	87.____	SECOND
13.____	28.____	43.____	58.____	73.____	88.____	EXAM
14.____	29.____	44.____	59.____	74.____	89.____	GRADE
15.____	30.____	45.____	60.____	75.____	90.____	____

Exam III

1.____	16.____	31.____	46.____	61.____	76.____	91.____
2.____	17.____	32.____	47.____	62.____	77.____	92.____
3.____	18.____	33.____	48.____	63.____	78.____	93.____
4.____	19.____	34.____	49.____	64.____	79.____	94.____
5.____	20.____	35.____	50.____	65.____	80.____	95.____
6.____	21.____	36.____	51.____	66.____	81.____	96.____
7.____	22.____	37.____	52.____	67.____	82.____	97.____
8.____	23.____	38.____	53.____	68.____	83.____	98.____
9.____	24.____	39.____	54.____	69.____	84.____	99.____
10.____	25.____	40.____	55.____	70.____	85.____	100.____
11.____	26.____	41.____	56.____	71.____	86.____	
12.____	27.____	42.____	57.____	72.____	87.____	THIRD
13.____	28.____	43.____	58.____	73.____	88.____	EXAM
14.____	29.____	44.____	59.____	74.____	89.____	GRADE
15.____	30.____	45.____	60.____	75.____	90.____	____